MOTOR LEARNING AND HUMAN PERFORMANCE

MOTOR LEARNING AND HUMAN PERFORMANCE

AN APPLICATION TO MOTOR SKILLS AND MOVEMENT BEHAVIORS third edition

ROBERT N. SINGER

The Florida State University

MACMILLAN PUBLISHING CO., INC.
New York

COLLIER MACMILLAN PUBLISHERS
London

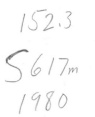
Copyright © 1980. Robert N. Singer
Printed in the United States of America

Earlier editions copyright © 1968 and 1975 by Robert N. Singer

Macmillan Publishing Co., Inc.
866 Third Avenue, New York, New York 10022

Collier Macmillan Canada, Ltd.

Library of Congress Cataloging in Publication Data
Singer, Robert N
  Motor learning and human performance.
  Includes bibliographies and index.
  1. Physical education and training.
2. Motor learning. 3. Physical education and training—Mathematical
models. 4. Motor ability. 5. Learning. I. Title.
GV436.S55 1980   152.3   79-14686
ISBN 0-02-410780-8

Printing: 4 5 6 7 8   Year: 5 6

To the many students and colleagues I have come to know and love.

PREFACE

When the second edition of this book was written in 1975, it was stated in the Preface that "the book had undergone a complete 'facelifting,' " as compared to the contents and approach taken in the first edition in 1968. Nothing as dramatic has occurred with this edition.

And yet, in only a short time between the last two publications, so many new ideas have emerged and research published on various aspects of motor behavior that a considerable amount of editing, adding, and deleting has been necessary. If there is one direction the field of motor learning is taking, it probably is toward sophistication. The advancement of models of motor behavior, topics addressed and experimental paradigms, methods, and statistics have paved the way toward sophistication. Today we witness, at least in the United States and Canada, areas termed *motor learning, motor control, motor development, sports psychology,* and *instructional methods for skills.* All have a common concern: motor behaviors, but according to certain scholars, each has an exclusive and unique domain of study.

What then should constitute the contents of a book on motor learning and human performance, geared as a text at the undergraduate or graduate level of study? After an analysis of alternatives, I have attempted to write the most comprehensive book in the subject area. This approach allows any instructor to select those topics that seem to fit best in a particular course. In many curricula at the same university, two or three different courses dealing with motor learning and the acquisition of skill may be taught. This book should provide sufficient flexibility to any instructor to cover content in any motor learning course.

Theory, research, and practical implications continuously permeate the pages of this edition. The writing style is intended to be relatively simple, the contents readily digestible. The topics are interesting, even exciting—at least to me! I hope they will be to you as well, be you teacher or student.

Furthermore, the book should be an excellent source for anyone interested in understanding processes and conditions involved in the learning of motor skills. Many additional references are provided for more extensive reading and comprehension. It is hoped that the contents will stimulate further experimentation, for scholars and practitioners alike. Whether learning about learning for the sake of gaining knowledge, extending research and theory on certain topics, or to becoming better instructors and learners of skills, the book is intended to fill a need.

The contents proceed from background material in Chapters 1 and 2, in which general foundational material is presented, to considerations about research methodology in Chapter 3. In Chapters 4 and 5 there is an overview of both traditional and recent theoretical developments, leading to the model of motor behavior prepared in Chapter 6. Information processing, cybernetic, and hierarchical control features are emphasized.

The nature of those abilities and capabilities that underlie motor learning and performance constitutes the substance of Chapter 7 and 8. Developmental considerations are discussed in Chapters 9 and 10, with heavy emphasis on learning processes and factors associated with the developing human organism. Chapters 11, 12, and 13 deal with instructional and training considerations, from pre-practice, to during practice, to post practice conditions. Finally, Chapter 14 concludes with a discussion of social and environmental influences on motor behavior.

Have I omitted anything? Not deliberately. There are always reservations about how to approach and interpret certain topics, and how much depth to treat each with. I sincerely hope that no major or glaring mistakes have been made in this regard. As was the case with the first two editions of this book, I will rely heavily on feedback from users of the book to determine the acceptability, usefulness, and overall quality of the different sections.

Consequently, I would like, once again, to express my sincere appreciation to my many students and faculty colleagues from all over the world for accepting and endorsing the first two editions of this book. I hope that this book will be even better due to the feedback I have received from them (and the non-endorsers as well!).

My appreciation is extended to those who have taken the time to make thoughtful and constructive suggestions while reviewing this manuscript. Drs. Robert Christina and Anne Rothstein kept me intellectually honest, and provided much practical and scholarly advice as to the format and content of the book. I wish I could have incorporated all of their suggestions, and where I have not, I am sure the book will suffer accordingly.

Special thanks are offered to Dr. Richard F. Gerson for his assistance in developing the human behavior model that appears in Chapter 6, as well as many constructive suggestions throughout the text; and to Mrs. Judith Chen for typing and retyping and retyping and . . . the manuscript. How could I possibly show my gratitude? Finally, to Mr. Lloyd Chilton, the Macmillan editor who has worked with me patiently and so helpfully during these three editions, what else can I say but to hope that we will continue our working and personal relationship through many more editions.

RNS

CONTENTS

---

7 ABILITIES AND INDIVIDUAL DIFFERENCES 181

8 OTHER PERSONAL FACTORS RELATED TO SKILLED PERFORMANCE 223

10 ADDITIONAL DEVELOPMENTAL CONSIDERATIONS 295

11 INSTRUCTIONAL AND TRAINING PROCEDURES: PREPRACTICE CONSIDERATIONS 325

13 INSTRUCTIONAL AND TRAINING
PROCEDURES: AFTER-PRACTICE
CONSIDERATIONS   449

15 EPILOGUE   527

1
BACKGROUND

The term *learning* is common to everyone's vocabulary. It is frequently used and may apply to numerous situations. During our lifetime we learn many things, including more directly observable behaviors, as required in motor and verbal performances, and less directly observable behaviors, which are associated with emotions, values, and attitudes. Habits, bad as well as good, are acquired. Learning does not even have to be intentional. It is demonstrated under such diverse conditions as performing athletic skills, remembering past situations, disliking opponents in a game, and believing in the team.

Interestingly enough, as one penetrates deeper into the concepts related to the study of learning, it is found that more and more questions are raised than are answered. How can one tell if learning has taken place? Is there actually more than one type of learning? What is the difference between learning and performance?

These questions are but a few of the many raised by persons bewildered by the learning situation. Learning is the concern of almost every individual, regardless of profession or primary occupation: from educators to mothers raising infants, from professionals to blue-collar workers, from scientists to coaches. Children in mathematics classes or physical education classes are involved in the process of learning. With so many and different types of people concerned with the way one makes adaptations in behavior to achieve standards presumably indicative of learning, it should surprise no one that many and various types of researchers, theorists, and educators have been actively involved in investigating the intricacies of the learning process. The *learner*, the *activity*, and the *learning situation* interact to produce behavioral changes. These three components, as they operate dynamically, comprise the major considerations and essence of research in learning.

THE STUDY OF LEARNING AND LEARNING PROCESSES

Learning phenomena were not studied through a formalized, scientific process until the end of the nineteenth century. When psychology became a distinct

1

discipline and broke away from philosophy, behavioral scientists began examining the learning process and learning phenomena in controlled situations. Data were collected. Research laboratories were initiated and developed. Research was also conducted in the classroom and in other real-life situations. Concepts related to the mind and casual observations of behaviors gave way to a science of learning.

From then until the present time, research efforts have intensified with regard to the study of all kinds of learning. The main goals, of course, are to improve instruction and to gain a better understanding of how people learn. A synthesis of research findings reveals a body of knowledge that indicates generalizations in the learning expectancies of students under specified conditions. Contrarily, equivocal data suggest our inability to neatly compartmentalize statements. Learning is a complex, dynamic process. Many exceptions exist to the rule. At present we have both reasonable, clear-cut directional statements as well as conflicting opinions in certain aspects of learning.

The study of learning entails the grasping of knowledge of the myriad of factors that contribute to changes in behavior. It means understanding the learning process and the acquisition of skill as regards this development. It includes an examination of environmental changes (e.g., situational, instructional) and how they might facilitate or impede learning. Furthermore, it involves an appreciation of individual differences in abilities, characteristics, development, aspirations, and the like—and how they affect learning rates and outcomes.

The understanding of learning is drawn from the efforts of educators, psychologists, neurophysiologists, biochemists, and others, and the field of learning is indeed broad. With so many factors to consider, it becomes apparent that to understand the nature of human behavior is an extremely challenging task.

Through the years, different schools of psychological and educational thought have reflected the contributions made in attempting to understand, explain, and predict behavior with a reasonable degree of certainty. One of the first and the most influential schools of thought affecting research on behavior was behaviorism. Stimulus-response (S–R) psychology, as it was also to be known, yielded many formal expressions of learning. Formalized, systematic measurements were taken on subjects in simplified and controlled situations by S–R psychologists who wanted to study behavior precisely. The research and theory were highly mechanistic, as contrasted with humanistic approaches to studying human behavior. Learning generalizations were made from group-collected data. They were nonindividual-centered. That is, it was felt that particular events in a situation would cause certain responses to occur, and that all persons would be generally affected in the same manner:

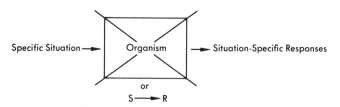

A number of other scholars opposed this simplistic viewpoint of explaining and understanding human behavior. Historically, the major opposition to behaviorism was Gestaltism, and these ideas were expressed by Gestaltists. Emphasis was placed on cognition and perception, as well as on attitudes and feelings. What soon became apparent was that there are great differences in the way individuals respond, behave, and learn but also many commonalities.

General and Specific Outcomes

The average person is interested in general "principles" of behavior. Information is sought that is broadly applicable to a variety of people and circumstances. As we attempt to become knowledgeable and scholarly in an area of interest, it becomes apparent that the assimilation of highly technical information is a time-consuming and laborious process. In other words, there are many specifics to which we have to attend. Therefore, the individual who transmits information can be a superficial discussant or a probing, penetrating analyst.

Similarly, some research efforts are attuned to answering more general problems; others are highly specific. Research on a specifically designed curriculum or course of learning experiences provides general guidelines for instruction. The analysis and comparison of premotor and motor reaction times is a highly refined process leading to understanding and to theory building in a very specific area. Research reported by educational psychologists, for example, is usually applied and general. Experimental psychologists, on the other hand, are usually involved in laboratory research that focuses on a highly specific problem.

Different Breeds of Scholars

During this century, educators and psychologists have made the greatest impact on instruction and contributions to a body of knowledge on learning. More recent breakthroughs by biochemists and neurophysiologists have contributed to a more complete understanding of the learning process. Thus, when we pool the concepts produced by Swiss psychologist Jean Piaget on the intellectual development of children; by Harvard emeritus psychologist B. F. Skinner on teaching models dependent on reinforcement and the shaping of behaviors; by Canadian Donald Hebb and Russia's Alexander Luria on the neurological bases of learning; by Professor David Krech of the University of California, Berkeley, on the biochemical bases of learning; and A. T. Welford of England (presently located in Australia) and the late Paul Fitts, last of the University of Michigan, on the nature of skill acquisition, we see representatives of different lines of research who all contributed in important and fundamental ways to a body of knowledge dealing with human motor behavior.

Because of the accumulation of research on a wide range of learning matter in which assorted conditions and procedures have been employed, an attempt must be made to relate the findings to a major concern of the instructor or trainer: the learning of motor skills. Besides learning how to teach, educators must understand how learners learn. Educators have, in recent years, demonstrated an increasing interest in this area, as evidenced by the number of investigations and writings in the motor learning literature. Fortunately, the combined efforts of all the researchers interested in the area of learning and its facilitation, from the experimental psychologist to the industrial psychologist, from the physical educator to the engineer, from the educator to the neurophysiologist, have produced a substantial body of scientifically oriented information that forms the known aspects of learning. That information is presented in this book, with necessary qualifications, as it applies to the learning of any kind of motor skill.

Laboratory and Field Situations

The fact remains that educators in general and psychologists in particular are the ones most concerned with advancing knowledge in the area of learning. Educational research undertaken directly in the classroom in order to work with the materials actually taught has been criticized as being too broadly defined and lacking in necessary research controls to be meaningful. Difficulty in controlling classroom investigations in the same manner as laboratory research, however, certainly does not negate the worth of educational research. Experimental psychologists have primarily used such lower forms of organisms as rats, dogs, chimpanzees, and chickens in their research. They have also been concerned with human learning, but in highly artificial situations and with such unusual learning material as nonsense syllables, mazes, pursuit rotors, and other novel fine motor skills, in order to provide more scientific control. Applications from such studies have been advanced to help explain and predict aspects of human learning.

These psychologists have been able to control effectively many extraneous variables in their research; however, the application of their findings to typical human learning situations leads to still further questions. Are nonsense syllables learned in a controlled situation mastered in the same manner as is prose studied by children in the classroom? Are the conditions prevailing in pursuit rotor tasks (maintaining a stylus on a moving target) comparable to those found related to other educational materials or to physical education skills?

Although there are objections to both educational and psychological techniques, there has emerged from them both a reasonable amount of scientifically verifiable information.

A *laboratory* can be almost anything. In the traditional sense, it implies an area away from the mainstream of activities where situations can be controlled fairly effectively. Freedom to control and to dictate circumstances that will occur from the initiation of testing to its completion is associated with laboratory conditions. Although *control* is optimal in the research laboratory, usually the realism of learning situations is lost. We give artificial learning tasks and we test students under artificial conditions. Behavior observed may or may not be the same as the real-life circumstance.

On the other hand, the *field situation* can include the classroom, gym, swimming pool, or athletic field. There is less artificiality here, but also a loss of experimental control over the subjects and conditions—although there is concern for control. However, the situation does not usually permit the same amount of control over circumstances as in the laboratory. Somehow the *control and artificiality of the laboratory* along with the *meaningfulness and realism with a loss of control in the field situation* must be resolved.

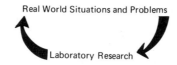

Both laboratory and field research are necessary for our understanding of human behavior. They should be complementary, not antithetical. It should not be laboratory versus field research. Some problems can be studied more effectively in one situation rather than in another. Findings in one area give rise to possible studies in the other area. The hope exists that findings will be somewhat verifiable in each area, even though different kinds of subjects, tasks, and conditions may be present. When this is not the case, specific parameters and their influences on behavior must be identified.

HOW MANY KINDS OF LEARNING?

In the early stages of learning theory development, it was widely believed that one theory could adequately explain any kind of learning. Although this is a desirable approach—and because the law of parsimony should prevail—efforts were generated toward this ideal goal. Indeed, depending on one's interpretation of processes underlying the different manifestations of human behavior, a single theory might be acceptable.

Yet, with a refinement of investigations and the identification of unique considerations in various behaviors, many scholars became disenchanted with the profitability of following this line of thought. From the early development of all-encompassing learning theories, most notably represented by behaviorism and Gestaltism, in recent years we have witnessed the emergence of a variety of models. Each is advanced to describe specific kinds of learning or behaviors.

Indeed, the experimental psychologist Arthur W. Melton (1964) proposed a taxonomy of human learning to order more systematically the vast amount of information produced on the topic. Seven categories, or kinds, of learning were identified:

1. Classical and operant conditioning.
2. Rote verbal learning.
3. Probability learning.
4. Short-term memory and incidental learning.
5. Concept learning.
6. Problem solving.
7. Perceptual-motor skill learning.

Strong similarities can be demonstrated among these categories of learning. But Melton felt that the identification of these seven types of learning was a necessity for theoretical integration and a more precise understanding of each. Interestingly enough, he concluded that any conclusion on the taxonomy of human learning is sure to be inconclusive! In any event, this procedure encourages a recognition of ways of ordering knowledge of human learning.

Educational psychologists like Benjamin Bloom have attempted a different approach. He and his co-workers categorized human behaviors into three domains: the cognitive, the affective, and the psychomotor. The first major publication on this topic (Bloom et al., 1956) produced eventful changes in educational practices and ways of looking at school learning situations. After that book in the cognitive domain was published, one in the affective domain followed, eight years later (Krathwohl et al., 1964). The least amount of work has been done in the psychomotor domain. One attempt has been offered by Anita Harrow (1971).

The convenience in categorizing behaviors according to the main type of behavioral component (to know, to feel, or to do) should not preclude the fact that most behaviors involve an *interaction* of all three components. Thus, high levels of tennis skill reflect effective integrated movements (psychomotor); the application of strategies, tactics, and knowledge of rules (cognitive); and appropriate attitudes, competitive feelings, and motivation (affective). Nevertheless, these taxonomic ventures include the identification of hierarchical behaviors in each category, encouraging a more thorough analysis of teaching approaches, expected outcomes, and appraisal.

From another point of view, educational psychologist Robert Gagné (1977) has proposed eight types of learning, each somewhat dependent on the other in a hierarchical sense. He has expressed the hope that the types of learning described will have particular relevance toward improved instruction. Gagné identified two basic forms of learning: signal learning and stimulus-response learning. He then described verbal and motor chaining (types 3 and 4). Continuing, he referred to discrimination learning (5) and concept learning (6), rule learning (7), and problem solving (8).

The preceding material developed by Gagné encompasses a hierarchical arrangement of types of learning specific to the domain of intellectual skills. The execution of simple motor acts (Gagné's type 3: motor chaining) obviously does not reflect higher-order behavioral activity. Yet we are primarily concerned with complex movement-oriented behaviors, and the attainment of high levels of skilled performance. In this context, perhaps it is more rewarding to examine another classification approach of Gagné's, that of identifying reasonably distinct domains of learning (Gagné, 1973).

The formulation of separate domains is intended to support the notion that all learning is not the same. Although a few similarities and general conditions may underlie a part or all of the domains, generalizations are presumably the most powerful as they are found to be unique from domain to domain. Consequently, Gagné has offered these five domains of learning:

1. Motor skills: movement-oriented, represented by coordination of responses to situational cues.
2. Verbal information: exemplified by facts, principles, and generalizations, referred to as knowledge.
3. Intellectual skills: represented by discriminations, rules, and concepts (the application of knowledge).
4. Cognitive strategies: internally organized skills that govern one's learning, remembering, and thinking.
5. Attitudes: affective behaviors, such as feelings.

The establishment of five domains of learning (or any other number) presumes their logically and empirically determined distinctiveness. When research findings are more closely allied to a particular domain, information can be more precise and instructional guidelines more adequate. Certainly it makes more sense to talk of learning domains in terms of processes rather than content. Content domains would include mathematics learning, science learning, and foreign language learning. Common sense indicates the utility in treating these areas in a similar way, for conditions of learning could generalize across them. Similarly, there are many examples of motor skills. Does each need separate consideration? No doubt there are certain basic similar factors operating when we learn to hit a baseball, to shoot a basketball, to operate machinery, to type, and to achieve in other behaviors that are primarily movement oriented.

As yet there is no agreement on how many kinds of learning or instructional processes exist. But the preceding descriptions of points of view suggest ways of looking at the problem. Some theorists still state that their laws and postulates can encompass all aspects of the learning process with all sorts of tasks. Others have deliberately tried to deal with specific types of learning and approaches toward behavioral changes. These assorted and somewhat unique interpretations of the nature of human behavior should provide intellectual stimulation and some interesting discussions for students of the learning process.

It is the viewpoint here, and one that will be developed later in the book, that many similar learning mechanisms and processes operate in so-called different learning tasks. After careful analysis, phenomena associated with verbal learning and motor learning, for example, appear to be not dissimilar after all. Perhaps different sense receptors are activated, decision processes occur under unique conditions, and the manifestations of behavior assume different expressions. Although there is value in examining the distinctiveness of behaviors, there is also value in determining commonalities. The learning of motor skills has much in common with the learning of other kinds of things, and yet unique considerations make it necessary to develop a body of knowledge especially oriented to the psychomotor domain.

LEARNING

As we have seen in the preceding discussion, there is a lack of agreement on (1) whether there is more than one type of learning, and (2) if so, how many types there are. Part of the problem lies with an acceptable interpretation of the word *learning*. What are the constituents and parameters of learning? While referring to the strong possibility of the existence of different kinds of learning, is it possible to present a definition of learning compatible to any situation and task?

Interpretation

Meditate for a second. How would you define learning? Consider the process, the nature of the task, and the expected results. If you are frustrated, discouraged, and disappointed, you have joined the ranks of established scholars who have attempted to sponsor a satisfactory definition, for one has yet to be proposed.

A variety of circumstances contributes to the problem. Part of the difficulty rests in the confusion about and failure to differentiate between the terms *learning* and *performance*. Another problem is the lack of separation between what occurs in learning in the early stages versus what occurs at the terminal stages. What of considerations for the process of learning and the final product; that is, the act of learning and the performance test that presumably reflects the level of learning? Should distinctions be made among tasks and behaviors as we attempt to define learning?

The process of learning will incorporate the features unique to the given circumstance. Learning motor skills, attitudes, or cognitive behaviors requires some degree of exposure to certain conditions that will result in changes in behavior or dispositions to act. No matter what the task or behavioral expression, learning refers to some change that occurs within the person and is usually reflected by observable behavior.

This change becomes relatively permanent. In other words, temporary performance states do not truly represent learning. Variable factors such as fatigue, influence of drugs, boredom, and such really affect performance, not learning. Growth and development factors are also variables considered to influence performance rather than to be true indices of learning. With increased maturation after infancy, greater capabilities to learn and perform can be demonstrated. All the variables mentioned reflect temporary states in the organism and as such are associated with learning, per se, only indirectly or not at all.

It should be emphasized that behavior is not really permanent, in a technical sense. Performance varies on different occasions as a function of the status of the organism and the nature of the environment. Learning is associated with changes in the internal state of the person, and this process can be handled through the acknowledgment of biochemical and neurological modifications. Or, psychological properties, such as habit strength (Schmidt, 1975) or abilities, may be changed that, in turn, affect performance. Allan Buss (1973) makes an excellent argument for considering the relationship of learning with ability factors. According to him, relatively permanent changes in ability factors should be used as indices of learning rather than behavioral changes. More specifically, Buss concludes that "relatively permanent properties of an organism brought about by changes in ability factors (as a consequence of experience or practice) [is] that which is meant by learning" (p. 277).

Performance, behavioral potential, habit strength, and associated abilities can be convenient, practical, or conceptual ways of talking about learning. In order to ascribe some relative value to a person's activity—in order to determine what amount of learning is taking place—however, an evaluation of behavior is necessary. Behavior is changed when learning occurs.

For the purposes of this book, *learning is reflected or inferred by a relatively permanent change in performance or behavioral potential resulting from practice or past experience in the situation.* A relatively permanent change implies that performance will not be represented by momentary fluctuations and inconsistencies. Also, well-learned acts usually persist for some time.

The process of *learning describes the acquisition of meanings.* With more learning, there are more meaning and meaningful, goal-directed behaviors. *Retention refers to the maintenance of the acquired meanings* and representations of meaningful behaviors. Usually, later availability (retention) is related to initial availability (learning). That is to say, the better something is learned initially, the more likely it will be retained reasonably well over time.

Practice and past experience underlie the learning process. Because increased capacity to perform may be due merely to developmental factors, or for that matter, an act may be performed by chance without experience, it is wise to disassociate changes in behavior resulting from maturation and chance and relate these changes more to practice and experience. In addition, changes in performance can be attributed to motivation or a lack of it. Any intention to assess learning level at a particular time should reflect optimal motivational conditions so that performance can more nearly reflect learning.

One of the distinct features in learning complex motor skills is the need for practice. Attitudes can be changed with one dramatic experience. Concepts, definitions, and facts can be acquired slowly or quickly. But high proficiency in motor performance can only be attained after repeated experiences, the necessary number and quality of each dependent on task complexity and skill level desired. The better learned the act, the more impervious it is to possible performance fluctuations. Therefore, a well-learned motor skill has most likely required a great number of experiences and is fairly consistently and predictably performed on request.

Learning and Performance

E. C. Tolman through his pioneer research and writings contributed much to the differentiation between learning and performance. His concept of latent learning indicates that learning may be taking place all the time during practice trials but is not demonstrated until reinforcement brings it out. Latent learning has been verified in many experiments in which rats were employed as subjects. A repre-

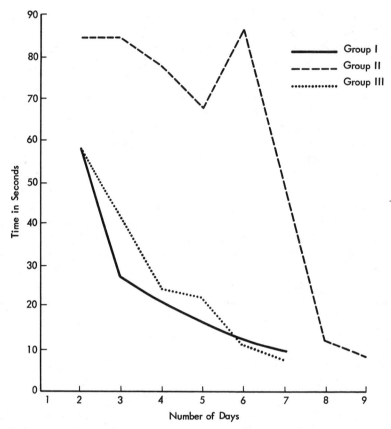

FIGURE 1-1. Time curves for rats learning a maze under different reward conditions. (*From Blodgett, H. C. The effect of the introduction of reward upon the maze performance of rats. University of California Publications in Psychology, 1929, 4, 113–134.*) Reprinted by permission.

sentative study is one completed by Blodgett (1929). His data are illustrated in the form of learning and performance curves in Figure 1-1. Rats were timed in their speed to traverse a maze, and three groups of the animals were tested under different conditions: Group 1 was rewarded with food each day of the investigation; Group II was not rewarded until the seventh day; and Group III was rewarded on the fourth day.

Tolman observed that differences in performance between the groups disappeared as reward was introduced. The nonrewarded rats were developing a latent learning of the maze—that is, they were learning the maze, but this was not evident until a reward was offered. At present, there is much conflicting evidence on the theoretical and practical implications of latent learning, even as there is in the distinction between learning and performance. Nevertheless, although the reward form of reinforcement may have little to do with the learning process, it certainly will account for differences in performance. *Performance may fluctuate from time to time because of the potential for many variables to operate, whereas learning is relatively more permanent.*

Obviously, though, in order to determine what learning has taken place, some measure is needed. We usually use performance to represent the amount of learning that has occurred, for the process of learning must be inferred on the basis of observations of change in performance. We can measure what a person does directly, but what is learned is subject to only indirect estimates. The limited value of this practice is reflected by the results of such studies as the one reported by Blodgett. Nevertheless, a truer measure of learning has yet to be devised, and performance scores reflect the best means available at the present time.

Behavioral Terminology

Often, different terms used by scholars may have similar meanings. Why, you may ask, do we have them? Are they necessary?

The answer to the second question is debatable, but an answer to the first question can be offered. Terms reflect the way scholars think, the way they can best communicate their ideas to others. Because scholars may represent different disciplines of study, a unique vernacular becomes established. Second, some expressions become more popular at different points in a century, as social-technical-cultural factors make their influence felt.

A case in point is the word used to describe what a person reacts to, that which precipitates behavior in a particular situation. A scientific word coined early in the formal study of behavior was *stimulus*. Later, the word *cue* became popular. *Input* has a logical association with developments in computer work. *Information* is a very popular term today, associated with information-processing theory, as is *stimulus* with behavioristic theory. All of these terms are in use today.

Similarly, terms used to explain what a person does in the situation include *response, performance, output,* and *behavior*. The relationship of the terms can be described as follows, with consideration for the theoretical frameworks in which they are usually associated:

Situation	Activity	Theory or Model
stimulus	response	behavioristic
input	output	systems
information	behavior	information processing
cue	performance	performance

Familiarity with these terms should help you to make sense of the literature dealing with learning. At the very least, you should understand them, for you will be introduced to many more terms and concepts that are far more challenging and difficult to explain.

MOTOR LEARNING

Although a certain number of similarities may be found in all "types" of learning, in this book we are interested in examining processes and factors related to the acquisition and performance of motor skills. As contrasted with other types of behavior the primary characteristic of motor behavior is movement. As can be readily sensed, the categorization of a form of behavior permits greater examination and understanding. Yet conflicts over terminologies and semantics can even plague this domain of behavior.

Descriptions and Terminologies

Scholars representing diverse professional backgrounds and personal research and theoretical interests have contributed to the growing body of knowledge surrounding motor learning and performance. It should be quite understandable that "pet" terms and expressions would be developed by these people. Often, similar tasks and learning phenomena are referred to in different ways. Although this situation is understandable, it is often confusing and frustrating for both student and scholar.

For instance, we have decided to use the term *motor learning* when relating the organismic and situational factors to the acquisition and performance of behaviors that are generally reflected by movement. Generalized patterns and highly specific skills are included in the study of motor learning. Athletic, secretarial, agricultural, dance, musical, and industrial activities include many motoric activities. Some activities seemingly involve many of the large muscles of the body; others require the coordinated precision of fine muscles.

Yet *motor learning* and *motor behaviors* appear to be terms favored by scholars in physical education, whereas psychologists, educators, and others have on many occasions used such descriptions as *psychomotor, perceptualmotor,* and *sensorimotor,* instead of *motor.* Aileene Lockhart (1964) has effectively addressed this persisting issue of semantics. Recognition of terms that often can be used interchangeably will assist you in reading literature relevant to the topics covered in this book. The obvious advantage in using *perceptual-* or *psycho-* in front of *motor* is that they more adequately suggest the true nature of the behaviors. *Motor* by itself implies muscular movement, as if reflexive or with little cognitive and perceptual involvement. But the truth is that the real-life skills we learn are usually somewhat complex and involve a high degree of cue detection, evaluation, and decision making. The actual response is only one feature of the entire act.

The terms *motor behavior* and *motor control* have become increasingly popular, as evidenced by their usage in the literature. Motor behavior encompasses learning factors and learner processes associated with performance in expressions of movement. Whereas motor learning is concerned with conditions that are related to improvement in learning (and performance), motor control seems to be associated with processes that operate under specified conditions. In the latter case, the interest lies in behaviors (processes underlying them) that are consistent from trial to trial. In the former case, changes in behavior (and the way processes operate) are analyzed. Motor control specialists study isolated tasks, and neurological, psychological, and biomechanical factors influential in the control of movement. Yet, you may interpret motor learning, motor behavior, and motor control as somewhat analogous expressions, as often distinctions in their usage are not made clear.

TASK CLASSIFICATIONS

Gross and Fine Motor Activities

Motor skills are often categorized as being fine or gross, and a distinction should be made between the two. The word *fine* denotes a delicate or sensitive quality. Certain segments of the body move within a limited area in order to yield an accurate response. The neuromuscular coordinations involved in fine motor skills are usually precision oriented and often refer to eye-hand coordination. Typing, tracking with pursuit rotors, and piano playing have been described as fine motor skills by psychologists in their investigations.

The term *gross* refers to a quality opposed to fine: large, whole, entire, or obvious. A gross motor skill involves contractions and use of the large muscles of the body. The whole body is usually in movement. Sport skills of all kinds may be considered as gross motor skills, and although reference is usually made to these skills without the term *gross,* it is implied.

From a theoretical point of view, we might successfully argue that there are certain fine elements to every sport skill. Acts must be placed on a continuum, for nothing is purely black or white, and certainly sport skills would be concentrated toward the gross motor-skill end. Such factors as strength, precision, and timing underlie gross and fine motor skills, with extreme emphasis on any of these factors distinguishing gross from fine skills.

Object and Person Motion

Motor tasks can be classified in four categories according to task and person constancies and dynamics. As proposed by Paul Fitts (1965) and developed further by M. David Merrill (1972), movement conditions of the body as well as an environmental object could be considered as a basis of a classification scheme. Table 1-1 summarizes this possible representation. Learning strategies will differ according to task category.

A type-I task is represented by the student being able to initiate the activity when ready. Typically, this brief behavior is associated with a student preparing to respond to a fixed object or static environment in a situation that permits movement at one's own rate of speed. Examples include playing a note on the piano,

TABLE 1-1 Task Constancies Relating Conditions of the Body and an Environmental Object During the Interval Prior to Initiation of Response

| | Environmental Object | |
	At rest	In motion
At Rest (Body)	*Type I* e.g. Drive golf ball Pick up pencil Thread a needle	*Type II* e.g. Hitting a baseball Aiming gun at duck Following rotary pursuit
In Motion (Body)	*Type III* e.g. Shooting a layup (basketball) Throw to first base (shortstop)	*Type IV* e.g. Aiming at aircraft from pitching ship Throwing a running pass to moving receiver (football)

(From Merril, M. D. Taxonomies, classifications, and theory. In R. N. Singer (Ed.), *The psychomotor domain: Movement behavior.* Philadelphia: Lea & Febiger, 1972.)

typing a letter, writing, starting a plane, and rolling a bowling ball. Because the environment and objects are stable, the learner needs to be concerned primarily with consistency of response.

A type-II or type-III task occurs where the situation is partially dynamic: (1) the performer is in motion but the object or situation is fixed (still), or (2) the performer is fixed (set) and the object is in motion. Dancing a sequence of steps in predesignated tempo represents a performance in motion on a stable (fixed) platform. The baseball batter, on the other hand, is in a state of preparation, while the baseball (object) is pitched. Many industrial skills, recreational endeavors, and military assignments require a mixed-pace strategy.

A type-IV task occurs when both the performer and the object are in motion during the performance of the activity. This highly complex and dynamic type of behavior is often witnessed in competitive sport, such as in rallying in tennis and handball. Another illustration would be a marksman on a boat being rocked by the waves while aiming at a moving target in the form of a bird. The complexity of this activity is apparent when one imagines how much easier it would be if it were a type-II or type-III situation—that is, if either the target were still or the boat were motionless.

The type-I strategy suggests that the performer be less concerned about quickness in perceptual adjustments toward the activity and more concerned about the appropriate sequence of responses. Because the stimulus or object is stable and the performer has time to be alerted prior to performance, "pressured intellectualization" of the task is at a minimum. When there are many variations of stimulus input, especially those unexpected in nature, response demands are great. This is not the case here. The type-I strategy permits a sensitivity to individual differences, and instructions can be developed accordingly. The performer has time to study the situation and to respond when ready (within reason). To the extent that the performer will perform in various situations that require the modification of responses, practice experiences should be planned accordingly.

As an example, learning to hit a golf ball is easiest from the tee, where the ground is level and the grass is low. However, in order to become a good golfer, one must practice with all the irons and woods, at different distances from the green, with various lies, confronted with assorted hazards, and under various environmental conditions (heat, humidity, cold wind). The response made in any given situation should have been so well practiced that it is habitual. Thus, there is heavy emphasis on the demonstrated movement. If the student will be required to perform the act in a variety of real-world situations, the opportunity to practice under several of these different conditions is necessary.

Because the type-I strategy can be applied to discrete or continuous tasks (see the discussion on page 19), there are certain unique, as well as common, practice considerations for both. In either task, sufficient practice time should be allotted to the students to reach the goal level. Practice conditions are easiest to control and manipulate for the type-I strategy. Because the performer and the situation are in fixed and self-dependent states, main emphasis in practice should be directed toward response consistency. The student has time to be prepared for the activity, the act itself is brief, and the main response requirements are conditioned.

In the type-II or III strategy, the more complex movement in either the performer or the object, along with uncertainties in the situation, dictates more possible alternative practice possibilities. Practice should initially occur under a standard, most probable situation. After an adequate amount of competence is shown, practice situations should be varied. In the type-II or III strategy, the variety of ways in which one might find oneself in motion or in which the object would be in motion should be experienced by the performer.

An accomplished baseball batter has trained with pitching machines or with ball players as pitchers, where balls are thrown in a predesignated and specified manner (fastball, curve, toward the middle of the strike zone, on the outside corner) or in the concealed way pitchers throw in the game. Experience with a variety of pitches, pitchers, and situations contributes to the batter's realization of his or her potential. When learning to drive a car, changing situational demands, either expected or unexpected, prepare the student to be better able to fulfill driving responsibilities.

In the type-II or III strategy, appropriate responses may be dictated by unexpected situational demands on the student. In other cases, a series of movements will be acceptable only if each was correctly executed in serial order, the response in one part of the activity acting as the succeeding cue for the next response, and so on. Because either the student or the object will be in motion, practice conditions become more complicated than for the type-I strategy.

The performer has usually learned more simple tasks leading up to those requiring the type-IV strategy. Readiness should therefore be present to pursue the present task with a model that attempts to simplify the complex components and yet is detailed enough (perhaps through verbal explanation) to adequately direct the learner. The ability to undertake a task requiring the type-IV strategy presupposes the maturation of the organism and the demonstrated mastery of enabling activities that might have involved type-II or III situations.

As both the performer and the object are in motion, a multitude of possible situations exists in which the performer might have to perform in real life. Suggestions expressed for the type-I and type II and III strategies apply here.

Successful behaviors can be demonstrated only after much practice under favorable practice conditions. Because specified timing techniques are designated between performer and object as the criterion for mastery, the type-IV strategy is primarily applied to acts that require skilled performance. Precision in response(s) to appropriate cues occurs in any skilled act. Thus, the ability to catch a ball while on the run, to perform tricks on water skis while being pulled by a boat, or to shoot at a moving target while running reveals high-level, sophisticated psychomotor behaviors. These skills do not come easily. Practice considerations lie in specific modeling procedures, precise cuing, simulation where appropriate, an emphasis on lead-up skills, and so on.

Self-Paced, Mixed-Paced and Externally Paced Tasks

Activities also can be classified according to their nature and the demands placed on the learner-performer. In other words, they may allow the person to self-pace the movement, or the person may be paced by the situational-task demands (externally paced).

Much of the discussion in the previous section pertains to any commentary that might be offered here. Because the self-paced task allows the learner to initiate an activity when ready, and the object is also not in motion, much of analysis made of type-I tasks and strategies applies to the nature of self-paced tasks. On the other hand, externally paced tasks are those that require the learner to perform at the right movement. They possess many of the characteristics associated with type-II and type-III activities and learner strategies. Table 1-2 highlights some of the key differential considerations in self-paced and externally paced tasks.

The concept of self-paced and externally paced tasks probably has its origin in the work of E. C. Poulton (1957). Although his model is geared for predictions in industrial work, it is certainly applicable to the learning of physical education and other skills. He distinguishes skills as being either closed or open. A *closed skill* depends on internal feedback—that is, on the kinesthetic feedback from the execution of the skill. Requirements of the act are therefore predictable, for the concern is with the body's operation in a fixed environment. Such skills can be performed with the eyes closed. Closed skills are probably similar to the notion of self-paced skills.

Poulton describes an *open skill* as one performed either in an unpredictable series of environmental requirements or in an exacting series, predictable or not. However, these skills usually occur in unstable environments. Feedback comes

TABLE 1-2 Differences Between Self-paced and Externally Paced Activities

| Variables | Activities | |
	Self-paced	Externally Paced
situational cues	predictable, static	nonpredictable, changing
response mode	time for anticipation, planning	quick perceptual decisions
movements	controlled, precision form	speed, adaptability
practice	response repetition (response emphasis)	repetition and alternative opportunities (situational emphasis)
aging process	minimal interference	maximal interference

from external and internal sources when open skills are performed, and these skills may be likened to the externally paced skills discussed in the context of self-paced skills. Most team and dual activities transpire in environments that are changing unpredictably.

Humans are systems, if we consider the interpretation of any system as one that contains wholeness, organization, interactive parts, and the potential to interact with other systems. A system can be closed or open. A closed system engages in repetitive activity and is rather limited. An open system demonstrates versatility and creativity: behaviors are redesigned to accommodate circumstances. Humans reveal the capabilities of both types of systems, the level of which depends on task demands and skill level.

The barriers to success are greater in skills performed in unpredictable situations and/or in skills composed of precision movements. According to Poulton, smooth movements in open skills can be made if (1) the requirements are not too exacting, (2) the requirements are presented when the individual is ready for them, and (3) the requirements are not separated by inactivity. These considerations are basic to not only industrial work, but to athletic performance, as well. A. M. Gentile (1972) has elaborated on the nature of open and closed skills, providing special practical considerations for the learning of physical education activities. This writer (Singer, 1972a) has offered similar suggestions for athletes.

In more recent developments, Gentile et al. (1975) have expanded (see Table 1-3) the original classification scheme of Poulton (1957); Higgins (1977), in turn, has made some modifications on it. Type of movement and nature of the environment are the primary measures of concern here. The situation places varying degrees of spatial and temporal regulation on performance, resulting in skills classified primarily as open or closed. Type of movement can be categorized according to body movement or stability, manipulative or nonmanipulative requirements.

Intentional variability is considered by Higgins for each type of skill. That is, from one performance to another, imposed environmental change may or may not occur (e.g., height of bar for high jump). Furthermore, Higgins has identified

TABLE 1-3 Taxonomy Based upon Environmental and Movement Requirements.

Nature of Environmental Control	Nature of Movement Required By Task			
	Total Body Stability		Total Body Transport	
	No LT/M[1]	LT/M	No LT/M	LT/M*
Closed (Spatial control: stationary environment)	Sitting Standing	Typing Writing	Walking Running	Carrying or handling objects during locomotion Javelin throw
Open (Temporal/spatial control: moving environment)	Standing on a moving train Log rolling Riding an escalator	Reading a newspaper on a moving train Skeet shooting Batting in baseball	Dodging a moving object Walking in a moving train Dancing with a partner	Run and catch a moving object Throwing on the run Dribbling in basketball

*LT/M = Independent limb transport and manipulation, usually involving maintaining or changing the position of objects in space.

(From Gentile, A. M., Higgins, J. R., Miller, E. A., & Rosen, B. M. Structure of motor tasks. *Mouvement, Actes du 7ᵉ symposium en apprentissage psycho-moteur et psychologie du sport.* October 1975, 11-28.)

independent temporal control as an important variable in his classification. It refers to those cues that regulate the beginning, length, and ending of certain skills. These are situational constraints independent of those described with regard to closed and open skills. Classification schemes such as these are helpful in studying movements and suggesting appropriate instructional techniques.

Barbara Knapp (1963) has pointed out that skills might be classified as predominantly perceptual or predominantly habitual. Such sports as tennis, basketball, and fencing would be *perceptually oriented,* whereas diving, shot putting, and trampolining would be habitually oriented. In other words, in some sports and activities the prime concern of the performer is the potential for the environment changing. Reactions cannot be fixed but, rather, depend on the circumstance. Other skills require repetitious practice until the act can be performed as a habit; perceptual need is minimized and the ability to reproduce the same act continuously and consistently is emphasized.

Habitual skills, those requiring a fixed response to a given situation, appear to be associated with S–R theory. The environment is relatively stable. Desired responses can only be achieved through constant practice, and the performer's attention is to the act itself. With successful practice, skill sets in, and the individual may execute the skill as if automatically, without any direct concern over the intricacies of the act. Self-paced skills, closed skills, and habitual skills possess many similar characteristics.

The diver's environment consists of a diving board and a pool, with the board a certain height over the pool. This condition is relatively constant, wherever competition is held. True, things are never quite the same day to day or place to place, but, then, no skill is purely habitual or purely perceptual. Elements of both are necessary for successful skill execution, but emphasis on each is dependent on the nature of the skill. Differences in diving-board structure, pool temperature, and spectators present, among many other factors, will contribute to an altered stimulus environment. In some cases, the diver must perform the same regardless of this change—for example, not paying attention to the crowd of people. In other situations, such as the board having more or less spring than the diver is accustomed to, perceptual and control mechanisms must be used to adjust the dive accordingly (or the board may be adjusted). But basically, the dive is an example of a habitual skill. The act is to be repeatedly performed under the condition in which it must ultimately be demonstrated for success to be probable. Any sport in which the participant initiates the action rather than responds to thrown objects or moving players can be identified as primarily habitual.

Common sense would dictate that a skill must be learned reasonably well under stable conditions before an individual can execute it regardless of unpredictable circumstances. But a fixed response is of no use to the performer reacting under varying conditions. The emphasis later would be on the environment, on understanding relationships and patterns. A tennis player might have beautiful form and execution when hitting against a ball-throwing machine. A game situation, however, requires much flexibility in response, for the ball now comes to the stroker at varying speeds, with curves and slices, and with indiscriminate bounces. Now one needs to demonstrate an awareness of spatial relationships and an ability to perceive and react according to changing stimuli. In team sports, the same condition exists. The basketball player must consider not only personal developed skill, but also position on the court with regard to teammates and opposing players. It is not enough merely to assume a definite response pattern each time a specific situation is present. The player who mistakenly fixates an offensive or defensive move, who reacts in an inflexible manner to cues, will certainly be discovered shortly and advantage will be taken of these conditioned patterns. It is much more desirable to have skills developed to be called into play at any time, regardless of the situation. Externally paced skills, open skills, and perceptual skills contain many similar characteristics.

Most motor acts require more than a conditioned reaction. Their complexity requires an understanding of many facets of the learning process on the part of the teacher and performer for the skill to be most effectively demonstrated. Therefore the instructor should be aware of the nature of both habitual and perceptual learning and know how an emphasis on one or the other might better facilitate the desired outcome.

Discrete, Serial, and Continuous Tasks

Psychomotor tasks can be designated as discrete, serial, or continuous. Discrete and continuous tasks can assume varied forms for any of the strategies just described. A discrete task contains one unit, with a fixed beginning or end. Often, in the literature, a task that contains a series of specified events, from beginning to termination, is referred to as a serial task, rather than a discrete task. A continuous task involves a series of adjustments of flowing movements, usually without an acknowledged termination point in time or specified movement. Feedback is often available during the performance of continuous tasks, if they are of a long enough duration and executed slowly enough. The attempt is to remedy errors during performance.

When a task is performed so quickly it cannot be deliberately changed in motion, it is referred to as a ballistic response. A fast movement aimed at a nearby target, usually taking .150 or .200 of a second, is voluntarily noncorrectable once initiated. During the short lasting response, no intervention of the central nervous system can occur.[1] It is, as we will see in Chapter 5, thought to be preprogrammed. A practical implication in sport is that one doesn't have to keep one's eyes on the ball during the last quarter of a second before hitting it or catching it, as the movement has already been committed. The last opportunity to amend the accuracy of the movement has passed. (However, it should be pointed out that movement of the eyes can alter the head, which in turn can influence balance, as well as spatial relations, which in turn can cause one to miss the ball.)

Discrete tasks in their most elementary form are binary-key presses, or the simple reaction-time test. The student is required to respond in a situation with a clearly defined beginning and end in an all-or-none manner. Some discrete tasks are repetitive and are performed in a specified rhythmic tempo. Other discrete tasks call for sequential steps without concern for tempo. As was mentioned previously, these types of tasks can also be referred to as serial in nature. The event may contain a predictable stimulus, in which case the response demand is not too taxing but fixed and stable. Where there are unpredictable stimuli, the response set must be more flexible.

Under laboratory conditions, the most widely used example of a continuous task, with potential implications for many real-life activities, is a tracking task. Typically, the subject stands or sits and attempts to "track" a moving target on an apparatus. The demands may be simple or relatively complex. The pursuit rotor, to be described in Chapter 3 and illustrated in Figure 3-1, represents a simple tracking task. Target sizes vary, as do speeds, paths, and instruments to be held and manipulated, thereby contributing to the relative simplicity or difficulty of the task. Tracking behavior is described thoroughly by Poulton (1966), who has made some cogent observations about human performance with tracking tasks.

Such complex serial tasks as tracking involves a series of decisions about which movements to make and when (movement action sequences). Contrary to popular belief, it appears from the research that tasks may be continuous but *adjustments to them are discontinuous.* As emphasized by Robert M. W. Travers (1977), when we initiate a movement in one direction, the movement cannot be changed for approximately one-fourth of a second. Then a new decision can be made and the action modified. In other words, about two or three adjustments in

[1] However, peripheral corrections can take place via the spindle reflex in 20 to 30 milliseconds, an indication of nonconscious motor control.

movement can be made every second. The more the situation is predictable and adjustments are anticipated, the more effective performance will be. Continuous tasks, especially those involving uncertainty and fast responses, require that learners learn to *anticipate,* as Travers suggests.

We will continually refer to this section of the book when we discuss learning phenomena and practice conditions. Obviously, unique considerations must be made according to activity classification. Effective performance in continuous tasks, for instance, will depend heavily on the type and appropriateness of the feedback present *during* performance. Self-paced tasks, where no time criterion is present, suggest the possibility of emphasizing fixed-pattern responses, with little concern for swift cue perception and reaction. Perhaps these examples suffice for now to indicate the importance of recognizing activity distinctions in the application of practice conditions and instructional techniques.

Task Analysis

A unified approach toward understanding the diverse number of performance tasks has been proposed by E. A. Fleishman (1975). As mentioned before, different types of activities are associated with occupational and recreational settings, and Fleishman suggests a taxonomy of human performance "which provides an integrative framework and common language applicable to a variety of basic and applied areas" (p. 1127). One major value is the application of instructional methods unique to specified classifications of activities.

Four conceptual bases currently used to describe and classify tasks have been described by Fleishman: (1) the behavior description approach, (2) the behavior requirements approach, (3) the ability requirements approach, and (4) the task characteristics approach:

1. behavior description approach: based on observations of what people do while performing a task (e.g., worker or performer functions and behaviors)
2. behavior requirements approach: processes identified as needed to successfully perform at a task (e.g., decision making, problem solving)
3. ability requirements approach: enduring attributes of the performer required to perform tasks, as identified through the factor-analytic statistical approach (e.g., manual dexterity, reaction time)
4. task characteristics approach: a task interpreted as a set of conditions that trigger performance (e.g., task features, procedures)

Fleishman's research has been oriented toward an analysis of psychomotor tasks and human ability requirements to achieve in them, and his conclusions, of course, hold much relevance for our thoughts about motor skills. He suggests that it is unlikely that one general taxonomy will suit all purposes. However, he is optimistic about empirical data, research, and evaluation, with experimental and correlational research approaches, serving as the basis for the formulation of meaningful taxonomies. The organizing framework may be one that ties together ability requirements and task characteristics.

History of the Study of Motor Skills

The first *Research Quarterly,* the research journal of the American Alliance for Health, Physical Education, and Recreation, was not published until 1930. Nevertheless, the psychological research literature included studies dealing with motor learning and performance as early as 1900. True, there were not many at that time, but very practical concerns were being considered, such as optimal practice conditions for archery shooting and the long-term retention of juggling skills.

Workers in the field of physical education examined the concepts of motor ability, motor capacity, and motor educability in the 1930s and 1940s. Many years later this area was to become highly controversial. Psychologists were refining laboratory studies and analyzed such behaviors as reaction time in great detail. But it was not really until after World War II, the time of the Korean War, and during the aerospace movement in the early 1960s that a number of psychologists interested in learning and ability made their contributions. Military and space operations called for information on the way people could best learn to perform tasks, many of which involved keen attention, performance under trying conditions, and high degrees of skill. Predictive test batteries were developed to determine possible success in such tasks. Industrial psychologists also devoted their energies to determining the most effective means for encouraging worker output in manual and operational tasks. Arthur Irion (1969) traces with precision the background of research movements in psychology.

More and more scholars have realized that the area of motor learning and skill acquisition has been virtually untapped. Research has been increasing at a fantastic rate and major contributions to a body of knowledge are being made. The directions of this work run essentially in two identifiable but not necessarily exclusive tracks: the formulation of theory and advancement of pure research and the application to instructional techniques.

THE PSYCHOMOTOR DOMAIN

A wide variety of movement behaviors is encompassed in the psychomotor domain. Previously in this chapter, a classification scheme was presented that categorized behaviors as being *cognitive* (knowing), *affective* (feeling), or *psychomotor* (doing). These distinctions are by no means pure. Considerable overlap often is exhibited among behaviors. As has been pointed out elsewhere (Singer, 1972b), it is primarily for the sake of convenience that such distinctions are made. Activities that are primarily movement oriented and that emphasize overt physical responses bear the label *psychomotor*. The psychomotor domain is concerned with bodily movement and/or control. Such behaviors when performed in a general way represent a movement pattern or patterns, and when highly specific and task-refined indicate a skill or sequence of skills. They include the following kinds of behaviors, all of which could be interrelated and any of which could be independent.

- Contacting, manipulating, and/or moving an object.
- Controlling the body or objects, as in balancing.
- Moving and/or controlling the body or parts of the body in space, with timing in a brief or long *act* or *sequence* under predictable and/or unpredictable situations.

Assuming the basis and validity of laws or principles of learning, the logical step is to use them in the psychomotor domain where applicable. Even research findings, not of sufficient quality and quantity to form the basis of a "principle," but strong enough to indicate a trend, constitute available support for action. Unfortunately, this "logical step" is not as easy as it sounds.

In the first place, acceptable principles of learning are usually so broad and generalized that they constitute nothing more than the obvious. Second, there is some question about the practical application of more specific learning principles, formulated on a conceptual basis from laboratory work in artificial situations. Third, and of most frustration, is the diverse nature present research takes in the various areas concerned with the acquisition of motor skills.

Military and industrial psychologists talk in terms of training factors. Knowledge of results, guidance and instructional techniques, cues in the display, task operations, and job analysis are basic concerns. Experimental psychologists still cling to concepts of conditioning. They are procedure and person-centered, studying instructional methods, practice variations, habit formations, and hypothetical constructs called intervening variables. Those interested in operant conditioning and the Skinnerian approach emphasize reinforcement and the shaping of behavior. Information or communication theorists research the processing and transmitting of information. The standard reference is *bits,* which refers to information the organism receives in a situation. Engineering psychologists stress task variables and closed-loop servosystems, where the main interest is the difference between input and output and the nature of the transmission system. Cyberneticians compare the human to a machine and provide a conceptual framework of control where feedback is of the utmost importance. Social psychologists analyze a person's behaviors in terms of attitudes, values, social systems, and family and peer influences. Physical educators, home economists, vocational educators, and special educators glean odds and ends from all these approaches but generally adhere to guidelines suggested by educational psychologists. Thorndike-type laws, terms, and research associated with the period before the 1940s and the explosion of sophisticated learning models and designs generally make this group of educators "comfortable."

Each of the previously mentioned groups is interested in skill development and modification in the psychomotor domain. The accumulation, consolidation, and syntheses of behavioral "facts" from so many diverse approaches may be beyond reconciliation. Nevertheless, anyone concerned with behavior in the psychomotor domain in general should at least attempt to confront and resolve all these conceptual and experimental approaches. Certainly B. Berelson and G. A. Steiner (1964) must be praised for their valiant effort to construct an inventory of scientific findings with regard to human behavior. Categories of behaviors were described succinctly and descriptive statements made within each as representative of research findings.

On the other hand, it can be legitimately argued that because of the unique complexities of each learning task area, research and theory whould be developed and applied to the specific situation. The present trend toward the formulation of miniature models of learning, applicable to unique problems associated within the area of interest, contrasts with the original goals of psychologists to describe all of learning in one theory. In the psychomotor domain it may be necessary for the physical educator, the vocational specialist, and the military psychologist each to attend to his or her own unique problems. Much depends on the degree to which we believe in task specificity. For that matter, the nature of the task (e.g., discrete, continuous, serial) might serve as a special consideration.

Thus, the problem of task-specific or area-specific research and theory versus a general-domain approach is a real one. Evidently, those concerned with instructional settings must consider situational-specific evidence and task-related information, as well as general behavioral knowledge.

J. A. Adams (1971) has very insightfully described the status of research and theory in the motor skills area until 1970. By way of contrasting efforts in verbal behavior with those in motor behavior, we can more easily identify the major problem for those who are concerned with the history and direction of scholarly work with motor skills. Adams writes

> The research on skills today is as many-sided as the definition of skills, about as McGeoch found it fifty years ago, with research being done on such diverse topics as sports, music, the factory, and military jobs. In their totality these fields can embrace a full span of human performance, from lifting a finger to flying an airplane or delivering a speech. In experimental psychology, topics like conditioning, for example, started out with a well-defined subject matter and paradigm and pursued a systematic search for variables, laws, and theory. Research on skills, by contrast, has studied anything that looks skillful to the commonsense eye. If the study of verbal behavior had gone the same way, we would have journals filled with studies on how to learn and remember novels, billboards, and theater marquees. Compared to the study of skills, the history of verbal behavior and conditioning over the same period is a scientific story to be envied (p. 112).

Going further, Adams calls for more basic research efforts. The focus should be on common elements and mechanisms in what is usually considered to be skilled behavior. He writes

> The villain that has robbed "skills" of its precision is applied research that investigates an activity to solve a particular problem, like kicking a football, flying an

airplane, or operating a lathe. This accusation sounds more damaging than intended, because applied research is necessary when basic science lacks the answers. Nevertheless, the overall outcome of applied research is a collection of answers on specific problems, practically important to someone at a particular moment, but not the steady building of scientific knowledge that can some day have power to answer all the problems. Instead of starting with ideas about the laws and theory of movements and then finding the best situations in which to test them, investigators of skills have often started with tasks that looked skillful and, by studying them, hoped to arrive at laws and theory. This approach is backward for scientific productivity because it results in disconnected pockets of data that lack the unifying ideas that are general scientific principles. The task-centered approach is justified when practical reasons require us to know about tasks and efficiency in them, but it is a limited way of achieving the larger scientific goals of laws and theory (pp. 112–113).

Many research and conceptualization efforts in the 1970s show much promise to alleviate Adams's concerns. Open-loop and closed-loop models of motor behavior have been refined and compared, as research efforts intensify in an analysis of human information processing and control processes (see, for example, Stelmach [1976, 1978]). These directions will be discussed in more detail later in this book.

THE IMPORTANCE OF STUDYING LEARNING

At the onset of this chapter it was pointed out that many people, with diverse backgrounds and interests, are concerned with learning. Questions they pose range from those reflecting a personal need to understanding how to learn and master material quicker and better, to those making a major contribution to research and theory. From your (the reader's) point of view, the study of learning dynamics may contribute to your (1) knowledge and ability to learn tasks, (2) helping skills (as a teacher or parent), (3) ability and interest in undertaking research, and (4) role as a designer of training and instructional programs.

The objectives in reading this text or any reference that encompass topics in learning can be quite diverse but not necessarily mutually exclusive. Most of us would like to know more about learning phenomena, simply because we spend a lifetime attempting minimally or maximally to master a great variety of materials, tasks, and activities. Any personal insights can be advantageous and rewarding. For potential or present parents, responsibilities rest in influencing and changing the behavior of the young.

A number of occupational roles require knowledge of human behavior and ways of constructively changing them. For motor skills, we may identify specialists in industry, military, aerospace programs, recreation, physical education, special education, elementary education, dance, and many more areas. Whether for personal or occupational purposes, the study of the nature of learning is a fascinating and rewarding journey.

CHAPTER HIGHLIGHTS

1. Learning is very complex and has been studied through the years from various educational and scientific perspectives, in real-world as well as in laboratory situations.

2. A recurring issue is whether there is one kind of learning or many, and whether different categories of behavior need to be identified. The trend seems to be in the direction of considering the unique features of motor learning, along with those in common with other types of learning.

3. Learning has been defined as a relatively permanent change in performance or behavioral potential resulting from practice or past experience in the situation. It is usually distinguished from developmental, transitory, and performance factors.

4. Performance is used as an indicant of learning, although there are many reasons why performance level may be suspect as representative of learning status or skill level.

5. Motor skills or tasks have been conveniently labeled, although without rigid and agreed on criteria. Gross and fine, continuous and discrete, motion of person and object, self-paced, mixed-paced and externally paced, and open and closed skills have been described, with the possibility that alternative teaching/learning strategies may be applicable for different kinds of tasks.

6. The psychomotor domain is broad and encompassing, and psychomotor behaviors are associated with many occupations, recreational endeavors, and daily routine occurrences.

7. Although the study of motor skills has been relatively atheoretical and without a strong conceptual base in previous years, much optimism exists today as we view the nature of contemporary research and the theories being developed.

References

Adams, J. A. A closed-loop theory of motor behavior. *Journal of Motor Behavior,* 1971, *3,* 111–149.

Berelson, B., & Steiner, G. A. *Human behavior: An inventory of scientific findings.* New York: Harcourt Brace Jovanovich, 1964.

Blodgett, H. C. The effect of the introduction of reward upon the maze performance of rats. *University of California publications in psychology,* 1929, *4,* 113–134.

Bloom, B. S., Engelhart, M. D., Furst, E. J., Hill, W. H., & Krathwohl, D. R. *Taxonomy of educational objectives, handbook I: Cognitive domain.* New York: David McKay, 1956.

Buss, A. R. A conceptual framework for learning effecting the development of ability factors. *Human development,* 1973, *16,* 273–292.

Fitts, P. M. Factors in complex skill training. In R. Glaser (Ed.), *Training research and education.* New York: John Wiley, 1965.

Fleishman, E. A. Toward a taxonomy of human performance. *American Psychologist,* 1975, *30,* 1127–1149.

Gagné, R. M. The domains of learning. *Interchange,* 1973, *3,* 1–8.

Gagné, R. M. *The conditions of learning*. New York: Holt, Rinehart and Winston, 1977.

Gentile, A. M. A working model of skill acquisition with application to teaching. *Quest, Monograph* XVII, 1972, 3–23.

Gentile, A. M., Higgins, J. R., Miller, E. A., & Rosen, B. M. Structure of motor tasks. *Mouvement, actes du 7ᵉ symposium en apprentissage psycho-moteur et psychologie du sport*. October 1975, 11–28.

Harrow, A. J. *A taxonomy of the psychomotor domain*. New York: David McKay, 1971.

Higgins, J. R. *Human movement: An integrated approach*. St. Louis, Mo.: C. V. Mosby, 1977.

Irion, A. L. Historical introduction. In E. A. Bilodeau and Ina McD. Bilodeau (Eds.), *Principles of skill acquisition*. New York: Academic Press, 1969.

Knapp, B. *Skill in sport: The attainment of proficiency*. London: Routledge & Kegan Paul, 1963.

Krathwohl, D. R., Bloom, B. S., & Masia, B. B. *Taxonomy of educational objectives, handbook II: Affective domain*. New York: David McKay, 1964.

Lockhart, A. What's in a name? *Quest*, Monograph II, 1964, 9–13.

Melton, A. W. (Ed.). *Categories of human learning*. New York: Academic Press, 1964.

Merrill, M. D. Taxonomies, classifications, and theory. In R. N. Singer (Ed.), *The psychomotor domain: Movement behaviors*. Philadelphia: Lea & Febiger, 1972.

Poulton, E. C. On prediction in skilled movements. *Psychological Bulletin*, 1957, *54*, 467–478.

Poulton, E. C. Tracking behavior. In E. A. Bilodeau (Ed.), *Acquisition of skill*. New York: Academic Press, 1966.

Schmidt, R. A. *Motor skills*. New York: Harper and Row, 1975.

Singer, R. N. *Coaching, athletics, and psychology*. New York: McGraw-Hill, 1972a.

Singer, R. N. (Ed.). *The psychomotor domain: Movement behavior*. Philadelphia: Lea & Febiger, 1972b.

Stelmach, G. (Ed.). *Information processing in motor control and learning*. New York: Academic Press, 1978.

Stelmach, G. E. (Ed.). *Motor control: Issues and trends*. New York: Academic Press, 1976.

Travers, R. M. W. *Essentials of learning* (4th ed.). New York: Macmillan, 1977.

2 SKILLED PERFORMANCE

Although there may exist a number of objectives in the learning situation, one of the immediate and ultimate goals is the mastery of the task and the attainment of skill. Different standards of achievement are established, but essentially the most efficient and effective ways of reaching goals should be sought. This implies a need to understand the nature of the task, the learner, the learning process, and the learning conditions.

Many factors apparently contribute to the skilled performance of any task. Genetics, childhood experiences, personal goals, environmental influences, and other interactions lead to the state of "excellence." Ideally, in order to determine potentials for developing proficiency in any task, genetic factors, familial tendencies, past experiences, and the individual's personality should be reasonably understood prior to the training of a given task in a particular situation. General learning principles and specific considerations, with appropriate environmental modifications and instructional techniques, should then be utilized.

WHAT IS SKILL?

The term *skill,* like the word *learning,* is difficult to measure and interpret. It may have various connotations, depending on what is to be defined and who is defining it. In the Webster dictionary it is stated that skill is "the ability to use one's knowledge effectively and readily in execution or performance."

Skill can refer to a particular act performed or to the manner in which it is executed. Many activities are considered to be skills or comprised of skills, and the degree of proficiency attained by an individual reflects a *level* of skill.

Skill is a relative quality, not to be defined in absolute terms. Performance displayed may be so outstanding that it warrants an individual being considered skilled, by comparison with a group of peers on the neighborhood football field. The same person, when placed with members of the varsity team, may appear relatively unskilled. Skill as demonstrated by performance is an indication of what has been learned. Skill and performance can be greatly influenced by a host of factors that may have psychological or emotional origins. However, it is usually thought that the highly skilled individual will be able to perform fairly consistently regardless of the factors present that might cause the "average" person's performance to fluctuate.

Requirements of various activities necessitate a complex development of both perceptual and motor facilities, with degree of emphasis dependent on the situation. In sports, physical processes must be developed before skill can be demonstrated. For example, gymnasts, wrestlers, and soccer players find their performances hindered if they have not shown concern for such underlying physical elements as strength, endurance, and flexibility.

Whereas the diver or gymnast primarily can concentrate on the act itself and display skill through a consistent performance, the team sport player must have mastered not only the basic skills but also an ability to react to changing, less predictable situations. Many people can shoot a basketball with a high degree of accuracy when called on to play 21, Horse, or other games not influenced by defensive players or players on the same team in a competitive situation. Their skills are limited to the given circumstance. Success may not be nearly as pronounced when these people have to demonstrate their skill in a game that requires a mastery of techniques, response flexibility, perception, and emotional stability.

High degrees of skill coincide with high degrees of spatial precision and timing. If certain actions are performed at the wrong time they can be disruptive. During skilled performance, responses to stimuli are set in an appropriate sequential order. Another aspect of skill is that the act is executed within a certain time limitation. The tennis player must stroke the ball at the proper moment and in a productive manner. There is no time to ponder the situation; the response must be appropriate and quick. Generally, in a given situation, a person who is skilled anticipates quickly and has more time to react.

The highly skilled individual demonstrates less variability in performance because responses are not made to every potential cue in the environment. Maximum information is received from a minimum number of identified cues. Skill is developed through constantly well-organized and informative practice, resulting in selective perception and reactions to appropriate cues.

With improved skill, the monitoring of available feedback becomes selective, and either proprioceptive control or central programming control may become more keenly developed, depending on task demands. Organizational factors operate, too. Units of information to be handled and controlled increase in size. The better-skilled performer can take in more information as a result of improved strategies for coping with available sources.

It appears that in order for skill to be present in most motor acts, at least four variables must be considered. These aspects of skill must be developed to a sufficient degree if the performer is to be called skilled. H. W. Johnson (1961) relates a colorful tale about woodchoppers in a contest involving skill. Through the story, he describes how each of the following factors plays a role in determining skill:

$$Skill = speed \times accuracy \times form \times adaptability.$$

Most skills have to be performed within a time limitation—hence, the importance of speed. Accuracy is also involved in acts of skill, for accurate movements will determine how successfully these acts are performed. Form refers to economy of effort, and certainly, skilled acts should be executed with a minimal amount of energy expenditure. Finally, a skilled individual is adaptive; performance is proficient under varying and even unpredictable conditions.

Therefore, it can be seen that the development of skill is highly complex. Consistency in excellent performance infers the activation and formation of good behaviors. But behaviors, if they are bad, can weaken skill. Perhaps an acceptable interpretation of *skill* as referred to in these pages is the *consistent degree of success in achieving an objective with efficiency and effectiveness*. The ease with which an act is performed is also part of the skill of the act. The objective in a baseball game for the outfielder is to catch a fly ball. Certainly there would be a great deal of difference in the method employed by Lou Brock to achieve this goal as compared with the writer of this book, even though both might succeed (the former with ease and grace, the latter with reckless abandon and prayer).

Skills, Patterns, and Abilities

At this point, it is wise to examine similarities and differences between the terms *ability* and *skill*. An *ability* is thought to be something that is general and enduring. It is a trait affected by both learning and heredity. A *skill,* on the other hand, is specific to given tasks and is attained with experience. Because it is task-oriented, skill usually refers to a highly developed specific sequence of responses. As an example, balance is an ability, and a person may demonstrate skill in trampolining, a sport that requires balancing ability. Balance is necessary for success in other sports, as well. However, although each sport may call for expressions of balancing ability, the skill demonstrated is specific to the situation in which it is practiced. Researchers have tried and currently are attempting to describe skills in terms of more basic abilities, with varying degrees of success. Edwin Fleishman (1972) has spent more than twenty years investigating the relationship of abilities to skilled performance and has provided meaningful distinctions and relationships for discussing skills and abilities.

Motor patterns and motor skills can be differentiated, as well. This is especially appropriate for scholars studying the developmental process. Barbara Godfrey and Newell Kephart (1969) write that:

Motor skill is a motor activity limited in extent and involving a single movement or a limited group of movements which are performed with high degrees of precision and accuracy. A motor pattern, on the other hand, is a much more extensive group or series of motor acts which are performed with lesser degrees of skill, but which are directed toward accomplishment of some external purpose. On the motor *skill,* movement is limited but accuracy is stressed. On the motor *pattern,* movement is stressed but accuracy is limited (p. 8).

An example offered of a motor pattern is locomotion. The child is free to select from alternatives to go from one place to another. He may run, jump, crawl, or use some other pattern to achieve the goal. Walking, however, is a specific skill. The child must learn the specific placements of the feet, how to shift weight, and how to function on various terrains and surfaces.

Skills are apparently refined from basic movement patterns, which in turn are related to the degree of presence of relevant abilities. Skills and patterns are acquired through learning. Some abilities depend more on genetic than learning factors, but it appears that all depend on both to some degree. Whenever the learner attempts to master a task, personal abilities are brought to the situation. The intricate relationship of abilities with successful task performance at various stages of development will be discussed later in the book.

Motor Skills

The word *skill* by itself might imply an art in writing, memorizing, acting, painting, talking, or playing. To delinate the confusion, muscular movement, or motion of the body required for the successful execution of a desired act is termed motor skill. It is difficult to isolate skill completely as being perceptual, motor, or verbal, but primarily the emphasis of each process on the skill will decide its nature.

Motor does imply movement. Various processes interact (e.g., cognitive, perceptual, affective, and motor) in order that the act may be integrated, meaningful, and successful. It is important to realize that presence of these factors is necessary to almost any skilled performance.

LEARNING CURVES

One leading method of depicting skill acquisition is through the use of the learning curves. The curve is a graphic illustration of practice trials versus performance and is an indicator of what one or more individuals accomplish from trial to trial. The abscissa line (horizontal) usually corresponds to trials or days of practice, and the ordinate line (vertical) represents the unit of measurement. Measurement might be in terms of points made, errors, or some other score. Typically, the vertical units are laid out to represent two thirds of the graphic dimension of the horizontal units. The appearance of the curves and their general interpretation can be influenced by the manner in which they are presented. Many factors, such as method of practice, administration of practice sessions, method of measurement, nature and level of skill, and age of the subjects, will result in different curves for the same practiced skill. Some curves reflect factors facilitating or hindering performance, and as such are not truly representative learning curves.

It is extremely difficult to obtain a true learning curve. Practice conditions, the nature of the task, and the learner's abilities and organismic state will be reflected in the type of curve obtained from the data. It should be emphasized here that typical examples of learning curves that are found in real-life examples have been smoothed out in order to make it easier to follow any apparent trends in skill acquisition. Actually, great irregularities usually exist from trial to trial and performer to performer.

Figure 2-1 presents four smoothed curves for a limited practice session. Curve A has been termed a negatively accelerated curve. Greatest gains are made in the early practice trials, with decreasing improvements in later trials. A leveling-off point appears to be reached, but positive gains, ever so small, still are occurring. This type of curve usually denotes both the learning of a skill that is relatively easy and where insight into the skill occurs quickly, as exemplified by the satisfactory performance on the early trials. As upper levels of skill are reached quickly, improvement diminishes, for little is left to be mastered.

Curve D is an example of a postively accelerated curve in which performance is poor in the early trials but increases from trial to trial. Although it appears to leave no upper limit, this curve would ultimately level off with practice. The example offered in Figure 2-1 represents relatively few practice trials, so the curve appears to be accelerating indefinitely. Curve B, the linear curve, is essentially a straight line. This curve has been obtained in a few cases where proportional increments are noted from trial to trial. It too would become asymptotic with increasing trials. Curve C, which is an S-shaped curve, indicates positive acceleration, approaching linearity, and finally negative acceleration. It contains many of the qualities of the other three curves.

It is important to note that no single curve of learning exists, that the nature of the task or the learner will be reflected in the manner in which skill is acquired. Some psychologists, L. L. Thurstone (1930) and W. K. Estes (1950), for example, have attempted to form mathematical equations in order to predict and fit learning curves. Varying degrees of success have been achieved in this endeavor. Certain data might very well be described by one of the equations, whereas this

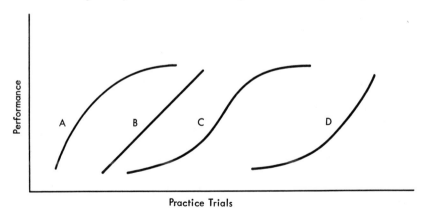

Practice Trials

A—Negatively Accelerated Curve   C—S-shaped Curve
B—Linear Curve   D—Positively Accelerated Curve

FIGURE 2-1. Representative but overly simplified learning curves with distinct features.

same operation would not be appropriate for other data. However, E. Culler (1928) and Culler and E. Girden (1951) present evidence that seems to indicate that complete learning curves are ogive (S-shaped). They employed a mathematical equation that is proportional to the product of the amount already learned and the amount remaining to be learned before the limit of learning is reached. As of the present time, there is no equation that would fit all types of data. Therefore, one concludes that the nature of the learning task (e.g., motor skill, nonsense syllables, prose, or puzzle), and its degree of difficulty, as well as the nature of the learner, determine the method in which the task is learned.

The method of measurement will often determine the smoothness or irregularity of a curve. Although a typical learning curve is obtained from practice trials completed in one or a few meetings, Figure 2-2 presents data collected on one discus thrower in competition during his four years at college. No doubt growth and development factors influence the curve, but it is presented for two reasons: (1) the similarity between this curve and a typical learning curve and, more important, (2) a comparison of three methods of measuring performance and each one's effect on the curve.

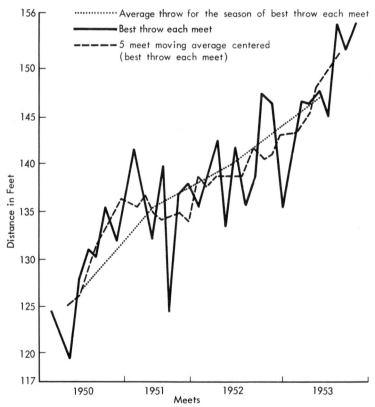

FIGURE 2-2. Three methods of analyzing performance, representative of one discus thrower's record for four years.

It can be observed that when more scores are averaged together, the lines become smoother. The most irregular line represents the best throw at each meet, a smoother line is obtained by averaging five throws per meet, and the smoothest curve is derived from the average throw each season. The athlete's record indicates fairly consistent improvement from meet to meet and year to year, although irregularities in performance are clearly apparent.

Because it would be erroneous to believe that every athlete's record is comparable to the preceding case and would improve so consistently, the performances of three other athletes, all javelin throwers, are recorded by the five-throw-per-meet-average method for comparison in Figure 2-3. Note the differences in the curves, many of which may be explained by such factors as a student getting married, loss or gain in motivation, proper or improper understanding of mechanics, poorer or better health, and, in general, a host of psychological and physiological variables.

If these curves were smoothed by such a method as averaging the throws per season, they would more nearly approach those curves found in Figure 2-2. Poorer records, caused by backache, marriage, or lack of interest are really factors in performance and not truly indicative of learning, as such. True curves of learning should reflect positive increments, even if they are so slight as to be outwardly un-

FIGURE 2-3. Individual performances of three javelin throwers during four years of competition.

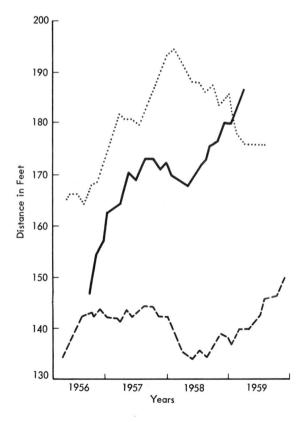

observable. The plotting of individual trials results in more noticeable trial increments and decrements and can serve a definite purpose. Without any major detrimental factors operating, averaged practice trials should yield positive learning performances.

Figure 2-4 illustrates learning curves for two different groups of subjects receiving 10 practice trials, each in the same time period on the stabilometer (an apparatus used to measure balance ability). The time in each trial in which the board was not ideally balanced is recorded; the curve decreases because performance was plotted against time off-balance. If it were plotted against time on-balance, the curve would go upward instead of downward. It should be observable in either case that there is improvement in performance—hence, learning—within the trials allocated for the experiment. If the curves are smoothed further, they would approach the typical negatively accelerated curve.

Estes (1956) supports the notion of group curves, or data averaged across subjects for each trial. They are useful for summarizing information and for theoretical interpretation. However, he is also against transferring inferences made from group learning curves to individual learning curves. Although the form of the averaged curve does not determine the forms of the individual curves, it does provide a means for testing hypotheses about them. The risks in making generalizations from group to individual learning curves are powerful, and Estes discusses them in particular, as experimental and statistical violations might be involved. It is important to remember that much information about individual learning rates is lost when data are averaged.

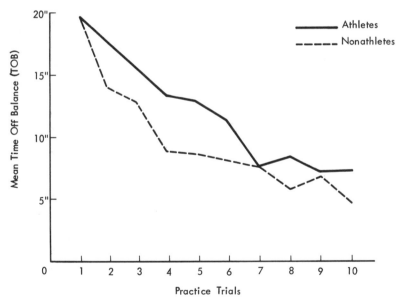

FIGURE 2-4. Stabilometer performance as a result of practice. (*From Singer, R. N. Effects of spectators on athletes and nonathletes performing a gross motor task. Research Quarterly, 1965, 36, 473–482.*) Reprinted by permission.

MOTOR LEARNING AND HUMAN PERFORMANCE

The shape of the learning curve is greatly dependent on the response measures utilized in the plotting of the data. The curve, as pointed out in an article by H. P. Bahrick, P. M. Fitts, and G. E. Briggs (1957), may be misinterpreted at various stages of practice, and effects deemed important are in reality confounded by the artifacts produced. These researchers used a tracking task to illustrate the effects of errors in the measurement of learning curves. However, they believe that their data have implications for a variety of tasks and conditions.

The shape of the learning curve is also influenced by *ceiling* or *floor effects*. When tasks are relatively easy to learn, and the range of potential improvement (as dictated by the scoring method) is rather restricted, asymptotes are arrived at quickly. When the upward swing of the learning curve (as in points scored in ten attempts at a target) or the downward swing of the curve (as in quickness to respond to a cue) is hindered, we speak in terms of ceiling or floor effects. Learning may be continuing, ever so slightly, but it is not detected in the performance when a high degree of skill is attained and the performance measure is insensitive.

Another aspect of learning and performance curves concerns practice to an asymptote as a criterion used in certain learning studies. A task is usually thought of as being "learned" when stabilization of performance becomes apparent. In real-life skills, as in sports, years of practice contribute to proficiency and consistency. Yet, in a few practice sessions, it is not unusual for researchers to expect similar occurrences with relatively simple laboratory tasks. James Bradley (1969) administered thousands of practice trials to one subject, and led him to conclude that asymptotes are not truly reached. A subject could still be learning or showing upswings or downswings in behavior, depending on situational and personal variables. Bradley favors doing away with practice to an asymptote as a means of eliminating unwanted learning effects in an experiment. He feels that group means might mask individual scores. Although precautions might be taken against unwarranted overgeneralizations, there are many types of learning experiments in which the analysis of specified learning phenomena depends on the learners' attainment of a relative degree of stability in performance. A plateau in performance, to be examined next, is an excellent example of a potential temporary asymptote (perhaps even a nontrue asymptote).

In summary, learning curves are influenced by:

1. the treatments (experiences) given to people.
2. performance artifacts and personal equations (fatigue, motivation, etc.).
3. the type of task used (e.g., difficulty).
4. the number of practice trials allowed and the duration of the study.
5. the type of measurement selected.
6. the number of scores used as the basis for each trial or block of trials.

Any learning curve must be viewed in the context of these considerations. Curves can be very helpful in gaining quick insight into learning progress over time, but they can be misleading, as well.

PLATEAUS

Almost everyone in a lifetime experiences a frustrating point of no apparent improvement in performance, though the task to be learned is practiced over and over—maybe it is a golf game that consistently stays in the low 90s, or perhaps a bowling average that always remains about 145. Specific skill acquisition or general sport performance appears to level off and may remain there seemingly forever or for a short period of time before an acceleration occurs in performance.

This phenomenon has been termed a plateau in the learning curve. A plateau represents stationary performance preceded and sometimes followed by accelerated learning increments. It is a condition that has not been found to occur in many experimental learning tasks, but the classic example of a plateau in the learning curve is the one obtained by W. Bryan and N. Harter (1897). The graphic illustration taken from their data and presented in Figure 2-5 refers to one's ability to learn to receive telegraphic signals in the American Morse code.

A hypothesis set forth to explain the plateau in learning is that there is a hierarchy of habits to be mastered by the individual when attempting to learn a complex task. After succeeding in the first order, the learner may be fixated at that level for some time before becoming able to integrate the patterns needed in the second-order habits. Information is consolidated and reorganized. An example of this situation is found in tennis. First-order habits might be the acquisition of basic strokes and skills underlying the sport, such as learning to stroke the ball from a stationary position. Second-order habits could include hitting the ball while the player is on the move, and a third-order category might include the integration of effective movement patterns in the game situation. Theoretically depending on the manner in which the sport is taught and the performer involved, a plateau could occur at any one of these transitional periods.

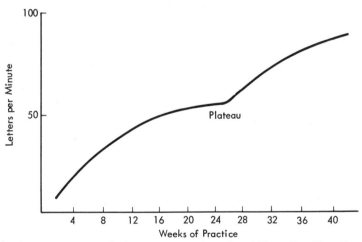

FIGURE 2-5. Learning curve with plateau representing telegraphic coding. (*From Bryan, W., & Harter, N. Studies in the physiology and psychology of the telegraphic language.* Psychological Review, *1897, 4, 27–53.*)

After a period of time in which one attempts to transcend from one hierarchy of habits to another, insight manifests itself in the form of an integration of past learned responses and new ones to be utilized. The curve accelerates sharply until the next plateau. Because actual plateaus are rare in experimental evidence, possibly because of the difficulty in setting up investigations that might demonstrate this phenomenon, we must draw more from theoretical implications and everyday experience. The latter evidence appears to indicate the reality of such an effect in the acquisition of skill, at least in some of the more complex sports. But damage to the concept of plateaus is presented by F. S. Keller (1958). From the title of his article, "The Phantom Plateau," one can surmise the content.

Two questions naturally arise concerning the plateau in the learning curve and its theoretical explanation: (1) Will the manner in which the skill is taught affect the learning curve and any possible plateaus? In other words, a complex activity may be treated in parts and learning directed toward gaining insight into the parts in a progressive manner. Will this method of approach lessen the possibility of a plateau occurring during skill acquisition more than if the skill is taught as a whole? (2) Is there really such a thing as a plateau in the learning curve? One reason for the leveling of performance may be a loss of motivation. If the learner is continually motivated, a plateau in performance might not be observable.

Concerning motivation, disappointment and discouragement when not improving in performance make it even more difficult to advance the learning cause. Perhaps all these factors—task complexity, hierarchy of habits, interest, and frustration—contribute to the plateau, if indeed it does exist. In addition, boring practice sessions may help to lessen motivation. Also, the elevation of anxiety, if risk taking becomes important, may cause stationary performance.

If, in fact, plateaus can occur in the learning of real-life activities (although this is not demonstrated in artificial laboratory tasks), several recommendations could be made to remediate the situation.

Cause	Remediation
1. Loss of interest Loss of novelty Loss of motivation	Make practice appealing; be creative; look for alternative approaches; be enthusiastic; be supportive and encouraging; use reinforcement.
2. Focus on wrong cues	Maintain the learner's attention to the appropriate cues so that practice is meaningful; provide knowledge of results.
3. Fatigue	Be alert to situation; stop practice or practice something else.
4. Emotions	Let learner progress slowly; provide security.
5. Lack of physical readiness	Analyze the task demands and the learner's physical development; he or she might possess physical capacities to perform a task at a certain level of proficiency but will need further development if higher-order skills are to be demonstrated.

Cause	Remediation
6. Low level of aspiration	Help the learner to establish realistically high but attainable goals.
7. Lack of understanding of directions Lack of ability to recognize and adapt skills	Make a task analysis, breaking down the activity into smaller units so that transistions are smooth and logical from one performance level to a higher level of expectation; allowing the learner to progress too fast in a complex activity places hardships on one's ability to apply lower-order learned skills to higher-order ones and to comprehend and use instructions and directions effectively.

THREE MAIN CONSIDERATIONS

Most of us find it hard to believe that so many factors can conceivably contribute to highly skilled performance. Two major categories of influence may be thought of as affecting the status of the learner: (1) personal or organismic, and (2) environmental and instructional. These vary with each learner and each instructional program. Because learners can differ in so many ways, it is desirable to prepare practice conditions that are sensitive to those differences. Yet, there are certain generalities, certain similarities, in the way we acquire skills, and this factor should be recognized along with the other two. The process of learning, of skill acquisition, reveals a number of consistencies among learners. Figure 2-6 indicates that consideration should be given to the three categories of variables as they relate to performance quality and help to explain performance: *the learner, the learning process, and situational factors.*

In the following chapter and in various sections of this book, the nature of the learning process and of skill acquisition will be introduced. Individual difference factors will be disregarded in these cases. It is important to understand

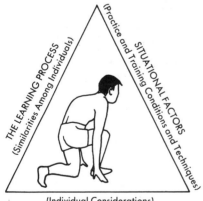

FIGURE 2-6. Three major considerations in skilled performance.

how, in general, people learn. A model or framework can thereby be created that provides guidelines for improved practice situations that work for most people.

Yet, learning-process explanations are incomplete by themselves for the serious student of motor learning. Knowledge of those personal factors that lead to successful performance, how they differ from individual to individual, and how and why they should be considered also lead to better instructional and learning environments. Furthermore, learning the ways in which the teacher or coach can modify learning situations for others so that the most productive results be realized in the time allotted is a necessity.

The Learning Process

Although it is trite but true to say that everyone is different, a search for similarities among people leads to fruitful, efficient means of instruction. Skill is a function of input (the reception and analysis of information), central processes (control and decisions), and output (motor functions). It is fair to say that structures and mechanisms operate similarly across people to permit the demonstration of the same type of behavior.

Theories and models have been formulated to suggest ways in which we react similarly to information (cues, stimuli) in the environment, process it, initiate control functions, and respond predictably. However, the nature of individual differences, a number of which will be briefly identified soon, serves to remind us how easy it is to punch holes in generalizations. Be that as it may, conceptual approaches, as expressed primarily in Chapters 4, 5, and 6, are indicative of efforts to explain and predict behavior in general.

Human control and processing systems are *likened in operation* to a computer. Computers are designed to handle so much information at one time and to produce an accurate output based on input and central decision-making processes. More elaborate operations can be demonstrated by more complexly designed computers. Similarly, more mature and experienced humans can produce a performance superior to that produced by inexperienced ones.

Information is received by sense receptors and processed (decisions are made) and then actions are made on the basis of decisions. The *integrated sequence of activities,* from mechanism to mechanism, is generally the same among people. Structures and mechanisms operate similarly in people, as activity goes on throughout the nervous system from input to output. *Plans of action,* based on prior experience and on any pertinent instructions, are developed to fulfill goals. They are more sophisticated and higher level with better-skilled performers, leading to a sense of automaticity in the execution of certain acts.

The information-processing *capabilities* of people are *limited.* There is just so much information that can be dealt with at one time. The use of *capacity* and the application of internalized *strategies* vary from individual to individual, resulting in performance differences. In addition, an *optimal level of arousal,* or motivation, is necessary for each activity if ideal performance is to be realized. An analysis of the activity demands on the performer suggests this level.

Finally, a person learns to become more *self-dependent,* instead of externally reliant, with the acquisition of skill. From signal detection to feedback, interpretations and decisions become more self-generated. That is to say, the novice requires assistance and looks to the guidance of the instructor for which cues to attend to and the nature of the response to be made. With the acquisition of skill, the learner learns to interpret situations for himself or herself and to make appropriate decisions about behaviors.

Because Chapters 4, 5 and 6 contain theories and models and subsequent chapters deal with a conceptual approach to motor behavior, no further isolation of descriptive statements about the learning process will be made here. Material in other chapters that is associated with developmental considerations, the effects of reinforcement, the uses of knowledge of results provided during and following performance, and transfer relationships indicates predictable outcomes in behavior for most people under specified conditions.

Personal Factors

Individuals differ from each other in obvious as well as in subtle ways. Personal characteristics influence potential for, and in fact the realization of, achievement in certain endeavors. In other words, although conditions can be identified that will affect many people in a similar fashion, there is a need to understand those factors that differ from person to person and are of major significance in determining learning and performance levels.

For instance, we can identify:

1. Sense acuity: the ability of the senses to register accurate representations of the stimuli.
2. Perceptions: the ability to make meaning of a situation.
3. Intelligence: the ability to analyze and problem solve situations and to make decisions related to motor performance.
4. Physical measures: the presence of the ideal level of those measures pertinent to successful performance in a particular activity.
5. Previous experiences: the extent and quality of prior experience related to the present learning situation.
6. Capabilities: abilities, skills, and knowledges developed as appropriate for the present learning situation.
7. Emotions: the ability to direct and control feelings as appropriate prior to and during performance.
8. Motivation: the presence of an optimal level of arousal for and performance expectations in a particular activity.
9. Attitudes: the presence of an interest in an activity, placing a value on it.
10. Other personality factors: the presence of extreme aggressiveness, need to affiliate, or other behaviors that may or may not be helpful, depending on the situation.

11. Sex: the effect of body composition, experiences, and cultural factors on activity performances and desire to achieve.
12. Age: the effect of chronological as well as maturational age on the readiness and ability to learn and perform certain tasks.

These individual learner considerations by no means exhaust the list of possible variables, but they certainly illustrate the complexity of learning situations in the psychomotor domain. They will be discussed in detail in Chapters 7 and 8 (motivation is elaborated on in Chapter 12). Now let us turn to a consideration of situational factors. Once the nature of the learning process is understood, with sensitivity to the unique characteristics of those learners in a particular situation, progress will be enhanced through the appropriate arrangement of the environment and the communication skills employed by the instructor.

Situational Factors

In any learning situation, the characteristics of the environment need to be identified and the demands imposed on the learners recognized. Coupled with a realization of the status of the learners, instructional conditions can be formulated to fulfill more readily program objectives. Learning environments, including the tasks and equipment, can be modified if deemed useful. Various practice strategies can be suggested, although it is hoped that the learners will acquire their own strategies for coping with circumstances.

The specific learning situation, or task, the individual is faced with is termed a display. A display refers to the equipment, cues, and task confronting the subject. In piloting a plane, it is represented by the flight conditions and response panel. The external information in a given situation, pertinent or not pertinent to the task, represents cues to which the organism may attend. The challenge in facilitating learning is to modify the display or situation in such a way that desired outcomes are best met. The teacher or instructor can serve as a potential display moderator or manipulator, making it easier for the learner to master the immediate task.

Merely changing the atmosphere from the previous practice can induce improvement. The Hawthorne experiments, performed in the 1930s, represent a classic example of this. Several secretaries were placed in rooms to work under various working conditions. Light illumination was changed, and the women were given free lunches, rest periods, and even allowed to go home early at times. Every time a change was made, for the better or worse, production improved. For example, when the rest periods were taken away, production still increased. Evidently, motivation was elevated with each situational change as the women were reminded that someone was concerned with what they were doing. A variety of experiences and environmental modifications can remove boredom and induce attention and motivation.

The previous discussion indicates the social aspects of changes in the working environment. The physical layout, in terms of the placement and nature of cues, the means to obtain feedback, and the actual involvement of the learner (active or passive, guided or nonguided) is more fully documented in the literature as to effect on performance.

With regard to cues, the *visual* aspects of the task display can be modified in numerous ways. At initial levels of motor learning, the visual modality is apparently of prime importance in contributing to success. When visual, verbal, and kinesthetic modalities are compared for early importance in skill acquisition, the visual sense is usually found to be most relevant. Therefore, anything the learner can contribute to the situation in already developed visual abilities (e.g., spatial orientation, depth perception, along with desirable specific modifications in the display) will be reflected in learning progress rates and achievement.

One of the problems a learner usually has when confronted with a new, reasonably complex learning task is that there is attention to too many cues or aspects of the situation. Selective attention to the most relevant ones, without experience and/or guidance, may not occur. A variety of cues can be distracting. Also, many tasks require a continual selective cue discrimination process. A basketball player in the midst of a fast break is bombarded with countless, ever-changing, potentially influencing stimuli. The dribbling and direction of the basketball, the awareness of the relative placement of opponents and teammates, the backboard, the rim, the spectators and noise, and the coach's screams constitute some major sources of input. Simultaneous attention to all these cues would obviously cause a breakdown in performance. High-level performance is demonstrated in part by concentration on the important cues of the moment, disregard for irrelevant ones, and perceptual awareness of possible immediate changes in the situation.

How does one reach that point in skill attainment? A good starting place is to examine the scope of the complex activity and to identify parts (mini-displays) of it that can be acquired separately. A mini-display can be left as it is in the "real" situation or modified according to emphasized desirable cues. The athlete must go through stages of mastering the skills that contribute to overall success. Consequently, dribbling the ball is learned so well that execution of this act is at a level not requiring conscious awareness. Shooting skills are perfected so that they are not disturbed by defensive maneuvers, off-balance positioning, crowd noise, and so on. Proficiency in mini-displays and combined display experience lead to overall competency.

Often certain visual cues are emphasized or *artificial ones* are introduced to promote the learning of various skills. Examples in sport of artificial visual cues are found in (1) basketball, where spots or marks on the backboard provide specific points at which to aim for backboard shots; (2) archery, where sometimes the point-of-aim method is employed (a marker placed before the target is sighted upon); and (3) bowling, where the spot method of aiming is often used (a spot placed on the alley is aimed at instead of the pins).

Artificial visual cues are used either as an initial learning technique, to be disregarded later, or as a continual performance aid. Although research is scattered and inconclusive on the value of these techniques, it does appear that many of them are of value in fulfilling certain objectives. Theoretically analyzing the problem, *specific and precise* visual cues are easier to attend to than general, vague ones. Furthermore, *nearer* cues should be easier to aim for than those more removed. However, not all learners will benefit equally from the identical cues in the same task.

Most of the work in the arrangement of displays can be found in the industrial and aviational psychology literature. Simplifying displays and rearranging them so that the perceptual information is more obvious and easier to attend to naturally results in greater insight into the task. In one study (Belbin, Belbin, & Hill, 1957), workers on complicated cloth weaves were subjected to special training techniques. Essentially it was discovered that an inadequate number of visual cues were present in the task. By reconstructing the task so that the weaves were enlarged, the cues were made more visible. With improvement in performance, the display was once again placed into its original dimensions. The efficiency of this technique was demonstrated in the study as well as in some subsequent research.

Beside the importance of cue arrangement in the display for understanding the task, *visual feedback* can function to motivate, reinforce, and direct behavior. In most tasks, a person can see what has been accomplished. In other ones, visual feedback is withheld or distorted. As is the case with all forms of feedback, immediate and accurate returns are desirable. Visual task cues, when compared to verbal and kinesthetic ones under systems of withholding or emphasizing, often have been found to be the most beneficial to skill acquisition. Therefore, motor tasks should contain visual information on performance returns (seeing the results of one's operations) as well as clear and specific visual cues for information processing.

Finally, displays have been adapted from real situations to artificial ones. In many industrial, military, and vehicle operations, equipment is expensive and an element of danger may be present. Simulated equipment permits the training of large numbers of individuals who otherwise might not have the opportunity to learn. Devices are thus specially made to simulate to a certain extent the actual performance conditions or, perhaps, to prepare the individual for the actual task via emphasized audio, visual, tactile, and kinesthetic cues.

These devices have been categorized according to their primary functions. A *trainer* is usually used as an aid in prompting the cues necessary for learning a skill. Films or specially designed equipment help the learner to gain greater insight into the nature of the real task, although they generally do not simulate it. The purpose of a *simulator* is to provide simulated practice on the skill in the way it is to be generally performed. For instance, in many parts of the country it is impossible to play golf all year. However, it is possible to simulate realistic golfing conditions. Regulation woods, irons, and balls are used with computerized apparatus, which simulates a golf course and true playing conditions. Golfers can improve their strokes, have the opportunity to play when outdoor weather does not permit it, and enjoy the competitiveness and reality of the golfing situation. Fake plane cockpits, automobile controls, and machinery displays also serve as simulators or trainers.

Not only can the display be manipulated to the benefit of the learner, but practice conditions can be imposed as well. There are so many variables that a brief description is all that is possible in this chapter. Most of these considerations are "old-hat" to psychologists and have been investigated extensively in the last century. Generally, research indicates that certain conditions produce the following results:

1. A skill may be practiced continuously (*massed conditions*), with rest pauses, or with interpolated skill learnings (*distributed practice*). For most skills, it is evident that distributed practice exerts a more positive influence than massed practice on performance, as compared to learning. Although immediate skill acquisition is favored under distributed practice, tests of retention demonstrate little difference in performance between initially massed and distributed practice groups.

2. *Practice* alone is not sufficient for improvement. Without *knowledge of results, interest and attention, meaningfulness* of the task to the learner, *understanding of goals, intent* to learn, *readiness* to learn, and some degree of *relationship* of practice conditions to real conditions, practice, for all practical purposes, is wasted.

3. *Overlearning*, or practicing past a criterion, results in better retention of what has been learned.

4. *Better-learned skills* are less prone to disruption by manipulated environmental conditions. Experiences in varying instructional or stressful conditions will contribute to high levels of skill.

5. Reinforcement increases the probability that the desired act will occur. Random reinforcement is a more effective continual form of motivation than constant reinforcement.

6. Very high *motivation* impedes progress in complex tasks. Highest performance is attained by individuals with intermediate motivation or drive, and as tasks increase in complexity, individuals with moderate motivation do better. Evidently, there is an optimal motivational level for each task.

7. Reasonably *difficult, specific, but attainable goals* produce better performance than easy goals or a general goal to do one's best.

8. Behavior is influenced by previous experiences. Greater resemblance between task elements, between their respective stimuli and responses, results in a greater amount of *positive transfer*. Transfer is determined by such factors as amount of practice on the prior task, motivation to transfer skill, method of training, and intent of transfer.

All of these and many more factors associated with the learning process, personal attributes, and situational considerations will be elaborated on in greater detail throughout this book. Their brief inclusion in this chapter should prepare you for recognizing the intricacies in studying motor learning and performance.

THE OBJECTIVE: PROFICIENCY

Although there may exist a number of objectives in the learning situation, one of the immediate and ultimate goals is the mastery of the task and the attainment of skill. Different standards of achievement are established, but essentially the most efficient and effective ways of reaching goals are sought.

A number of factors contribute to proficiency. They are described generally in Figure 2-7. Genetics, childhood experiences, personal goals, environmental influences, and other interactions lead to the state of excellence. Ideally, to determine potentials for developing proficiency in any task, genetic factors, familial tendencies, past experiences, and an individual's personality would be reasonably understood prior to training on a given task in a particular situation. General learning principles and specific considerations, with appropriate environmental modifications and instructional techniques, would then be utilized. The instructor is thus the ultimate determiner of the learner's productivity. Personal factors of the learners are incorporated in the instructor's plan in directing practice sessions.

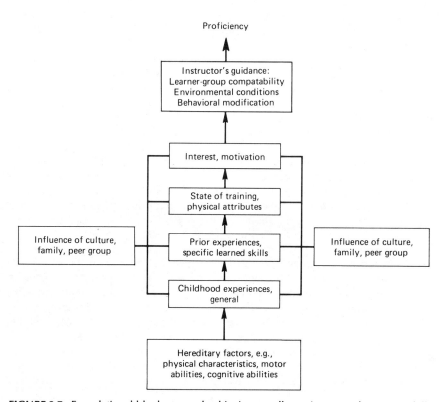

FIGURE 2-7. Foundational blocks toward achieving excellence in a complex motor skill.

CHAPTER HIGHLIGHTS

1. Skill can be described in terms of speed, accuracy, efficiency, and adaptability, or any combination of these. It has been defined as the consistent degree of success in achieving an objective with efficiency and effectiveness. A skill consists of a specific set of responses to particular cues in certain situations, whereas an ability is a general trait that contributes to success in the performance of a number of skills.

2. Learning curves are graphic representations of changes in behavior over time, as a result of practice under designed conditions. Great irregularities usually appear from person to person and from task to task when learning curves are examined. However, when averaged out over many people and possibly blocks of trials, any one of four different types of curves may be obtained: negatively accelerated, linear, S-shaped, or positively accelerated. Learning curves are influenced by: (a) the treatments (experiences) given to people; (b) performance artifacts and personal equations (fatigue, motivation, etc.); (c) the type of task used (e.g., difficulty); (d) the number of practice trials allowed; (e) the type of measurement selected; and (f) the number of scores used as the basis for each trial.

3. Plateaus have been defined as relatively stationary performances preceded and sometimes followed by accelerated learning increments. The true existence of plateaus is debatable because they have not been verified with laboratory research. But real-world acceptance of their existence in many activities suggests a reexamination of the problem. If in fact they can, and do, occur, plateaus should be analyzed for possible causes, and remediated accordingly. Possible causes might be (a) loss of interest, loss of novelty, loss of motivation; (b) focus on wrong cues; (c) fatigue; (d) emotions; (e) lack of physical readiness; (f) low level of aspiration; and (g) lack of understanding of directions and lack of ability to reorganize and adapt skills.

4. The understanding of learning and performance encompasses three major categories of factors: the learner (and consideration for individual differences); the learning process (and similarities among individuals); and situations (and how practice and training conditions differentially influence the average learner and different types of learners).

5. People possess similar mechanisms for learning and performance that need to operate properly in sequence or in parallel fashion, although these mechanisms may be trained to function more effectively by some rather than others.

6. There are too many personal (or individual difference) factors to describe here, as they can potentially influence learning and performance levels. Many influence all forms of learning, and some are more uniquely associated with psychomotor behaviors. Body build, physical measures (strength, endurance, speed, etc.), motor abilities, previously learned skills, and fear of danger in performance are factors associated with psychomotor behaviors.

7. Learning environments can be modified in many ways if consideration is shown for learning-outcome objectives, the nature of the activities, and the characteristics of the learners. Physical environments can be varied, cues and feedback manipulated, and training procedures altered. Practice conditions can be consistent with what appear to be "accepted learning principles."

8. Proficiency in any complex activity depends on genetic factors, childhood experiences, the learning of specific skills and knowledge related to the activity, state of training, motivation, and guidance.

References

Bahrick, H. P., Fitts, P. M., & Briggs, G. E. Learning curves—Facts or artifacts. *Psychological Bulletin,* 1957, *54,* 256–268.

Belbin, E., Belbin, R. M., & Hill, F. A comparison between the results of three different methods of operator training. *Ergonomics,* 1957, *1,* 39–50.

Bradley, J. V. Practice to an asymptote? *Journal of Motor Behavior,* 1969, *1,* 285–296.

Bryan, W., & Harter, N. Studies in the physiology and psychology of telegraphic language. *Psychological Review,* 1897, *4,* 27–53.

Culler, E. Nature of the learning curve. *Psychological Bulletin,* 1928, *25,* 143–148.

Culler, E., & Girden, E. The learning curve in relation to other psychometric functions. *American Journal of Psychology,* 1951, *64,* 327–349.

Estes, W. K. Toward a statistical theory of learning. *Psychological Review,* 1950, *57,* 94–107.

Estes, W. K. The problem of inference from curves based on group data. *Psychological Bulletin,* 1956, *53,* 134–140.

Fleishman, E. A. Structure and measurement of psychomotor abilities. In R. N. Singer (Ed.), *The psychomotor domain: Movement behavior.* Philadelphia: Lea & Febiger, 1972.

Godfrey, B., & Kephart, N. *Movement patterns and motor education.* New York: Appleton-Century-Crofts, 1969.

Johnson, H. W. Skill = speed < accuracy < form < adaptability. *Perceptual and Motor Skills,* 1961, *13,* 163–170.

Keller, F. S. The phantom plateau. *Journal of the Experimental Analysis of Behavior,* 1958, *1,* 1–13.

Thurstone, L. L. The learning function. *Journal of General Psychology,* 1930, *3,* 469–493.

3
DESIGN AND MEASUREMENT

In order to derive a scientific body of knowledge about behavior, data must be collected. This information should not be expressed casually but rather recorded with care and in detail. Research, conducted through a scientific method of analysis, provides a reasonably objective means of answering questions about animal and human behavior. Problems are studied and procedures are designed for their solution. Inferences to large numbers (a specified population) are often made from the results of data collected on sample subjects.

Most of the research reported in this book will be experimental in nature. Investigations in the motor learning area tend to be experimental, for researchers are attempting to determine antecedent and consequential relationships. What kinds of effects will a particular condition produce on behavior? If we were to help learners set reasonably high but attainable goals for themselves before and during the practices of a task, would performances be any more proficient than when learners practice without such assistance? Experimental projects would help to solve this issue. Motor learning specialists often compare different treatments (situational modifications), as administered through practice, in their quest to ascertain the best practice or training techniques.

Motor skills researchers also look at relationships among variables. One example of a study of interest might be the relationship between the age of a person and ability to learn a moderately difficult motor task. How about the association of personality traits, intelligence scores, and motor performance? Further study might be done on the learning process itself: e.g., the generality of rates of learning across a variety of learning tasks, the relationship of initial level of success with later task proficiency, or abilities underlying achievement in particular activities at different stages of practice.

Motor behaviors can be observed under artificial and manipulated conditions as well as in natural situations. The research laboratory or the gymnasium may provide the appropriate data for the problem of concern. Regardless of the task used, the variables of interest, and the setting, the scores of the subjects are typically recorded and analyzed in some way in order to reach conclusions about the stated problem. Thus, scores—how they are obtained and how they are used— become the essence of the report. In experiments where the effects of some variable on learning are to be determined, a crucial decision must be made with regard

51

to a score that constitutes learning. In this chapter, various approaches to the measurement of learning will be reviewed, with implications made for researchers and practitioners alike.

DECISIONS IN MEASURING LEARNING

Scientifically accepted methods for studying motor learning can easily be decided on, on some occasions, but not so on others. Certain procedural aspects in the design of investigations require careful deliberation, as the consequences of these decisions can be quite dramatic. With this thought in mind, let us identify problems and decisions in the experimentation of motor behaviors. This discussion should help you to recognize and to be sensitive to these problems, thus aiding in the interpretation of research findings or the undertaking of research. Major decisions must be made in the following areas:

1. Selection of appropriate learning tasks.
2. Determination of the number of learning trials and the duration of the study.
3. Selection of a dependent variable (what and how to measure).
4. Determination of a learning score or scores.

Selection of Appropriate Learning Tasks

The selection of the "right" task in a particular experiment is by no means easy. The researcher must consider the purposes of the study, the nature of the subjects who will be tested, and the various tasks that can be used. More specifically, tasks are usually selected on the basis of

1. reliability.
2. validity.
3. novelty.
4. ease of administration, practicality, and control.
5. purpose of the study.
6. degree of difficulty.
7. compatability with subjects' maturational level and physical abilities.
8. availability.
9. degree of inherent interest.

Reliability refers to the consistency of the subjects' scores when the subjects are tested on the same test on more than one occasion. Consistency will be obtained when (1) test conditions are identical, including the experimenter's directions and overall role; (2) the apparatus has been calibrated or examined carefully, preferably before usage on each occasion; and (3) the learners are controlled as to consistent treatment when they are tested.

Whether the task measures what it is supposed to measure is indicative of its *validity*. If the intention is to employ a test of balance, how do we know it measures that characteristic? Arm strength? Speed of movement? In most learning studies, we are interested in tasks that can be used to demonstrate a learning effect when certain conditions are introduced by the experimenter. In many of these cases, face validity, or common sense, suffices.

If the investigator wants to study the learning process or the effect of situational changes on the acquisition of skill, the typical concern is for subjects who are *naive* to the task that will be practiced and learned. Said another way, the task should be *novel,* or new, to the subjects. Because there is difficulty in finding real-life activities that are novel to a group of subjects, the usual recourse is to select an artificial laboratory task or a contrived athletic task for a study.

Once a nonfamiliar task has been selected (assuming this is desirable), the investigator must consider its *degree of difficulty.* Difficulty will be a function of input demands (the number of cues needed to be attended to and under what conditions), processing demands (speed to initiate response), and response demands (number of movements, refinement of movement, and so on). The nature of the learning phenomenon to be studied will suggest the type of task that might be used. As the reader will see, many of the tasks employed by motor learning researchers are of the laboratory variety and are relatively simple to perform, at that. That is, they are easy relative to the dimensions of athletic activities, like learning to fence, to play tennis, or to perform gymnastic routines. The laboratory tasks may be fairly well learned after ten or twenty trials, whereas it takes years to become a good tennis player. However, simpler tasks often permit the study of a learning variable(s) if taught in purer settings under good control and in a brief time span.

If the task is learned too quickly, however, it is probable that learning variables of interest might be camouflaged. The effects of an imposed condition might go unnoticed. For instance, if one selected task is simple to learn well and we want to study the differential effects of reward and punishment on task proficiency, the two groups might not show any difference in performance, primarily because of the simplicity of the task. A related problem exists where a criterion of task mastery is predetermined and it turns out to be unrealistically low or easy to attain.

Tasks are often selected on the basis of ease of *administration* and *availability.* Practical reasons may encourage the selection of one task over another. By all means, the experimenter should be able to exert full control over the operation and administration of the task.

All things being equal, the more desirable learning task is one that can be measured with a minimal amount of interference and bias. Response measures are never pure. The challenge is to obtain measures that reveal "true" scores. Disturbing environmental cues, subjective experimenter observations, direct experimenter interactions with the subject, and uncalibrated and unexamined equipment will produce artifacts contributing to nonvalid data. Finally, a task should be appropriate for the *maturational level* of the subjects. Inability to perform because of immaturity of the nervous system and the musculature would certainly be a factor contributing to confounded data.

Types of Learning Tasks

The most commonly used laboratory tasks in motor learning research, reported in one form or another, are pursuit rotors, star-tracing tasks, positioning tasks, and stabilometers. They are invariably novel tasks to the subjects and yet can be acquired to a reasonable degree in a relatively short time. A wide range of learning phenomena can be studied with these tasks and implications are made about motor behavior activities. A pursuit rotor, illustrated in Figure 3-1, is com-

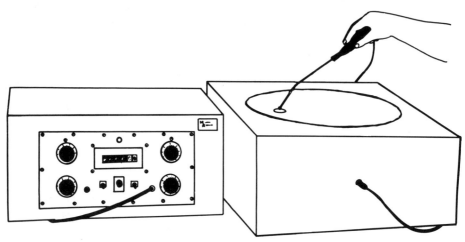

FIGURE 3-1. A pursuit rotor with a control unit with which test periods and rest periods can be preset.

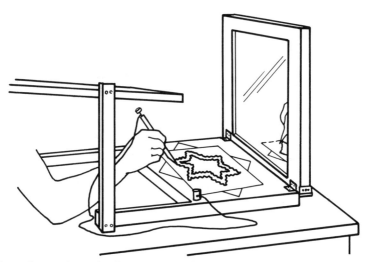

FIGURE 3-2. Star-tracing task. The star is traced as accurately as possible with the subject viewing it in the mirror. (*From Fulton, R. Speed and accuracy in learning movements.* Archives of Psychology, *1945, 300.*)

posed of a moving turntable on which a small disk must be pursued by the subject with a stylus. Time on target is usually recorded to 0.01 or 0.001 of a second. The star-tracing task (Figure 3-2) requires a subject to trace the pattern with a stylus as quickly as possible but while making a minimum of errors (an error being determined by the stylus touching the side of the tract). Viewing the mirror instead of the actual pattern makes it a reversal task and increases the task's difficulty. A more difficult tracking task is illustrated in Figure 3-3.

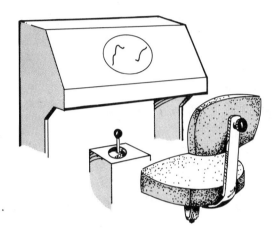

FIGURE 3-3. A tracking task in which a dot appears on the subject's display (a cathode ray tube); as the dot moves across the tube, the subject has to track it with a joy stick. Uncertainty about direction and position, velocity and acceleration make this a challenging task. (*From McLeod, P. D. Recovery strategy during temporary obscuration of a tracked target.* Ergonomics, *1972, 15, 57–64.*) Reprinted by permission of *Ergonomics* and Taylor & Francis Ltd.

Positioning tasks make demands on the subject to replicate predetermined movement speeds and distances. Judgment and timing are important. A stabilometer is a movable platform that the subject attempts to stabilize. During a prescribed testing period, one must maintain the platform as horizontal as possible. This balancing task is shown in Figure 3-4, and balance within the designated range is usually timed to 0.01 of a second.

Creative investigators have devised other kinds of laboratory tasks as well as field tasks. Furthermore, far more complex tasks have also been reported in the literature. For instance, Figure 3-5 indicates the complex coordinator, an apparatus that demands the appropriate timing of leg and hand responses to specific cues. Task difficulty increases when investigators develop tasks that contain a variety of cues that in turn require complex decision making and a variety of response possibilities from which the subject must select the correct ones.

Another type of task frequently found in the literature is one involving reaction time and/or speed of limb movement. Many situational variables can be manipulated to determine how an individual processes information and responds. Although the tasks are relatively simple, much of what we know about human behavior has been determined from data collected in reaction-time experiments. A choice reaction-time task and timer are illustrated in Figure 3-6.

The increased availability and diminishing costs of computers and solid-state programming equipment have researchers turning to them to manage the administration of performance tasks. Greater precision is attained in the process, and the

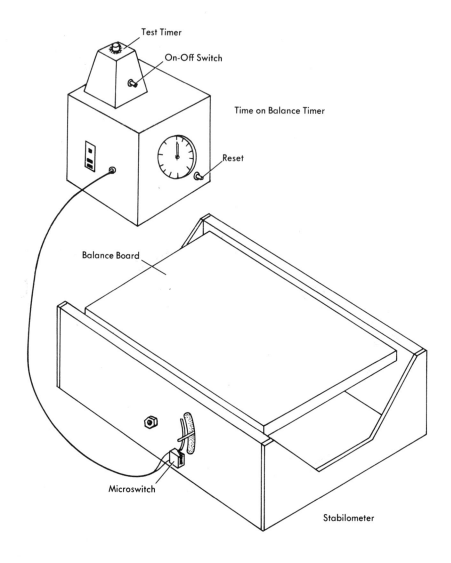

Test Timer

On-Off Switch

Time on Balance Timer

Reset

Balance Board

Microswitch

Stabilometer

(Stabilometer and Timer Not to Scale)

FIGURE 3-4. A stabilometer.

data collected are recorded with minimal chance of errors, often a problem when the experimenter is in a more active role with less sophisticated equipment.

Motor and Sensory Measurements

The instruments and tasks described in the preceding section, as well as many others, have been used for the experimental analysis of behavioral change, or learning. Yet, there may be other purposes for conducting research in the motor

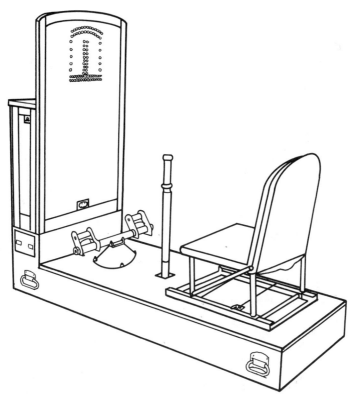

FIGURE 3-5. Complex coordination test. The subject is required to make complex motor adjustments of stick and pedal controls in response to stimulus light patterns. (*From Fleishman, E. A. A comparative study of aptitude patterns in unskilled and skilled psychomotor performances.* Journal of Applied Psychology, *1957, 41, 263–272.*)

learning area. Specific motor behaviors may be of interest, either for the establishment of norms or to determine the effects of such factors as fatigue or drugs on them. Sensory measurements, on the other hand, are primarily used to detect phenomena associated with perceiving physical stimuli (psychophysics). The level of functioning of the sense organs may be related to proficiency in various motor skill endeavors.

Instruments to evaluate motor responses or performance of the sense organs are found in many motor learning laboratories. A dynamometer measures exerted force, or static strength. There is equipment to measure hand steadiness or body sway. Pieces of equipment used in the testing of learning changes can also be used for measuring motor responses—e.g., pursuit rotors for hand–eye coordination and stabilometers for balance.

In regard to sensory measurements, there are apparatuses to analyze depth perception and field of vision. Visual perception is evaluated with a tachistoscope, in which presentation times in sequences of visual displays are varied. An audio-

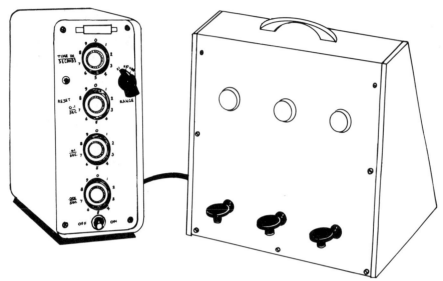

FIGURE 3-6. Choice reaction timer *(Marietta Apparatus Co., Marietta, Ohio)* and Hunter Klockounter, which measures to 0.001 of a second *(Hunter Manufacturing Co., Iowa City, Iowa).*

meter measures hearing acuity, weighted cylinders help to detect the sensitivity of tactile sense receptors, and positioning tests require proprioceptive involvement. An excellent source book on biomedical instrumentation—an introduction to various apparatuses, their design and usage, and applications to the measurement of body functions—is *Biomedical Instrumentation and Measurements,* by Leslie Cromwell and his colleagues (1973).

Duration of the Study

Most published research studies on learning reveal data collection that extends over a relatively brief time span. One reason for this is that the tasks used are not too difficult and the ceiling effect is noticeable before long. That is, potential maximum performance is attained easily and quickly. Performance scores with such tasks are insensitive to improvements as they approach the upper limits set for the task. Upper limits in performance are set by the experimenter or by the very nature of the task and the length of practice or test periods. Quick gains in performance are observed in about the first five trials and an asymptote is approximated after about fifteen or twenty trials on such tasks as the pursuit rotor, stabilometer, and star-tracing apparatus. Thus, a study may be completed in from one to four days. Such constraints in laboratory settings bias the data, although relatively "clean" data can be observed otherwise, as environmental and personal variables can be controlled in a reasonable manner. In contrast, a ceiling effect is nearly impossible to reach in athletic skills. The criterion of excellence is difficult, if not impossible, to ascertain. There is always room for improvement.

Of course, if long-term retention is under study, an experiment may last a few months or a year. By the same token, long-term retention is not studied only with long retention intervals. If retention of information from long-term memory is of interest, it could be that a retention test is administered only five minutes from the original learning in some studies. An advantage to a short-duration study is the general lack of subject mortality, a fancy term for the loss of subjects that is usually found to be proportional to the length of the project. The longer a study goes on, the better the chance subjects will miss testing occasions for one reason or another. Consequently, long-term experiments should include more subjects than might be included in short-term ones, to compensate for expected subject mortality.

An experiment must be of long enough duration, in terms of trials, experiences, or days, for behavior to be altered as a result of specially designed practice conditions. If too much experience is provided, it is equally possible that special treatment effects will not be revealed when a treatment group of subjects is compared to a control group of subjects. More practice does not necessarily result in better data. Careful consideration must be given to the purpose of the study, and along with a review of previous research completed in related areas, decisions can be arrived at in a meaningful and logical way.

Sometimes the question of *warm-up trials* is an issue. Should any warm-up, or task-familiarization, experience be given to the subjects? Once again, the answer is not simple. If the task is very unusual, there may be good reason for allowing a few task-familiarization trials. Sometimes warm-up trials can confound data, especially if the task is rather easy. Once again, the purpose of the study must be reviewed critically, the advantages and disadvantages of warm-up trials evaluated carefully, and decisions made accordingly.

The Dependent Measure(s)

Experiments contain independent and dependent measures. The independent measure is the variable of interest; the dependent variable represents the recorded data. For instance, we might be concerned with the effects of motivation on performance. The independent variable, motivation, would be introduced in some form and compared to a control situation. An example might be one group of subjects experiencing the learning of a task where verbal encouragement is constantly offered. Another group of subjects, the control, would learn the task without any comments offered. The dependent measure would be the method of recording the behavior observed. If the task were a pursuit rotor, the dependent measure would probably be the time the subject maintained the stylus in contact with the moving disc during a particular trial. If the task involved archery shooting, the dependent measure would be the subject's score.

The assessment of motor behavior is usually made with regard to (1) speed, (2) accuracy or error, or (3) magnitude. Sometimes, combinations of these measures or different forms of the measures are obtained in the same experiment. As long as various measurements are not merely "saying the same thing," learning processes and outcomes can be analyzed more thoroughly with the use of more than one dependent measure. We will return to this problem shortly.

Speed of response in the laboratory has usually been analyzed in reaction-time experiments and/or movement-time experiments. *Reaction time* (RT) is the interval between the presentation of a stimulus and the *initiation* of a response. *Movement time* (MT) encompasses the time it takes a subject to complete the act *after* it has been initiated. Further descriptions and illustrations of apparatus will appear later in this book. It is important to note, however, that these movements are usually found to be independent and unrelated. That is, a person who has a fast reaction time provides us with no assurance that a fast movement time will be emitted when compared to others. The opposite is, of course, true, as well. Typically, in practical situations *response time* is recorded, such as with the runner covering a specified distance. Response time is the composite score of reaction time and movement time.

Accuracy can be determined in the real world by hearing the number of correct notes played by the piano player, seeing the number of correct keys pressed by the typist, or seeing the number of serves that are within the boundaries of the tennis court. In the laboratory, accuracy through time-on-target scores (TOT) is indicated with the pursuit rotor, through traversing a maze without errors, with the star-tracing task, or with a positioning task, where a subject attempts to relocate the distance and location of a previous response.

Response magnitude refers to effort yield, such as jumping as high as possible or exerting maximal force against a hand dynomometer to measure grip strength. Such measures are often observed in the sports world but are rarely taken in the laboratory.

Although the dependent measure may be an obvious decision in a number of tasks, it is often controversial in others. When a variety of possibilities exists for recording data, the experimenter's dilemma is increased. The severity of the consequences in selecting an inappropriate or less desirable measure from the alternatives should never be understated. Conclusions based on the selected dependent measure may be more or less valid, depending on the experimenter's wisdom.

In a classic article, referred to in Chapter 2, Bahrick, Fitts, and Briggs (1957) demonstrated the effects of changing the response-sensitivity measures used for subjects performing a tracking task. The size of the target zone (variously sized scoring zones) resulted in varying shapes in the learning curves. The arbitrary selection of a cut-off point (what is considered on-target or off-target) can significantly affect the data and the conclusions derived from them. The magnitude of the errors in performance, for example, seems to be a more justifiable measure than a gross recording of time on- or off-target. The latter score has limited value in research. Any task that is scored with an all-or-none performance measure instead of considering a continuous and normal distribution of scores is subject to experimental artifacts.

With many tasks it might be wise to record and analyze more than one dependent measure. The acquisition of skill, especially in more complex tasks, usually encompasses the mastery of a number of task components. The analysis of more than one dependent variable may provide additional insight into learning progress. As an example, the oft-employed star-tracing task calls for the performer to trace a pattern as quickly as possible with a minimum of errors. What, then, should constitute the subject's score? A number of techniques have been suggested, and John Drowatzky (1969) has compared five scoring techniques, arriving at interesting conclusions. The methods were

1. time required for the completion of each trial.
2. number of errors committed during each trial.
3. the product of task completion time and number of errors per trial.
4. the number 1,000 divided by the product of completion time and errors per trial.
5. the sum of completion time and number of errors per trial.

Drowatzky's conclusion was that "no one . . . performance measure appeared to fully meet all requirements of an optimal measure of skill, and . . . that evaluation of star-tracing performance should include the measures of completion time, errors/trial, and product of time and errors" (p. 229).

Sometimes the reporting of too many performance variables is redundant and unnecessary. Obviously, if two measures are really measuring the same thing, there would be little gain in analyzing both of them. For instance, it is fairly common to see three dependent variables—(1) algebraic error, or constant error (CE); (2) absolute error (AE); and (3) within-subject variability, or variable error (VE)—presented in experiments dealing with positioning tasks. These tasks require the subjects to match movements against standards, with error or deviation scores as the variable of interest. The less the deviation, the better the performance.

AE indicates the amount of *magnitude* of error made in one performance, with no indication of the direction of overshooting or undershooting (+ or −) the mark. Magnitude of error is calculated by adding all the subjects' scores over trials and dividing by the number of trials. An average error in magnitude is thereby devised.

CE scores provide information about the *direction* of the error. CE is calculated in the same manner as AE, except that the direction of the scores is recorded, and this reveals an individual's *response bias*.

VE is an indicator of the subject's variability in performance, and conversely is an indicator of response *consistency*. It is calculated by taking the CE score for all trials and subtracting the error score from it for each trial. The score is then squared. All the trial scores are divided by the total number of trials, and the square root is taken.

Robert Schutz and Eric Roy (1973) have questioned the assumption of the independence of CE, AE, and VE scores and, in turn, the wisdom in using all of them in the same experiment. Using their definitions:

Error: The algebraic difference $(X_{ij} - Y)$

Constant error (CE): The mean algebraic error

$$\frac{\Sigma(X - Y)}{k} = \frac{\Sigma(e)}{k}$$

Absolute error (AE): The average error or mean deviation

$$\frac{\Sigma|X - Y|}{k} = \frac{\Sigma(e)}{k}$$

Variable error (VE): Intravariance, intraindividual variance, and within-subject variance [1]

$$\frac{1}{k}\Sigma\left[(X - Y) - \frac{\Sigma(X - Y)}{k}\right]^2 = \frac{1}{k}\Sigma[e - CE]^2$$

Or because Y is a constant and therefore does not affect the variance:

$$\frac{1}{k}\Sigma(X - \bar{X})^2$$

Reworking data published in other studies and applying mathematical theory, Schutz and Roy arrive at the conclusion that both AE and VE are quite interdependent and that, therefore, it is unwarranted to report both variables. It has been recommended by Jerry Thomas (1977) and others that if AE and VE measures are used, they should not be analyzed with a multivariate statistical model because of multicollinearity. AE is determined by Shutz and Roy to be completely dependent on CE and VE, and thus can be predicted from them. The authors call for the elimination of AE as a dependent measure in experiments, for CE and VE are statistically independent and can adequately describe most data.

On the other hand, F. M. Henry (1974) has made a persuasive argument to show that a composite error score (E) is most appropriate. E should be squared and would be equal to $\sqrt{\epsilon e^2/k} = \sqrt{V^2 + C^2}$. Henry claims that AE is definitely inadequate as a dependent measure. Also, the absolute rather than the algebraic constant error (C^2) should be made. E would reflect the contributions of both the variable error and constant error components correctly. R. W. Christina and W. J. Merriman (1977), terming E as total direction error, used it as the dependent measure in their study.

The latest and one of the most comprehensive attempts to analyze the effectiveness and appropriateness of AE, CE, VE, and E scores has been reported by M. J. Safrit, J. A. Spray, and G. L. Diewert (1979). Rather than favor one particular measure, they state that the choice of dependent measures should be based on

---

[1] Variable error is usually expressed as the standard deviation of a person's score about the individual mean performance score ($\sqrt{VE}$).

the behavioral dimensions which these measures reflect. Furthermore, due to the nature of the distribution of these scores, an analysis of them should require different statistical procedures.

The Learning Score

Another difficult decision is related to the measure or the score that best represents learning, or the effects of practice. In most studies of learning, repeated measures are collected on subjects over trials or time. Returning to the hypothetical study on motivation, with two groups, one a control and one experimental, what should be used as the achievement measures with which the groups can be compared to determine if verbal encouragement indeed resulted in increased learning over no verbal encouragement in either the pursuit rotor task or in archery shooting? Perhaps twenty trials of thirty seconds' duration each were interspersed with thirty-second rest periods in pursuit rotor performance. Do we compare both groups on their scores attained on the twentieth trial? Would it be better to work with gain scores—that is, the difference scores between the last and first trials? How about the best score reached by each subject on any one trial? What about the average score for each subject across all twenty trials? Is there a particular formula that might be more sensitive and valid than any of the preceding formulas measured?

As we become more familiar with the research literature dealing with motor learning, it will become apparent that a wide variety of approaches has been described in an attempt to make comparisons between learning situations. As is the case with any step in an experiment, more appropriate decisions will lead to more valid conclusions. Unfortunately, there appears to be no easy answer to the question of how learning should be determined. Probably the most widely accepted techniques include some form of arriving at a (1) gain or difference score, (2) average score, or (3) final score(s). The use of the average, or mean, score across all trials administered to the subjects can be defended if no trend is present. Walter Kroll (1967) supports this notion with the use of reliability theory. If a trend appears, alternatives for a criterion measure might include (1) a search for a measurement schedule free of systematic measure-error variance, or (2) the use of the high or low score for each subject, with necessary cautions.

The argument of whether to use the best score or average score of subjects on trials appears frequently in the literature. Although Kroll (1967) and Henry (1967) generally favor the use of the average score, Hetherington (1973) has taken issue with their statistical rationale used in support of their positions. He favors the best score obtained on any trial whenever the measurement error is believed to be small, relative to within-subject variation. He raises the question of whether the between-trial variation is normally distributed about the "true" score, especially in cases where an estimation of maximum performance is derived. The relative advantages of the best or average score as "the score" are still being debated, and certainly a number of factors must be considered before a choice can be made for one or the other.

In certain kinds of experiments it might be advisable for the experimenter to establish a criterion performance measure that the subjects are expected to achieve. In many laboratory motor learning studies, data are usually analyzed in terms of three different measures:

1. The total time taken by the subject to reach a given criterion of performance.
2. The total number of errors made in reaching the criterion.
3. The total number of trials taken to reach the criterion.

These three measures of learning performance are confounded by several factors, notably:

1. The learning ability of the subject.
2. The subject's initial skill level.
3. The criterion of achievement established by the experimenter.

A satisfactory resolution of these factors that influence data deserves considerable attention.

There are various methods of analyzing changes within practice. Measurement of these changes usually associated with differences between initial and terminal performances indicates the degree of learning that has occurred. L. W. McCraw (1951, 1955) has compared many of the possible ways of measuring and scoring tests of motor learning. In each of his two studies, McCraw obtained data from subjects who performed two novel motor skills. Learning that has occurred because of practice can be measured by considering such factors as initial status versus final score, difference between first and last scores, and percentage of improvement. Also, there is the problem of ascertaining the number of trials that should represent the first score as well as the final score. How many trials are necessary for warm-up and task familiarity are open to question, but most authorities agree that at least a few should be provided before an actual initial score is recorded.

In attempting to reconcile these problems, McCraw (1955) formulated eight methods, based on those found in other experiments, to score the practice effects on learning two tasks. Some of these procedures were:

1. *Total Learning Score Method:* consisted of cumulatively adding all the trial scores during practice.
2. *Difference in Raw Score Method No. 1:* required finding the difference between the final and initial trials.
3. *Per Cent Gain of Possible Gain Method No. 1:* represented by the formula:

$$\frac{\text{(Sum of last } N \text{ trials) minus (sum of first } N \text{ trials)}}{\text{(Highest possible score on } N \text{ trials) minus (sum of first } N \text{ trials)}}$$

where N = number

4. *Two Per Cent Gain of Initial Score Method:* depicted by the formula:

$$\frac{(\text{Sum of last } N \text{ trials}) \text{ minus } (\text{sum of first } N \text{ trials})}{(\text{Sum of first } N \text{ trials})}$$

The number of trials should be kept constant for all portions of the formulas. Thus, if the sum of the first two trials is used for the initial score, and the sum of the last two is the final score, then the highest possible score would be two times the highest score that was made on any trial during the practice period. The following example is an application of the formula to ten trials on a rope-skip test in which each trial is the number of times the subject can skip the rope in 10 seconds (see formula 3, which precedes):

Scores on Ten Trials: 6,5,8,7,10,12,16,12,14,13

Initial Score: $6 + 5 = 11$

Final Score: $14 + 13 = 27$

Highest Possible Score: $2 \times 16 = 32$

Per cent gain $= \dfrac{27 - 11}{32 - 11} = \dfrac{16}{21} = 76\%$

McCraw reported considerable variability in the scores as yielded by the diverse means of measuring improvement. As to a comparison of methods, he states that the most acceptable appear to be those that relate gain to possible gain, while the least desirable are those that interpret gain in relation to the initial score. The Total Learning Method and the Three Per Cent Gain of Possible Gain Method were the most valid measures in comparing individuals with dissimilar initial scores. McCraw generally found little relationship between the various scoring methods—i.e., each yielded different results.

Thus, it can be seen that varying the techniques for measuring improvement results in dissimilar outcomes and interpretations of the data. The nature of each study must be scrutinized before the procedure of data analysis is selected, although some methods are apparently more acceptable than others. One of the difficulties in determining laws of learning pertaining to any factor is the variation in design from investigation to investigation, including the selected method of data analysis.

Change or gain scores probably should not be calculated unless necessary. If subjects are truly randomly placed into groups and are statistically equal in initial skill status, then the computation of gain scores is not necessary. Posttest analysis of scores is sufficient (Cronbach, Gleser, Nanda, & Rajaratnam, 1972). However, if necessary, gain scores can be computed quite laboriously, as we will see, to obtain the truest measurements possible.

In the typical case of measuring change that is the result of practice, the "raw" change score is computed, which consists of the difference between a pretest and a posttest on the variable of concern. The definition of this measure from variable A to variable B (e.g., pretest A and posttest B) is $B - A$. The usual contaminant in this methodology is that $B - A$ is negatively correlated with A. That is to say, the higher the pretest score, the smaller the gain score. If a person had had no experience with the task and was beginning at a zero level of proficiency, any achievement later would be a gain. This assumption is reasonable with very unusual tasks, such as learning nonsense syllables and mazes. In real situations, however, everyone comes to the "new" learning situation with some previously related experience. Consequently, subjects start at different skill levels. If we measure progression in a task where thirty points is maximum, we cannot at all assume that the gain from zero to twelve is the same as from twelve to twenty-four points. As the potential ceiling (score limits) are closer to being reached, gains are much more difficult to demonstrate. The same gain score for any two people, in this case twelve, does not truly reveal enough information when starting points are dissimilar.

There is no clear-cut answer to how many trials should be averaged to constitute the pretest score or the posttest score (Schutz, 1975). Tasks, characteristics of subjects, and learning phenomena studied differ from study to study, and unique considerations must be made. Nevertheless, Schutz makes a good case for some form of average score over the selection of only one score when initial learning status is compared with final level of attainment.

In particular situations it is of advantage to have a change score that is independent of the pretest. An alternative to the raw change score is the *residual change* score, also known as a base-free measure, where final scores are uncorrelated with initial scores (see, for example, Tucker et al., 1966). The portion of the posttest that is linearly predictable from the pretest is eliminated. The residual gain procedure yields estimates of deviations from the expected scores of individuals (or groups). A zero residual gain means that the actual gain for the individual or group was identical with the gain that was predicted from a knowledge of the pretest score by linear regression techniques.

Henry (1956) used three motor learning experiments with the tasks in each involving (1) jumping, (2) speed of arm movement, or (3) balancing. As expected, he found raw learning scores to be unrelated to final skill accomplishments but negatively correlated with initial performance. He shows how the use of the residual method can alleviate this circumstance. It estimates the individual learning that would have occurred had all subjects begun at the same initial skill level.

Another model with a number of variations that has been supported in the literature is the *true change* approach. If the pretest and posttest are measured without error (experimental contamination), then a true change score is observed. Because this is rarely the case, some estimate must be made of the observed gain in performance attributable to measurement errors so that an estimate of true gain is possible. Regression equations have been proposed to handle this problem, and these models as well as other approaches are summarized by Chester Harris (1963).

An excellent summary of the many residual gain and true change models is offered by Lee Cronbach and Lita Furby (1970). Relative strengths and weaknesses are discussed. Interestingly enough, after laboriously representing the various measures of change, these writers argue against their usage. Assuming equality between groups of subjects at the start of the experiment, as well as errors of measurement on the posttest that are randomly distributed, *a simple posttest comparison would do*. Other suggestions are made for specific situations.

When using raw gain scores, the assumption is made that the groups of subjects to be compared are equal at the start of the experiment on the parameters that might be influential on the performance outcomes. This may occur, at least theoretically, when large enough samples of subjects are randomly placed into groups and the groups in turn randomly assigned to specific treatments. But there are instances when it is known that the groups are in fact dissimilar prior to any administered treatments. For instance, it is conceivable that one group of subjects might show a lower pretest score than another group in the same experiment. Or, one group might, for some reason, possess a greater prominence of an influential factor, say desirable body builds, for the learning of a particular activity. In many cases, an *analysis of covariance* is the statistical tool that can adjust posttest scores according to pretest differences or differences on a variable(s) of influence. Yet, the limitations of covariance should be recognized. If differences exist between the groups prior to the experiment other than in the covariate (e.g., pretest), confounded data will still occur.

In Table 3-1, the various measures that have been used to assess changes in motor behavior are presented and compared. The table provides a good overview and summary of the material presented in this section of the chapter.

Some general recommendations to be made in determining the learning score follow:

1. Assuming that an adequate number of subjects are placed into groups according to acceptable procedures such as randomization or blocking of scores, a final score (preferably based on a few trials for reliability, if the learning phenomenon under study permits it) will suffice. The learning score is derived simply. But care must be taken to assure that the subjects are placed properly into groups.
2. If the subjects differ in characteristics and performance at the onset, analysis of covariance, true change, or residual gains will be appropriate.
3. If an analysis of learning over trials is desired, with between and within group comparisons made at various points, analysis of variance can be appropriate if statistical assumptions are met. Multivariate analysis of variance should be used instead if more than one dependent measure has been obtained, and those measures are relatively independent of each other.

TABLE 3-1 The Measurement of Learning: Learning Scores for Group Comparisons[1]

Subject's Measure	Strengths	Weaknesses
1. Average score (total score divided by number of trials) or Cumulative score across trials	a. smooths out data and provides representative scores for subjects and groups b. uses all data	a. assumes equality of subjects at the beginning of the experiment b. no analysis of trends in the data c. no indication of improvement at the final stages versus initial task performance d. assumes similar number of trials for all subjects
2. Best score[2]	a. because terminal score may be depressed temporarily, the best score may truly reflect level of learning	a. may be "chance" effect due to faulty experimental control (overemphasis on contribution of one score) b. no consideration for reliability c. assumes equality of subjects at the beginning of the experiment
3. Final score[2]	a. assuming initial equality of subjects, provides easy-to-assess indication of terminal achievement	a. may be lower than "true" score due to experimental artifacts b. assumes equality of subjects (in performance level and in learning ability) at initial testing c. assumes errors of measurement are randomly distributed
4. Trial or blocks of trials scores (repeated measures ANOVA or MANOVA)	a. can observe trends in the data, interactional effects, and group differences at different stages of learning b. reduces measurement errors	a. ANOVA may violate certain statistical assumptions b. little information about *form* of change over time c. assumes equality of subjects at the beginning of the experiment
5. Raw gain (difference) score[2]	a. simple to calculate b. indicates degree of improvement	a. assumes equality of subjects (in performance level and learning ability) at initial testing

[1]This assumes the analysis of one dependent measure, although a number of appropriate dependent ones can be handled through MANOVA designs.

[2]Although reference is made to only one score, in any of these cases scores could be averaged over a few trials (e.g., three-trial average to determine the final score). Shutz (1975) for one, favors average score over a one trial score in these cases.

Subject's Measure	Strengths	Weaknesses
		b. favors starting low to show great gains c. is gain really the same in different cases (e.g., 10–15 versus 1–6)? d. final score may be lower than "true" score due to experimental artifacts e. nonreliability of score
6. % gain of possible gain	a. accounts for differences among subjects at initial testing	a. maximum gain possible not always known b. use of difference score in calculation; therefore, possesses weaknesses listed in 5
7. True change	a. measurement errors on pretest and posttest are determined and accounted for b. overcomes many of the weaknesses of the raw-gain method	a. laborious procedure b. data may not meet statistical assumptions
8. Residual gain	a. final scores are uncorrelated with initial scores b. regression technique partials out any relationships between initial and final scores c. overcomes many of the weaknesses of the gain method	a. laborious procedure b. data may not meet statistical assumptions
9. Final scores adjusted on basis of initial scores (analysis of covariance)	a. considers individual differences on pretest	a. individuals may differ on important variables not identified and adjusted with the analysis of covariance

MOTOR LEARNING LABORATORIES AND EQUIPMENT

In order to investigate learning processes, the effects of training manipulations, learning and performance correlates, and other related considerations, decisions must be made about space, subjects, and learning tasks. A laboratory, in the formal sense of the word, connotes an isolated area in which extremely controlled testing can occur. Motor learning laboratories exist in many physical education departments, experimental and engineering psychology areas, and military and aerospace programs. Often they are equipped with a minimum amount of expensive equipment (much handmade apparatus) or, at the other extreme, computerized controlled operations are available. Depending on the sophistication of the experimenter, the equipment, the testing conditions, and the type of learning phenomenon investigated, the data will usually be handled in a technical manner, contributing to theory and knowledge, with implications for practical conditions.

If we expand our interpretation of the laboratory or consider field testing environments, subjects are tested under conditions that are more like real life and with more familiar motor tasks, often not involving equipment. These data are usually more directly applicable to programmatic or instructional concerns. As we will see, studies in the area of motor learning range considerably regarding testing conditions, learning phenomena, and performance variables investigated.

With the assumption that you can readily comprehend how research might be conducted in gymnasiums, classrooms, and other familiar situations, let us discuss the nature and use of more formal established laboratories. Because one of the major thrusts in the motor learning area is to determine how we learn skills and how we can learn them more effectively and efficiently, the identification of the "right" task is of paramount concern. As was mentioned earlier in this chapter, the need is for novel and unusual tasks, those with which the learner is unfamiliar, so that processes and the effects of situational manipulations can be examined in a technical manner. These tasks can be purchased, but in many motor learning laboratories they are constructed to fit the needs of the experimenter and the particular area of investigation.

Such tasks so commonly used as pursuit rotors or star tracers can be purchased or made. Stabilometers and positioning tasks can be made easily. (See the illustrations and discussion earlier in this chapter, but especially the laboratory manual developed by Singer, Milne, Magill, Powell, and Vachon [1975] for a much more intensive description of a variety of purchased and constructed tasks.) Simple tasks can effectively provide answers to problems in the motor learning area. Because the usual data are recorded in the form of speed of performance and/or accuracy, timers and counters are often hooked up to constructed or purchased equipment. It is quite usual to see motor learning laboratories heavily armed with workshop tools and materials as well as electrical and electronic accessories. Learning experiments usually make innovative demands on the researcher in a variety of forms, one of which is task development and utilization.

Besides those already illustrated, another versatile piece of equipment is the Automatic Performance Analyzer (Figure 3-7), which can be used to time a variety of events. Various stimuli and response modes can be adapted with the Analyzer. One possible application of the Analyzer is illustrated in Figure 3-8. As described elsewhere (Singer, Llewellyn, & Darden, 1973), the Analyzer has been used with an interval timer, a 0.01 of a second performance timer, and a photoelectric relay system. The subject began the test (to determine reaction- and movement-time scores under specified conditions) seated in a ready position with the index finger of his dominant hand depressing a key. Upon illumination of a light on the interval timer (randomly timed following the preparation signal) the sub-

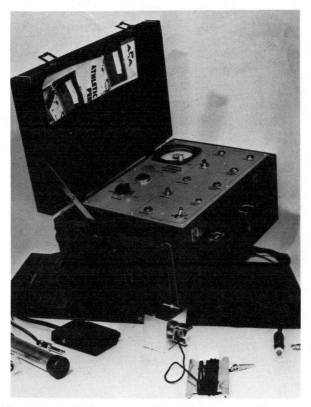

FIGURE 3-7. The Automatic Performance Analyzer (*Dekan Timing Devices, P. O. Box 712, Glen Ellyn, Illinois*).

ject, as quickly as possible, removed his finger from the starting key and moved his hand through the ray of the photoelectric relay system in a prespecified direction. The elapsed time from the illumination of the light stimulus to the release of the starting key was recorded as the subject's reaction time. Upon release from the key, another timer was initiated. When the subject's hand passed through the ray, the second timer was deactivated, providing a measure of movement time. Note in Figure 3-8 that the experimenter and subject were separated with the use of a divider, to minimize any experimenter and subject interaction effects.

Space is needed in any laboratory to store testing equipment and shop tools and materials. Space is also needed to construct equipment and to arrange various testing configurations. Another space consideration is testing privacy through the use of separate rooms or isolation booths. Distractions can contaminate data. An illustration of how pursuit rotor testing can occur without the noticeable presence of the experimenter appears in Figure 3-9. The subject operates the rotary pursuit apparatus in an isolation booth. The interval timer connected to the rotor provided the subject with a five-second warning in the form of an illuminated light prior to the initiation of each trial. A series of trials, with tests and rests of 20 seconds' du-

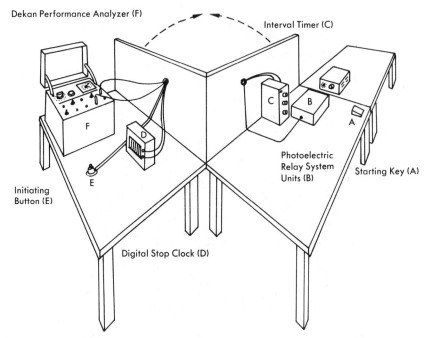

Dekan Performance Analyzer (F)

Interval Timer (C)

Photoelectric
Relay System
Units (B)

Starting Key (A)

Initiating
Button (E)

Digital Stop Clock (D)

FIGURE 3-8. Arrangement for testing reaction time and movement time. (*From Singer, R. N., Llewellyn, J., & Darden, E. Placebo and competitive placebo effects on motor skill.* Research Quarterly, *1973, 44, 51–58.*)

ration, was administered. Performance was measured by time on target for each trial, using a 0.01 of a second timer located outside the isolation booth. The experimenter recorded the time on target for each trial and then reset the timer.

The apparatus and testing situations described thus far are relatively simple. Expense is minor and testing arrangements are not difficult to formulate. With increasing experimenter sensitivity for control of extraneous sociopsychological variables, as well as advances in technology and lowered prices of computers and solid-state systems, behavioral data are being collected more validly under improved testing conditions. Small-scale computers and solid-state programmers are becoming more widely used in behavioral laboratories, resulting in controlled cue presentations and response recordings.

For instance, the model presented in Figure 3-10 is very versatile and inexpensive. The experiment can be programmed on a plugboard, which is inserted in the console control panel with the appropriate stimuli input and response output accessories. The subject's performance data can be recorded with timers or counters. The user must be familiar with digital logic. Preprogrammed experiments free the experimenter's time and usually contain more precision and control than nonprogrammed experiments.

In an experiment done at Florida State University to determine relationships of factors associated with reaction time and movement time, R. A. Magill and F.

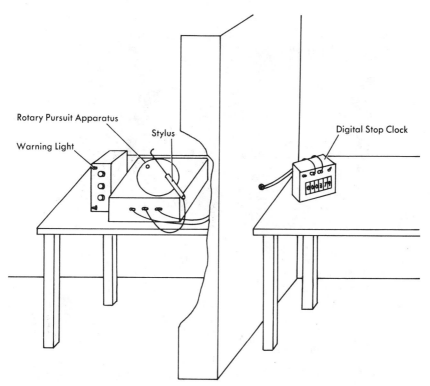

FIGURE 3-9. Arrangement for testing pursuit rotor performance. (*From Singer, R. N., Llewellyn, J., & Darden, E. Placebo and competitive placebo effects on motor skill.* Research Quarterly, *1973, 44, 51–58.*)

M. Powell (1975) used the Foringer model. Two millisecond timers were used to record RT and MT latencies to a visual stimulus. The stimulus warning light, stimulus light, random presentation (one to four seconds of the stimulus light following the onset of the warning light), intertrial interval, total experimental time, number of stimulus presentations, and number of subject responses were controlled and recorded by a BRS Foringer DigiLab (DLC-002). The DLC is a portable solid-state digital logic system that allows great flexibility in programming. Because the experiment was controlled from a room adjacent to the testing area, the experimenter communicated with the subject by means of an intercom. A white noise generator provided a masking noise to the subjects at an intensity of 72 decibels at ear level. During verbal interaction, the ambient noise level was automatically attenuated to 66 decibels. Task instructions were prerecorded on magnetic tape and presented to each subject via the intercom. The experimenter's display is presented in Figure 3-11.

Regardless of the available financial and apparatus resources, the crux of any model experiment rests with the researcher's talents and abilities. Being aware of experimental control factors and understanding the nature of the learning phe-

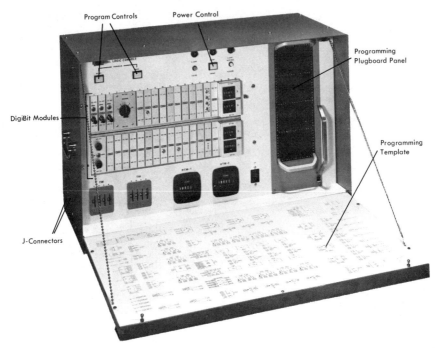

FIGURE 3-10. The Digilab, a portable solid-state system for programming experiments. (*From BRS Foringer, 5451 Holland Drive, Beltsville, Maryland.*)

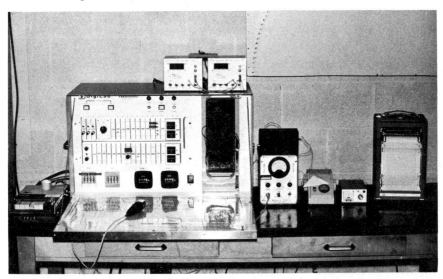

FIGURE 3-11. Experimenter's display, with the BRS programmer and appropriate accessory equipment, for reaction-time-movement-time experiment. (*From Magill, R., & Powell, F. M. Is the reaction time-movement time relationship essentially zero? Perceptual and Motor Skills, 1975, 41, 720–722.*)

nomenon under investigation lead to a quality research project. We can all be envious of working in the most elaborate settings and with the finest and most expensive apparatus. But there are many examples of experiments that have made outstanding contributions to learning theory and practice with a minimal amount of costly equipment.

RESEARCH METHODOLOGY AND EXPERIMENTAL DESIGN

The scientific study of learning and behavior is based on research evidence. *Research* refers to a product completed in a systematic, controlled way, using a formalized type of process and following a scientific method. *Systematic* means that there is a definite arrangement of the processes used. They are not undertaken in a haphazard way. Certain generalized rules must be followed in order that confidence can be held in the results of the study. And the use of the word *formal* implies a similar interpretation. There are formal rules governing the conduct of research. The planning and execution of the study do not transpire solely out of logic, intuition, and reasoning. There is a set of concrete interrelated steps followed.

The word *control* means that the investigator has control over the situation. The investigator is the one who selects the subjects and the content matter. If it is an experimental study, the researcher chooses the task and the way the subjects will be manipulated and tested. Control is thus exhibited in numerous ways. There is never, of course, total control as to how the subjects will perform in the experiment. Nevertheless, valid, or true, measurements are, one hopes, obtained. The researcher tries to exhibit control by succesfully manipulating variables that will result in true results—not in chance, haphazard outcomes.

All of these procedures have to do with scientific methods of analyses. At one time, researchers spoke of *the scientific method* of analysis. Books on research methodology consistently inferred that there was only one scientific method. Well, that is simply not true. There actually are a number of acceptable ways in which one can conduct research, and a given scientific method may be applicable in a particular situation. Distinctions may be made in the nature of research projects (e.g., historical, descriptive, and experimental), although there is a certain amount of formalized routine that is followed from study to study. Thus, the novice should be aware that there are distinctions within research and acceptable types of procedures and techniques, as well as overlapping.

Gaining Information

Research is not the only way to gain information about the universe or behavior. Other techniques besides a scientific approach may be reasonably acceptable. Knowledge can be obtained through at least three approaches.

Intuition and reason are used by all of us every day. Perhaps some of us do not use them enough. Some who are involved in research, it is argued, should call on reason more when designing experiments or interpreting results. Nevertheless, by only reacting according to rationale, we are in danger of being too subjective in the way we view things. Objectivity is tossed aside. One must consider this when appraising or evaluating anything. When you say you know something—how do you know it? Through belief, reason, feeling, thought? How accurate is this process? Is there a better way? At any rate, reason and rationale are approaches to understanding and gaining information.

A second technique employed fairly often is the acquisition of beliefs through *authority:* a person directing another's thoughts or actions. We listen to individuals who are in positions of power and have a tendency to go along with everything that is said. Are their statements all truisms? It is true that authorities provide a way to learn. Is it the best arrangement? You have to decide for yourself if being told what is right and wrong is desirable. Naturally, some knowledge can be assimilated through the authoritarian approach. However, the danger exists of being misinformed or misled. Furthermore, to discourage probing, questioning, and problem solving can also be detrimental to the learning process.

Finally, the third avenue to knowledge is *a scientific approach,* in which some sort of formalized system and more objective ways are used for obtaining answers to questions that disturb us. Who discovered the game of baseball? I can tell you who I think invented it. The answer can also come from a book. But perhaps you are not ready to accept these sources and the information offered. So you take a year and examine all possible resources in the archives and determine that Abner Doubleday probably did not invent the game of baseball after all, as is popularly thought. The circumstantial evidence would lead us to believe that he could not be responsible for its origin, although, for some reason, scattered evidence has been passed on through the years suggesting that he did invent the sport.

Nonacceptance of "factual" material or the viewpoints of authorites can be countered by a personal undertaking of scientific processes to establish the "truth." In the case of baseball, you did not accept an established "fact." Much time and effort was spent in order to come closer to the truth. Of course, each of us would not care to utilize such a lengthy and precise process to ascertain the answers to our questions. But we can scrutinize the means by which others have arrived at their conclusions and determine their credence.

There is danger at times in accepting statements based on belief and intuition, or materials unquestionably passed on through the years, as was the case with Doubleday and baseball.

But there is nothing wrong with probing, questioning, and searching. In other words, then, the product of a sicentific method enables us to have greater objectivity and affirmation of the thoughts we hold on a given topic. To advocate scientific processes does not exclude other means that might yield solutions. Solutions may be found through logic and reasoning or words written or spoken by authorities. But our greatest strength will come from answers that we actually have to find for ourselves, by using scientifically acceptable techniques in the search.

The Experiment

Experimentation is crucial in scientific research. Most of the research data to be reported in this book were collected in experimentally designed studies. In the classical sense, an *experiment* is a way of formulating and testing hypotheses. We begin with a hunch. Hunches provide direction for our thoughts on problems, and an experiment allows us, in a formal setting, to see if our hunches are confirmed. With the experiment, a planned attack is made on a particular problem. Typically, through well-constructed operations, changes are induced in natural events and results are observed, recorded, and analyzed. This is the outstanding feature of experimental research, as contrasted with descriptive research; there must be some manipulation or change in at least one variable under study.

Historically speaking, concepts and implications of experimentation have been diverse and misunderstood. At one time people expected miraculous answers from experiments but were, instead, disapppointed and disillusioned. It is now understood that experiments do not provide once-and-for-all answers. "Facts" are not necessarily permanent, and numerous experiments, constantly being refined in technique, provide tentative solutions to problems.

This is especially true of experiments dealing with human behavior. The degree of control and sophistication in an experiment in physics or chemistry is potentially far greater than in the human behavior experiments of psychology, sociology, physiology, or physical education.

The experimenter needs a spirit of curiosity, or *inquiry*. A search for the truth, a dissatisfaction with the present state of knowledge, and a desire to resolve an issue in a scientifically acceptable manner are all involved. *Background* information is necessary before an experiment is attempted. Experience, reading, and communication contribute to the investigator's level of understanding of the problem, enabling that person to raise legitimate questions, conceive of reasonable hypotheses, and formulate adequate experimental designs.

Because statistics and experiments often go hand in hand, an understanding of mathematics is most helpful. Statistics aid in various steps from the initial to the terminal stages of the experiment. Finally, good old-fashioned common sense is needed at all points throughout the experiment. The investigator must make numerous decisions along the way, not all of which can be guided by directives. Evaluation of suggested procedures, analysis of the particular experimental conditions, and competencies to handle unpredictable and unexpected occurrences all require common sense. Through these and other personal qualities, the experimenter examines theories and statements, formulates workable hypotheses for a particular problem, and executes the investigation.

IMPORTANCE OF RESEARCH IN MOTOR LEARNING

As can be seen, research, and more specifically experimental research, is primarily associated with information gathered about the acquisition and performance of motor skills. Consequently, great care must be shown in planning studies, collecting data, and drawing conclusions from the data. It is a tremendous challenge to meticulously design an experiment that yields valid data, further advancing our state of knowledge.

Such knowledge can increase the understanding of (1) learning processes similar among most people, (2) individual differences in learning and in the factors that contribute to those differences, and (3) learning situations that are most beneficial for learners in general or for those who need special considerations. Research can be oriented toward the resolution of more practical questions or more theoretical issues. But a relationship usually exists between both lines of research. A body of knowledge is needed in order to construct a solid scientific foundation of motor learning. By the same token, instructional decisions and learning procedures should reflect scientific evidence.

These points will become evident as we continue through subsequent chapters of this book. The next three chapters deal with theories of learning and theoretical issues. The remaining chapters contain many practical considerations within a scientific framework. It will be shown how researchers attempt to design studies to investigate learning phenomena and many times address the pragmatic concerns of instructors and learners as well. You are a potential researcher and user of research. Whether you undertake your own research or attempt to interpret and apply existing findings, it is helpful to develop an understanding of and appreciation for research methodology and statistics.

CHAPTER HIGHLIGHTS

1. Research in motor learning is crucial to our understanding of behavior, and consequently, important decisions must be made about research designs, the selection of appropriate learning tasks, the duration of studies, the number of learning trials, the use of one or more dependent measures, and the technique or measurement that should be used to "represent" learning.

2. The selection of a particular learning task depends on the purpose of the study, the phenomenon to be investigated, and the inferences to be made. Furthermore, task reliability, validity, and novelty should be considered. Other factors to be considered include ease of administration, availability, degree of difficulty to learn, and compatability with the subjects' maturational level.

3. An enormous array of tasks has been used to study learning phenomena related to personal and situational factors. Perhaps the most typical have been tasks involving simple and choice reaction time, tracking, and positioning. Mazes and stabilimeters serve as tasks to be mastered.

4. The duration of a study must be sufficient to demonstrate trends in the data but not so long that ceiling effects for the particular selected task will mask those trends. A warm-up trial for task familiarization may be desirable in some cases but not in others, depending on the purpose of the study.

5. Dependent, or recorded, data measures in learning research usually include movement speed, accuracy or error, and/or magnitude. The particular selection of one or more dependent measures, and how each is recorded, will influence data analysis and the ultimate conclusions.

6. In the measurement of learning, to assess changes in motor behavior, the following scores have been used: (a) the average; (b) the best; (c) the final; (d) individual trials or blocks of trials; (e) raw gain (difference); (f) per cent gain of possible gain; (g) true change; (h) residual gain; and (i) final scores adjusted on the basis of initial scores (by the analysis of covariance statistical method). There are values and criticisms in each approach, but generally, the following recommendations are offered:

(a) Assuming that an adequate number of subjects is placed into groups according to acceptable procedures, such as randomization or blocking of scores, a final score (preferably based on a few trials for reliability, if the learning phenomenon under study permits it) will suffice. The learning score is derived simply. But care must be taken to assure that the subjects are placed properly into groups.

(b) If the subjects differ in characteristics and performance at the onset, analyses of covariance, true change, or residual gains will be appropriate.

(c) If an analysis of learning over trials is desired, with between-and within-group comparisons made at various points, analysis of variance can be appropriate if statistical assumptions are met. If not, multivariate analyses of variance might be more appropriate.

7. Motor learning research laboratories differ widely in research orientation, available equipment, and general mode of operation. From simple mazes to computerized systems, from the self-constructed to the purchased, the range in type of testing apparatuses is considerable from laboratory to laboratory. Considerations for the initiation and maintenance of a laboratory include: (a) overall space available; (b) money available; (c) priority objectives (class and research); (d) equipment to be made or purchased; and (e) the division of available space for equipment storage and ready access, testing areas, class usage, a workshop, office space, and a miniature resource center.

8. The study of learning needs to be built upon a solid foundation of research evidence; experimental and descriptive data collected with a scientific approach (formal, systematic, and controlled) contribute to this endeavor.

References

Bahrick, H. P., Fitts, P. M., & Briggs, G. E. Learning curves—facts or artifacts. *Psychological Bulletin*, 1957, *54*, 256–268.

Christina, R. W., & Merriman, W. J. Learning the direction and extent of a movement: A test of Adams' closed-loop theory. *Journal of Motor Behavior*, 1977, *9*, 1–10.

Cromwell, L., Weibell, F. J., Pfeiffer, E. A., & Usselman, L. B. *Biomedical instrumentation and measurements.* Englewood Cliffs, N.J.: Prentice-Hall, 1973.

Cronbach, L. J., & Furby, L. How we should measure "change"—or should we? *Psychological Bulletin*, 1970, *74*, 68–80.

Cronbach, L. J., Gleser, G. C., Nanda, H., & Rajaratnam, N. *The dependability of behavioral measurements: Theory of generalizability for scores and profiles*. New York: John Wiley, 1972.

Drowatzky, J. Evaluation of mirror-tracing performance measures as indicators of learning. *Research Quarterly*, 1969, *40*, 228–230.

Fleishman, E. A. A comparative study of aptitude patterns in unskilled and skilled psychomotor performance. *Journal of Applied Psychology*, 1957, *41*, 263–272.

Fulton, R. Speed and accuracy in learning movements. *Archives of Psychology*, 1945, 300.

Harris, C. W. (Ed.). *Problems in measuring change*. Madison: University of Wisconsin Press, 1963.

Henry, F. M. Evaluation of motor learning when performance levels are heterogeneous. *Research Quarterly*, 1956, *27*, 176–181.

Henry, F. M. "Best" versus "average" individual scores. *Research Quarterly*, 1967, *38*, 317–320

Henry, F. M. Variable and constant performance errors within a group of individuals. *Journal of Motor Behavior*, 1974, *6*, 149–154.

Hetherington, R. Within-subject variation, measurement error, and selection of a criterion score. *Research Quarterly*, 1973, *44*, 113–117.

Kroll, W. Reliability theory and research decision in selection of a criterion score. *Research Quarterly*, 1967, *38*, 412–419.

Magill, R. A., & Powell, F. M. Is the reaction time-movement time relationship essentially zero? *Perceptual and Motor Skills*, 1975, *41*, 720–722.

McCraw, L. W. A comparison of methods of measuring improvement. *Research Quarterly*, 1951, *22*, 191–200.

McCraw, L. W. Comparative analysis of methods of scoring tests of motor learning. *Research Quarterly*, 1955, *26*, 440–453.

Safrit, M. J., Spray, J. A., & Diewert, G. L. Measures of error in short-term motor memory research. *Journal of Motor Behavior*, 1979, in press.

Schutz, R. W. *Possible solutions to the problems of measuring change in motor behavior*. Paper presented at the annual meetings of the American Alliance for Health, Physical Education, and Recreation, Atlantic City, N.J., March 1975.

Schutz, R. W., & Roy, E. A. Absolute error: The devil in disguise. *Journal of Motor Behavior*, 1973, *5*, 141–153.

Singer, R. N., & Llewellyn, J. K. Effects of experimenter's gender on subject performance. *Research Quarterly*, 1973, *44*, 185–191.

Singer, R. N., Llewellyn, J., & Darden, E. Placebo and competitive placebo efforts on motor skill. *Research Quarterly*, 1973, *44*, 51–58.

Singer, R. N., Milne, C., Magill, R., Powell, F, & Vachon, L. *Laboratory and field experiments in motor learning*. Springfield, Ill.: Charles C Thomas, 1975.

Thomas, J. R.. A note concerning analysis of error scores from motor-memory research. *Journal of Motor Behavior*, 1977, *9*, 251–253.

Tucker, L. R., Damarin, F., & Messick, S. A base-free measure of change. *Psychometrika*, 1966, *31*, 457–473.

4 GENERAL LEARNING THEORIES

Psychologists, educators, and other scholars have been formulating and modifying theories of learning during most of this century. Extensive research has been the basis for these theories, as well as a means for questioning them. Learning theories are far from fully developed or clearly defined, and as a result of the complexity of human behavior, may never be.

Familiarity with learning theories should encourage intellectual stimulation and thought, provide better understanding of learning phenomena and the laws regulating them, and promote methods of teaching consistent with scientific evidence. A theory provides the guidelines within which one may work. It suggests a frame of reference, a means of achieving objectives. Basically, a theory deals with a particular area of knowledge in which large collections of facts and information are explained and interpreted in a limited number of words. It is an ordered and formal presentation of data. Theory helps to explain relationships within the body of knowledge and permits deduction of new relationships or new facts. It is, as Fred Kerlinger (1977) suggests, a "systematic presentation of phenomena and relationships, in order to explain and predict phenomena" (p. 5).

Scientists interpret data, and theorists use these facts as well as logic to formulate theories. Facts, which represent reality and actuality, alone do not satisfy many individuals; hence, there is a need for a theory to organize the data into meaningful and unifying systems. Systems of laws explain the regularity of events surrounding us, and a theory contains an integration of those laws. A few facts do not constitute a theory in themselves, for the quality and acceptability of a theory is determined by the scope of the scientific facts it represents.

Scientific inquiry, based on the search for the truth, serves as the foundation for theory formulation. With the accumulation of facts, laws are constructed that pertain to and govern isolated events. A behavioral law usually is derived on the basis of a sequence of events observed to occur with great consistency or conformity under the same conditions. The term *law* is often used interchangeably with *rule, principle,* and *postulate.* The explanation of many events allows us to interpret and predict behavior in given situations and the final result is a system of

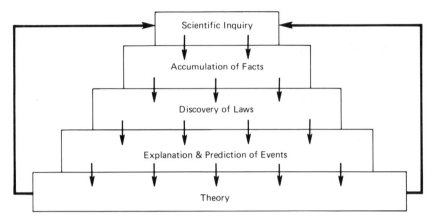

FIGURE 4-1. Scientific inquiry leads to the development and formulation of a theory and, in turn, generates further inquiry and research.

laws or theory. This state of transition in theory construction is depicted in Figure 4-1.

There are two levels in science: observable, or empirical, relationships; and theoretical, or inferred, relationships. The implicit assumption in theory construction is that it is formed as a basis of scientific activity and stimulates further activity. The fruitfulness of theory is that it enables a person to deduce a large number of empirical relationships. Facts should support theory, which in turn should generate research and new hypotheses, resulting in a reformulation of theory.

VALUES AND CRITICISMS

Actually, theories should arise after the relevant variables have been studied extensively. Because it is debatable whether scholars have met this responsibility, the noted psychologist B. F. Skinner (1965) has questioned whether we are ready for learning theory. He has stated that we may best understand learning from research not designated to test learning theories. His view, although not without foundation, is not the dominant one.

One of the major criticisms of early learning theories is that they attempted to explain all learning on the basis of fragmentary information. Another problem arose—that persists—associated with the conflicting results obtained with different learning materials when investigating certain learning phenomena. Theories have also presented problems in communication. Some theories have been written in clear language, whereas others are represented by statistical symbols. Actually, theorists may talk about the same thing in different ways, a practice that serves to confuse the issue.

MOTOR LEARNING AND HUMAN PERFORMANCE

The meaningfulness and utility of theories have stirred controversy. Learning theories exhibit many questionable features, and these must be reconciled before they will meet with more acceptance. They are as follows: (1) generalizations beyond actual scientific evidence; (2) selective use of facts and interpretation for convenience; (3) social problems not usually considered; (4) impractical and unrealistic application to everyday life; (5) scope too broad; (6) disregard for developmental factors; and (7) too much concern for mass behavior rather than individual behavior.

Beyond their limitations, theories, if based on the scientific approach, serve a number of purposes. A scientific system meets the following criteria:

1. Material is presented in a systematic and orderly fashion. It is not a haphazard collection of statements or facts.
2. Material is essentially based on the most accurate available scientific information. There is evidence or proof for the existence of statements.
3. Material is such that it allows us to understand behavior better. It explains and predicts behavior in all its forms in relatively few principles.
4. Material is offered in a conceptual form. It allows a person to generalize over a series of related events regarding expected occurrences.
5. Material is pertinent to given situations; it allows for predictions in these situations.
6. Material is of such a nature that it encourages further research.
7. Material is applicable to practical situations.

The last criterion, practical application, holds the greatest meaning for the average person. Unfortunately, as of the present time, it must be frankly stated that the present stage of theory development does not permit an easy transition from theory to practice. Theorists disagree on certain points, although many of them are actually reconcilable on the larger issues. Theory can be helpful in governing instructional practices, but a number of problems still cannot be handled because of the lack of many well-established principles. Yet, as instructional theory and psychoinstructional design are advanced, dependence and interrelatedness with psychological research and learning theory must be reached (Snelbecker, 1974). Nevertheless, some theories appear to apply to certain situations better than others, and this chapter contains the highlights of better-known theories, as well as examples of potential applications to the teaching of skills.

Modern theorists no longer explain performance solely through simple conditioning processes. Singer (1966), for one, has attempted to offer some alternative approaches to teachers of physical education. There is a tendency to go to miniature theories (models) in place of the broad theories, and thus to a more fine-grained analysis of particular areas of interest. We will follow the transition from earlier association theories to the contemporary performance models, which hold so much promise for the understanding of skilled performance.

THEORIES

Of the many theories attempting to explain and predict learning and behavior, some have unique differences but have managed to remain in existence despite the scrutiny of researchers. Although earlier theories have been modified as a result of certain contradictions from more controlled and extensive research, they should be studied for a number of reasons: (1) for the impetus to research that would at a later date uphold or refute the theories; (2) for an understanding of how theories have developed through the years and the direction in which they are going; and (3) for any possible direct application the educator might be able to make to a specific teaching situation.

At the beginning of this century, the behaviorists, led by Watson, battled against the idea that behavior was caused by preformed connections called instincts. Behavior, according to this group, was accounted for by S–R conditioning. No other factors, including reinforcement, were thought to be important, except that the S–R occur together (contiguity). A stimulus can be any cue, direction, or event to which a particular association, in the form of an appropriate response, is to be made.

From this beginning, the reinforcement theorists exerted great influence on education and psychology under Thorndike's leadership. The necessity of some form of reinforcement occurring to secure learning after the response was thus recognized. Many theories were formed in the 1930s and 1940s, from Gestalt (cognitive and field) theory, to Tolman's sign-learning theory, to Hull's drive-reduction theory, to Skinner's operant-conditioning theory. The earliest theories did not account for mentalistic actions (intervening variables), processes that occur within the organism between the onset of a stimulus and the execution of a response, as they were based on the S–R conditioning approach made so famous by Pavlov and Watson. With more research and greater consideration for human as well as for environmental conditions, theorists tended to become more aware of factors beyond an S–R occurrence and the mere repetition of this event that contribute to behavior.

For convenience, the traditional theories have been classified as being associative (S–R) or cognitive-perceptual (Gestalt). Some theorists believed in intervening variables occurring between the S–R, others did not. Still other theorists combined elements from both theories. There was agreement that S–R theories were more exacting and led to greater research, whereas cognitive-perceptual theories were more general and elusive, emphasizing the perceptual and intellectual processes. The traditional behavioristic theories emphasized the contiguity of stimulus and response, as well as the role of reinforcement. Let us first briefly examine some major traditional theoretical approaches in studying behavior, although they have been presented in much greater depth by such authors as Hilgard and Bower (1975) and Sahakian (1970). We will then examine other approaches that seem to hold more promise for the analysis of human motor behavior. In a sense, we have here a historical overview of theoretical developments. In another sense, the potential contributions of these positions toward an understanding of motor behavior will be implied or expressed, leading us to Chapter 5, in which other positions will be presented, and then to Chapter 6, in which an integrated conceptual approach will be presented for the study and analysis of human motor behavior.

ASSOCIATION THEORIES

Thorndike's Laws

For many years Edward L. Thorndike (1931) was the leader in the formulation of learning theory. He was the forerunner in the stimulus–response, or S–R, psychology of learning. His theory has been termed *association theory, bond theory,* or *connectionism.*

These terms simply imply that there are no intervening ideas between the stimulus and response, that the connections are strengthened automatically when they occur. Thorndike gave much impetus to knowledge in the area of problem solving and contributed his famous laws of readiness, exercise, and effect. Even though many of his laws had to be revised in later years because of research findings that contradicted his theory, his laws are still acknowledged for their impact on education.

For example, he stated in his original *law of exercise* that during repetition the S–R connections are strengthened and the probability of the desired response is increased. However, it has since been shown in many instances that mere repetitions of an act are not enough to demonstrate learning. Thorndike modified his position and stated that for more effective learning the desired connection should be rewarded by praise, knowledge of right or wrong, or some other means.

The law of effect, another example of a famous Thorndike postulate, was modified in his later years. Generally speaking, this law was concerned with what happens after an act. If the response is followed by a satisfier—i.e., it is pleasant and rewarding—the tendency is for that response to be strengthened. When an annoyer such as punishment occurs, the response is weakened. At first Thorndike felt that both conditions had an equal effect on the individual, but later he adjusted this law to give greater importance to satisfiers than annoyers. He was among the first to emphasize the value of reinforcement, for this is what the law of effect is concerned with.

In his famous *law of readiness,* Thorndike was interested in a person's preparatory adjustment to a particular situation. Satisfaction and frustration depend on a personal state of readiness when responding or when blocked in responding. In other words, when things go right as an objective is reached, the act is satisfying. If the act is not fulfilled or it is blocked, the situation is annoying.

Another part of Thorndike's learning theory dealt with transfer, and it was referred to as the *identical-elements theory of transfer.* Basically, he stated that all learning is specific and may appear to be general only because new situations or acts contain elements similar to elements of old situations or acts. It is in this area of transfer that Thorndike made one of his most significant contributions to education. He attacked the then popular belief in the generalized theory of transfer—that logic, memorization, reasoning, and the like transferred from specific school subjects to everyday life experiences—and emphasized specific training and education for desired behavior.

It is important to remember that in Thorndike's theory the emphasis was on the learner and his or her motives, readiness, and needs. Also considered were the rewards and effects that "stamp in" or imprint the portions of a random activity that bring chance success. All parts were regarded as singular and isolated. This emphasis is in contrast to the holistic concepts of Gestalt theory, as will be seen later. Finally, the importance of the need or intention to learn was stressed by Thorndike. To learn well, the learner must participate actively; to do that, drive must be present.

Hull's Drive Theory

Clark L. Hull (1943) developed many postulates and described definitively the effect of intervening variables on behavior. For example, Hull's theory of a performed act would be represented by the symbols $_sE_R = [_s\overline{H}_R \times D \times V \times K - (I_R + _sI_R)] - _sO_R - _sL_R$. Interpreted in an oversimplified manner, this means that the momentary effective reaction potential is equal to the number of reinforced trials × drive × incentive × intensity of stimulus—(reactive inhibition + conditioned inhibition)—the fluctuation of the individual from moment to moment—reaction threshold.

Hull's theory was one of the most formal, precise, and elaborate of all behaviorist theories to be proposed. He mathematically arrived at figures that were used as constants and helped to quantify his postulates. Hull talked mainly in terms of needs and drives, and this theory often has been referred to as a drive-reduction theory. His efforts encouraged much research and his many disciples continued his work.

An important consideration of Hull's theory for skill instructors is the effect of mere practice on performance. Hull demonstrated that repetitive practice led to what he termed *inhibition,* a sort of depressant variable that is built up during non-reinforced trials and that offsets the strength of the performance. Reactive inhibition dissipates with rest. This would explain why a basketball player who attempts one hundred consecutive foul shots would most likely perform best in the middle trials and worst near the termination of the trials. Yet, the following day, the player is able to begin again at a greater skill level than had been observed at the end of the previous practice session. This is a perfect example of the effect of practice on performance, rather than on learning. Obviously the performance level of the participant can be raised or hindered, depending on the manner in which skills are practiced. However, the true extent of learning may be disguised, as was explained in Chapter 1.

Gagné's Motor Chaining Hypothesis

Many of the ideas William James expressed in 1890 were incorporated in Robert Gagné's (1970) motor chaining model, one of the eight different types of learning he proposed. The model represents behavioristic, or S–R, thinking (or an open-loop approach, as contrasted with a closed-loop model). Central in any response chaining model is the concept of proprioceptive information as stimuli (response-produced feedback), functioning as other kinds of stimuli to influence subsequent behavior.

For Gagné, chaining is the sequencing of a set of individual S–Rs. Chainlike skills include, among countless other examples, buttoning, tying, using scissors, and throwing and catching balls.In order for the complete act to be successful, each individual link (S–R) in the chain must be mastered. An example of chained behavior is unlocking a door with a key. Each S–R, or link, when completed, serves as the cue or stimulus for the next one, until the act is terminated. For instance, in the act of opening a door with a key:

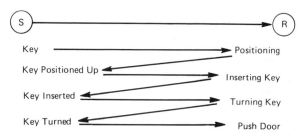

Verbal cues assist the learner in the appropriate chaining of events. These cues can be provided by the person learning, for most likely the learner "talks to himself or herself" when initially learning the routine. Nonspoken, internal cues direct behavior for a while, but well-learned acts probably flow without any need for additional control. In order for chaining to be effectively demonstrated, certain conditions must be present.

1. Each link should be fully learned. Because each link is related to the preceding one, any breakdown in one would probably hamper the entire activity.
2. Each link should be demonstrated in the proper order. This can be encouraged with proper cuing techniques, or else a backward chaining technique termed mathetics (starting from the last link and working backward) can be practiced.
3. Individual links should occur appropriately in time. The principle of contiguity is relevant here, for responses should be made on receipt of the right stimuli. Delays in the performance of certain links might ruin the goal of the activity, for timing and association lead to successful executions.
4. Sufficient repetitious practice should occur if the chain is to be well learned.
5. Reinforcement, in the form of successful completion of the act or satisfaction at the end of the act, is necessary; otherwise, chaining behavior is extinguished.

It should be emphasized that Gagné's motor chaining model is not really a theory for motor learning. Rather, it is one of the steps, or tasks, he proposes in the hierarchical development of cognitive behaviors. Nevertheless, there are a number of people who would view behavior as a series of discrete and related acts. Gagné's model serves to represent this viewpoint and to offer an alternative mode of looking at behavior.

Skinner's Concepts of Operant Conditioning

Of all the psychologists prominent in the study of learning and behavior in this century, B. F. Skinner has had the most impact. He is interested not only in predicting behavior, but also in controlling it—an idea objected to by many people.

Among his other contributions, Skinner has written *Walden Two,* a novel about the development of a Utopian society made possible by the control of human behavior. He invented the Skinner Box, where animal behavior could be observed and data produced visually and made readily comprehensible. He developed the "baby box," an enclosed compartment in which the baby lives and the temperature is maintained. Skinner's promotion of the teaching machine caused the method of programmed instruction to gain wide theoretical and practical acceptance and has had an enormous impact on industry and education.

Skinner's theory of operant conditioning contrasts with respondent conditioning (S–R standard theory—e.g., Pavlov's works). In respondent behavior, the subject has to respond in a certain way to a given stimulus. Standard laboratory experiments have been used to demonstrate such specific S–R connections, which were termed reflexes in the early years. Operant learning is reflected by the behavior emitted by the organism, instead of elicited by external stimuli. Most human behavior is of the operant kind (for example, playing in sports), and Skinner has been concerned mainly with responses instead of stimuli.

Perhaps Skinner's theory can be represented best by the widely used *shaping concept.* If there is a desired response and the possibility of occurrence is quite remote, the chance for success will increase if the act is reinforced in some way whenever it occurs. However, there is an alternate possibility: to provide reinforcement for a general response in the direction of the desired response. This is the procedure followed by animal trainers, who administer reinforcers more frequently, or in greater magnitude, as the displayed behavior comes closer to matching the behavior of interest. Shaping consists of reinforcing closer and closer approximations of a desired terminal behavior.

For example, the desired response might be for a novice bowler to execute a four-step approach and roll a hook ball into the appropriate pins. Reinforcement (verbal acknowledgment) is offered increasingly as the ultimate goal is approached. According to Skinner, the effect of reinforcement is central in the shaping of behavior. The bowler, instead of achieving the desired movement by chance in trial-and-error performance, is channeled into the correct groove through the appropriate provision of reinforcement. Concern would first be focused on the skill in the approach and ball release, later on accuracy and score.

The teaching machine, or programmed text, apparently is an extension of this shaping concept and may have great implications for educators. The teaching machine discourages any wrong responses throughout learning. It shapes learning from the simple to the complex. If a child is learning to read, he or she must first know about forms. Matter becomes more complicated as the child learns about forms, letters, simple words, more complex words, and finally sentences. Continuation is not permitted until all the information presented up to that point is mastered. The learning of errors along the way is minimized, as incorrect responses are rejected, requiring those responses to be repeated. Students can progress at their own speed while the teacher assists those who are having difficulties, an important consideration of individual differences.

Perhaps the entire concept of the teaching machine can be applied to the teaching of skills (Neuman & Singer, 1968). When learning a skill (hitting a tennis ball with a forehand stroke, for example), each element of the movement would be taught and correctly executed before the learner advanced to additional or more complex movements. The student learns the correct stance, the correct movement, and, in a stationary position, strikes a ball thrown from a ball-tossing machine. Balls are not hit on the run until this act is performed successfully.

The tennis student learns to hit balls accurately when running sideward, then forward, then backward. It is important to remember that complex movements are building on simpler ones. No advancement is allowed until reasonable mastery is shown at a particular level of skill. Later on in the course there will be no competing responses (wrong and right), for only the right ones will have been learned.

How many of us as youngsters learned a sport skill incorrectly? Trying to execute that skill in good form later in life presents a difficulty. The situation is a consequence of the effect of competing responses. Is it not easier to learn a skill correctly for the first time than to undo past error-filled experiences?

Skinner is a firm believer in the power of reinforcement in promoting learning, advocating the principle that a response followed by reinforcement increases the probability of the occurrence of that response. His classification of reinforcement manipulations, or the schedule of reinforcements—concerning *ratio* and *interval, fixed* or *variable*—has permitted a better understanding of reinforcement and the relative values of the different kinds of reinforcement. Skinner states that behavior should be determined by scientific principles, not chance. Behavior is related to environmental manipulation, and teachers can manipulate the movement patterns of students. How much behavior and performance can and should be controlled is a matter of conjecture, as, in fact, we really do not know the relative value and costs of controlling behavior versus directing it in a more subtle fashion.

EARLY COGNITIVE-PERCEPTUAL THEORY

The Gestalt movement had its greatest impact on American learning theories in the 1930s and is usually associated with the names of Max Wertheimer, Wolfgang Kohler, Kurt Koffka, and Kurt Lewin. The German word *gestalt* means "form" or "shape." It is suggested in Gestalt theory that the learner perceives meaningful relationships in the environment and thereby gains insight into the understanding and solving of problems.

Gestaltism was perhaps the earliest form of cognitive theory and developed as an alternative to behaviorist theory. Gestalt psychology came into prominence as educators, primarily because of the Dewey influence, were more concerned with the individual and one's own ability to determine outcomes in a situation. To these educators, Thorndike was too mechanistic and his theory too laboratory oriented. Gestaltists believed that learning is not random and accidental, but instead, a result of organized, meaningful, and perceived experiences. The learner perceives the environment as a whole; personal experiences are constantly reorganized, and eventual insight is inevitable. The theory goes beyond the simple S–R explanation of learning. Whereas S–R theorists were concerned with overt behavior, the Gestalt theorist was more interested in the cognitive process, in what the learner understands. A greater understanding of Gestalt psychology may be obtained by reading *The Principles of Gestalt Psychology* by Koffka (1935).

Perhaps one of the greatest contributions of Gestalt theory to education is the concept of emphasizing the holistic manner of teaching material, as contrasted with an atomistic relationship of parts. It is felt that the learner strives to make sense of each task, to search for significant relationships between tasks, until progressive change occurs through the discovery of insightful wholes. Basically, it is important to comprehend the Gestaltist belief that during practice changes go on within repetition, not as a result of repetition (S–R associations). Also, transfer from one skill to another takes place not because of identical elements, but because of similar patterns.

Because of the difficulty in testing a number of Gestalt ideas, the impact of Gestaltism gradually waned. However, in more recent years, a revival of interest in cognitive psychology has come about. Although, once again, a number of scholars have become distressed with behaviorist approaches and directions, new experimental methodologies have been developed this time. The new methodologies will provide much greater clout to the concepts forwarded by cognitive psychologists. The efforts of cognitive psychologists are often flavored with humanistic approaches in the study of behavior, with implications for instructing groups of people as well as individuals, all of whom possess different information processing and organizational capabilities. In Chapter 5 we will describe these developments, along with their implications for theory and instruction in motor learning.

MATHEMATICAL AND STATISTICAL MODELS

It is probably evident in reviewing the theories of learning presented thus far, with the exception of Hull's, that their formulation lacked precision. The introduction of mathematics to theory construction produced a new wave of statistical models in about 1950. This emergence of more specific, restricted theories solved many problems but created others.

The use of mathematical equations actually dates back to an earlier portion of this century, with Thurstone as one of the primary contributors. There were attempts to deduce curves of learning mathematically, to fit the best curve to data already available. The learning function via the learning curve was analytically defined on the basis of simple probability theory and differential equations. How a measure of performance improved with practice was mathematically described.

Hull was the first proponent of formal theory, and he was a pioneer in mathematically translating certain learning phenomena. Later, the work of Estes, Bush and Mosteller, and Miller and Frick resulted in models successful in demonstrating the great impact of mathematics on psychology and learning.

The shape of learning curves is predicted in these models, but they have limited value because they cannot describe all the conditions that influence learning. Most of these efforts have encompassed the process of knowledge acquisition, of how something is learned in a choice situation. Models have been developed to answer the question: Why is a certain response made in a given situation, and how long does it take before that response is stabilized? Probability theory is important here and is applied to the stimulus population in a given situation. The number and nature of stimuli associated with an act are of central importance in some models.

W. K. Estes (1959) has probably formulated the most widely accepted statistical model, a probabilistic response model. The approach is better understood when one realizes that his definition of learning is a systematic change in response probability. Unfortunately, most statistical models appear to describe the acquisition of verbal material better than motor skill learning; indeed, the concern of most psychologists has been in the former area. Because of this, other models and theories have been developed, especially by those interested in industrial and military performance, to explain aspects of motor behavior.

PERFORMANCE MODELS

The dissatisfaction of industrial engineers and psychologists, as well as military psychologists, with the traditional theories of learning was evidenced by the new approaches taken to theorize about the learning of motor skills in the 1940s. World War II brought about a great involvement of psychologists in assisting the armed forces to develop better training devices and techniques, and of course, more effective trainees. The revolution in industry, which led to the development of sophisticated computer models, promoted an interest in comparing machine methods of operation with human operational techniques. The concern in industry and the military for maximum efficiency in the performance of motor tasks led to the computer-human analogy.

These operational and theoretical factors caused a departure from theories that were geared mainly to describe verbal learning or the performance of rats to those intended to explain and predict human performance in the motor skill area. It should be realized that the motor skills considered in these concepts were of the positioning or tracking type, not the athletic skills so familiar to physical educators. However, it does appear that sports activities might have more in common with the military and industrial tasks than with verbal learning or subhuman performances.

The concept of *signal detection,* or *vigilance,* which is associated with the perception of above-threshold events during a period of time, is of great interest to military personnel. After all, rare events are important to detect during war. A vigilance situation, which requires continual attention and monitoring, is very boring, due to infrequent and irregular signals and silence.

As well, the practice and performance of athletic skills can often be repetitious and monotonous. Vigilance is the attentiveness of a subject and the capability of detecting changes in stimulus events during a lengthy period of observation. Although vigilance does not apply directly to the performance of most athletic skills, the concern for maintaining motivation and perceptibility is certainly there. Evidently, motivation and vigilance are decreased very little if (1) the task is complex, (2) knowledge of results is provided, (3) many cues are present, (4) the period of involvement contains some break or recess, and (5) the stimuli are of greater intensity and longer duration.

Theories have been developed to explain vigilance. D. E. Broadbent's (1958) filter theory, which is actually an attention theory, represents a classic attempt to explain more than just performance decrements. He states that there is a *filter* in the nervous system that permits some classes of stimuli to pass but not others. The priority of selection is given to stimuli that are physically intense, that are of greater biological importance, and that are novel. Decrements in performance are attributed to competition of the stimuli.

According to Broadbent, the person is selective in what is taken in from the environment. Some stimuli are attended to and others left out, and the selection varies from time to time. The uniqueness of signals or cues will result in better attention; but after a long time period, attention is lost with the absence of a unique signal. With practice on a task, fewer cues are needed and the capacity required for performance is reduced, freeing neural mechanisms for other tasks.

Broadbent's work in its entirety is actually a communication or information theory. The S–R approach of simply considering the presence or absence of particular stimuli is not satisfactory to information theorists. They feel that the whole ensemble of stimuli has to be considered, as well as the coding of input into output. Patterns, situations, and temporal sequences of stimuli, rather than simultaneous patterns, are central to information theory. The evolvement of information theory and its characteristics are described in Chapter 5.

Detection theory (Swets, 1964) provides a framework for understanding human behavior in a variety of perceptual tasks. Statistical decision theory has been translated into signal detection theory. The detection or perceptual process is based on the observer's detection of the goal and the information present about probabilities and values concerning it. One does not merely passively reflect about environmental events but instead makes a substantial contribution to what is perceived. A decision process depends on the stimulus condition, as well as the instructions to the observer.

The concept that a human samples stimuli from the environment in a predictable manner is relevant to military warfare operations, athletic competition, and a host of other situations. Theoretically, if you have sufficient data on an enemy or opponent, you can know his or her cutoff point for making a decision or executing an act. Thus far, though, the theory has had limited application for all types of behavior and has been restricted mainly to visual experiences.

This theory, which is concerned with the decision-making process, contradicts previous theories in which it was advocated that stimuli are only detected where a certain threshold level is present. Perceptual decisions, which preclude purposeful motor acts, are based on rewards and expectancies, according to signal-detection theory. In other words, a person makes a decision after considering payoffs from the possible outcomes of responses, as well as estimating the actual stimulus. Perhaps an example in sport will serve to demonstrate the theory in actual practice.

Consider the batter in a baseball game. Any pitch can be perceived to be a strike or a ball, and in fact, the pitch may be a strike or a ball. There are two kinds of possible mistakes in this situation: (1) if the pitch is a strike and the batter does not swing, or (2) if the batter swings when a pitch is not a strike. The batter is actually faced with several alternatives, as we can see in Table 4-1. Decisions are made on costs and payoffs, as perceived by each person.

TABLE 4-1 The Decision-Making Process as Faced by the
Baseball Batter, Showing the Outcome of Responses

Event	Swing	No Swing
Strike	Possible hit	Possible strike out
Ball	Possible strike out or badly hit ball	Possible walk

The applicability of signal-detection theory to the prediction of basketball shooting performance was examined recently by R. J. Jagacinski, P. D. Issac, and M. W. Burke (1977). Experienced players shot at the basket, and before each attempt, they, as well as passive observers, attempted to predict the outcome. Although the results were not conclusive, the investigators suggest the promise of the theory to test hypotheses, with implications for training and screening purposes. As we will see shortly, the trend in the study of behavior is away from an associationistic framework and more toward an understanding of perceptual and cognitive processes that influence behavior.

The respondent has to weigh the possible payoffs of a response in terms of rewards and penalties. Past experiences and the present situation will influence expectations and payoffs. Although the precise methodology for predicting signal detection will not be discussed here, signal detection theory does permit specific predictions of stimuli detection and behavioral responses when alternatives are present in the situation.

AN OVERVIEW

The material presented in this chapter sets the stage for the directions in theory described in the next chapter. We saw the powerful influence of behaviorism on research and teaching, its different forms and unique contributions to our understanding of human behavior. Gestalt theory, too, made its impact felt in psychology. In many ways, this school of thought can be viewed as the precursor to the current development of cognitive psychology and the popularity it is enjoying in many circles. Information-processing theory is often viewed as an integral part of cognitive psychology, and this relationship will be shown in the following chapter.

The brief introduction to signal-detection theory reveals changing concepts about people, with acknowledgment given to their active role in processing information and evaluating circumstances to influence behavioral outcomes—instead of acquiring conditioned responses to environmental controls. The study of complex behavior requires the analysis of many variables, from situational constraints and task demands to the organizational processes used by individuals to control their behaviors.

CHAPTER HIGHLIGHTS

1. Theories are formulated on the basis of research and help to provide conceptual directions to subsequent research, as well as practical implications for instructional and training programs. Scientific inquiry leads to research and the accumulation of facts and then to the discovery of laws that can be used to explain and predict events. A theory evolves from these efforts, which in turn leads to further scientific inquiry, and the cycle continues. Theories are described or modified accordingly.

2. Theories have values as well as liabilities. On the debit side, they have been criticized on occasion on the basis of their being (a) generalizations beyond actual scientific evidence; (b) selective in the use of facts and biased interpretations; (c) difficult to apply to practical situations; (d) broad in scope; (e) unmindful of developmental factors and social considerations (unless explicitly directed to either of these fields); and (f) oriented toward average behavior, with little consideration for individual differences. On the positive side, theories contain material that (a) is presented in a systematic and orderly fashion; (b) is based on scientific evidence; (c) promotes understanding of behavior; (d) is conceptually based, permitting generalizations across situations; (e) allows for predictions in particular situations; (f) encourages further research; and (g) is applicable to practical situations.

3. Behavioristic (associationistic, S–R) theory represented the foundations of psychological learning theory in the early part of this century. That and Gestalt (cognitive-perceptual) theory provided alternative frameworks in which to view behavior. The basic difference between the two schools of thought was that the behaviorists tended to stress environmental control and conditioning processes and the Gestaltists, individual cognitive and perceptual processes. Thorndike's, Skinner's, and Hull's works illustrate early behaviorist approaches and Gagné's work is contemporary.

4. Mathematical and statistical models gained favor in the 1950s as psychologists attempted to study behavior with more precision. The thrust was toward the quantification of behavior, often with probabalistic models. The impact of these approaches gradually tapered off and led the way to other models, some of which contained certain elements of mathematical prediction.

5. Performance models, such as signal-detection theory, generated interest in the decisions people make about their pending behaviors. Possible outcomes of responses are weighed against rewards and penalties. In vigilance theory, attentiveness, alertness, and motivation are examined as people pursue monotonous tasks for a long time, and have to detect and respond to unexpected and infrequent signals. These types of performance models help us to recognize the importance of such processes as attention and decision making in the study of human behavior.

References

Broadbent, D. E. *Perception and communication.* Elmsford, N.Y.: Pergammon Press, 1958.

Estes, W. K. The statistical approach to learning theory. In S. Koch (Ed.), *Psychology: A study of a science* (Vol. II). New York: McGraw-Hill, 1959.

Gagné, R. M. *The conditions of learning* (2nd ed.). New York: Holt, Rinehart & Winston, Inc., 1970.

Hilgard, E. R., & Bower, G. H. *Theories of learning* (4th ed.). Englewood Cliffs, N.J.: Prentice-Hall, 1975.

Hull, C. L. *Principles of behavior.* New York: Appleton-Century-Crofts, 1943.

Jagacinski, R. J., Isaac, P. D., & Burke, M. W. Application of signal detection theory to perceptual-motor skills: Decision processes in basketball shooting. *Journal of Motor Behavior,* 1977, *9,* 225–234.

Kerlinger, F. N. The influence of research on education practice. *Educational Researcher,* 1977, *6,* 5–12.

Koffka, K. *The principles of Gestalt psychology.* New York: Harcourt Brace Jovanovich, 1935.

Neuman, M. C., & Singer, R. N. A comparison of traditional versus programmed methods of learning skills. *Research Quarterly,* 1968, *39,* 1044–1049.

Sahakian, W. S. *Psychology of learning: Systems, models, and theories.* Chicago: Markham, Publishing Co. 1970.

Singer, R. N. Learning theory as applied to physical education. *National College Physical Education Association for Men Proceedings,* 1966, *69,* 59–66.

Skinner, B. F. Are theories of learning necessary? In H. Goldstein, D. L. Krantz, & J. D. Raines (Eds.), *Controversial issues in learning*. New York: Appleton-Century-Crofts, 1965.

Snelbecker, G. E. *Learning theory, instructional theory, and psychoeducational design*. New York: McGraw-Hill, 1974.

Swets, J. A. (Ed.). *Signal detection and recognition by human observers*. New York: John Wiley, 1964.

Thorndike, E. L. *Human learning*. New York: Appleton-Century-Crofts, 1931.

5 CONTEMPORARY APPROACHES TO THEORIES AND MODELS

Perhaps it does an injustice to those theories and models just presented and those to be discussed to classify them arbitrarily as "older" and "newer," if not chronologically, then in orientation. There is no doubt that many of the older traditional concepts are still in existence, only modified to be more consistent with the latest knowledge. That is, many new concepts about behavior have their roots in traditionally accepted psychological laws and principles.

However, the conceptual orientations described in this section are associated with different approaches to describe and predict behavior than the standard S–R and perceptually oriented theories. Their prominence and impact on research, education, and skill learning can be traced back twenty or so years, and therefore can be categorized as recent. One can readily perceive unique terminology, methodology, and intent of application, as well as some resemblance to the standard and well-known theories.

In recent years, we have witnessed the formulation of models and theories that are specific to motor skill acquisition. These developments are exciting to those interested in motor skills, for they indicate that serious scholarly thought is being given to the skills area. Some developments are highly theoretical. Others appear to be quite practical and applied. The ones described here are not necessarily unique from each other or independent of previous efforts in theory and model construction. They do, however, reflect the latest thinking in regard to skill acquisition.

For convenience, these models are characterized in the following manner:

1. General descriptive: emphasis on general characteristics of skilled performance, usually for practical consideration.
2. Information processing: emphasis on perception, decision making, capacity to handle information, and information-retrieval capabilities.
3. Cybernetic: emphasis on personal control through self-regulating mechanisms.
4. Adaptive or hierarchical control: emphasis on higher-order and lower-order

97

routines and person-computer analogies for the organization of information and control of behavior.

The concepts and terminologies in these approaches tend to represent technological advancements. The models evolved out of similar histories and are very much interrelated, as A. W. Smith (1974) indicates. Many ideas applied in technology have also been applied to human behavior. For example, cybernetic models were advanced to explain the way in which a person exhibits control in behavior and behavioral changes. Information-processing models have tended to describe the capabilities and limitations of an individual's perceptual, memorial, retrieval, and decision-making abilities. Both of these kinds of models, along with adaptive ones, are extremely popular today, especially in the skills area, where they appear to be more relevant in describing movement-oriented behaviors than do association and older versions of cognitive-perceptual theories.

The key concepts of these three models, as related to personal control over behavior, are presented in Table 5-1. Although it is possible to focus on cybernetic, adaptive, and information-processing models independently, the understanding of complex motor behavior requires the integration of these three types of approaches. As a result, it is easier to deal with more concepts and events associated with skill learning. This task will be taken in this book, as will be seen in Chapter 6, with the proposed model for the study of motor behavior.

TABLE 5-1 The Human Behaving System: Information-Processing, Cybernetic, and Adaptive (Hierarchical Control) Considerations

Variable	Information Processing	Cybernetic	Adaptive
Control systems	Sense registers, perceptual mechanisms, short-term memory store (limited capacity), long-term memory store (unlimited capacity), information transformation, evaluation, storage, usage	Response-produced feedback, ongoing performance regulation, modification, and adaption, closed loop (peripheral control)	Programs, plans schemas, schemes, higher-order and lower order routines, (hierarchical regulation of behavior), conscious and subconscious behavior, open loop (central control)

As a final introductory note here, there is great excitement today in a branch of psychology called cognitive psychology. Cognitive processes are studied as they influence the processing of information that leads to effective behaviors (e.g., Posner, 1973). The main view is that the person is an active processor of information rather than a passive receiver of responses that are stamped in through practice (Ellis, 1978). Cognitive psychologists have tended to advance information-processing models, to contrast with the older associationistic models.

The person does not totally influence any situation; nor is it probable that the reverse occurs. Whereas behaviorists might lead us to view human behavior as passively controlled by situational dictates, cognitive psychologists suggest that we actively control our environments. The truth probably lies somewhere in the middle. Behaviors are not produced without cues or stimuli. Behaviors are directed accordingly. But all people do not respond similarly to the same events, thereby demonstrating a pseudoprinciple of self-determination. In a sense, then, associationistic behaviors are indeed developed, but in a person's own way. Because we have already dealt with the nature of behavioristic approaches, let us examine in more detail the salient features of the models indicated in Table 5-1.

GENERAL DESCRIPTIVE MODELS

A number of models of skilled acquisition seem generally to describe involved processes, without leaning to cybernetic, associative, information-processing, or adaptive camps. Sometimes the approach is toward a specific aspect of performance, such as the ability to transfer previous experiences to present demands, or the quality of skills retention. An interesting model, leading to much research on the ability of subjects to perform generally well in a number of tasks, versus specifically in task performance, was developed by Franklin Henry. The value of this model is the fruitfulness in encouraging research efforts, especially in the relationship of reaction-time and movement-time performance in various laboratory tasks.

Bryant Cratty's model is a three-level approach at suggesting the organization categories of variables that influence learning and performance. He suggests that general human abilities and characteristics as well as task-specific factors be considered as determiners of level of achievement. The Fitts–Posner model of skill acquisition indicates three stages of development in the learning process, going from learner helplessness and dependence on many sources of information to independence and self-controlling operations. It is particularly appealing as a general descriptive overview of the nature of the acquisition of skill, from initial performance level to the most proficient. Ann Gentile's flow model of the mechanisms involved in the early learning of skills is derived from research and theory, with special direct applications to instruction. It is especially useful for teachers involved in instructing students how to learn skills.

In many respects, the models presented here and throughout this chapter are quite complementary. In other words, similar operational mechanisms and processes are indicated within the models, although at times different terminologies are employed by the proposers. Emphasis also differs. We should expect similarities among the models when they are reduced to their simplest forms to describe similar aspects of behavior. On occasion, however, data may be interpreted in a variety of ways for the purpose of model construction; incomplete data will lead to alternative hypotheses.

Henry's Memory-Drum Theory

The method by which a human functions in motor performance is likened to a computer, in the memory-drum theory offered by Henry (1960). That is, the computer contains stored programs, ready to function in a desired fashion upon the appropriate signal. Humans also store specific, well-learned motor acts in the form of neural patterns in the higher centers of the nervous system. This *unconscious motor memory* is retained as programmed movements on a so-called *memory drum*. Particular stimuli cause the arousal of a neuromotor center, resulting in the execution of an act.

A well-coordinated skill will be performed in an efficient manner because it has been stored on the drum. It can be initiated effortlessly at a point just above the unconscious level. A complicated less-learned or unlearned task is performed continuously at the conscious level in uncoordinated style. This is because of the lack of stored, organized information. An important concept of the theory is that *only specific* acts are stored, and even generally similar movement patterns will not correspond to the same program. Henry emphasizes this point through his research. One of his conclusions is, "Individual differences in speed of arm movement ability are predominantly specific to the type of movement that is made; there is only a relatively small amount of general ability to move the arm rapidly" (Henry, 1960, p. 457).

This statement summarizes an analysis of data obtained from subjects who performed three similar but distinct arm movements. Low relationships from task to task were observed—individuals were not consistent on these tasks, with regard to each other, in the time it took them to execute the prescribed movements. In other words, Henry did not find a general speed ability.

These results lead to the conclusion that, in a practical situation as in the sports world, abilities to perform in the various sports are, perhaps, independent. Success in more than one skill is to be explained by means other than general abilities. Some plausible explanations are as follows. The person who is highly motivated to succeed, especially in sports, will put a greater effort into such undertakings. This general motivation may carry across many skill learning situations. The athlete who has acquired skill and success in one sport may be struck with the urge to make a good showing in other sports.

Second, past experiences are of tremendous importance in determining present motor performance status. When an individual performs a new skill well, with little apparent practice, perhaps it is due to previous experiences in highly related movement patterns. Sports demand certain skills, and initial ease in demonstrating success in some sports is dependent on these developed skills. According to Henry, past experiences contributing to proficient acts are stored on the memory drum, ready to be unlocked and put into action when the situation demands. Of course, the situation must be related specifically to the situation in which the skills were learned. Memory–drum theory, in this regard, is related to the behaviorists' restricted view of the nature of transfer of learning, which has been termed the concept of identical elements. Much research has been completed on the specificity–generality problems of motor performance, directly or indirectly, by psychologists and physical educators. We will deal with this topic in Chapter 7.

Cratty's Three-Level Theory

B. J. Cratty (1966) has incorporated in his theory three levels of factors that presumably influence learning and performance. Level 1 is represented by general factors in human performance, including level of aspiration, task persistence, and ability to analyze task mechanics. This level contains attributes associated with a wide range of motor tasks. Specific ability traits associated with success in motor performance are presented in level 2. Examples of these abilities are trunk strength, arm–leg speed, and extent of flexibility. At the third and highest level are found factors specific to the given task, such as practice conditions, past experience, and the unique movement patterns required by the task. Figure 5-1 illustrates this theory. Cratty calls for the teacher of skills to be aware of all three levels and their interactional effects on skilled performance. According to Cratty's conceptualization, general and specific factors operate in the learning of all tasks. Cratty's second level, which he calls perceptual-motor ability traits, appears to include only abilities that are primarily physical in nature. In fact, the traits he

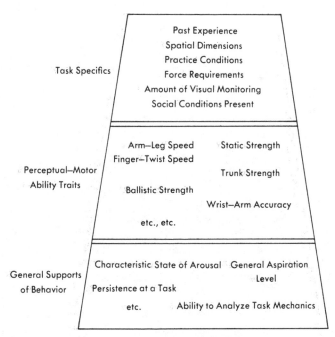

FIGURE 5-1. A theory of motor behavior. (*From Cratty, B. J. A three-factor level theory of perceptual-motor behavior. Quest, 1966, 6, 3–10.*)

lists have been proposed by E. A. Fleishman (1967) as representing physical proficiency.

There are other abilities that may account for performance levels, and Fleishman has extensively researched these possibilities, as well. From his experiments, he suggests eleven psychomotor factors (Fleishman, 1967) that seem to appear consistently in the tasks he utilizes. Their labels are manual dexterity, control precision, multilimb coordination, reaction time, arm–hand steadiness, wrist–finger speed, aiming, speed-of-arm movement, response orientation, finger dexterity, and rate control. Certainly psychomotor abilities and physical proficiency measures unique to achievement in a particular skill should be considered.[1]

Cratty suggests that the effective teacher should consider the three levels of factors and their mutual influence on motor performance. As the teacher becomes aware of their relative influence on the activity to be learned, and which are modifiable in a short period of time and which are not, instruction can be organized in a more meaningful manner. Developmentally, the three levels of factors probably change in import.

The Fitts-Posner Model

Paul Fitts and Michael Posner (1967) have described skill learning as occurring in three phases. Although described in a general way, there is intuitive acceptance for these phases, with evident implications for more effective instructional techniques and an understanding of the learning process. The three phases are

Phase I: Early, or cognitive.
Phase II: Intermediate, or associative.
Phase III: Final, or autonomous.

In the earliest stages of skill learning, the cognitive, the individual is burdened to understand directions, to attach verbal labels to movement responses. The thought processes are extremely active: What is the learner to do? How? The learner attends to the variety of cues that surrounds the situation and attempts to reduce the number that is useful. Written directions, verbal instructions, and/or live models might be provided, and this information must be translated into personally effective movements.

In the intermediate, or associative, stage, primary concern is for practice conditions and requirements. Which kind of training schedules should be followed? Should practice be continual or spaced with rests? Should the emphasis be on speed, on accuracy, or both in the execution of movements? Should whole or partial methods of practice be followed? The learner understands what is supposed to be done and now the concern is for those practice conditions that will most efficiently and effectively lead to proficiency.

---

[1] However, Fleishman has only analyzed performance on laboratory-type tasks. If more real-world tasks were analyzed, it is indeed probable that other psychomotor factors, or abilities, would emerge.

The third and final stage, according to Fitts and Posner, would be the autonomous stage. The highest level of skill is demonstrated with a minimal amount of conscious involvement. Acts performed in this stage are almost impervious to distractions and stress. The soccer player dribbles the ball without attention to this activity; instead, thought is directed ahead about the impending situation: where to go, whether and when to pass or kick to the goal. The gymnast executes routines with little apparent attention to the specific details of the movements. In addition, it should be pointed out that inappropriate aspects of performance are very difficult to correct when they have been well learned.

Thus, the learner progresses from an extremely conscious role in the activity, where verbalization and understanding are crucial and where, of course, the movements are quite crude and probably inappropriate on many occasions, through an intermediate phase, in which the emphasis is on practice conditions. The learner then goes on to an autonomous stage, where execution occurs with a minimal amount of conscious involvement.

Gentile's Model

In one of the few attempts to apply a skill acquisition model directly to teaching, Ann M. Gentile (1972) has delicately balanced a concern for neurophysiological and psychological experimental data, behavioral concepts, and the relatively naive teacher of skills. This model is presented in Figure 5-2. It indicates the factors involved in the initial stage of skill acquisition, and the illustration is clear enough so that further discussion of it is probably not necessary. The model is of special value to teachers of skills, as they can incorporate the basic concepts in their teaching.

Gentile differentiates closed and open skills (see Chapter 1) and suggests alternate teacher strategies for dealing with them. Two stages of skill development are suggested: (1) general ideas of the act and (2) fixation and diversification. Stage 1 would involve accomplishing a goal with a general movement pattern; stage 2 is associated with a particular level of skill. The demonstration of excellence in closed skills suggests a fixation process; that is, the movement patterns become refined and stable. For open skills, a diversification of patterns must be mastered because situational cues vary easily and often unpredictably. The con-

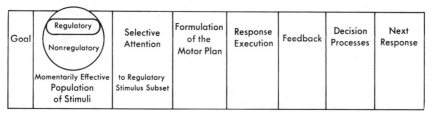

FIGURE 5-2. Initial stage of skill acquisition. (*From Gentile, A. M. A working model of skill acquisition with application to teaching. Quest, 1972, 17, 3–23.*)

trast of open and closed skills, in terms of their characteristics and appropriate learning strategies, represents a major contribution of Gentile's work. The notion of how decision processes may work and how teachers may facilitate them also represents a significant contribution.

INFORMATION PROCESSING (COMMUNICATION) MODELS

Traditionally, information-processing models tend to provide the framework for examining limitations of attention, perceptions, memory, and decision making in the performance of skills (see, for instance, Posner, 1966). The proficient execution of simple or complex movement behaviors depends greatly on the organism's capacity for discriminating effectively among a variety of cues. The capacity of the learner to deal with a number of cues, to transmit information at a fast rate, and to retrieve derived information from memory is of interest to information-processing theorists.

An understanding of one's capacity to attend to a number of stimuli simultaneously leads to applications that might be made for useful instructional techniques. This is also the case when we learn about limitations in one's capacity to register and code information in storage, as well as to retrieve it at the right time—although appropriate organizational processes will help make best use of this capacity. The ability to anticipate events is an outstanding feature of the skilled performer, who responds to the fewest possible cues. The system is thereby freed to think ahead and anticipate circumstances while it executes acts, as if in a programmed state. Attempts made by information-processing theorists have been the most fruitful in describing internal organizational variables of influence on skilled performances. Actually, many information-processing models are cybernetic as well, because self-control and regulation systems are considered. Often there is great difficulty in describing a model as strictly cybernetic or information processing, for these approaches to understanding and explaining skill learning overlap considerably.

Information theory, also called *communication theory,* in its original form, is an example of probability theory serving as a basis for a model. C. E. Shannon and W. Weaver are credited with its development in 1948; their publication (1962) describes the formulation of the theory and contributions to it. This descriptive and quantitative theory has been used mainly for verbal learning, with visual displays, and tracking, but it is inviting to speculate on its application to gross motor skills, as Harry Kay did in 1957.

The capacity to transmit information is determined by assigning numbers to various magnitudes of stimuli. *Uncertainty* and *information* are terms used interchangeably, for the more uncertainty in a situation, the greater information can be of assistance. In other words, information removes or reduces uncertainty. George Miller (1956) compares variance to amount of information, because greater variance indicates more uncertainty. In any communication system, person, or machine, there is a great deal of variability in what goes in and what comes out. Naturally, a good system will show some relation between input and output. The amount of overlap between input and output, whether expressed as variance or amount of information, is illustrated in Figure 5-3. In this case, the relationship between input and output would not be great. Performance output would not be of a high caliber, as there is only a small area of overlap between A and B (variance in common).

FIGURE 5-3. The relationship of output to input.

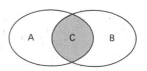

A — Input, Stimuli
B — Output, Response
C — Overlap, Transmitted Information

The binary digit (two possibilities—yes or no), a bit, is the unit used in the measurement of information and uncertainty. The object, then, is to determine the number of bits (the power to which 2 must be raised to equal the number of alternatives) needed to solve a particular problem. Fred Attneave (1959) presented the simple illustrative case where, of sixty-four square cells in a large square, the learner must guess the predesignated cell. With the formula $M = 2^H$, where $M =$ the number of alternatives and $H =$ binary possibilities, we substitute $64 = 2^6$ for example. Six questions, or six bits, are needed to find the cell in question. The first question might be whether the cell is in the right thirty-two cells. (1) Yes. It is in the upper half? (2) No. Is it in the lower half? (3) Yes. In this line of questioning, the correct cell could be discovered in six statements. One bit of information is needed to make a decision between two alternatives, two between four alternatives, four between sixteen alternatives, and six bits for sixty-four alternatives.

We often talk about the uncertainty in stimuli (termed information in information theory) and responses. How much can we remember in a given situation; how many objects or words can be recalled after a short exposure to them? Information transmission is another way of talking about accuracy, and Figure 5-4 serves to represent the information-processing system in simplified form. The sensory processes begin the encoding process; information is then processed further and transmitted in the organism, decoded, and translated into muscle movements that reflect purposeful behavior. No mechanism, machine, or person, is perfect; *noise* (amount of interference or uncertainty) may be present anywhere in the system—in the encoding and decoding or transmission mechanisms—that is, any-

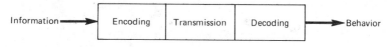

FIGURE 5-4. Information processing.

where processing takes place. Therefore, it is a rarity when the response is exactly appropriate in complex motor behavior.

Every person has a *channel capacity* above which information cannot be transmitted. This capacity can be determined by increasing the input and measuring it with the responses, for if the material can be handled accurately, there will be few errors. With too much of an increase, more errors are expected. Greater input results in increased output, to a point, as there is an asymptotic value for every channel. For example, it is not difficult to distinguish among a few tones. When more tones are presented to the observer, a limited number of them will be recognized and distinguished. This number can be increased, however, with the use of better organizational strategies. This is one way in which individuals differ.

It has been found that 2.5 bits is the average channel capacity of the typical listener making judgements in pitch. This number of bits is equal to about six alternatives. In other words, if an infinite number of alternate pitches is presented, the average listener can only distinguish about six of them. Other studies indicate that for unidimensional judgments, for individual sensory attributes, 6.5 bits is average. More dimensions increase the total channel capacity but decrease accuracy for any particular variable. In this case, the person makes rough judgments.

It has been shown that an individual can increase the amount of information stored. When the object is to memorize a series of numbers, more can be remembered if these numbers are recoded. If the channel capacity of the learner of motor activities could be determined, the appropriate amount of information would be provided at one time. Too much material would be wasted and not monitored, too little would not promote maximum use of the time allotted. The search for the number of bits that could be transferred in a motor learning situation certainly is worthwhile.

One of the most valuable contributions of information theory has been the analysis of processes associated with selection, perception, memory, and decision making in skilled performance. Previously in theory and research, emphasis had been on the observation of the response alone. It is recommended that the reader examine Kay's (1957) article to understand better the relationship between information theory and skilled performance.

One of the more interesting phenomena called to our attention by information-processing theorists concerns storage and retrieval processes related to information. When learning written material, knowing how to "chunk" information is extremely important. That is, if we had to learn a serial listing of fifteen different numbers, progress would be slow indeed if we took one number at a time. By chunking them—that is, grouping them perhaps in groups of two or three—learning, memory, and retrieval are vastly improved. We can only process so much material at one time. But we can improve on the efficiency of the system. Instead of fifteen separate numbers to learn, chunking (a coding system) in groups of three results in five "numbers" to be acquired. Let us say that the list was as follows:

1 8 2 9 0 4 6 3 8 7 1 9 5 9 2

Try to memorize the list with each number in correct order, one by one. Now try chunking:

182 904 638 719 592

Easier? It should be. The point is that we can improve on our learning when we know how to organize stimuli in a meaningful and more simplified way. Chunking and making associations help.

Welford's Model

For many years, one of the most impressive scholars in the area of skilled performance has been A. T. Welford. He has researched the mechanisms that operate between sensory input and motor output, primarily using relatively simple laboratory tasks that involve reaction time or the tracking of moving targets. His concept of these mechanisms as composing a "communication channel of limited capacity" indicates a desire to determine which mechanisms function, how, and with what restrictions during human performance.

Motor performance for Welford is illustrated in Figure 5-5. Of major interest is how information is perceived and translated into action, with special reference to short- and long-term storage systems in response control. He advocates (1) quantifiable behavioral theories and improved psychometric techniques, (2) person-machine comparisons to study similar operations, (3) close ties between neurophysiology and psychology in the study of mechanisms, and (4) the study of the components of complex behaviors within the appropriate broad and natural context.

Mathematical formulas and logic, along with extensive data, have enabled

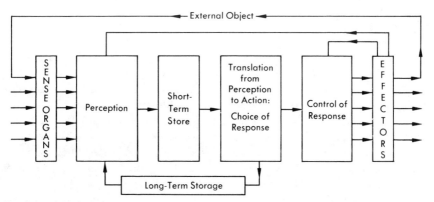

FIGURE 5-5. Hypothetical block diagram of the human sensorimotor system. Only a few of the many feedback loops that exist are shown. (*From Welford, A. T.* Fundamentals of skill. *London: Methuen & Co. Ltd., 1968.*) Reprinted with permission.

Welford to propose "laws" about a person's channel capacities. One of the most famous of his proposals is the single-channel operation of the human organism. An examination of an individual's ability to process information presented simultaneously and to perform on dual tasks led Welford to postulate limitations in the channel capacity to attend to cues, process information, and respond effectively in a number of ongoing acts. Welford has also suggested a formula for predicting speed of arm movement as reflected by the nature and distance of the target and other variables. Space does not permit a summary of all of Welford's contributions to theory and research, but the reader might very well want to examine Welford's major and comprehensive book, *Fundamentals of Skill* (1968).

Limitations in processing information are provided in the following example. The single-channel hypothesis predicts that the central mechanisms can handle only one signal or set of signals at one time. If a second signal occurs right after a first signal, response to the second one takes longer, as it has to wait until the central mechanisms are free (Welford, 1976). Welford theorizes that movement time is determined more by central processes controlling movement than by the factors of muscular effort involved. Choice reaction time is primarily affected by the translation mechanism. Performance is limited by the phasing and coordinating movement of the central mechanisms.

In the writings of Welford and other scholars concerned with skill acquisition and motor performance, there tends to be agreement on the fact that the learner responds to both external, or situational, demands and internal (self-controlling and regulating) mechanisms that operate as response-produced stimuli. An understanding of how a person processes situational or response-produced information, with what capabilities and rapidity, suggests instructional techniques that would be favorable to the learner. Redundant information or too much information could be a waste of time or overtax the channel capacity. Too little information might result in inadequate cues and poor performance. It also might indicate that the channel capacity is not being used to its fullest advantage.

Whiting's Model

One of the more popular models developed in recent years is attributed to H. T. A. Whiting (1969, 1972). His work is an excellent example of how a relatively simple systematic model can lead to greater perceptivity of the relationships of subsystems associated with motor performance. Structural components, functional components, central mechanisms, and a composite are shown in Figure 5-6. The composite model reflects not only the general processes all persons use in performance, but also the effects of individual differences in body capabilities and in environmental influences. As we have seen thus far, very few models have taken into account individual differences (such as those referred to in Chapter 2) and their effects on performance. The same is true for the effects of various practice conditions and environmental situations on learning and performance (also briefly alluded to in Chapter 2). Although Whiting is primarily interested in the similar mechanisms by which most individuals acquire skill, at least his model reflects

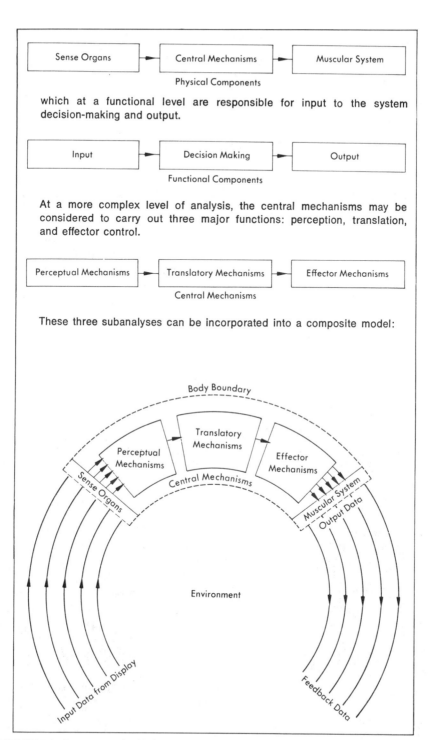

which at a functional level are responsible for input to the system decision-making and output.

At a more complex level of analysis, the central mechanisms may be considered to carry out three major functions: perception, translation, and effector control.

These three subanalyses can be incorporated into a composite model:

FIGURE 5-6. Systems analysis of perceptual motor performance. (*From Whiting, H. T. A. Overview of the skill learning process.* Research Quarterly, *1972, 43, 266–294.*)

factors influencing differential outcomes in human performance. But primarily, his model falls into the information-processing category. The emphasis of Whiting's work has been directed to the neurophysiology and psychology of the central mechanisms involved in performance, on such factors as selective attention, arousal, and decision making.

CYBERNETIC (CONTROL) MODELS

Cybernetics deals with control and communication. In the cybernetic viewpoint, biological evidence is considered in terms of mathematical precision; cybernetics cuts across many disciplines, namely, biology, psychology, communication, engineering, mathematics, and physiology. Actually, the origin of the word *cybernetics* is Greek: it is based on *kybernetes,* meaning "steersman; one who operates a ship and has to keep it on course." The human brain and machine computer are both types of control systems—hence, the descriptive term to describe and compare them.

An analogy to describe cybernetics exists between a human organism and emitted behavior and an electronic transmission system and transmitted events. The digital computer contains an input and output system, a control, and a storage system. The human organism receives situational cues and responds, has a brain as a controlling process, has a storage system in the form of memory, and receives response-produced feedback, which helps to regulate subsequent actions. Cybernetics explains human behavior as a flexible internal model where actions are dependent on flexibility and the adaptability of the response. Consequently, responses will be adjusted according to the availability and utilization of feedback.

The idea that a person and a machine might be compared on the basis of their activities and means of functioning is by no means new. However, it took the work of Norbert Wiener in 1948 to crystallize the relationship and formulate *cybernetics*. Formally defined, cybernetics is the study of control processes and mechanisms in machines and human organisms. The theory in its original presentation as well as developments in this area was presented by Wiener (1961).

The most important concept in cybernetics is *feedback.* It occurs when some of the output from the system is isolated and fed back into it as input. The potential to use feedback is available to humans as well as closed-loop control machine systems. Another name for the feedback system is a *servosystem.* A servosystem is a closed-loop control system operating on the principle of feedback. Information, in the form of errors, is sent back to the device that controls the output; the input is then modified, and the output is corrected. Every human organism must have information about or see the results of actions, otherwise, improvement will not occur. In a skilled act, responses cause input from the proprioceptors, eyes, and other sense organs to be sent back to the system, and this feedback is informative to the person. When errors in movement are made, feedback informs us about the nature and extent of the correction needed. In other words, performance output is constantly modified through the use of information feedback when it shows a discrepancy with the input information. Many motor skills can be thought of as continuous closed-loop system interactions between performance and the sensory effects of each performance. Continual activity is controlled and regulated by means of this sensory input.

Learning situations, writes K. U. Smith (1968) are dependent on space-time patterns of motions. Basic body movements are space structured, and learning is a process of establishing new spatial relationships in patterns of motion. The human organism is not a "victim" of the environment, responding passively to environmental stimuli, but rather dynamically, with the resultant activity processed in the form of feedback for control and guidance. Smith, with his interest in realistic learning problems and a concern for motor patterns and skills learned outside the laboratory, has demonstrated but another of the recent attempts to move away from an S–R viewpoint of learning, which he calls artificial and restricting, to our acquisition of knowledge on the learning process.

Adaptive behavior is modified through experience. George (1965) suggests that feedback brings about simple adaptation, whereas complete adaptation is the outcome of learning. The typical example of a device that operates on the principle of feedback is the thermostat. This is a self-controlling, self-regulating device, for temperature itself controls the change of temperature. When the temperature is low, the thermostat turns on the heating unit, causing the temperature to rise. When the temperature reaches the desired level, the thermostat turns off the unit, the temperature will eventually fall, and the process will be reversed. Room temperature is the input, furnace activity the output, and the difference between the thermostat and the room temperature is fed back into the system as input.

In cybernetics, the descriptive phrase often referred to is closed-loop systems. That is, certain types of apparatus and apparently many kinds of human behaviors appear to be self-regulating. Adjustments are made according to the detection of discrepancies within the system. The primary mechanism is feedback, which encourages and permits detection and correction. Feedback, in this type of theory, refers to the sensory aftereffects of responding. This information is then used by the learner to make adjustments in behavior until the goal and behavior are matched.

By contrast, an open-loop system does not make adjustments, as no error regulator or feedback mechanism is postulated. Typically, association (S–R) theories might be thought of as open-loop systems. The orientation is to external control over the learner, that adjustments made in the environment can influence the learner's actions. Such researchers as K. U. Smith and Jack Adams have attacked association theories as not describing motor behaviors as adequately or appropriately as closed-loop models. Smith has written extensively for many years in this area and has undertaken much research to support his notions about cybernetic theory (Smith, 1972). A theory that has produced a considerable amount of attention recently is Jack Adams' closed-loop theory of motor learning, to be discussed shortly.

Bernstein's Model

From a perspective different from many of those reported in the literature, N. Bernstein, the late renowned Russian physiologist, contributed many cybernetic and biomechanical notions about coordinated and skilled activity. A number of his prominent papers have been translated in English (Bernstein, 1967), although of special consideration here is the one entitled "Some Emergent Problems of the Regulation of Motor Acts." As in any cybernetic model, the emphasis in this one is on the role of feedback for control and self-regulation. Differences are apparent as well, however, for Bernstein incorporates a heavy emphasis on physiology. A main point of Bernstein's is that the performer's changing and adaptive movements cannot be described only by efferent impulses. The prominent role of, afferent feedback (stimuli produced from responses) was recognized by Bernstein for controlled movement in his closed-loop model.

Those of us who deal with skilled movements are obviously concerned with the integration of movement of the parts of the body involved. We have an enormous number of *degrees of freedom* (Bernstein's term) that we must control in successfully completing activities. There is great internal flexibility and elasticity. The more degrees of freedom one has in an activity, the more complicated the system and the greater the difficulty in controlling it. Thus, to Bernstein, coordination in movement "is the process of mastering redundant degrees of freedom of the moving organ, in other words its conversion to a controllable system" (p. 127). It is the organization of control. Which mechanisms are involved and how in this process? Let us examine Figure 5-7.

This diagram is typical in cybernetic theory in that it reveals a closed-loop interaction among the mechanisms to describe coordinated movement. It is unusual in some respects in regard to terminology and the conceptual relationship and the framework presented. The acquisition of skill suggests the stabilization of movements. Bernstein uses the term *motor structure of movements* to mean style in the execution of sports skills. According to him,

> the process of practice toward the achievement of new motor habits essentially consists in the gradual success of a search for optimal motor solutions to the appropriate problems. Because of this, practice, when properly undertaken, does not consist in repeating the *means of solution* of a motor problem time after time, but in the *process of solving* this problem again and again by techniques which we changed and perfected from repetition to repetition. It is already apparent here that, in many cases, practice is a particular type of repetition without repetition and that motor repetition, if this position is ignored, is merely mechanical repetition by rote, a method which has been discredited in pedagogy for some time (p. 134).

Interesting comments for sure! Through practice we learn how to solve problems. Bernstein emphasizes the intellectual involvement of the individual achieving skill, not only the response itself. These and other explanations of movements are to be found in his writings.

MOTOR LEARNING AND HUMAN PERFORMANCE

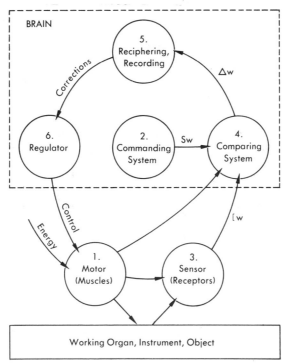

FIGURE 5-7. The simplest possible block diagram of an apparatus for the control of movements.

1. *effector* (motor) activity, which is to be regulated along the given parameter
2. a *control element,* which conveys to the system in one way or another the *required value* of the parameter which is to be regulated
3. a *receptor* which perceives the *factual* course of the *value* of the parameter and signals it by some means to
4. a *comparator device,* which perceives the discrepancy between the *factual* and *required* values with its magnitude and sign
5. an *apparatus* which encodes the data provided by the comparator device into correctional impulses which are transmitted by feedback linkages to
6. a *regulator* which controls the function of the *effector* along the given parameter

(*From Bernstein, N.* The coordination and regulation of movements. *Oxford: Pergamon, 1967.*) Reprinted with permission of Pergamon Press Ltd.

Adams' Closed-Loop Theory

J. A. Adams' notions of closed-loop theory were first presented in an article in the *Psychological Bulletin* (1968) and then in the *Journal of Motor Behavior* (1971). Perhaps the basic difference between closed-loop and open-loop theory is, in the words of Adams (1968), that the latter holds that "proprioception is stimuli which can be the cues to which relatively long sequences of motor responses can be learned, and by secondary reinforcers. Closed-loop theory would say that proprioceptive stimuli can guide well-learned responses because current proprioceptive stimuli from our movements are compared against their reference levels from past learning and are recognized as correct (p. 499).''

Adams' conceptualization is oriented toward an explanation of simple, self-paced, graded movements. An example would be learning to draw a line of specified dimensions. Due to inadequacies in S–R theory, Adams has suggested that his theory offers an alternative approach to explain many of the fundamental variables and various mechanisms not touched on previously. He has proposed a reference mechanism, a *perceptual trace,* as central to closed-loop theory. Previously executed movements presumably leave a trace, or image, and are used by the learner to modify subsequent actions. Knowledge of results (KR) of the movement is compared to the trace. The sense of the movement (proprioception) is a major contributor to knowledge of results, and in turn to the perceptual trace. Other types of sense receptors, such as tactile and visual, are sources also. According to Adams, the perceptual trace is based on response-produced feedback stimuli.

Early in learning, knowledge of results provided from someone else is extremely important, as the learner continually must adjust the trace accordingly. This stage has been termed the verbal–motor stage. The final stage, where skill is demonstrated at the highest levels, is referred to as the motor stage. When appropriate responses are continually made, knowledge of results reveals very little discrepancy with the perceptual trace. Essentially, knowledge of results is ignored and the perceptual trace is strong. In principle, the description is likened to volitional or willed behavior that ultimately becomes automatic.

Whereas a perceptual trace serves as the comparison base for knowledge of results, especially in early learning, a *memory trace* is posited as the selector and initiator of a response. Although both fast and slow movements are initiated by a memory trace, the perceptual trace and KR are used in different ways. In a fast movement, the response is over before KR can be used effectively during its execution. The KR match with the perceptual trace occurs after the movement and is valuable for the adjustment in the next response, if an adjustment is appropriate. During slow, continuous movements and in the verbal–motor stage, trace matches occur frequently and assist in correcting performance for its duration.

Many aspects of knowledge of results—e.g., delays and removals—are discussed by Adams. Presumably, without KR in the beginning stages of skill acquisition, the perceptual trace, which is weak, undergoes forgetting. As was mentioned previously, with high task proficiency, additional learning occurs without KR and is based on internal information. To summarize, the most unique concepts in the closed-loop theory are:

1. the identification of two traces in motor learning: the memory trace and the perceptual trace.
2. the heavy reliance on peripheral rather than central feedback mechanisms, where a person's performance output is compared against a reference model for the detection of errors.
3. The association of error correction with the selection of a new memory trace that yields a response to match the perceptual trace.

ADAPTIVE (HIERARCHICAL CONTROL) MODELS

Behavior can be viewed in terms of activities and subactivities. Certain enabling tasks must be mastered before higher-ordered ones can be displayed. The identification of all the activities, in sequential order, that must be performed if the goal is to be realized is an aspect of sound instructional procedures. Similarly, skilled behavior can be explored through the identification of higher- and lower-order operational processes. It is important to know how these processes, or routines, exist in relation to each other and at different levels of skilled mastery.

Assume that a person, like a computer, functions with higher-order (executive) programs or routines and subroutines or subprograms. It would appear logical that executive routines function with higher-order subroutines, at early levels of learning. However, they "delegate" their authority to lower-order routines in later skill development, thus freeing the system to attend to other matters. As an example, the boy learning to play basketball for the first time concentrates very hard on dribbling the ball. There is little choice or chance for him to do anything else. Yet, once the skill has been mastered, he apparently dribbles with very little conscious control over his activity and attends to such matters as previewing the game situation, thinking ahead about alternatives, and making decisions. The executive routines of control for dribbling have been freed, and other lower-order subroutines are activated for this role. Additional subroutines for other movements are operative. The executive program can be broadened—that is, expanded to encompass a higher-order goal.

An executive program contains subroutines that often operate in sequential fashion. Many skills involve sequential activities that, when properly timed, indicate optimal performance. In other words, the executive program, or master plan, contains the necessary subroutines when the act is well learned. In order for the executive program associated with serving the tennis ball with a twist to the opponent's backhand and rushing to the net to be operational, subroutines (parts of the executor) must already be mastered. Figure 5-8 presents a superficial and partial example of this discussion.

The subroutines can be observed as foundational building blocks, mastery at each level helping to ensure goal realization. They can also be viewed in sequential format, with each one, from initial to terminal, contributing to the overall quality of the execution. The hierarchical concept of control over movement with increased skill helps to explain why certain acts, such as walking, appear to be automatic. There is little need for conscious control over routinized and well-learned responses. The *executor program* can be thought of as the *plan, idea,* or *goal* in a situation. The *subroutines* are the *processes*—e.g., movements, that enable the plan to be executed.

Also associated with the concept of the hierarchical development of control and organization is the notion of open-loop control. Movements become smoother when not under the constant monitoring of peripheral sensory feedback. Open-loop control means that a movement must run its course, once initiated, for approximately 200 to 400 milliseconds (Schmidt, 1975). A new program cannot be

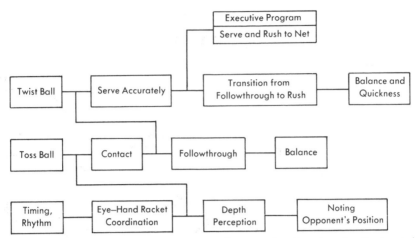

FIGURE 5-8. The relationship of subroutines to the executive plan of serving the tennis ball with a twist and rushing to the net.

initiated by a peripheral cue during this time. As we will see, this is a major argument posed by Schmidt and Keele against Adams' closed-loop concept of ongoing peripheral control during movement.

Some scholars have gone beyond the descriptive terminology of human-computer comparisons and have attempted to demonstrate the hierarchical functional organization of the nervous system. Jacques Paillard (1960), for instance, talks in terms of two levels of nervous systems structures as he analyzes skilled movements: the lower motor-neuron keyboard and the upper motor-neuron keyboard.

Skilled movement patterns depend on the role of the corticomotor-neural tracts in conveying messages, according to Paillard. The lower motor-neuron keyboard consists of the medulla and spinal cord and directly controls peripheral activity. The upper motor-neuron keyboard is associated with critical involvement and represents highest-level control. The activities within and between these keyboards are integrated in a manner depending on functional requirements. Less complex or better-learned responses would be performed in a nonvolitional manner and be under control of the lower keyboard. Complex routines are under the control of the upper keyboard. The ability to perform highly skilled acts would depend on the internal organization of the entire motor arrangement. The lower keyboard will respond accurately to the signals of the upper keyboard as a function of the upper keyboard as well as the close connection between the two boards. Using neurological terminology and concepts, Paillard has attempted to identify executive programs and subroutines, discussing ways in which they work dependently and more or less independently.

We will examine some representative models in which the controlling mechanism for movement behavior has been expressed as a plan, motor program, or schema. The development and refinement of such a mechanism leads to higher-level performance, as the executor changes in nature and level of control.

Plans

The idea that a plan guides behavior is analogous to the notion of a program that guides a computer's operations. Dwelling heavily on cybernetic concepts, George Miller, Eugene Galanter, and Karl Pribram (1960) developed their notions about the hierarchical nature of the organization of behavior. The basis of human activity is what these authors term plans. A plan is conceived to be a hierarchy of instructions. More specifically, "A Plan is any hierarchical process in the organism that can control the order in which a sequence of operations is to be performed" (p. 16).

Instead of talking about reflex areas as the basic elements of behavior, Miller and his colleagues introduced the Text-Operate-Text-Exit (TOTE) unit. A reflex is one of the many possibilities in a TOTE pattern, which is itself a feedback loop. A simple TOTE unit follows:

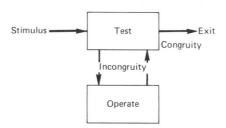

Where the person initiates an action, and if his or her state and the one being tested for are congruous, it is satisfactorily completed. If the states are incongruous, the action will persist until incongruity vanishes. Feedback allows for comparison and testing, and it may be in the form of information that can be used to control behavior. When a desirable state is achieved within the organism, the operations are satisfactorily performed and the test is satisfied, the organism exits and moves on to the next activity or continues the activity with increased probability.

Complex plans of activities are hierarchies of TOTE units. The baseball batter will swing, make good contact with the ball, and run speedily to first base. The whole action appears like a simultaneous series of events, controlled by a single plan. It is composed of a number of distinct phases, each with its own plan, and, in turn, subplans and more subplans. The planning stage for any activity consists of constructing a number of alternative tests (plans for action), attempting to select one that appears to fulfill the desired outcome. The operational stage contains the execution of the plan, with both tests and operations (TOTE units).

When a learner attempts to master a skill, it is assumed that there is some notion of what is supposed to happen and what strategies need be used. There is a plan. Complex tasks require integrated strategies, which are developed through extensive practice. The construction of these subplans enables a person to deal "digitally" with an "analogue" process. This comparison of human behavior to computers in the chapter entitled "Motor Skills and Habits" [Miller et al. (1960)]

is most insightful. Digital operations are discrete—yes–no, on–off. Analogue devices produce qualitative data—variations, magnitudes, and so on. The skilled performer appears to make desirable operations to continuously varying input. The baseball pitch (speed, location) is responded to by a swing or no swing. The superb batter has learned how to translate this type of information like an analogue device because plans are formulated symbolically and digitally. A hierarchy of learning–performance strategies occurs. In the words of Miller, Galanter, and Pribram (1960), "planning at the higher levels looks like the sort of information processes we see in digital computers, whereas the execution of a Plan at the lowest levels looks like the sort of process we see in analogue computers" (p. 91). A motor vocabulary is established whereby well-learned skills are represented digitally. The authors feel that association and chaining theories inadequately describe this type of behavior. Skilled behavior is viewed as ongoing actions, directed toward specific situations that guide them. This behavior is organized hierarchically into units with varying levels of complexity.

Keele's Motor Program Model

The belief in a motor program that governs a sequence of movements, allowing this sequence to be executed without any peripheral feedback, is in contrast to closed-loop theory. Within closed-loop theory, the memory trace as the central mechanism of control was hypothesized. But the mechanism is limited in application to motor tasks, as it is easier to explain its involvement in slower rather than faster executed acts. Yet, it is always of interest to speculate how skilled motor performance, when it is rapidly and accurately demonstrated, occurs in a short time period.

Brief movements, usually taking a fraction of a second, are typically referred to as ballistic acts. The notion of the existence of motor programs is especially helpful, as attempts are made to explain how such rapid responses occur. Because this kind of response cannot be corrected during a brief period of time, it is rationalized that it must be governed by some kind of program. It is as if there needs to be a preestablished sensory awareness in order to enact a motor program. Steven Keele (1968) believes that motor programs exist for predictable and well-learned events, such as when a person aims at and hits a target a short distance away. Such a program would act to control the direction, extent, and speed of the movements.

Movements can be controlled with the use of visual feedback and/or kinesthetic feedback if the movements are slow enough. Keele indicates that movements may be preprogrammed in that the particular muscle fibers to be activated and the timing of their innervation are determined prior to the actual movement. A motor program would exert control until a certain period of time has elapsed, at which point peripheral feedback could influence a change in the movements. Control in a series of well-established and predictable movements most likely shifts from visual and kinesthetic feedback to preprogrammed conditions. Preprogramming would suggest:

1. reduced necessity to attend to cues.
2. increased anticipation of successive stimuli.
3. faster possible movements.

Keele also feels that the research evidence demonstrates that movement control may become internalized, and free from visual influence for briefly timed tasks. But can good performance be shown without kinesthetic feedback? Adams speculated that movement generated a trace and that timing is based on kinesthesis. Keele (1968) raises the question of "whether the individual movements within the series are initiated by feedback from the previous movement or whether kinesthesis is used only intermittently in correcting a motor program" (p. 398). He concludes that the ability to perform movements probably depends on a motor program, as well as other cues. To Keele, Adams's memory trace is a small-scale motor or movement program. It only helps to select and initiate responses, not to monitor a long sequence of learned responses that might be executed in continuous activity.

Further elaborating on these thoughts, Keele (1973) has reported experiments that might support the notion that kinesthetic feedback functions in certain ways in skilled performance and yet not necessarily in directly controlling the patterning of movements. Insisting against a closed-loop theory (e.g., Adams') as well as against the S–R chaining concept (e.g., Gagné's motor chaining hypothesis), Keele has written that the skilled performer constructs a motor program for an activity that contains a series of predictable and perhaps rapidly executed movements. The activity is open loop in nature.

Feedback in this case does not and cannot monitor, control, or regulate such movements. It would appear, though, that feedback helps the learner to formulate motor programs. It also might initiate programs and help in the adjustment of movements in certain ways until the movements are well learned. In those movements where it is necessary continually to make adaptations and modifications to cues, learner attention is necessary for their correction. In predictable situations where corrections will not be necessary, attention and feedback need not operate for the governance of a sequence of movements.

Peripheral Versus Central Control Issues

To this point, models have been described as prepared by various scholars in which there has been a general attempt to analyze skill acquisition and performance (1) similarly across all kinds of tasks, or (2) for a particular kind of task. In the latter case, some models have been prepared to deal with continuous and fast adjustment movements. In the former case, the same model is used to describe mechanisms or processes involved in all motor performances.

It would seem logical that great similarities exist in the way we function in the learning and performing of a broad spectrum of learning tasks. The law of parsimony suggests that we look for commonalities and attempt to describe behaviors in their least common denominators. But inaccuracies occur in some cases and data are "forced" to fit the model. Why not different models for different task classifications? One might be developed to describe the processes involved in undertaking a continuously performed, externally paced task. Another model might best describe a discrete, self-paced activity. It is conceivable that other models could be developed for other categories of tasks. However, these suffice for the purposes of demonstrating similarities and dissimilarities among models that might be used to explain two different types of activities.

The externally paced continuous task requires constant selective attention to cues and perceptual anticipation of events. Perceptual anticipation includes the ideal intermix of arousal level and set for oncoming unpredictable cues. Selective attention and perceptual anticipation work together, leading to recognition and identification processes. Long-term memory, the result of previous experiences in similar situations, influences the work done by all these processes. Decision making must usually occur instantaneously. Based on situational analysis, previous experiences in similar situations (retrieved from the storage system), and the feedback of information as to the match of performance to the situation, movements are continuously adjusted for appropriate action. The long-term memory system contains stored movement programs, with executive and subordinate routines that correspond to them. The degree to which acts have been learned will be reflected by the ability to respond as instantaneously and accurately as the situation demands, with alternative plans ready and available for use when necessary. The importance of feedback for the ongoing performance as a performance regulator is underscored.

Yet, success in self-paced, brief tasks appears to be governed by carefully made analyses of the situation, dependent on factors similar to those in the previously described task. There is much more time, however, to formulate the plan and to put it into action. Feedback in this case is in the form of knowledge of the results of performance, rather than knowledge of ongoing performance. As such, the act may be completed without any immediate function of feedback, except as an additional source of stored matter to be called on when and if the act is repeated.

There are cases where feedback can be of some value in adjusting performance in these tasks. Think of the pitcher throwing the baseball or the tennis player hitting the serve. These are relatively discrete acts in which results of performance are of no value for those events but can be employed as useful information for subsequent events. But during these acts it is possible to respond to visual or proprioceptive cues that inform the performer to some extent whether movement adjustments are necessary. A particular plan for serving the tennis ball may have to be modified upon recognition of a poorly tossed ball. While throwing the baseball, slight slippage should result in compensating movements so that the pitch is still effective. A more rapid and briefly timed movement is less apt to be regulated by feedback processes.

The emphasis on certain processes for excellence in performance in some activities and on other processes in other activities is useful information for the learner and the teacher. Instructional procedures should be geared to reflect these considerations.

A comparison of Keele's and Adams's models might lead us to accept the possibility that both types can indeed explain motor performance, especially if we categorize tasks as involving (1) extremely fast movements without time for the performer to benefit immediately from feedback, or (2) movement slow enough that feedback can assist the individual during task performance. Thus, the availability of feedback during performance becomes the central issue between the two models.

Although it is true that Adams proposes the memory trace as an open-loop motor program, operating without feedback, it is not presented and developed to the extent that Keele considers movement control to occur. Adams suggests a motor program that only selects and stimulates a response. Keele stresses its function in controlling longer sequences of behavior, as well. The position taken by this writer throughout this text is that the execution of different categories of tasks will contain commonalities for explanatory purposes as well as distinctions. In the Keele–Adams issue, preprogrammed plans could conceivably operate in case 1 and closed-loop control in case 2. This point has been elaborated on, with an extensive review of pertinent research, by Eric Roy and Ronald Marteniuk (1974).

Although Adams' and Keele's models have been compared on numerous occasions by their creators and by others in scholarly presentations and articles, and many apparently contrasting views have been resolved somewhat, still others persist. The nature of movement representation and error correction is one such instance. As Neill (1977) illustrates in Figure 5-9 and states, Keele postulates a "template" (a referent model) analogous to Adams' "perceptual trace," which represents the sensory consequences of the ideal movement sequence. Adams suggests that a "memory trace" initiates a movement, whereas Keele believes that a "motor program" specifies all components of the movement sequence. Feedback from the response would be compared against the template, and the motor program would be corrected if error is determined. In essence, then, a dual representation of movement is proposed by Keele: in the template and in the program. In open-loop tasks, Neill (1977) points out that theorists disagree about whether feedback is intermittently and optionally sampled or it is detected automatically to modify a planned movement. Movement programs can be executed with or without feedback, argues Neill.

Stuart Klapp (1976) makes the point that a movement may appear to be programmed or under feedback control, depending on the level of analysis. For instance, programs are probably maintained under gamma-efferent (the spindle-receptor system) feedback control. It is probably true, as Klapp (1975) writes, that "long movements are under feedback control whereas short movements are predominantly programmed and ballistic in nature" (p. 151). Feedback controlled and programmed movements are "mutually exclusive forms of movement control" (p. 152), at the general level of analysis. Yet, both forms of control may operate in either type of movement. In longer movements, for example, programs may

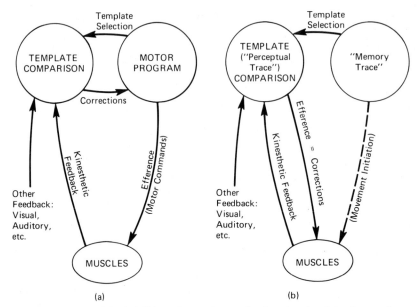

FIGURE 5-9. (a) A model of skill learning and a mechanism for the detection and correction of errors (*adapted from Keele and Summers, 1976*). Note dual (but not necessarily redundant) representation of the movement. (b) Adams' closed-loop theory, similarly represented for comparison. Details of movement are incorporated only in the "perceptual trace." (*Fom Neill, W. T. Input and output coding in motor control: A review. Unpublished paper, University of Oregon, Eugene, Oregon, 1977.*)

operate. Feedback control in shorter movements is not continuous but occurs periodically in program implementation. As we can see, interpretations of what is meant by a program, or central control, and feedback, or peripheral control, encourages the analysis of movement to take differing perspectives.

Further analysis of the problem—whether skilled, rapidly performed complex movements are exhibited as a result of closed-loop (*peripheral*) control or open-loop (*central*) control—has been made by Dennis Glencross (1977). Following a thorough analysis of the literature that deals primarily with such topics as feedback latency, deafferentation and the ischemic nerve block technique, serial organization, the control of positioning movements, and delayed and augmented feedback, Glencross suggests that the evidence does not strongly favor one position over the other. He calls for an integrated approach to incorporate the notion of a central control system and a sensory feedback system.

In this two-stage adaptive-type model, Glencross proposes that in the early stage of learning a skill, the performer is dependent on feedback (closed loop). With skill, the performer uses a motor program (open loop), which can be run off without any sensory or central intervention. There is an advancement of hierarchical control as progress is shown. The executive program control in the first stage is at a "lower level" than the executive control in the second stage. Obviously,

MOTOR LEARNING AND HUMAN PERFORMANCE

there are many phases of development that must take place before the executive program is established and well honed.

Schmidt's Schema Theory

Schema theory, as proposed by Richard Schmidt (1975), contains points of view expressed earlier by others, as well as departures, in order to more adequately resolve some limitations in open-loop and closed-loop theories. In schema theory, Schmidt deals with discrete, rapidly executed tasks, rapid ballistic tasks, and (externally paced) and closed (self-paced) tasks. He does not cover tasks of a continuous nature.

The heart of his theory is with the concept of schema, as opposed to program. Theorists usually posit a one-to-one relationship between stored programs and generated movements. Perhaps this is too much of a storage problem in the limited capacity that we possess. On the one hand, the existence of schema implies that there are "generalized motor programs for a given class of movement" (Schmidt, 1975, p. 232). These schema, or this set of rules, would not take up so much storage space, and could help to explain one's ability to perform somewhat novel tasks or in novel situations. This ability would be related to the degree to which a schema is developed for a particular movement category and the width of the category.

As was the case with Adams' work, Schmidt's theory has been instrumental in stimulating much research by motor behaviorists. As was indicated at the

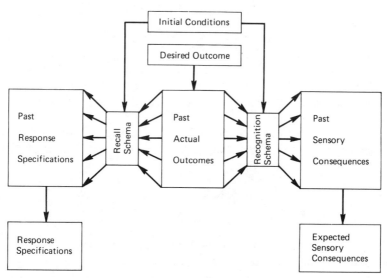

FIGURE 5-10. The recall and recognition schema in relation to various sources of information. (*From Schmidt, R. A. A schema theory of discrete motor skill learning.* Psychological Review, *1975, 82, 225–260.*) Copyright 1975 by the American Psychological Association. Reprinted by permission.

beginning of this chapter, the mark of a good theory is that the hypotheses in it are testable. Many researchers have attempted and are still attempting to determine the validity of these hypotheses with various tasks and under varying conditions.

Schmidt (1975) proposes that four sources of information are stored together by a person after a purposeful movement is attempted. A schema is developed from the arrays of information from these sources as movements become more effective. Schmidt refers to such stored sources as: (1) knowledge of the *initial conditions* (state of the organism and environment), which is used preparatory to activity; (2) knowledge of the *response specifications* (movement requirements), which is used before executing an act; (3) *sensory consequences* (response-produced sensory information without a value judgment); and (4) *response outcome* (the relationship of the performance to the intention), derived from internal and/or external sources of feedback. These sources of information, which contribute to the formation of schema, are presented in relationship form in Figure 5-10.

Recall and recognition schema also identified in Schmidt's theory (see Figure 5-10). *Recall schema* are formed from the relationship between previous response outcomes and response specifications and help the performer to determine what should be done to complete an act successfully. The relationship between the actual performance outcome and the sensory consequences represents the *recognition schema*. The recall and recognition schema presumably involve distinct processes, although Schmidt has combined both of them in Figure 5-11 for presentation purposes.

Both forms of schema are dependent on the actual outcome and the initial conditions, but while the recall schema depends on the response specifications, the recognition schema uses obtained sensory consequences. Knowledge of results affects the recognition schema, not the recall schema. Both these schema will develop in relation to the experiences had with these variables. Increased amount and variability of practice will lead to the formulation of increasingly strong recall schema, as well as recognition schema (Schmidt, 1976). Therefore, the schemas may not involve totally distinct processes.

It is instructive to read Schmidt's works for his own criticisms and questioning of his theory, as well as Adams' (1976) for his arguments in favor of his closed-loop theory. In this way, a greater appreciation can be realized of the many considerations that need to be addressed on an empirical basis if motor behavior concepts are to be accepted fully.

AN OVERVIEW

As we have noticed, the trend in theory and model development associated with motor skills has indicated less reliance on association (S–R) models and more dependence on adaptive, communication, and control models to describe the nature of skill acquisition. Nevertheless, each approach emphasizes factors that the other does not. Some are deeply embedded in behavioral science, highly dependent on experimental findings, and intended to contribute to basic theory. Others

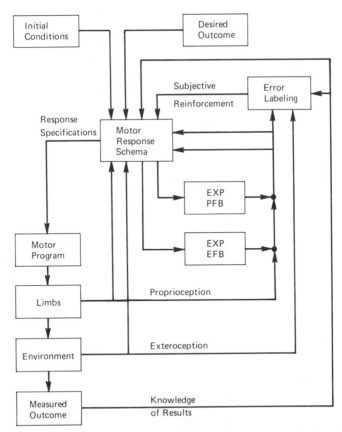

FIGURE 5-11. The motor response schema in relation to events occurring within a trial (recall and recognition schemata are combined for clarity). Abbreviations: KR = knowledge of results; EXP PFB = expected proprioceptive feedback; EXP EFB = expected exteroceptive feedback. (*From Schmidt, R. A. A schema theory of discrete motor skill learning.* Psychological Review, *1975, 82, 225–260.*) Copyright 1975 by the American Psychological Association. Reprinted by permission.

are far more general and descriptive, with obvious ramifications for teachers and learners.

The purpose of this chapter was to discuss what theories and models of behavior are, how they contribute to our knowledge, and how they have been derived. As dissatisfaction with general learning approaches to explain processes involved in skilled acquisition increased, other ways to examine them were developed.

Although the distinction often is not clear, and the terms theory and model have been used interchangeably in the literature, theories have tended to be associated with more general attempts to explain more of behavior than have models. Models have usually been more restricted in scope and concentrated in effort. Conceptual trends in understanding behavior reveal that the popularity of general learning theories has given way to the much needed development of models and more constrained theories that can specifically deal with aspects or particular types of learning and performance.

Theories overlap or are distinguished by emphasis on unique features. For some scholars, it is the contiguity of the correct response to a given stimulus. Skinner, although nontheoretical in experimental procedures and admittedly against the notion of theories of learning, is associated with reinforcement, the Gestaltists with perception and cognition, and cybernetic theorists with feedback loops. Theories differ in vocabulary. Stimulus–response, input–output, reinforcement–feedback, and other terms serve to distinguish methods of analyzing the learning process.

Both generalized and specific theories have their respective values. The more general theories provide general laws of learning, consistent over a wide assortment of learning materials. Specific theories are concerned with particular situations and therefore apply more adequately to those unique problems associated within the area of interest. Learning theorists have been interested primarily in verbal learning and classroom methodology. More recent developments indicate trends in which dissatisfaction with traditional theories has resulted in theories of communication and control.

The current emphasis on going beyond S–R analysis, on identifying those intervening variables that influence performance, and on determining the relationships of mechanisms and processes is healthy and fruitful. Systematic approaches to model development clarify such considerations.

It needs to be reiterated, however, that the true value of theories and models lies in their ability to generate workable and testable hypotheses for research efforts. Naturally, the more data that are available to support a particular set of beliefs, the more acceptable the models or theories. They should stimulate and generate research. If not, much of their value is lost. Many of the theories and models presented in this chapter help us to understand behavior more adequately, but by the same token, a number of them are so vague and general that they cannot be proved wrong. They do not encourage specific testable research hypotheses. They are logical and interesting approaches for the analysis of behavior but need to be laid out in a more specific and sophisticated fashion. If that is done they will be meaningful for practical purposes and at the same time act as a stimulant for research efforts (e.g., to see if behavior can be predicted from them).

Adams', Schmidt's, and Keele's models can be contrasted with Gentile's and Cratty's models, for instance, in the following way. The first three have been developed with scientific scrutiny and allow and encourage experimental work that might substantiate or refute their basic tenets. The latter two are more general and descriptive and are geared primarily for the teacher of skills. From these perspectives, each has an important role to play.

I have deliberately avoided taking a stand on evaluating the work of each approach described in this chapter. My purpose has been to familiarize the reader with early and contemporary efforts in theory and model development. The serious scholar will readily see that many of the conceptual approaches contain statements and descriptions that are quite elusive, evasive, and general.

As we will note in the next chapter, the approach taken in this book is to integrate even further the leading concepts from adaptive, cybernetic, and information-processing models in order to put forth a more adequate description of motor behavior in a variety of activities and situations.

CHAPTER HIGHLIGHTS

1. A number of proposed models of motor behavior have been stated more generally and have served different purposes. Henry's memory-drum theory stirred much interest in the relationships among behaviors and the degree to which they are distinct versus general. Cratty's model is broadly descriptive. The Fitts-Posner three-phase model of skill acquisition is referred to in many sources and serves to emphasize the stages learners go through from beginning to advanced levels of skill. Gentile incorporates research in her model of skill acquisition and makes it practical for the teacher.

2. Advanced technological developments in the 1940s paved the way for the formulation of models of human behavior based on the operations of computers and other types of hardware. Those models gained increasing acceptance in the study of behavior, cognitive as well as psychomotor. The three major theoretical thrusts have been cybernetic, adaptive, and information processing. Overlap is evident in these approaches, along with unique features and emphases.

3. Information-processing theorists have also been concerned with control processes, but primarily those involved in the transmission, storage, and retrieval of information. Ways to improve the functions of capacities have been studied. It is important for motor behaviorists to realize that skilled performance depends not only on knowing the mechanisms of the movement, but also on recognizing cues, processing information quickly and correctly, and making appropriate decisions with reference to movement location, amplitude, speed, distance, and other parameters. The works of Fitts, Welford, and Whiting stand out in this regard.

4. Cyberneticians stress the capabilities of a person's control over personal behavior through the availability and effective utilization of feedback. When activities are continuous and movements slow enough to be monitored under conscious control, performance output is constantly modified through the use of information feedback; when there is a discrepancy between the output and intended goals, corrections are initiated. Cyberneticians view humans as possessing closed-loop systems; behaviorists sponsor the notion of open-loop systems. Such scholars as Smith, Bernstein, and Adams have been recognized for their work in this area, with applications to motor behavior. Adams has been most notable for his impact on research efforts in motor learning.

5. Adaptive models also have been termed hierarchical control models, and the emphasis here is on higher-order and lower-order programs (processes, plans, routines, activities) and how their relationship is advanced with the acquisition of skill. Some scholars, such as Keele and Schmidt, have attempted to explain open-loop control (control monitoring) of rapid movements through the changes that occur in hierarchical control, allowing certain acts to be executed as if automatic. An earlier but still popular version of an adaptive model is one proposed by Miller, Galanter, and Pribram; their discussion centers around plans and TOTE units.

6. What does the future hold for the formulation of motor behavior theory? One possibility is the classification of tasks and models developed for unique considerations and applications. In many ways, it would appear that Schmidt, Adams, and Keele, for example, have oriented their theories to different types of tasks. Then again, there may be attempts to strengthen and expand present ideas, following the law of parsimony, to present one all-encompassing theory of motor behavior. As we have seen, terminology and interpretations can help to bring together, as well as pull apart, the various approaches.

References

Adams, J. A. Response feedback and learning. *Psychological Bulletin*, 1968, *70*, 486–504.

Adams, J. A. Issues for a closed-loop theory of motor learning. In G. Stelmach (Ed.), *Motor control: Issues and trends*. New York: Academic Press, Inc., 1976.

Adams, J. A. A closed-loop theory of motor behavior. *Journal of Motor Behavior*, 1971, *3*, 111–149.

Attneave, F. *Applications of information theory to psychology*. New York: Holt, Rinehart & Winston, 1959.

Bernstein, N. *The coordination and regulation of movements*. Elmsford, N.Y.: Pergamon Press, 1967.

Cratty, B. J. A three-factor level theory of perceptual-motor behavior. *Quest*, 1966, *6*, 3–10.

Ellis, H. C. *Fundamentals of human learning, memory, and cognition* (2nd ed.). Dubuque, Iowa: W. C. Brown, 1978.

Fitts, P. M., & Posner, M. *Human performance*. Belmont, Calif.: Brooks/Cole, 1967.

Fleishman, E. A. Development of a behavior taxonomy for describing human tasks: A correlational-experimental approach. *Journal of Applied Psychology*, 1967, *51*, 1–10.

Gentile, A. M. A working model of skill acquisition with application to teaching. *Quest*, 1972, *17*, 3–23.

Glencross, D. J. Control of skilled movements. *Psychological Bulletin*, 1977, *84*, 14–29.

George, F. H. *Cybernetics and biology*. San Francisco: W. H. Freeman & Co., 1965.

Henry, F. M. Increased response latency for complicated movements and a "memory drum" theory of neuromotor reaction. *Research Quarterly*, 1960, *31*, 448–458.

Kay, H. Information theory in the understanding of skills. *Occupational Psychology*, 1957, *31*, 218–224.

Keele, S. W. Movement control in skilled motor performance. *Psychological Bulletin*, 1968, *70*, 387–403.

Keele, S. W. *Attention and human performance*. Pacific Palisades, Calif.: Goodyear Publishing Co., 1973.

Klapp. S. T. Feedback versus motor programming in the control of aimed movements. *Journal of Experimental Psychology: Human Perception and Performance,* 1975, *104,* 147—153.

Klapp, S. T. Short-term memory as a response preparation state. *Memory and Cognition,* 1976, *4,* 721–729.

Miller, G. A. The magical number seven, plus or minus two: Some limits on our capacity for processing information. *Psychological Review,* 1956, *63,* 81–97.

Miller, G. A., Galanter, E., & Pribram, K. H. *Plans and the structure of behavior.* New York: Holt, Rinehart & Winston, 1960.

Neill, W. T. Input and output coding in motor control: A review. Unpublished paper, University of Oregon, Eugene, Oregon, 1977.

Paillard, J. The patterning of skilled movement. In J. Field (Ed.), *Handbook of physiology: Neurophysiology* (Vol. III). Baltimore: Williams & Wilkins, 1960.

Posner, M. I. Components of skilled performance. *Science,* 1966, *152,* 1712–1718.

Posner, M. I. *Cognition: An introduction.* Glenview, Ill.: Scott, Foresman, 1973.

Roy, E. A., & Marteniuk, R. G. Mechanisms of control in motor performance: Closed—loop versus motor programming control. *Journal of Experimental Psychology,* 1974, *103,* 985–991.

Schmidt, R. A. A schema theory of discrete motor skill learning. *Psychological Bulletin,* 1975, *82,* 225–260.

Schmidt, R. A. The schema as a solution to some persistent problems in motor learning theory. In G. Stelmach (Ed.), *Motor control: Issues and trends.* New York: Academic Press, 1976.

Shannon, C. E., & Weaver, W. *The mathematical theory of communication.* Urbana.: University of Illinois Press, 1962.

Singer, R. N., & Dick, W. *Teaching physical education: A systems approach.* Boston: Houghton Mifflin, 1974.

Smith, A. W. Information theory and cybernetics. *Journal of Cybernetics,* 1974, *4,* 1–5.

Smith, K. U. Cybernetic foundations of physical behavioral science. *Quest,* 1968, *8,* 26–82.

Smith, K. U. Cybernetic psychology. In R. N. Singer (Ed.), *The psychomotor domain: Movement behavior.* Philadelphia: Lea & Febiger, 1972.

Welford, A. T. *Fundamentals of skill.* London: Methuen, 1968.

Welford, A. T. *Skilled performance: Perceptual and motor skills.* Glenview, Ill.: Scott, Foresman, 1976.

Whiting, H. T. A. *Acquiring ball skill: A psychological interpretation.* London: G. Bell, 1969.

Whiting, H. T. A. Overview of the skill learning process. *Research Quarterly,* 1972, *43,* 266–294.

Wiener, N. *Cybernetics.* New York: M. I. T. Press & John Wiley, 1961.

6 A MODEL OF MOTOR BEHAVIOR

The statement that people do some things in the same way and other things differently is self-evident. Of concern in this chapter are the processes and subsystems within us that operate somewhat similarly as we attempt to acquire skill or maintain high levels of it. The approach taken here is to integrate many conceptual approaches—primarily those with an emphasis on information processing, cybernetics, and hierarchical control—to develop the descriptive model of motor behavior presented on these pages.

The underlying thoughts that pervaded this effort were that (1) cognitive processes have a tremendous impact on the learning and performing of complex motor tasks, and (2) there is a need to integrate various conceptual approaches to gain a more comprehensive view of motor behavior as to how and why events occur. Previous efforts in the analysis of motor skill learning have been geared to relatively simple tasks that place minimal demands on a learner's organizational and decision-making capabilities. The acquisition of complex skills requires a learner to utilize cognitive processes in a more extensive manner than heretofore realized. In the proposed model, of particular interest is the way learners select, manipulate, transform, make decisions about, and, in general, utilize information to acquire skill.

The strategies learners use to process information to achieve a high level of skill are of concern to many contemporary cognitive psychologists. In the psychomotor domain, the primary emphasis has been on the response itself. Yet, a skilled response is one in which the receptor-effector-feedback processes are highly organized, both spatially and temporally, under conscious or semiconscious (programmed) control, to fulfill some specified goal. A central problem for those who study the process of skill acquisition, then, is how such organization or patterning comes about. There are great similarities as to the processes and mechanisms involved in motor learning and verbal learning, and a thorough analysis of the current literature on the learning of cognitive matter is instructive in our understanding of such factors. There are unique considerations and distinctions as well in the learning of motor skills and verbal material.

The potential usefulness of a model of motor behavior lies in its ability to allow adequate descriptions and explanations of scientific data, as well as in its ability to bridge the gap (at least for our purposes) between research and practical concerns. Mechanisms, real or hypothesized, in the human system through which the flow of information progresses will be identified and described. These "structures" in the nervous system permit the identification of cognitive processes that a learner may activate during the acquisition of skill. The model was developed primarily to tease out mechanisms that are conceptually sound so that processes and strategies that are helpful for training could be identified. The distinguishing feature of any cognitive activity is that a learner is able to self-generate and to invoke any process and strategy that is deemed appropriate for the situation. Such processes may actually govern and control the transmission of information within and between mechanisms in the system.

The intention behind the model proposed in this chapter is not only to depict a flow of information from input to output, but to demonstrate the role of instructor-imposed or self-generated strategies in maximizing the functional use of the limited capacities we possess. An understanding of relationships among mechanisms, processes, and strategies can promote the learning of complex motor skills, by suggesting techniques that will eventually contribute to the improved operation of pertinent processes and, hence, learning. This information can provide a meaningful basis for instruction designed to assist learners in the formulation and the selection of the best one of alternative strategies applicable to the acquisition of different categories of motor tasks.

As we examine the model, we must be cognizant of the fact that errors in performance may be due, according to K. B. De Green (1970), to (1) the act being performed incorrectly (no goal is known); (2) a failure to perform the desired act; (3) the sequence of actions being performed incorrectly; or (4) the performance of the act not being executed within the allotted time.

These failures can be remedied as we become more familiar with the material in this and subsequent chapters. Other performance failures may be attributed to structural and functional limitations, misunderstandings, motivation, stress and arousal, and the lack of presence of the potential to execute the mechanical aspects of the act.

A SIMPLIFIED MODEL APPROACH

Before describing in detail the series of events that occurs in the model of human motor behavior, let us analyze some simplified and common considerations. These basics should make easier the transition to the more elaborate model. Remember that the behaviorists (associationists) described behavior in essentials: S→R. A particular stimulus led to a predictable (an associated) response. Later, the position was modified to: S→ organism →R, giving credit to the way a person functioned between being administered a stimulus and then responding.

In more contemporary language and broadened interpretation, the sequence of events would be:

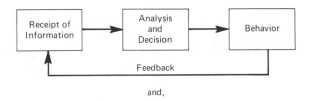

and,

the basic neurological mechanisms would be:

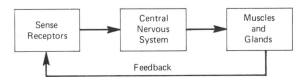

with information flowing from the peripheral nervous system to the central nervous system and back to the peripheral nervous system.

Obviously, something occurs between stimulus recognition and response execution, between sensory register and performance generation, or input and output, depending on your favorite terminology. What happens? A sequence of events or operations follows logically; the events or operations are more logical and productive in highly skilled performers. The learner/performer is confronted with a problem that needs a resolution. A number of *information-processing stages* unfold in order, represented by a set of operations and transformations. In each stage, as we will see, a different set of operations take place. Each stage takes time to transform the initially received information further, to make it available for the next stage.

When we talk in terms of structural stages, we refer to the nature of the information at each stage. Functionally speaking, internal operations occur sequentially or in overlapping fashion. Perhaps our introductory analogy between the human system and a computer system best provides an understanding of operations. The computer performs in a prescribed manner and yields appropriate data, the output of which depends on the input. It generates voltage patterns that result in a series of operations, which appear complex but nevertheless can be broken down into relatively simple steps. In essence, the typical computer contains an input system, a transmission system, a central data processor with a permanent and temporary storage system, and an output system. With this brief description in mind, let us now examine the operational and mechanism similarities between the computer and the human nervous system.

Let us think of the computer as consisting of an orderly arrangement of wires that permits data to be processed accurately. The cabling organization is such as to interconnect certain wires with other wires and, in turn, certain mechanisms with other mechanisms. With the input of instructions, or *coded words,* electronic operations begin, and appropriate wires and mechanisms are activated in order that the response, or output, is consistent with the input.

If the output is not consistent with the input, there then exists a state of incongruity. The machine is reprogrammed; the organism continues to respond until the desired response occurs.

Input-output comparisons are dependent on energy, information, and control. Energy is represented by neural impulses, information related to that which is transmitted from one place to another, and control gives order to the way an act is executed. The notion of feedback helps to explain the relation between what is received and the resulting action. With appropriate feedback and motivation, the human system repeatedly performs until congruence is attained between input (the desired goal) and output (the actual performance).

All forms of life contain wiring arrangements of neural circuits with structures that permit particular behaviors to occur. The forms of behavior to be displayed by living organisms will depend on many factors, not the least of which will be the complexity of the arrangement of the neural pathways and associated structures. The computer accepts coded words and transforms them to electrical currents for processing. In the same way, the organism receives various types of environmental stimuli and may respond by immediately transforming them to electrical impulses, which will travel in the transmission system or neural network. In organisms, however, not all inputs are automatically transformed to impulses. The modulation of generator potential is affected by the nature of the input, in many cases not leading to an action potential.

The potential capabilities of the central data processor, or brain, will often determine the resultant action. Specific and generalized areas of the nervous system are involved in every complex act, and without the appropriate structures, or at least without these structures becoming activated at the proper time, responses to given stimuli will not be appropriate. At the same time, the input must not exceed the amount of data to be processed at any one time. A live creature can sample and respond to just so many surrounding stimuli, a situation that has advantages and disadvantages, as we will see.

We may, therefore, extend the simple models a little bit more by making the computer-human analogy more obvious, as Dominic Massaro (1975) and many others have attempted. Figure 6-1 illustrates the relationship. Some new terms have been introduced. Encoding and decoding refer to transformation processes

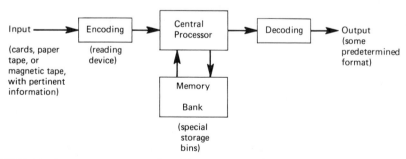

FIGURE 6-1. Computer system, with evident corresponding structures and processes in the human system.

MOTOR LEARNING AND HUMAN PERFORMANCE

applied to information in the system in order to speed up transmission and have accurate output as a result.

These, then, are the basics. Information is received and transmitted in the human behaving system for action, with processes operating in these mechanisms. Obviously, actual behavior is far more complex, involving more processes and mechanisms that interact in complex ways. Let us examine them, step by step, and then attempt to put the pieces together. Be forewarned: There is no model or theory in existence that has gained unanimous support. There are some aspects of the proposed model that are not in dispute, but in others it is very difficult to gain confirmation, for certain processes are literally impossible to study directly. The model proposed here represents a serious intention to "put it all together," adhering to available research findings, with liberty taken to extrapolate and implicate from indirect evidence.

NEED FOR AN INTEGRATIVE MODEL

The major emphases of the cybernetic, information-processing, and adaptive models are identified in Figure 6-2. Do not worry about the boxes, forms, and arrows now. Each will be elaborated on in the pages that follow. It is interesting to note that specific mechanisms in the system can be associated with a particular approach. The features in the model of motor behavior, to be proposed shortly, most associated with information-processing models are incorporated in the perceptual, short-term storage (STS), and long-term storage (LTS) mechanisms. The mechanisms associated with hierarchical control models that contribute to the

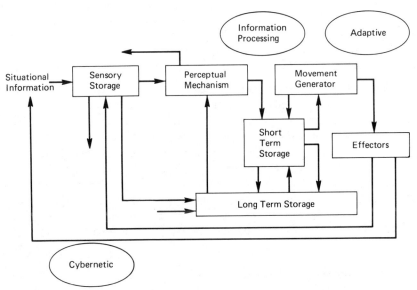

FIGURE 6-2. The major emphases of information-processing, adaptive, and cybernetic models in understanding motor behavior.

selection, storage, and execution of motor programs are the short-term store, the movement generator, and the effectors. Various sources of feedback are available during or following a motor response, and the emphasis in cybernetic models is on how this information from the effectors is returned to the system and processed for future use. The unique and overlapping major contributions of the various conceptual directions oriented to the study of motor behavior must also be considered, with respect to the differing capabilities of individuals.

Although it might simplify instruction and learning if all persons acquired and utilized information similarly, this is obviously not the case. People possess characteristics that lead to dissimilarities in ways of processing information and behaving in the same situation, and a model of behavior must account for these potential individual differences.

Many influences contribute to such differences: culture, environment, instruction, developmental considerations, past experiences, structural and functional capabilities, emotions, personality, and cognitive style. These primary factors interact differentially to affect how individuals learn motor skills. Throughout this book, these kinds of factors will be discussed.

Differential behaviors associated with various personal characteristics will not be analyzed here. Instead, a general conceptual model of motor behavior will be proposed and described in depth (Figure 6-2 will be elaborated on). The model will be used as a framework for the study of the sequential stages of processing information that occur from the receipt of stimuli to the exhibition of purposeful motor behavior. A clearer understanding of the cognitive processes any learner employs to become proficient at a motor task can be obtained through the identification and the explanation of the association between the control of information transmission and the hypothesized stages in the model.

ENERGIZING THE SYSTEM

A person, as an active processor of information, continuously interacts with a transient environment. The stimulation of the various sense receptors (e.g., auditory, visual, kinesthetic, tactile) by environmental or internal cues stimulate the human behavior system to be functionally operative. The activation of the system is evidenced in a series of transformations that ultimately results in a conversion of the stimulus input into a selected, observable response. Although the previous diagram of the model may lead one to infer that incoming stimuli pass uncontrolled from one mechanism to another, the ensuing description of the mechanisms and their associated cognitive processes will serve to illustrate the intricacies involved in the processing of information during skill acquisition.

Situational and Internal Cues

Any system lies dormant until it is activated. Except when we are sleeping, an infinite number of cues bombards our system. These may come from the immediate environment or from the internal state of affairs; cues potentially serve as activating forces on and in the system. A ball thrown to us, words from another person, temperature, a stomachache, an itch, and the like, are potential cues. Any cue must overcome a certain threshold in order to be attended to, and consequently the vast majority of them go unattended.

An organism must have a means of receiving and transmitting a stimulus, thus allowing it to respond meaningfully to this stimulus. Actually, the entire nervous system, which permits this activity, is built up of independent units called *neurons*. Although all nerve cells are structurally similar, certain ones are responsible for the input of information, others function in the output, and yet others act as *connectors* between two nerve cells. *Sensory* or *receptor* neurons play the role of transducers; that is, they convert the information input into electrical signals capable of being transmitted to other parts of the nervous system. The amazing quality of these transducers is their ability to change a specific kind of stimulus (e.g., visual, tactile, or auditory) to the same common transmission: the impulse. Each receptor is specific to one stimulus form only. Not only do they transform various types of inputs, but sense receptors function to code information, too.

The senses serve as the interface between stimulation (from internal or external sources) and the transmitting and interpreting systems. A phenomenon called *sensory adaptation* occurs under certain conditions. The sensitivity level of receptors to a given stimulus condition is lowered with continuous experience with that condition. For instance, when we first place a hat on our head, it is quite noticeable. We feel its placement and position. After a while, and with sensory adaptation, we become unaware of its presence. Another example is going into a dark room—a movie theater, for instance—which requires adaptation to the darkness.

The Sensory Store

Any behaving system becomes activated and functionally operative when sense receptors are stimulated by environmental and/or internal cues that become briefly stored as internal representations of the impinging stimulus field (Sperling, 1960). The information from the task or situation is stored briefly, along with information from the performer's own efforts, in the sensory stores. In Figure 6-3, it is shown how these two sources of information impinge on sensory mechanisms to be stored for a brief period of time. The organism conducts a preattentive analysis (Neisser, 1967) that results in some stimuli that are below threshold being unattended to and fading from the system. At the same time, other inputs that are above threshold are made ready for processing. This pre-processed information, as it may be termed, is transmitted forward to the LTS to make memory contact with previously stored, similar, internal representations. The sensory store functions as a repository that accepts inputs without regard to feature differentiation. The receipt of inputs can be thought of as analogous to a vacuum cleaner that ingests all objects in its path, impervious to article distinction.

The arrival of environmental cues into the sensory stores prompts the learner to conduct a precategorical analysis (Neisser, 1967). U. Neisser has suggested that the preattentive process involves discriminations based on relatively crude physical distinctions (e.g., location, shape, size). Additionally, R. M. Shiffrin and W. Schneider (1977) have emphasized the importance of previous experience (acquired through training and/or practice) as a mediator of the preattentive process.

As can be seen in Figure 6-3, stimuli can be transmitted from the sensory storage to either the LTS (the stimuli are not really being processed at the point) or directly to the perceptual mechanism. The specific pathways of the stimuli are contingent on a distinction between detection and/or recognition of the incoming signal. Detection is the process by which the human behaving system becomes aware that a new stimulus has been received without meaning being applied to that stimulus. Thus, it is detection that may initiate the first of multiple transformational processes that ultimately will lead to the selection of a response by the organism.

The determination that a change has taken place in the environment does not always necessitate that the particular stimulus be recognized. "Specific memory for a stimulus need not be involved at all in this [detection] process" (Massaro, 1975, p. 292). For example, in a crowded room amidst numerous conversations, an individual may hear a sound (signal) that does not match the environmental noise. Although the sound is too faint to be recognized, the individual can still be said to have "detected" that signal. As illustrated in Figure 6-3, a given stimulus may be detected without contracting LTS for recognition purposes, and the stimulus may then proceed onward to the perceptual mechanism. In essence, there can be detection without the process of recognition.

To summarize, the sensory store serves two functions within the human behaving system: (1) it receives incoming stimuli, storing it briefly; and (2) it transmits the stimuli immediately to the perceptual mechanism for detection or to the LTS for memory contact.

With regard to the mastery of motor skills, visual and proprioceptive sources of information are probably the most important, as compared to possible sources of available sensory information. I. G. Temple and H. G. Williams (1977) make

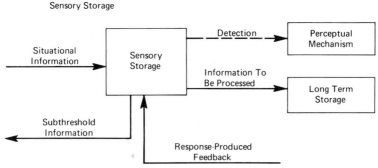

FIGURE 6-3. Activation of the human behaving system by information reaching the sensory register.

MOTOR LEARNING AND HUMAN PERFORMANCE

the point that achievement in any motor activity may be a function of (1) an individual's preference for or capacity to process the most relevant information and (2) the nature of the demands of the task itself. These researchers studied children classified as better or poorer processors of visual information and those classified in the same way with regard to proprioceptive information. The tasks used differed in the relative importance of visual and proprioceptive components. Levels of task mastery, rather than rate of mastery, were evidenced by the differential trends in the data, as a function of task type and processor type.

The Long-Term Store

Although stimulus cues impinge on the sensory stores, the inputs have not yet acquired meaning within the context of the particular situation. Therefore, "preprocessed information" must be transmitted to the LTS to activate memory contact with previously stored, similar representations. In addition to the arrival of external inputs, the organism provides internal cues representative of developmental characteristics, structural and functional capabilities, present arousal state, thoughts, personality factors, and individual cognitive style (see Figure 6-4).

Although there are other viewpoints, it would appear that the access and structure of memory must be based on sensory signals if recognition is to occur (Norman, 1976). If the contention was not plausible, how else would the organism know immediately what it didn't know? The suggestion here is that the incoming sensory signals contact LTS and are internalized in the form of a representation that achieves access to the memory structure (Atkinson & Shiffrin, 1968; Atkinson & Wickens, 1971). Similarly, H. A. Simon (1976) has concluded that there already exists information in LTS (acquired through experience) that permits the identification of incoming stimuli. These interpretations lend particular credence to the contention that the neurological code momentarily stored in the sensory regis-

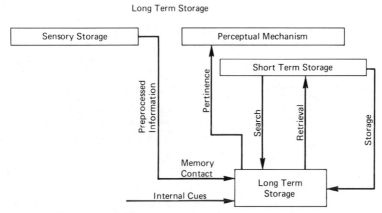

FIGURE 6-4. The long-term store as a mechanism that provides pertinence levels, referents, and a storage space for information.

ter must be transmitted to the LTS, where it can be matched with previously stored representations.

It is conceivable that while all past events may reside in LTS, the person places differential importance on the knowledge with respect to variables such as recency and frequency of occurrence and familiarity. The information that occupies the memory structure is stored in an organized fashion. The organizational structure is based on the pertinence value allotted to each item by the organism, such that the most salient events are the most accessible. The significance of pertinence can be derived from two distinct sources, such as stimulus identification and an analysis of inputs (Lindsay & Norman, 1977; Norman, 1968, 1976). Previous experiences and present stimulus inputs are combined to establish the pertinence value of all "items" that contact the LTS. It would logically follow that more experience with a particular stimulus results in a greater pertinence value assigned to that stimulus. Illustrative of this point is that fact that individuals, regardless of specific attentional demands, react instantly upon hearing their name (Cherry, 1953). The cocktail party phenomenon has been offered as evidence that frequently experienced items (e.g., an individual's name), or very familiar items, achieve higher pertinence levels within the LTS, which facilitates access to the perceptual mechanism. The facilitatory process has been termed "automatic processing" by Shiffrin and Schneider (1977).

An automatic process can be defined as parallel pathways of information transmission through the cortical centers that become activated in response to a *particular* well-learned stimulus and that require little or no conscious attention on the part of the learner. The initiation and subsequent completion of the automatic process, whether externally or internally generated, is contingent on the strength of the initial input.

The suggestion is that the greater the potential pertinence value derived from the stimulus that contacts memory, the greater the probability that an automatic process will be initiated by the learner. Additionally, it appears that detection is also an automatic process, as evidenced by the fact that it does not require much active control or attention by the learner.

The implementation of a subconscious automatic process enables the learner to immediately activate representations in LTS similar to the stimulus input (LaBerge, 1973, 1975; Norman, 1976). However, it is implausible to suggest that the human behaving system is capable of automatically matching all inputs to its internal representations. The indication is that a need exists for a second type of processing that enables the organism to actively control transmission of inputs through the system. The advantage for a learner to engage in controlled processing rather than automatic processing is that more cognitive control is exerted in the situation, so the learner has greater adaptability to novel situations. Thus, there are some situations in which an automatic detection process may best suit the learner's needs; at other times, a controlled, sequential search will be more desirable.

The activation of either an automatic or controlled process based on contact with the LTS is dependent on the pertinence value (e.g., previous experience) assigned to the incoming stimuli. The higher the pertinence level of an item, the greater the probability that it will be processed automatically, or detected, without the necessity of conscious control. Contrarily, the lower the pertinence value, the more likely the learner is to invoke a controlled process activation of the LTS. It may be concluded that pertinence value as well as the particular information expectancies derived from the confirmation of previously experienced inputs of similar situations (Hochberg, 1970; Norman, 1968) will determine whether an automatic or a controlled process is initiated by the learner.

In Figure 6-3, it can be seen that information in the sensory store can be detected and *automatically* transmitted to the perceptual mechanism. Other information, termed preprocessed, is forwarded to LTS to make memory contact and to be assigned a pertinence value for controlled transmission to the perceptual mechanism where recognition will occur.

Thus, the function of the LTS can be dichotomized. One provision is as a pertinence value to information that contacts memory so that the information can be recognized in the perceptual mechanism; a second provision is as a storage space for information that is transmitted from the STS for learning. In this sense, the LTS preserves the modified internal representation of the information for future use. This latter function will be discussed more fully following a description of the role of feedback.

The Perceptual Mechanism

The detection process, and the level of pertinence, or information expectancy set, alerts the perceptual mechanism to anticipate the ordered arrival of specific information (see Figure 6-5). The sequential arrival of information enables the individual to attend selectively to the most relevant inputs, usually those stimuli that enter the perceptual mechanism first. However, although the pertinence items have acquired relevancy through contact with LTS, they have not yet gained meaning within the context of the present situation. Therefore, the perceptual mechanism must recognize the present cues so that the information may be rendered meaningful.

FIGURE 6-5. The perceptual mechanism provides more meaning to situations and tasks after receiving information with pertinence value from long term storage or information directly from the sensory storage.

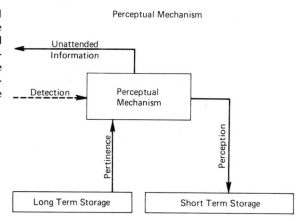

The application of meaning to stimuli can be viewed as the unitization of similar features into recognizable patterns (Estes, 1970; LaBerge, 1976). For example, the sensory features of a human face or a word may have contacted singular representations in LTS (e.g., nose, mouth, eyes, ears). The identification of the features as a face, however, requires the analysis and subsequent consolidation of the individual characteristics into one recognizable unit. Herein lies the differentiation between detection and recognition. Through the process of detection, the organism merely acknowledges the existence of an object. The process of recognition, however, requires a more complicated analysis of the specific features leading to the rather sophisticated judgment that the eyes, ears, nose, and mouth form a face. It is the face that is "recognized" as a whole unit. As LaBerge (1975) contends, if these patterns were transmitted to the STS as just a list of features that were processed either serially or in parallel, the system would have to operate on each feature separately.

The unitization (combining process) of similar features in the perceptual mechanism reduces the number of items sent to STS for decision-making purposes. It is conceivable that, during the process of unitization, items may be lost from the system due to dissimilar features within the present context or lack of attention by the organism. Similarly, the detection of a signal may not necessitate a response on the part of the organism. Thus, signals that are detected, but not acted on, also exit from the perceptual mechanism.

In marked contrast to the view that a functional perceptual mechanism exists within a behaving system, numerous information-processing theorists have excluded a perceptual mechanism from their models (e.g., Broadbent, 1971; Deutsch & Deutsch, 1963; Shiffrin, 1976; Shiffrin & Schneider, 1977). Designers of these models have allocated the processes that underlie a perceptual mechanism to either the sensory mechanism (Broadbent, 1971) or to the STS (Shiffrin, 1976; Shiffrin & Schneider, 1977) or to an attentional mechanism (Kahneman, 1973). The general viewpoint has been that an attention mechanism or filter (Broadbent, 1971; Deutsch & Deutsch, 1963; Treisman, 1964) becomes activated directly after information passes through the sensory stores. The purpose of the filter is to distinguish relevant from irrelevant information and to allow only the relevant information to receive continued processing through access to memory stores.

Perhaps it is too impossible a task to determine a specific location point for attention. Instead, attention is viewed as influencing all information-processing behaviors, from decisions about which information to focus on, to decisions about what aspects of the inputs should be rehearsed. The concept of attention and its relation to memory processes may very well be the central issue in cognitive psychology. It is not suggested here that an attentional mechanism does not exist. Rather, attention is such a pervasive behavioral phenomenon that it probably cannot be located within one hypothetical structure in the human behaving system. It is proposed, therefore, that a perceptual mechanism, located at the beginning of the system, can control the process of selective attention, which is a subsidiary of all attentional behavior. Furthermore, it is contended that selective attention in the perceptual mechanism cannot occur before LTS contact because the representations have not yet acquired contextual or situational meaning. Without meaning, a learner cannot know which information is relevant.

There is an alternative position. Shiffrin and Schneider (1977) have suggested that the STS simultaneously functions as organizer, analyzer, and appraiser of incoming information. However, to assign all these functions to the STS would appear to negate the widely accepted notion of limited capacity associated with it. Thus, there would appear to be a necessity for the inclusion of a perceptual mechanism within the human behaving system.

Although perception as a process is conveniently conceived of as an operation that occurs after sensation and before decision making and as located in one part of the human behaving system, it is more likely that it and selectivity occur from the beginning to the end of information processing (Erdelyi, 1974). In other words, there are many potential points in the system where selectivity occurs. It encompasses a sequence of events. For instance, selectivity occurs during sense reception, encoding from sensory storage to short-term storage, rehearsal for transfer of information from short- to long-term memory storage, retrieval of information for usage, and the like.

One of the major functions of the perceptual processes is to deal with information overload. Many skilled movements demand an efficient system, one that can quickly and expediently deal with a minimal amount of task-relevant cues. Therefore, effective perceptual processes must contain a useful filtering mechanism.[1] It appears that

1. irrelevant and meaningless information is filtered out, leaving the person to attend to the bare necessities.
2. a priority is established with regard to incoming information and information to which the person will attend. A theoretical buffer zone is established.

A person possesses a limited channel capacity, and so it is imperative that the system be used intelligently. Capacity limitations suggest that one cue is handled a fraction of a second before a second cue can be attended to, under most conditions.

Upon completion of the perceptual process, the human behaving system has analyzed the relevant features, consolidated these features into recognizable units, and applied meaning to the incoming information. It is the combined result of these activities that stimulates the transmission of information to STS, where a decision about the course of action will be made. Before discussing the further flow of information, it is important to note that the state of arousal will potentially influence the processing of information at any stage.

---

[1] Earlier and more established theory credits the filtering system with operating between sense reception and the activation of central processes. More recent theory questions this stance, and there is a suggestion that the filter system works later when the memory system is activated.

Arousal

The state of the voltage waves in the brain is associated with the level of activation within the individual. The optimal state of arousal is necessary for skilled performance, for obvious reasons. It is one thing to have the necessary paths and an orderly cabling arrangement as well as neural structures, but perhaps more should be said about attentiveness to certain situational cues and selection of appropriate responses. In other words, the action of certain parts of the nervous system determines consciousness, alertness, and preparedness for activity and has a bearing on response. Appropriate arousal levels are responsible for activation, direction, and persistence in behavior.

These functions have been attributed to the *reticular formation* of the brain stem, also known as the *reticular activating system*. The reticular formation is a mesh of motor nerve cells, distributed from the top of the spinal cord to the thalamus and hypothalamus, that receives and distributes impulses to the lower as well as the highest centers of the central nervous system (see Figure 6-6). The main function of the formation appears to be that of alerting the individual, of placing the person in a condition of arousal.

When an individual is in a sleeping state, little activity occurs in the reticular formation. However, stimulation of this center has an effect on the cortex and results in its awakening. Many of the afferent pathways feed into the reticular system, and if the impulses are strong enough, they will pass on to the hypothalamus, thalamus, and, finally, the cortex. Damage to the upper portion of the reticular system may result in extensive sleepiness or even pathological sleep.

Stimulation of the reticular formation facilitates or inhibits ongoing motor activity by increasing or decreasing activity in the *gamma efferent system*. Gamma motor neurons (efferents) are responsible for the control of sensitivity of the muscle spindles. When the gamma neurons are stimulated, reflex contractions and voluntary movements are encouraged.

Some scholars have attributed great significance to this formation. In fact, it has been termed a program-selection mechanism that determines the nature of a response. As a response selector, the reticular system assigns priorities to messages, determines which are important, and selects the appropriate responses in order of importance. Nearly all of the incoming and outgoing impulses of the brain pass through the reticular formation.

With the influence of the cerebrum, cerebellum, reticular formation, and other areas of the brain, the output of the nervous system, displayed in the form of complex coordinated movement, is made possible. Selective input is partly dependent on attention processes, or an optimal level of activation of the system. Optimal arousal suggests the ability to discriminate and select from many available situational cues the most relevant one or ones to which to respond.

Fatigue causes an overload of the system, and understimulation or underload results in boredom. There is a tendency not to respond to appropriate cues as practice time increases and there are fewer behavioral adaptions to the display. Attention is increased with greater stimulus intensity, fewer repetitious acts, personal

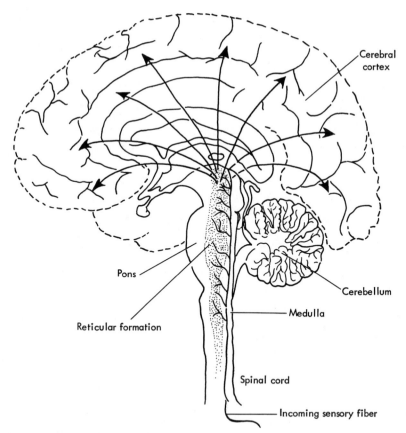

FIGURE 6-6. Section of brain showing the reticular formation. It is composed of interlacing fibers and nerve cells that form the central core of the brain stem. Incoming fibers from the spinal tracts send collaterals into the reticular formation. Arrows indicate the general arousal of higher brain centers that the reticular area controls. (*From Kimber, D. C., Gray, C. E., Stackpole, C. E., Leavell, L. C., & Miller, M. A.* Anatomy and Physiology *(15th ed.). New York: Macmillan Publishing Co., Inc., 1966).* Copyright 1966 Macmillan Inc.

motivation, and stimuli that contrast with other available stimuli. Warnings are likely to help performance, especially if the stimulus event is going to be weak or brief.

According to activation theory, the relationship between behavioral outputs and state of arousal assumes the form of an inverted U. Too little or too much arousal impedes the system; somewhere in the middle for most tasks, although the level varies for different tasks and different people, is most desirable. Some tasks require more inhibition and control over movements than others, and vice versa. Tasks requiring much information processing would be impeded by high arousal levels. The relation of exercise-induced changes to activation level and motor performance has been analyzed by Bernard Gutin (1973).

The arousal state may be controlled by the system itself, a sign of a skilled performer. Nondesirable fluctuations in arousal in task performance indicate a relatively new experience for the learner. One has to learn how to optimize arousal levels for the task demands if effective cue selection and decision making are to occur. The energizing of the system to fit the task requires experience and familiarity with the situation and outcomes associated with various states of arousal. Activation is dependent on emotional levels and motivational levels, such as level of aspiration. The goals we set for ourselves in task performance will be reflected in the way the system is geared for the activity and the manner in which it attempts to handle it.

DIRECTING THE SYSTEM

The Short-Term Store and Retrieval from the Long-Term Store

Activation helps to provide direction to the system's output. So does the use of information stored in the memory banks. The speed with which we learn something and learning efficiency in general depend to a large extent on what is remembered from previous similar experiences. Events are stored for future use. The location and nature of memory traces are difficult to ascertain, but they appear to be widely dispersed throughout the brain.

Breakthroughs in understanding memory and intelligence have been made from the findings of recent research concerned with these problems. Studies on rats, fish, and flatworms indicate an increase in ribonucleic acid (*RNA*), which is the genetic material in each brain cell's nucleus, in the cells, as learning takes place. Neurons produce RNA, with more cell activity resulting in more of this substance. RNA has been termed the memory molecule by some scientists, even though research is still scanty in this area. Memory traces may be stored permanently in the form of new protein molecules (Maggio, 1971). Rats trained at problem solving, besides demonstrating an increase in their RNA and protein contents in the brain cells, also have heavier and larger brains. If RNA is the learning secret, there are great implications for improving the learning abilities and performance of those individuals who previously were thought to be hopeless as learners. Possibly, the administration to them of additional amounts of this substance would benefit their learning potential.

No one part of the brain can be called the central repository of stored information, and, as we have just seen, neuronal activity increases the RNA in all brain cells. However, as indicated by research evidence, the temporal lobes of the cortex are involved in the recall of many previous experiences. W. Penfield and L. Roberts (1959) write that in the processes of recall and comparison and interpretation the interpretive cortex of the temporal lobes plays its specialized role. Electrical stimulation of portions of these lobes sometimes results in the sudden remembrance of events that occurred many years earlier.

In contrast, Maggio (1971) has summarized the curent thought on the matter by stating that

> It seems that memory traces are made by entrance into the function of patterns of neuronal units, which are widely represented throughout the cerebral cortex of both hemispheres. They are interconnected with each other and with some subcortical structures, especially those of the reticulolimbic system, which also contribute to the emotional color with which the memory traces are reexperienced during the recall (p. 143).

E. Roy John (1967) has written a scholarly and well-documented book in which he refutes the idea that learning and memory are associated with neural pathways involving specific brain cells for receiving certain inputs and triggering certain outputs. He expresses the belief that ''learned behaviors are motivated by systems which are anatomically extensive and involve many brain regions'' (p. 418). John doubts that any one structure or set of neurons is responsible for storage of the memory of a particular experience, that no specific set of cells must discharge for memory to operate. John proposes that stored information is associated with ''spatiotemporal patterns of organization in enormous aggregates of neurons'' (p. 417).

In a recent book, R. W. Thatcher and John (1977) extend this position, suggesting that a stimulus initiates a broad distribution in the brain that is organized into a representational system. There is information representation about (1) the external world, (2) internal occurrences, (3) information (memory, awareness), and (4) complex mental operations that can be performed on information (thinking, planning, and creating). And, write Thatcher and John, the response of many different anatomic regions of the brain to a signal is dramatically altered by learning. Change does not occur in one place.

The later performance of once-learned skills is also dependent on the physical condition of the neural system. What happens when there is damage to a nerve cell or two? Regeneration of nerve cells is believed to be possible only if at least the cell body (and its nucleus, which is the center of repair) is intact and a neurilemma sheath surrounds the fibers. Because neurons in the central nervous system lack a neurilemma, regeneration is only possible in the peripheral nervous system. Nerve cells that are completely destroyed cannot be replaced, but other neurons may be able to take over their function, to certain degrees. This ability will be dictated by the period in the individual's life when specific nerve cells are destroyed, as well as the specific cells involved. Cells may die because of such factors as injury or disease, and if certain patterns of movement have been established before this occurs, there is a better chance neurons in surrounding areas will be able to compensate for their loss of function. Thus, a baby will be handicapped to a greater extent than a more mature child or adult, as a baby will not yet have had the opportunity to develop skilled motor patterns. Greater experience and education result in more and varied learning patterns. As a result, less behavioral deterioration might be expected to occur after brain damage in older and/or highly educated people.

Memory is theorized to be of two types: long term and short term. Apparently, information is rapidly lost in short-term memory when there is no sustained attention or rehearsal. With adequate rehearsal, information is sent on to long-term memory storage, ready to be called forth at a later date. It is interesting to speculate why we remember so well certain things we did in childhood and yet have forgotten others and also why motor skills are often retained for a lengthier period of time than once-learned literary passages. Are there different memory mechanisms involved in the operation of, say, long-term retention versus short-term retention? One fact remains sure at the present time: we cannot isolate or localize a memory trace, regardless of its nature. It does appear, though, that during the retention process of whatever is to be retained, a multiple representation in the cortex is established. That is to say, various portions of the cortex are capable of relaying previously gained information to the individual when it is needed.

Stored memory will affect judgments, for consideration of the costs and payoffs for certain decisions are based on previous experiences in similar situations. Previous successes, risk taking, and the ability to isolate and attend to certain cues reflect input from the memory system and the ability to retrieve effectively from it. Speed and accuracy of retrieval for the immediate task demands reflect learning and experience. All of the components discussed so far lead to the activation of an appropriate plan of action, which can be called a movement plan or program and will be discussed shortly.

The STS (see Figure 6-7) is the most significant mechanism in the human behaving system because all the mechanisms transmit information to the STS for rehearsal, organization, and decision making. The mechanism, in turn, transfers this information to the LTS for learning to occur. Upon completion of a movement, the response outcome is transmitted through the sensory storage and the LTS and then back to the STS, where error correction can occur. It appears from this rather global description that the processing capacity of the STS is limitless,

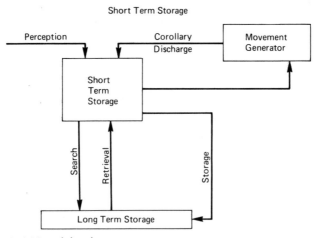

FIGURE 6-7. Activities of the short-term store.

MOTOR LEARNING AND HUMAN PERFORMANCE

but this is not the suggestion at all. Results of investigations into the area of immediate recall (auditory and visual) have consistently been supportive of the individual's inability to process numerous, differential stimuli concomitantly (e.g., Massaro, Cohen, & Idson, 1976; Sperling, 1960). The capacity limit of the STS, then, has a strict upper limit, based on the complexity and quantity of the information that can be handled within the mechanism, as reported by Miller (1956). It will be beneficial at this point to discuss the parameters within which the STS operates, as well as the processes carried out by the mechanism.

The memory structure of the STS serves three distinct functions within the human behaving system. First, the STS furnishes the learner with a temporary storage area ("working memory") for information currently important to the organism. Second, the STS is responsible for a majority of the decision-making, problem-solving, and thinking behaviors of the human organism. Third, the STS integrates the first two functions to determine which information is transferred to long-term storage. These functions are carried out, based on the storage capacity the mechanism. Miller (1956) has proposed that the amount of information that can be stored in the STS is contingent on the familiarity of the items. In this sense, the less familiar items would require additional time and space for processing to take place. As such, and with respect for differences in individual processing capabilities, Miller quantified the amount of information held in STS as being 7 ± 2 chunks (units of information). Thus, individuals were viewed as being able to handle as few as five or as many as nine units of information at one time, although these numbers have been shown to vary (e.g., Glanzer, 1972).

The differences in processing capacity among individuals are not the result of structural deficiencies. Rather, differences in the functional capabilities of the STS are the causes of performance differences. This functional deficit has been related to inexperience in strategy usage (Brown, 1978; Chi, 1976) across age groups. Although mature learners show greater processing ability because of a more sophisticated use of stragegies than their less mature counterparts, performance differences resulting from an inability to apply appropriate strategies have also been evidenced by learners who differed only in their level of experience with the material to be learned (Brown, 1978). It can be concluded that the functional capability, and therefore the available processing capacity, has a direct relationship to the type of strategy the learner invokes to acquire and to organize information.

Through the use of various learner strategies, incoming information is transformed into more organized units, which allows additional processing space to become available (Chi, 1976; Dansereau, 1978). The more automatic the sequence becomes, the less need there is for the learner to attend consciously to the process. A decreased necessity for conscious control by the organism frees the system so that the learner is able to process input cues while working on information already in the mechanism. Within this context, the efficiency of a continuation of automatic processing from LTS is apparent. As situations become more familiar or redundant, a simple repetitive sequencing of the processing operations is all that is required.

Although familiar information may be processed automatically and directly transferred to the LTS, less familiar information must be rehearsed in the STS. A major function of the STS during rehearsal is to provide greater meaning to the inputs, so this information can be easily transferred to the LTS. Perhaps the most efficient method of information transfer a learner would use involves organizational strategies to recode information or to transform it so that it can be incorporated within a previously established stable internal code.

The provision of an organizational structure to information in the STS results in a greater learning of that material, because the information is now more meaningful. The transfer of the learned items from the STS to the LTS proceeds rather easily at this point, as the present material has been related to and grouped with stored knowledge. The reconstruction of newer, more meaningful chunks of information leads to the inference that memory function between mechanisms is an interactive process. Although the functions can be described independently, it is the interaction of the functions tht leads to effective behavior. Thus, while the major function of the LTS is as a storage unit, the interactive nature of memory is exemplified by the extraction of information from and the transference of information to the LTS. This process is necessary for the STS to conduct all of its active processing operations.

In addition to serving as the mechanism in which a majority of the processing of information occurs, the STS also functions as the mechanism in which decisions are made about movement selection and execution. The decision process requires the retrieval of information from the LTS, a comparison of this information with the learner's present knowledge of the surrounding environment, a knowledge of the goal to be achieved, and finally, the selection of an appropriate motor program that can be used to control the upcoming movement. It is this decision-making process for motor program selection and movement generation that uniquely distinguishes the model of the human behaving system from other models of memory and behavior.

The Multistore versus Depth-of-Processing Approaches Contrasted

One of the major issues that has developed in psychology research on memory is how memory is to be viewed within an information-processing context: according to depth of processing or to stages of processing. In contrast to the present multistore, or stage, theory of information processing, F. I. M. Craik and R. S. Lockhart (1972) have proposed a unitary, levels-of-processing model of memory functions. The emphasis in this approach is that the durability of the memory trace is a function of the depth of processing, or the amount of meaning applied to the information. More simply stated, the degree to which a stimulus is semantically analyzed is the major determinant of the quality of memory performance. As Craik and Lockhart have suggested, the more elaborate the encoding process, the greater the probability of retention.

Recently, Craik (1977) and Craik and E. Tulving (1975) revised the original model with the suggestion that it is the degree of stimulus elaboration rather than the depth of processing that is the critical determinant for the establishment of a durable trace. In this view, retention is a function of spread of processing within a particular level or depth, and memory can be considered on a continuum ranging from simple sensory analysis to semantic-associative operations. Additionally, instead of distinguishing between short-term and long-term memory, Craik and Lockhart (1972) proposed type-I and type-II processing. Type-I processing is merely maintenance rehearsal in STS, so that information can be retained beyond the normal decay period. Type-II processing involves a deeper analysis of an item, which should result in more efficient storage (in our LTS) and thus lead to improved memory performance.

To summarize the levels-of-processing approach, it can be seen that the learner progresses through a series of hierarchical processing stages, such as an analysis of physical features, a match of input to stored abstractions, and an extraction of meaning. From the ensuing discussion of the activities of the system's human behaving mechanism, it can be easily seen that feature analysis is equivalent to our detection and recognition processes; matching inputs with stored knowledge is similar to our internal representational match within LTS; and the application of meaning is the function of our perceptual mechanism.

It would appear that the levels-of-processing approach is an extension of stage theory based on a semantic argument, rather than an opposite viewpoint. This contention was supported recently by M. Glanzer and L. Koppenaal (1977), who employed variations of encoding structures (a standard procedure in levels of processing investigations) in an examination of the serial position curve (standard procedure in stage-theory investigation) to separate output performance assigned to LTS and STS respectively. Utilization of the combined approaches enabled the authors to investigate whether the two theories were in conflict. They determined the effects of encoding instructions on performances previously associated with the LTS and the STS.

Results of the investigation were not supportive of two contrasting approaches. Glanzer and Koppenaal (1977) concluded that a single approach existed, and the difference was only in the semantics of the labeling process (stage versus level). In a final note, the authors suggested that the levels-of-processing approach extended rather than replaced the stage model by placing more emphasis on the encoding and retrieval processes in memory. It appears that, aside from differences in the labeling of particular mechanisms, the levels-of-processing approach and the stage approach are similar. In both, emphasis is placed on the central role of cognitive processes and strategies employed by the learner for effective control during skill acquisition and information retrieval.

Motor Program Selection

A motor program is a predetermined set of neural commands that controls muscular activity (Klapp, 1976). The uniqueness of the motor program lies in the fact that the response is structured before the movement sequence begins (Keele,

1968). The execution of the movement is often dependent on the present environmental conditions. Thus, it is not always the availability of certain programs that prescribe the movement to be executed; rather, it is the situational context within which the movement must be performed that influences program selection by the STS, based on information extracted from the LTS. There is justification, then, for the STS to receive ordered and meaningful inputs from the perceptual mechanism that convey information about the relationship of the organism to the current state of the environment, as well as to search and to retrieve from the LTS any previous knowledge that pertains to a particular situation. Once these sources of information have been integrated, the STS selects the appropriate motor program to achieve the desired goal.

At this stage of processing, the person has searched the LTS for the potentially appropriate motor programs and has used the STS to select the one that best matches the environmental conditions and the demands of the skill to be performed. Although there is intuitive appeal to assume that a *perfect* match between previous experience (learned motor programs) and present conditions (perceived information) can be obtained, this does not often occur. Recent biomechanical and electromyographical analyses of movement sequences have led to the conclusion that individuals do not execute movements in identical fashion each time the movement occurs (e.g., Higgins & Spaeth, 1972). Similarly, F. C. Bartlett (1932) stated that a movement is never performed twice in the same way. Therefore, to produce an effective movement, the problem that the learner must overcome is how to modify a stored motor program so that previous response specifications can be adapted to meet the demands of the present task.

The specifications or the parameters of the motor program that a person will use must account for variables such as speed of movement, terminal location of the movement, distance to be moved, force and timing of the movement, and the effort required to execute the movement properly. Klapp (1977) has provided some recent evidence in which the suggestion is made that these response-programming variables occur independently of the muscles that are chosen to effect the response. It is not the purpose here to determine whether response programming and muscle selection occur separately; however, it should be noted that if these two stages are independent, the latency of the decision process for movement probably increases.

Decisions must be made about the activation of appropriate movements to meet environmental demands and the demonstration of effective patterns of movement. Two kinds of error have been identified in this regard: errors in response selection and errors in response execution. In the first case, the person improperly perceives the task demands or his or her own bodily orientation to the task. The wrong movement, although properly executed, is initiated and completed. In the second case, the best of intentions may be useless if some occurrence within the system causes the execution to falter or if instantaneous adaptations are not made to accommodate situational variations. Improper execution may be the result of a misinterpretation of a state of fatigue or an inability to actually perform the act, caused by any one of a myriad of reasons.

The cognitive processes a person uses to reach a movement decision are also shown in Figure 6-7. The operations of search and retrieval of information from the LTS and the modification of a stored motor program in the STS are essential to produce a goal-directed movement. Once the motor plan has been decided on, the STS transmits the results of the decision to the LTS, where the information can be stored for future use. Simultaneously, the STS transmits the motor program to the movement generator, where it is loaded in preparation for the movement to occur.

The Movement Generator

Although it can be expected that at least one motor program will be selected by the STS and entered into the movement generator to control a discrete movement, it is incorrect to assume that a single program would be capable of regulating a long sequence of responses. The exact duration of a program is unknown, but there is evidence to support the contention that several motor programs can be called up to control a sequence of movements (Shapiro, 1976). This conclusion served as the basis for Klapp's (1976) contention that several motor programs can be loaded at one time into an output mechanism (movement generator) to effect a series of movements. Upon completion of the loading process, the individual must organize and initiate the programs in the appropriate order to achieve the movement goal.

The loading and the organization of the sequence of motor programs in the movement generator symbolizes the completion of the response-programming stage of movement. The motor plans are merely abstract representations of the intended goal of the movement (Klapp, 1977). Therefore, it is necessary for the movement generator to select the appropriate musculature to perform the activity. When the muscle group or groups that can best achieve the goal have been determined, the generator mechanism initiates the motor program or programs through the transmission of a sequence of efferent neural commands to the chosen muscles to cue them to perform the response (Keele & Summers, 1976). Simultaneously, the movement generator emits a feed-forward signal, corollary discharge, to the STS to prepare the system for the sensory consequences of the forthcoming motor act. These processes are illustrated in Figure 6-8.

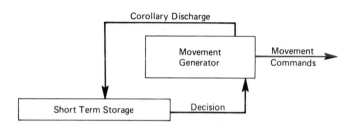

Movement Generator

FIGURE 6-8. Movement generator as it operates to produce a motor response.

Corollary discharge is essentially a "carbon copy" of the efferent commands sent to the effector mechanism. In addition, the corollary discharge serves much the same function for the STS as the pertinence value serves for the perceptual mechanism. Both processes facilitate the transmission of information through the human behaving system, based on the anticipation of the arrival of particular inputs. Furthermore, although pertinence value is only a hypothetical psychological construct, the existence of a corollary discharge, although not firmly established, has recently received strong support from investigations of preselected and constrained movements. Results of these studies have been almost unequivocal. When blindfolded individuals initiated volitional movements (preselected), which had to be replicated, considerable enhancement of reproduction performance occurred relative to conditions where individuals moved to an externally determined end point (constrained) (cf. Kelso, 1977; Kelso & Stelmach, 1976; Marteniuk, 1973). The performance differences were attributed to the corollary discharge associated with the production of an active, voluntary movement, thus providing some support for the existence of this neuropsychological process.

For corollary discharge to be beneficial to a learner, the muscle-selection process based on the loaded motor programs must be carried out. If muscle selection and response programming (STS) are independent processes, there is a need for a mechanism in the human behaving system to carry out the muscle-selection process. It is proposed that a movement generator exists to execute this function. Therefore, the movement generator not only loads, stores, and organizes selected motor programs, but it also determines which efferent impulses are discharged to a particular muscle or muscle group.

Plans or programs may be under volitional or nonvolitional control, by or without intent. The human organism is capable of demonstrating an assorted array of motor patterns, from the most elemental motor acts to the most complicated stunts. As an example of the nervous system's efficiency, sensory information is usually rearranged in lower levels of the system. There is an interconnection and rearrangement in the interneurons of the spinal cord and brain stem before the data arrive at the cerebral cortex. Not all responses or movements need be mediated by past experiences and thought processes. Not all stimuli need be recorded in the cortex.

Some simple receptor–effector loops located outside and inside the brain free the cerebrum for other work. These circuits are associated with certain body activity, which transpires as if automatic. Consider, for example, the reflex, the most simple of motor movements. Reflexes do not usually require the attention of the higher levels of the nervous system and represent the most elementary movement plan.

Simple Movements

Reflex arcs constitute the pathways involved in a simple reaction to a stimulus, usually not requiring the functioning of the higher centers of the nervous system. In the beginning of the twentieth century, the outstanding physiologist Sherrington (1858–1952) experimented on reflex transmission and the reflex at the spinal level; his efforts are still having a tremendous impact on our thinking about the nervous system. Reflex arcs may contain two, three, or more neurons in any case, these reflex arcs result in somewhat consistent responses, usually unconscious, to the same stimuli. Because a reflex is an unconscious response, it can be conditioned to be highly predictable.

The reflex arc, in its simplest form (two-neuron), contains five parts:

1. *Receptor:* specialized sensory nerve ending.
2. *Afferent neuron:* sensory transmitter of impulse from the receptor to the gray matter in the spinal cord.
3. *Synapse:* a gap in the anterior horn of the cord, where an afferent and efferent neuron are in functional proximity.
4. *Efferent neuron:* motor neuron, passing the impulse from the cord to an effector.
5. *Effector:* organ responsible for response.

Examples of a two-neuron reflex arc are the *postural reflex* and *knee-jerk reflex* (see Figure 6-9), both of which are classified as stretch reflexes. In the stretch reflex, or postural reflex, inhibiting impulses are sent to antagonist muscles, while appropriate muscles contract in order to maintain body stability. When an extensor muscle contracts and the flexor relaxes, or vice versa, we have a con-

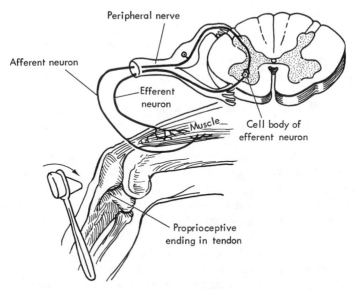

FIGURE 6-9. Simple reflex arc (knee jerk). The four fundamental parts of a reflex arc are shown: (1) a receptor—proprioceptive ending in muscle (2) a sensory transmitter—the afferent neuron; (3) a motor transmitter—the efferent neuron; and (4) the effector—the muscle. (*From Grollman, S.* The Human Body. *New York: Macmillan, 1964.*) Copyright 1964 The Macmillan Publishing Co. Inc.

dition known as reciprocal innervation. The process of the actual stretch reflex can be described in the following way: Stretch reflex: spindles stretched → afferent impulses to spinal cord → innervation of alpha neurons → reflex contraction of the appropriate muscle fibers.

The knee-jerk reflex involves the stimulus of tapping the patellar tendon and response of leg extension. During stimulus application, the quadriceps muscle is stretched, causing the stimulation of receptors in the muscle and resulting in a reflex shortening of this muscle. Basic reflexes such as the knee-jerk reflex can be used for diagnostic purposes: if there is some disturbance in the reflex pathway, the reflex will not be produced normally. Some reflex acts can be facilitated intentionally. A clenching of the fists before the patellar tendon is struck would result in a greater response—hence, the reason for an examining doctor to insist on complete relaxation of his patient before the test.

Certain reflexes are inborn: those needed for chewing and swallowing, simple defense reactions, defecation, micturition, and the like. Previous learning experience is not necessary for these responses; hence, they are unconditioned. Others are *conditioned* or *acquired* (learned) reflexes. An example of the latter is best represented by the research of Pavlov, who contributed extensively by developing methods by which new responses mediated by the cerebral cortex could be studied. Salivation accompanies food as well as its anticipation in a hungry animal. Pavlov rang a bell on each occasion that he fed the dog involved in his experiment. After a number of trials in which the bell and food were presented together, the food was eliminated; however, each time the bell rang, the animal salivated: a conditioned reflex.

Other reflexes are concerned with body protection via withdrawal and are termed flexor reflexes. The quick withdrawal of the foot from contact with a sharp object is an example of a flexor reflex.

The complex reflex arc is exemplified by the withdrawal reflex. Figure 6-10 illustrates foot withdrawal from a painful stimulus. Although only a few localized receptors are involved, it is interesting to note the *spread of effect* (a generalized reflex response involving many effectors). Notice how many parts of the body actively respond to a stimulus that activates but a few skin receptors. This startle reflex appears to be a "stored program" reflex, as an organized set of reactions occurs without consciousness.

Incorrect withdrawal reflexes have been obtained in a series of experiments by R. W. Sperry (1959). After crossing the sensory nerves of rats and frogs, extensive training still had no effect in re-educating their motor systems. During the rearrangement of nerve connections, rats would withdraw the right foot in response to an electric shock to the left foot. These results seem to indicate that although higher nervous system centers are capable of extensive learning, the anatomical arrangement of the lower ones are not plastic. They cannot be modified much by use or training. Spinal reflexes do recover to some extent following disease in or injury to the spinal cord. Damage to the spinal cord, however, will cause a total loss of sensory input and voluntary physical movement.

Simple reflexes are wired-in nerve circuits; the action is not premeditated,

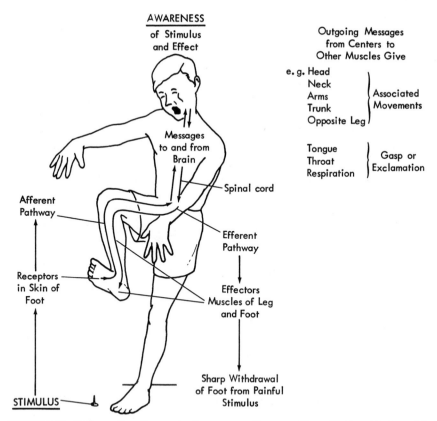

AWARENESS
of Stimulus
and Effect

Outgoing Messages
from Centers to
Other Muscles Give

e. g. Head
Neck
Arms   Associated
Trunk   Movements
Opposite Leg

Tongue
Throat   Gasp or
Respiration   Exclamation

Messages
to and from
Brain

Spinal cord

Afferent
Pathway

Efferent
Pathway

Receptors
in Skin of
Foot

Effectors
Muscles of Leg
and Foot

Sharp Withdrawal
of Foot from Painful
STIMULUS   Stimulus

FIGURE 6-10. Reflex action demonstrating many reflex arcs. (*From McNaught, A. and Callander, R. Illustrated Physiology. Baltimore: Williams and Wilkins Co., 1963.*) Reprinted by permission.

nor has it been learned. Other reflexes are learned and are associated with more complex behavior than heretofore discussed. Certain movements in sports situations, although termed reflexive, go far beyond the simple processes discussed thus far. Take, for instance, the almost automatic responses needed for success in sports. After slight deliberation, responses must be made quickly to given stimuli: (1) the batter interprets the pitch, its accuracy, and its type in less than a second; (2) the wrestler under control attempts to escape when the referee blows his whistle, before his opponent can react to impede his sudden movement; (3) the hockey center must decide whether to pass the puck to a forward or shoot it at the goalie himself, all in a fraction of a second; and (4) the football quarterback decides, in the face of onrushing linemen and while he is on the move, if it is wiser to hand-off, run, fall down, or pass and, if so, to whom.

These responses and many more are required in dynamic sports situations. The total situation is ever-changing and unpredictable, but the performer must react almost instantaneously. Except under conditions of high certainty, there is always some temporal lag in performance. In other cases, the environment is relatively stable. The athlete is prepared for his task, and he attempts to perform a series of acts in a skillful fashion. The diver, the gymnast, and the trampolinist condition themselves to display routines that appear automatic. If we define a reflex as an automatic performance of a complex sequence of spatially and temporarily related motor patterns (Wooldridge, 1963), then sports contain examples where reflexes are demonstrated. Then again, other writers find fault in explaining any form of human behavior, let alone reflex action, in reflex arc terms. Perhaps even reflex action is far more complex than we think. Behavior may be controlled in terms of the order in which a sequence of operations is to be performed. All action may be guided by a ''plan,'' like a computer program.

If we define reflex in traditional terms, as we did a few pages ago, it is doubtful that the athlete's performance is usually based on reflexive behavior. An athlete's reaction time or movement time should not be confused with reflex time, as these events might pertain to a particular task. As a point of interest, there are no data demonstrating that an athlete's reflex time is any faster than a nonathlete's.

Athletic situations are filled with examples of seemingly predetermined performances to predetermined stimuli. Perhaps there are stored programs (organized memory traces) in the brain. When sensory data are filtered into the nervous system, the appropriate program would be activated. Evidently, these programs become effective with repetition (practice). Most daily and athletic activity does not involve simple movements and responses, for frequently we have to select an appropriate response for a given stimulus. Because these actions go beyond the complex reflex stage, or what appears to be somewhat automatic responses, the highest levels of the nervous system become involved.

Complex Movements

The development of the cerebral cortex is correlated with a person's intellectual superiority over other animals. This structure of the highest order is necessary for refinement of movements, for precision, and for effectiveness. The cortex itself is not necessary in all motor activity, for gross body movements are but slightly interfered with by the loss of cortical function. However, we are referring here to the most gross movements, such as walking, crawling, and moving a hand in prescribed directions, and obviously the learning and often the performance of athletic skills demand cortical involvement. We now address ourselves to the notion of complex movement plans.

The cerebrum contains motor, sensory, and association areas, which interact during most coordinated complex movement. Between various species, structural differences in the brain are related to differences in physical characteristics. For example, a bird has large-sized optic lobes but small olfactory lobes; vision, not smell, is important to the bird. There is a relationship between the number of cells in the motor area allocated to a particular portion of the body, the number of motor units in an effector, and the complexity of movements related to that area.

Hence, relatively few cells control foot and leg movements; a much greater motor area is related to finger and lip motions.

The upper part of the motor region stimulates the lower extremities; the middle sends impulses to the trunk; and the lower part is concerned with facial and head movements. Although the motor cortex exerts influence on the various parts of the body, integrated functioning will occur only if surrounding cerebral areas are in place. The nervous system is extremely complex and integrated, requiring coordination between the neural structures involved in a particular act.

The cerebral cortex plays an important role in voluntary movement, in contrast to reflex movement, which is usually regulated at lower levels of the nervous system. The function of the motor cortex in willed movements and the effects on the body if damage occurs have been confirmed.

One side of the motor area controls movement in the opposite side of the body. If, for example, there is damage to some cells in the left cerebral hemisphere's motor area, possible paralysis may be inflicted in the corresponding muscles on the right side of the body. The reason for this is that nerve pathways cross over at the medulla or spinal cord level on their way down to specific effectors. Although it is possible for some recovery to take place in the form of gross movements, finger skills very rarely, if ever, return.

The various sense areas of the cortex are just as important as the motor cortex in skilled movement. Sense impulses for vision are distinguished in the occipital lobe, whereas those for audition are distinguished in the temporal lobe. Muscle sensations are interpreted in the somesthetic or sensory area of the parietal lobe, located posterior to the motor area. Representation of the different parts of the body in the somesthetic area is similar to the representation of the motor area. The somesthetic region is concerned with such sensations as touch, pain, pressure, and body position. Although a habit abolished by the removal of certain areas in the cerebral cortex can be relearned, damage to the sensory areas of the brain cannot be compensated for by any amount of retraining.

Association areas, which comprise the bulk of the cortex, are thought to be responsible for memory, speech, reasoning, intelligence, and thought and are not as localized as the other areas described. These functions are not usually designated to specific areas of the brain, as evidenced by the fact that such a process as discrimination learning is thought to be controlled in the posterior association areas, which include the parietal, occipital, and temporal sectors. There is a great interdependence when most acts are performed between motor, sensory, and association areas of the cerebrum.

The cerebellum offers an automatic control function, for it is responsible for smooth and coordinated movement. It receives information from muscles and the semicircular canals on body position and rate of movement and produces a stabilizing effect on the body. The cerebellum and cerebrum work closely on all forms of coordinated motor acts.

After input, the impulse travels along a preestablished path to the appropriate part of the brain. Typical sensory pathways include a three-neuron relay:

neuron I going to the spinal cord, neuron II extending from that point to the thalamus, and neuron III communicating with the sensory area of the cortex. One of the most important of the sensory tracts is the *spinothalamic tract,* responsible for feeling pain and temperature changes.

Following sense activity, certain areas in the brain issue orders to the various parts of the body. Voluntary activity is initiated in the higher centers, although the site can only be conjectured. It has been found that stimulation of any part of the motor cortex does not result in skilled acts, leading Paillard (1960) to speculate on the presence of an intermediary system, capable of controlling the motor cortex but receiving its stimulation from some other area of the nervous system. Involuntary or reflex movements have their origin at lower levels of the central nervous system. A method of classifying motor pathways is based on the way their fibers enter the spinal cord. Two motor systems, pyramidal and extrapyramidal, are distinguished in this manner. These two systems are responsible for volitional movements.

Assuming that well-learned acts do not require conscious control—or at least much of it—perhaps something akin to these behaviors becoming almost like reflex acts is a plausible interpretation of the situation. Movement plans contain built-in mechanisms for the continuance of activities. For instance, the response from a just-performed act (part of the total activity) triggers the next act. Response feedback stimulates appropriate sense receptors to initiate subsequent movement. It has been suggested that "different anatomical structures or areas are involved in the acquisition of a motor skill and its final performance" (Isaacson, Douglas, Lubar, & Schmaltz, 1971, p. 180). These authors speculate further that, "A given area might be necessary for the trial-and-error process of mastering a given motor skill but no longer be involved once the skill has become automatic or reflexlike. If this were the case, it would account for the finding that very complex motor behaviors often remain intact after extensive damage to prime motor areas in the cortex" (p. 180).

A well-developed movement plan seems to be associated with highly skilled performance. In an act demanding instantaneous and extremely rapid and continuous movements, the plan must be well-constructed beforehand. Externally paced acts suggest the refinement of a number of plans, any one of which might be called into action with the appropriate cue. The ability to switch plans while action is occurring will be dependent on the time available and adaptability of the performer to change channels. Task familiarity, repeated experiences, and the capabilities of the person will influence the refinement of movement plans and their effectiveness.

The learning of complex motor skills reveals a similar syndrome for both children and adults. Obviously, these skills are performed best when the person need not think about or plan for the sequence of actions. Yet, in the early stages of learning, the most elementary form of practice shows gross and often unnecessary movements. Precision occurs later. Successive experiences bring the learner closer to the goal of appropriate movement. With all learners, the transition is apparent from crude and uneconomical behaviors, as well as from heavy reliance on external cues, to automatic, smooth behaviors. *Automatic* implies no need to attend deliberately to the various components of the whole movement or series of activities.

Effectors

Although R. G. Marteniuk (1976) has combined the processes of the movement generator and the effectors into a unitary mechanism, it is proposed here that effectors exist within the human behaving system distinct from the movement generator (see Figure 6-11). The effector mechanism consists of the muscles that control the limbs that produce the desired response. Once the muscle-selection process has been completed in the movement generator, the effector mechanism executes the movement in the proper sequence. The execution of the movement leads to response-produced feedback, as indicated in Figure 6-11.

An effective movement plan directs the activation and inhibition of various muscle fibers of the body. In a fast sequence of movements, it appears as though the activation and inhibition of responses are preplanned. In slower and continuous movements, control and adaptations can occur as a result of ongoing performance feedback. Skilled performance reflects the sensitive balance between activated and inhibited tissue. One of the most challenging tasks for a young child is to learn how to inhibit movements, to control them.

Coordinated movement encompasses the selection and stimulation of appropriate muscles (spatial control), their activation at the right time (temporal control), and gradual muscle inhibition (quantitative control).

With repetitious practice and mature enough neurophysiological structures, the organism begins to demonstrate structure movements, or complex movement plans. A sequence of body movements involved in a goal-oriented behavior is initiated with the onset of a particular cue. The nature of the task—discrete or continuous, self-paced or externally paced—will dictate the possibility of flexibility in the programming during the actual activity. Variability in performance decreases with practice, and the motor programs in the repertoire of programs yield the responses appropriate for the situations in which they are initiated. Practice helps

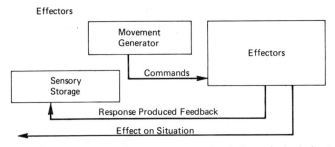

FIGURE 6-11. Effectors and the transmission of feedback through the behaving system.

to develop the programs essentially needed for the solution of problems. Learning how to solve motor problems, how to integrate impulses effectively that will innervate or not activate certain muscle tissues, is the key to successful performance. Movement in terms of direction, force, and velocity must be under conscious control or so well learned that subconscious volitional activity serves its intended purpose.

There are many cases in which movement plans must be restructured during the course of activity, presuming time is available for an alternative. Plans are often disrupted because of an unpredictable change of events or the excitation of inappropriate muscle tissues. Feedback, which serves as a comparator, is useful in many activities as the source of performance information that will stimulate a modification of plans. A program established in advance of an act and in anticipation of cue occurrence may work effectively. Then again, adaptive restructuring of the program in progress is often called for as well, and the ability to modify is one aspect of skilled performance. The hierarchical system of behavior possessed by a person indicates that many immediate changes in ongoing performance occur at subconscious levels of control.

Reflex activity can be seen as involving a feedback loop that operates within the skeletal muscle system. Alpha motor neurons, which function between the ventral horn of the spinal cord and muscles, affect the quality of movements in the body. Sensory receptors in the skeletal muscles make smooth and coordinated movements possible. Extrafusal fibers form one type of muscle bundle and contract when stimulated by the alpha motor neurons. Intrafusal fibers are a second type and are activated by gamma motor neurons, which, like the alpha neurons, have their origin in the ventral horn of the spinal cord. The gamma motor neurons also affect the contraction of extrafusal fibers because of the physiological and functional arrangement of the system.

The state of contraction and relaxation is monitored by the feedback loop. Central facilitation and inhibition is possible through this means. Muscle groups involved in the same body movements must cooperate. Synergist muscle groups work together and antagonist muscle groups produce opposite body movements. Two sets of muscle groups are involved in a motor response: one set contracts while the other set relaxes. When the spindle organs in a muscle are stimulated, increased activation occurs. When stimulated, the Golgi tendon organs have an inhibitory influence on extensor muscle contraction. The gamma motor neurons (efferents) are responsible for the control of sensitivity of muscle spindles and in turn control muscle contractions. The highly skilled performer will probably demonstrate a greater ability to utilize the gamma system to advantage, for many postural and movement adjustments require adequate functioning of the gamma neurons.

Alpha motor neurons mediate all reflex and voluntary movements in the body. Complete destruction of the pathway to a particular limb is reflected by a complete loss of movement in that limb. If the alpha motor system is intact but the afferent system is destroyed in a given area, no more reflex movements will occur there, but movement can still occur voluntarily.

With the upward progression of skill, changes occur in intramuscular and intermuscular mechanisms. The study of types of muscle fibers indicates that they respond differentially according to the nature of the task and the performer's level of skill. Electromyographical analysis permits a greater understanding of the pattern changes in motor units, and, in turn, the intramuscular changes, with the development of skill. Although it is true that the agonist (prime mover) musculature is important in coordinated movements, the antagonistic musculature plays a major role in motor control. Antagonistic musculature involvement needs to be conscientiously attended to in the early stages of learning. Gross motor activities involving speed, strength, and accuracy are refined and appear skilled when adequate control is present. Negative acceleration of a limb at the appropriate moment will make the difference in refined performance.

Highly skilled patterns of movement appear effortless and under subconscious control. Antagonist muscle spindles most likely contribute heavily to this feeling and the ability to perform proficiently. At the present time, it appears that the cerebellum coordinates alpha and gamma neurons and, in turn, excitatory and inhibitory processes in selected muscle groups. Motor behavior is under the control of alpha and gamma neurons, which are linked to numerous descending pathways. The coactivation of these neurons and their involvement in movement is not clearly known as yet, although scholars have attempted to shed light on limb control when actions are slow and continuous, in contrast to extremely rapid movements. It appears that linkage of the alpha and gamma neurons at the supraspinal center is fundamental for coordinated moderately rapid movements, and that the gamma loop contributes to precision in the temporal patterning of alpha neurons.

Motor units can be trained to respond in certain ways and therefore be under the control of a person with the proper training techniques. Efforts by J. V. Basmajian and others have led to breakthroughs in this area in recent years. Fine control over single motor units has been demonstrated. Even tonic motor unit activity normally not under voluntary control (the external sphincter is in a state of continuous contraction and is considered a tonic muscle) can be suppressed following motor unit training (Gray, 1971). In order for specific motor units to be activated, it appears that descending pathways are controlled in the spinal cord by proprioceptive input. With conscious efforts and appropriate feedback in the form of sensory information, motor units are activated. After training, volitional control is lessened.

The selective initiation of specified motor units and muscle fibers at a subcortical control level may help to explain complex movement patterns demonstrated by the highly skilled. Inhibition control, the timed role of antagonistic musculature in selected movements, influences the quality of performance. Excellent resource material on the topic of movement control from a neurophysiological frame of reference can be found in books by J. Maser (1973) and R. Granit (1970).

The Role of Feedback

Feedback is any response-produced information a person may receive through the various sense receptors as a result of his or her own efforts. When it is provided through an external source, such as an instructor, it is referred to as augmented or supplementary feedback. As an example of feedback, a person who shoots a ball at a basket receives kinesthetic feedback associated with the execution of the response, as well as visual feedback about the outcome of the response. Thus, feedback is informational in regard to the "feel" of the movement, as well as to situational changes that occur because of the movement. Either source of outcome information is usually available without being supplied by an external source. Should outcome information be provided for the learner, it would be transmitted through the human system in the same way as any other environmental information. These processes are illustrated in Figure 6-11, where it is shown that response-produced feedback enters directly into the sensory stores, and feedback resulting from the effect of behavior on the environment is considered as situation-outcome feedback. This information, although not externally supplied, also enters the sensory stores from the environmental display.

Regardless of how feedback enters the system, either intrinsically or extrinsically, the information flows through the system in much the same way as any other stimuli. The difference between the processing of feedback and the processing of any other inputs that may enter the system at this time is that the corollary discharge has alerted the cortical centers of the brain to anticipate the arrival of the response-produced information. The anticipatory state prompts the learner to activate a search of the LTS for a specific portion of the knowledge base (i.e., the movement goal) that should match the feedback. Thus, when the feedback contacts memory, the pertinence value of the response-produced information will be high, and that leads to the rapid transmission of that information from LTS through the perceptual mechanism to the STS.

One point must be clarified. Feedback information must contact the LTS and be recognized in the perceptual mechanism to be rendered meaningful, before it is transmitted to the STS. A simple detection process is necessary, but not sufficient, for the feedback to be utilized by the system, because detection does not involve a comparison with stored referents. Feedback can only be used to determine the existence of an error when there is a standard to which the feedback can be compared. Additionally, feedback can only become meaningful after it has been detected and recognized, at which time the processes of error detection, error correction, and learning begin to occur.

The processes of error detection and error correction are associated with the STS. The learner interprets the feedback information and extrapolates what modifications, if any, are necessary in the motor program so that future performances can achieve the goal. The change in the response specifications of the program is transferred to the LTS, along with information about the current state of the environment. The stored knowledge will then serve as a referent for future performances.

Concurrently, with the transfer of information related to the movement decision from the STS to the LTS, the learner adapts upcoming responses based on the correction of errors. The modified motor program is then determined, and the movement plan is transmitted to the movement generator in the same manner as the initial program information was loaded. When the response is run off, feedback is again sent through the system to continuously update the referent of the correct movement. The process continues until there is little or no discrepancy between actual and intended performance, at which time the information in the STS is placed into the LTS for permanent storage. It is at this time that learning has occurred.

Learning occurs through the use of two types of feedback. The performance of a slow, graded response enables a learner to detect and to correct errors that may occur during the response through the use of continuous feedback. The learner utilizes this form of response-produced information to modify activities while they are being performed. The response occurs slowly enough to allow the available feedback to be attended to and processed before the motor act has been completed.

In contrast, certain motor skills are performed too rapidly for feedback to be attended to and processed during the activity. Although feedback is available throughout the performance of these ballistic movements (those movements that occur in approximately 200 msec or less), the learner is unable to use response-produced information until the termination of the movement because of processing delays associated with information transmission (see Keele, 1968, 1973; and Schmidt, 1975, 1976, for reviews). The learner then uses terminal feedback information for error detection and error correction in a manner similar to the one in which continuous feedback information functions.

Both types of response-produced information contribute to better performances. The difference between the two is the availability of each type during the acquisition of a motor skill. Learners must be taught an awareness of which feedback information is most appropriate for a particular motor skill, so that attention can be properly directed for the feedback to be correctly interpreted and made functional. However, feedback is not only available for error detection and error correction; it also influences other conscious cognitive activities.

The integration of feedback information with other information about the response (e.g., corollary discharge and program selection criteria), both of which are in the STS, serves as the basis for the learner's establishment of performance expectancies and causal attributions. These cognitive motivational factors have a greater influence on motor learning and performance than previously acknowledged. Although feedback is often quantitative information about errors in performance, feedback may also be qualitative and provide information relative to the success or failure of a movement. The learner's perception of and interpretation of this qualitative information will lead to inferences about present and future performances.

Based on the learner's attributions for a performance, shifts in expectancy formation will occur. The typical shift is that expectancies for success will increase following a successful performance, whereas these same expectations will decrease following failure. This conclusion was reached by several researchers (see Weiner, 1974, for a review) and shifts in expectancies of success have been related to stable attributions (Weiner, Nierenberg, & Goldstein, 1976).

The relationship between stable attributes and future expectancies of success is the preferred pattern of causal inference. Similarly, if success were expected, but failure occurred, future expectations would remain high if the performance were attributed to unstable and external factors. However, if the performance were attributed to stable and internal factors, expectancies of success would decrease. If failure continued, and attributions remained stable, success would be perceived as impossible (Dweck, 1975). Therefore, the implication for any training program is to have the learner activate cognitive processes to interpret feedback so that failures are attributed to unstable and external factors and success is attributed to stable and internal causes (Weiner & Sierad, 1975). In this way, the future expectancies of success will be higher and performance will be enhanced (Brickman, Linsenmeier, & McCareins, 1976) through the conscious use of feedback.

Feedback information also can be obtained through means other than the use of conscious cognitive processes. Outcome information can be received by a learner through a nonconscious means of control depending on the depth, or level, at which one investigates the mechanisms and control processes involved. A learner may apply cognitive processes to direct the transmission of feedback within the system during skill acquisition. At a different level of analysis, the learner's use of feedback may involve the implementation of the gamma-efferent, or spindle-receptor, system to control the execution of the motor program (Keele & Summers, 1976; Klapp, 1976), and this control may become refined with the development of skill. The refinement of the lower, nonconscious level of feedback control may serve as a partial explanation of the performance differences between beginners and highly skilled performers, as well as account for the apparent automaticity in the execution of skilled movement.[2]

Through previous experience and practice, the execution of skilled movement becomes automated. The degree of automation is related to the level of conscious control required by the organism. Thus, the more "automatic" a movement becomes, the less need there is for conscious involvement by the learner. As a result, less conscious control leads to the faster processing of other incoming information. Thus, feedback can affect motor performance at both a conscious, cortical level and at a subconscious, spinal level, both of which contribute to motor learning and motor control.

The influence of feedback on subsequent performance is an integral part of motor behavior. Motor programs are modified and updated based on the information provided by the feedback display. Feedback is a major determinant in the learning process. A learner who can make use of outcome information continu-

---

[2] It should also be pointed out that deafferentation techniques do not permit the learner to use sensory feedback during the performance of a skill (see Kelso & Stelmach, 1976, and Taub, 1976, for reviews), but reasonable movement can occur, based on previous information feedback stored in the long-term memory. These movements are crude and can approximate the skill to be performed.

ously increases the sophistication of the stored referents for movements, which leads to the establishment of higher pertinence values in the LTS. These processes then aid the functions of other mechanisms in the system. With increased learning and higher pertinence values comes an increase in anticipation skills and a decrease in processing time. Additionally, because the system is prepared for the receipt of certain information, the arrival of that information leads to the learner increasing performance expectancies of success. The expectancies are related to attributions about the performance, which, in turn, influence subsequent expectancies. Therefore, the feedback information constantly fulfills its roles of facilitating error detection and correction (motor program modification), learning, goal-image formation, expectancy formation, and patterns of causal inference.

In summary, then, the learner is able to use feedback information to (1) stimulate the peripheral organs to regulate ongoing behavior; (2) adapt behavior to situational demands; (3) activate or to lower emotions; and (4) evaluate the performance through the formation of attributions. Therefore, the enormous contribution of feedback to motor learning must be considered if an instructional program is to be successful.

OVERVIEW OF THE MODEL

Mechanisms and processes with unique considerations for motor behavior have been identified systematically in a model of the human behaving system. The complex sequential and parallel cognitive operations a learner uses to acquire, to select, and to execute a motor response have been described at both pragmatic and theoretical levels. Skilled performance occurs as a result of the serial or simultaneous flow of information through the mechanisms of the system, whereas an inefficient performance can be attributed to a functional deficiency somewhere in the system. Therefore, it would be instructive to summarize briefly the processes of information transmission that lead to efficient learning and skilled performance.

Information must be transmitted through the system for effective learning to occur. Inputs are received and briefly retained in the sensory stores. If the response can occur without further processing, then the stimuli need only be detected by the perceptual mechanism before the inputs are forwarded deeper into the system. In contrast, if stimuli require more elaborate processing, the inputs are sent to the LTS to contact previously stored representations and to establish a pertinence value.[3] The pertinence value alerts the perceptual mechanism to anticipate the arrival of information in a sequential, priority order based on the degree of familiarity acquired during contact with the LTS.

Information in the perceptual mechanism is recognized by the learner, who then begins to apply meaning to the inputs. When the inputs are perceived, they

[3] It has been argued in other sources that all input needs to be processed in the STS before it can go to the LTS. But if this were the case, a person would not know immediately if the stimulus were familiar. It would pass through the STS to the LTS without undergoing processing, then be sent back to the STS for processing. This seems like an inefficient use of time and processing capacity.

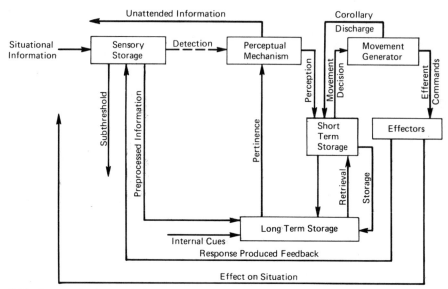

FIGURE 6-12. The human behaving system: Mechanisms and control processes associated with the transformation and transmission of information.

are transmitted to the STS, where all active processing occurs. Through the STS, the learner is able to rehearse information for temporary maintenance or future storage, to search and to retrieve additional information from the LTS, to make decisions about movements, and to select motor programs that will effectively achieve the desired goal. These cognitive processing operations serve to make the STS the primary mechanism in the human behaving system. However, it must be remembered that the STS is a limited capacity mechanism, and to require too much processing would overload the system.

Information that has been processed effectively leads to the selection of the appropriate motor programs, which are then loaded into the movement generator. The program commands are sent to the effector mechanism, where the musculature is activated to perform the movement sequence. As a result of the movement, the system begins to receive response-produced feedback, either through the proprieceptors, or through the other sense receptors as the performance effects a change on the environment. The feedback is used to update the stored knowledge base, to attribute causes for performance outcomes and to influence future performance expectancies, to influence the emotional state, and to modify the selection of subsequent motor programs so new goals can be achieved, or so the old goal can be reached again.

When the desired goal has been obtained, the learner stores the pertinent information in the LTS to increase the existing knowledge base. The information may then be used to aid the establishment of pertinence values, to provide referents for error detection and correction, and to serve as a standard from which current attributions and future expectancies can be established. The learning process has completed a full cycle of information transmission through the human behaving system, and the learner is ready to encounter new situations. Figure 6-12 contains the entire model.

How a person functions with regard to a program of action can be examined from a simplified perspective. In Table 6-1, an analogy is made between the operations of a record on a phonograph and those an individual undergoes in meeting task demands.

TABLE 6-1 The Phonograph and Human Behaving System Analogy

1. Sensory and perceptual mechanisms:	present phonograph (ready the system)
2. Long-term storage:	record storage (programs in existence)
3. Short-term storage:	record selected (learner decides how it should be played based on situational parameters)
	How to put it on?
	How fast to play it?
	How long to play it?
	OR
	no available record for purposes (have to combine available aspects of available records, make a "new record")
4. Movement generator:	record played (movement initiated)
5. Feedback	record good for purposes or, if inappropriate, record is changed

STRATEGIES, PROCESSES, AND MECHANISMS

Real and hypothesized *mechanisms* have been conceptualized that appear to be activated sequentially in stages or in parallel as information is processed leading to complex motoric behavior. *A mechanism has been defined as a real or hypothesized "location" or "structure" associated with the nervous system in which specified unique control processes and functions occur.*

Similarly, *cognitive processes* (also referred to as cognitions or control processes by others) have been identified as to type and location in the previous pages and are associated with the proposed mechanisms. A cognitive process is *a control process that is a self-generated, transient, situationally determined conscious activity that a learner uses to organize and to regulate received and transmitted information, and ultimately, behavior.* Alternative strategies are usually available to learners/performers to help facilitate the processing of information and benefit performance. The goal for the learner or instructor is to determine the most beneficial strategies, considering task demands and individual differences in capabilities and performances. *A strategy is a self-initiated or externally imposed way of directing information that leads to decisions for purposeful behavior.*

Whereas previous efforts in the analysis of motor skill learning have been geared to relatively simple tasks that place minimal demands on a learner's organizational and decision-making capabilities, the acquisition of complex skills requires a learner to utilize cognitive processes in a more extensive manner than has been realized. The identification and the subsequent effective manipulation of these control processes by learners will enable them to use personal information-processing capabilities to develop appropriate strategies for learning and performing a variety of psychomotor activities, in order to be able to problem solve and to adapt to new, but related, situations with minimal guidance.

An understanding of the processes that may be under the control of the learner can lead to a more thorough analysis of potential alternative strategies that the learner can activate to meet task demands. In turn, this information can provide a meaningful basis for instruction designed to assist learners in the development and selection of the best strategies applicable to the acquisition of different types of tasks.

Although organizational processes have been frequently investigated in studies of verbal memory by examining the input-output relationship of to-be-remembered material, the concept of organization has been virtually ignored by researchers in motor learning. However, interest in the organizational variables that may affect motor skill acquisition has increased. This is evidenced by the concern for central or peripheral mechanisms of motor control (Keele, 1968; Kelso & Stelmach, 1976; Schmidt, 1975), the processing characteristics of spatial information (Jones, 1972, 1974; Kelso, 1977) Laabs, 1973; Marteniuk, 1973; Stelmach, Kelso, & McCullagh, 1976; Stelmach, Kelso, & Wallace, 1975), and the general encoding properties of movement information (Nacson, Jaeger, & Gentile, 1973).

Without providing a detailed description of these studies, it will suffice to say that the general conclusion has been that *a learner imposes some type of structure on movement information* so that it is learned and retrieved more efficiently. Performance is either dependent on the experimental structuring of the task, in which the totality of the relations among the movement cues is emphasized (Gentile & Nacson, 1976), or on the subjective organization of the information, in which a structural context corresponding to the learner's cognitive capabilities is imposed on the movement cues. Thus, the development of the organizational strategies occurs in one of two ways.

The behavioral processes that a learner uses to select and to govern attentiveness in a learning situation, the management of information storage and retrieval skills, and the construction of a problem solution are directed by the implementation of associated strategies. These strategies may be external, instructor-imposed strategies, or internal self-generated strategies. These types of instructional strategies have been found to facilitate both verbal and motor learning.

An instructional strategy that is imposed by the instructor on the learner can be designed to help the learner acquire a skill as quickly as possible or to facilitate transfer effectiveness or problem solving in the future. Although some imposed strategies may increase the rate of initial skill acquisition, they may not facilitate learning in transfer situations in which no instructor is present. In the latter case, this can only be achieved when a learner becomes capable of self-generating learning strategies, whether initially they were externally directed or self-generated.

Within the restrictions of the model, the following relationships can be realized. As a learner enters a particular situation, potential alternative strategies may be activated to deal with available information. The learner has a choice in the possible methods for processing information at different stages of its transmission. The particular strategy that is chosen corresponds to and influences the activation of a cognitive process, which regulates the activities performed on the information at a particular point in time (see Figure 6-13).

1. A situation activates potential alternative *strategies*
2. A particular *strategy* influences a corresponding *cognitive process*
3. A particular *cognitive process* is associated with a corresponding *mechanism*
4. Situation → strategy → process → mechanism

FIGURE 6-13. Relationship among strategies, cognitive processes, and mechanisms.

An example of the proposed relationship involves the act of hitting a pitched baseball (see Figure 6-14). The task goal has been determined, and the learner needs a strategy that will facilitate the accomplishment of the task. Because concentration is a key factor in batting, the learner decides to focus attention on a narrow stream of inputs, mainly the location of the ball. The cognitive process that is activated is selective attention, and the dominant mechanism for this task is the perceptual mechanism.

In general, strategies are produced by an individual in conjunction with the information-processing system to facilitate (1) storage and retrieval of information, (2) a comparison of incoming information with referents previously stored, (3) transformation of information, and (4) decision making about the movement that will result in achieving the desired goal. The learner's appropriate use of strat-

FIGURE 6-14. Example relationship.

Hit a Baseball
↓
Narrow Focus (Concentration)
↓
Selective Attention
↓
Perceptual Mechanism

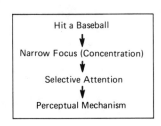

egies in these cases and many others is a significant determinant of motor learning and performance.

The manner in which a learner develops and utilizes cognitions and strategies becomes evident in the acquisition rate and performance level of motor skills. An incorrect cognition, such as selecting the wrong motor program, or an inefficient strategy, is sufficient to retard the learning process and lower the performance quality. Instructional procedures must be designed so that appropriate learning strategies can be identified, methods for enhancing the *self-production* of these strategies within a learner can be taught, and the content of these strategies can be made applicable to a wide range of motor behaviors.

DIFFERENTIAL INFLUENCES ON THE SYSTEM

If all human systems were exactly alike, then we could expect all to respond in exactly the same way in similar situations. Such is not the case, but we can attempt to posit similarities in behavioral manifestations for the "average" person under certain conditions (laws of learning and behavioral modification). Countless research publications and theoretical notions provide us with some security in making general statements about behavior. In fact, most of the content of this book includes statements about how the average system works and how it is affected by external systems, such as peculiar environmental conditions.

Nonetheless, a recognition of individual differences (such as with the use of strategies) suggests special considerations, for both general understanding and practical implications (see Figure 6-15). Not only do individuals behave dif-

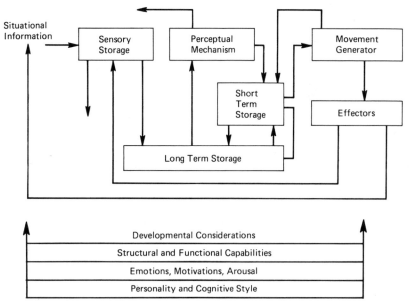

FIGURE 6-15. The effect of individual differences on the human behaving system.

MOTOR LEARNING AND HUMAN PERFORMANCE

ferently when present in the same circumstance, but it is conceivable that the same person might elicit varying behaviors in that same circumstance, as well. In order to attain a better understanding of how systems function, we must be familiar with commonalities as well as distinctions.

The design of many systems favors some to the disadvantage of others. Motor and intellectual abilities, physical characteristics, temperament, and personality traits vary from person to person, the product of hereditary and experiential factors. Extreme distinctions among human systems in any one or a combination of these characteristics may dissimilarly affect the learning of and performance in activities. Abilities are personal traits that underlie potential for success in specific skills. The ideal presence of abilities and capabilities suggests a system to be favored in skill acquisition and performance.

More elaborately structured systems have a greater probability of performing more complex tasks. Actually, with development and sophistication, each of the subsystems in the system can function at a higher level. Performance output is, among other things, a function of the complexity and performance capabilities of the system. The human system undergoes noticeable maturational changes, especially in the early and formative years. These changes affect the functioning possibilities of the sensoriperception process, memory and retrieval processes, cognitive processes, and motor mechanisms. At an older age, the system is also undergoing some change, usually influencing performance output in a negative manner.

Systems of instruction and training affect performance output as well as the learning processes associated with every subsystem in the model along the way. So is the case with immediate environmental conditions: noise, temperature, lighting, and other variables. On the broadest scale, human behavior is shaped by the sociocultural system. This system infiltrates the human behaving system by manifesting itself in the form of interests in and attitudes toward activities, motivation and reinforcement, and outlet possibilities.

Figure 6-16 depicts the learner or performer more formally, as a system within a system. This much larger system describes the relationship of the human to factors other than internal ones that influence behavioral output. As we can see,

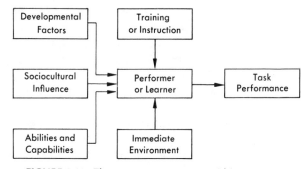

FIGURE 6-16. The person as a system within a system.

sociocultural variables influence the attitudes, interests, motivations, and general predispositions of those who want to participate in certain activities, as well as to excel in them. Differential factors, such as developmental characteristics, abilities, and capabilities, cause each human system to operate in different ways. Also, it is important to acknowledge that there are broad-based abilities and capabilities that will influence a person to succeed in a wide variety of tasks, as well as task-specific demands. The quality and extent of instruction and training a person has, with consideration of immediate environmental factors, will help to produce behavior in specified situations. Viewed in this way, a person is but one subsystem, along with others, with a role in influencing behavior. He or she influences, and is influenced by, the situation.

If we want to know how the *average* person will perform in a newly introduced task, a fairly good estimation can be obtained from an analysis of task characteristics (e.g., number of response alternatives, magnitude of response, timing, sequence, cue alternatives, cue predictability). But if we are after knowlege of an *individual's* performance with a newly introduced task, the task and the individual's unique characteristics must be known. Although practice techniques can be geared for the average or the individual, in general, learning will occur to some degree through practice as capabilities improve. Environmental characteristics (temperature, noise, illumination), as well as training techniques, can affect learning and performance.

The complex human behavioral system can be modified through instruction and training and must be if excellence in skilled performance is the goal. Specific practice regimens can influence one's ability to discriminate among and attend to relevant cues, to process information quickly and accurately, and to formulate, enact, and execute effectively appropriate movement plans. Thus, training systems can modify the human behaving system. There are many practice considerations that will be dealt with later. Among them are speed-accuracy trade-offs; massed and distributed practice trade-offs; simulated versus real practice decisions; the availability of reinforcement, incentives, and knowledge of results; whole versus part task practice; and the use of principles of the transfer of training. An ample discussion on practice systems is presented later in this book, in Chapter 12. An instructor, or a learner, can do much to modify the behavioral system with appropriate learning techniques.

The situation in which the human performs no doubt has some impact on behavior. The most influential environmental factors surrounding performance might be regarded as stressful. Audiences, noises, extreme temperatures, and the like require adjustments on the part of the human system, although we usually think of the skilled performer as one who can accommodate to changed and even noxious-appearing environments. The interplay of environment with performer is most obvious with the relatively unskilled. But regardless of skill level, all environmental factors constitute a system of considerations that should be recognized and understood in order to (1) analyze human behaviors more adequately, and (2) design environments to be more compatible with learner competencies and characteristics.

Often neglected or taken for granted is the sociocultural impact on those activities we tend to participate in and in which we want to excel. This influence is more obvious when we observe that, in different societies and countries, relatively more craftsmen of one kind than another can be counted. Recreational pursuits differ. Forms of athletic competition, in variety and intensity, also vary from culture to culture. It is not within the scope of this book to analyze the philosophical ramifications of the effect of culture on behavior. However, it would be remiss not to acknowledge the association, as B. F. Skinner has so powerfully done in his book *Beyond Freedom and Dignity* (1971).

NEUROLOGICAL PROBLEMS AND PERFORMANCE

So far, the assumption has been made of a nervous system intact, not in disarray. Obviously, some human systems have disorders that may influence performance, the practice of a skill, and subsequently, learning.

Many learning disorder syndromes and corresponding defects in the nervous system have been identified with the learning of cognitively oriented behaviors. Others are associated with the decomposition of movement—for example, dyssynergia. It is thought that this syndrome includes a loss of postural tone of the muscles and appearance of irregular movements, perhaps caused by the inability of the cerebellum to coordinate inhibiting and facilitating impulses. Tremor is another disease of the cerebellum and can be detected with purposive movements. Tremor and other unnatural movements are no doubt reflective of problems in the motor cortex as well as the cerebellum.

Damage to the extrapyramidal system could result in Parkinson's disease. Muscle tone is disturbed, and voluntary movement is characterized by rigidity. The rigidity paralysis in resisting movements may only be part of the syndrome, as tremor may be seen in the same muscle groups when the person is at rest.

Damage to the vestibular system impairs the maintenance of equilibrium. Vertigo gives one the feeling of rotation, a sense of movement of the person or the environment. Like many diseases, vertigo may involve disease of the cerebellum or the cerebrum. Or, for that matter, a problem with the visual sense receptors, a nystagmus, may be associated with vertigo. A loss or impairment of proprioception may be reflected by a disease of the posterior spinal column, called ataxia. There is difficulty in gauging direction, and there is a loss of proprioception from the joints.

Motor impairment may be assessed from parent or teacher observations or clinical (neurological examinations, an electroencephalograph) or motor performance tests especially designed to diagnose disorders. Correct diagnosis is no easy matter. Obviously, though, the more accurate the diagnosis, the easier it is to suggest remedial activities. Performance expectations are more realistic, and the learner will benefit most from activities most compatible with his or her condition.

Various tests of motor impairment are described by P. R. Morris and H. T. A. Whiting (1971), as are a variety of compensatory activities.

CHAPTER HIGHLIGHTS

1. A model of motor behavior has been proposed that emphasizes features from information-processing, cybernetic, and adaptive approaches to the study of human behavior.

2. Orientation has been toward the information-processing aspects of performance, with cognitive (control) processes emphasized as they might influence the successful execution of a motor act.

3. The human system is potentially energized upon the receipt of information (cues, stimuli) from internal (inside the person) or external (situational, environmental, task) factors by sense receptors. A certain amount of information will proceed through the system, to be processed and reacted to, while other information will be below the threshold value necessary for reaction.

4. Upon the activation of the sensory store, information proceeds directly to the perceptual mechanism for detection or to be transmitted to the long-term memory store to make contact with previously stored, similar representations, to provide initial meaning to the preprocessed information.

5. Once information enters the perceptual mechanism, it is provided with additional meaning. Patterns of recognition unfold, relevant features of selectivity attended to cues are determined, and this information is forwarded to the short-term memory store.

6. The arousal state of the person as information is organized in the system will determine the effectiveness of the processing.

7. Information stimulates a broad distribution in the brain that is organized into a representational system. Changes do not occur in only one place in the brain. The short-term store (STS) is the most significant mechanism in the system for operations performed on the information, and it is referred to as the working memory. It is there that information is rehearsed and organized and decisions are made about what to do with it. STS provides a temporary storage area for information, and decisions are made about immediate responses and/or the transfer of information into long-term storage for (LTS) for future reference. Because there is a limited capacity of the functioning capability of the STS, much depends on the use of appropriate strategies to cause maximal usage of this mechanism. Most information processing occurs in the STS. More and better processing transmits information in the LTS. Programs of action are selected, based on situational analysis and reference to pertinent information in the LTS.

8. A movement generator initiates a goal-directed movement. The STS transmits the motor program to the movement generator, where it is loaded in preparation for the movement to occur. Plans of action may be simple or complex, under nonvolitional or volitional control.

9. The effector mechanism executes the movement and produces response-produced feedback, to be used during the movement to help regulate and control it, or afterward, in future situations, depending on the speed and brevity of the movement. Feedback about performance outcomes also provides information that leads to future performance expectations. Attributions are formed and related to expectations.

10. The real and hypothesized mechanisms identified in the model of motor behavior suggest the cognitive processes that operate in serial or parallel fashion to control and direct learning/performance. Alternative strategies are available to learners to help promote the processing of information, and, in turn, the quality of the performance. A situation activates strategies to deal with information; they correspond to particular cognitive processes, and these processes are related to particular mechanisms.

11. Human systems operate differentially because of differences in abilities and capabilities, genetics, structure, emotional reactivity, developmental factors, previous instruction and experiences, motivations, environmental conditions, and sociocultural influences.

References

Atkinson, R. C., & Shiffrin, R. M. Human memory: A proposed system and its control processes. In K. W. Spence & J. T. Spence (Eds.), *The psychology of learning and motivation* (Vol. 2). New York: Academic Press, 1968.

Atkinson, R. C., & Wickens, T. D. Human memory and the concept of reinforcement. In M. Glanzer (Ed.), *The nature of reinforcement*. New York: Academic Press, 1971.

Bartlett, F. C. Remembering: *A study in experimental and social psychology*. Cambridge: Cambridge University Press, 1932.

Brickman, P., Linsenmeier, F. A. W., & McCareins, A. G. Performance enhancement by relevant success and irrelevant failure. *Journal of Personality and Social Psychology*, 1976, *33*, 149–160.

Broadbent, D. E. *Decision and stress*. New York: Academic Press, 1971.

Brown, A. Knowing when, where, and how to remember: A problem of metacognition. In R. Glaser (Ed.), *Advances in instructional psychology*. Hillsdale, N.J.: Erlbaum, 1978.

Chi, M. T. H. Short-term memory limitations in children: Capacity or processing deficits. *Memory and Cognition*, 1976, *4*, 559–572.

Cherry, C. Some experiments on the reception of speech with one and with two ears. *Journal of Acoustical Society of America*, 1953, *25*, 975–979.

Craik, F. I. M. Depth of processing in recall and recognition. In S. Dornic (Ed.), *Attention and performance* (VI). Hillsdale, N.J.: Erlbaum, 1977.

Craik, F. I. M., & Lockhart, R. S. Levels of processing: A framework for memory research. *Journal of Verbal Learning and Verbal Behavior*, 1972, *11*, 671–684.

Craik, F. I. M., & Tulving, E. Depth of processing and the retention of words in episodic memory. *Journal of Experimental Psychology: General*, 1975, *104*, 268–294.

Dansereau, D. The development of a learning strategies curriculum. In H. F. O'Neil, Jr. (Ed.), *Learning strategies I*. New York: Academic Press, 1978.

DeGreen, K. B. *Systems psychology*. New York: McGraw-Hill, 1970.

Deutsch, J. A., & Deutsch, D. Attention: Some theoretical considerations. *Psychological Review*, 1963, *70*, 80–90.

Dweck, C. The role of expectations and attributions in the alleviation of learned helplessness. *Journal of Personality and Social Psychology*, 1975, *31*, 674–685.

Erdelyi, M. H. A new look at the new look: Perceptual defense and vigilance. *Psychological Review*, 1974, *81*, 1–25.

Estes, W. K. *Learning theory and mental development*. New York: Academic Press, 1970.

Gentile, A. M., & Nacson, J. Organizational processes in motor control. In J. Keogh & R. S. Hutton (Eds.), *Exercise and sport sciences reviews* (Vol. 4). Santa Barbara, Ca.: Journal Publishing Affiliates, 1976.

Glanzer, M. Storage mechanisms in recall. In G. H. Bower (Ed.), *The psychology of learning and motivation: Advances in research and theory* (Vol. 5). New York: Academic Press, 1972.

Glanzer, M., & Koppenaal, L. The effect of encoding tasks on free recall: Stages and levels. *Journal of Verbal Learning and Verbal Behavior*, 1977, *16*, 21–28.

Granit, R. *The basis of motor control*. New York: Academic Press, 1970.

Gray, E. R. Conscious control of motor units in a tonic muscle. *American Journal of Physical Medicine*, 1971, *50*, 34–40.

Gutin, B. Exercise-induced activation and human performance: A review. *Research Quarterly*, 1973, *44*, 256–268.

Higgins, J. R., & Spaeth, R. K. Relationship between consistency of movement and environmental condition. *Quest*, 1972, *17*, 61–69.

Hochberg, J. E. Attention, organization, and consciousness. In D. I. Mostofsky (Ed.), *Attention: Contemporary theory and analysis*. New York: Appleton-Century-Crofts, 1970.

Isaacson, R. L., Douglas, R. J., Lubar, J. F., & Schmaltz, L. W. *A primer of physiological psychology*. New York: Harper & Row, 1971.

John, E. R. *Mechanisms of memory*. New York: Academic Press, 1967.

Jones, B. Outflow and inflow in movement duplication. *Perception and Psychophysics*, 1972, *12*, 95–96.

Jones, B. Role of central monitoring of efference in short-term memory for movements. *Journal of Experimental Psychology*, 1974, *102*, 37–43.

Kahneman, D. *Attention and effort*. Englewood Cliffs, N.J.: Prentice-Hall, 1973.

Keele, S. W. Movement control in skilled motor performance. *Psychological Bulletin*, 1968, *70*, 387–403.

Keele, S. W. *Attention and human performance*. Pacific Palisades, Calif.: Goodyear Publishing Co., 1973.

Keele, S. W., & Summers, J. J. The structure of motor programs. In G. E. Stelmach (Ed.), *Motor control: Issues and trends*. New York: Academic Press, 1976.

Kelso, J. A. S. Planning and efferent components in the coding of movement. *Journal of Motor Behavior*, 1977, *9*, 33–48.

Kelso, J. A. S., & Stelmach, G. E. Central and peripheral mechanisms in motor control. In G. E. Stelmach (Ed.), *Motor control: Issues and trends*. New York: Academic Press, 1976.

Klapp, S. T. Short-term memory as a response preparation state. *Memory and Cognition*, 1976, *4*, 721–729.

Klapp, S. T. Response programming, as assessed by reaction time, does not establish commands for particular muscles. *Journal of Motor Behavior*, 1977, *9*, 301–312.

Laabs, G. E. Retention characteristics of different reproduction cues in motor short-term memory. *Journal of Experimental Psychology*, 1973, *100*, 168–177.

LaBerge, D. Attention and the measurement of perceptual learning. *Memory and Cognition*, 1973, *1*, 268–276.

LaBerge, D. Acquisition of automatic processing in perceptual and associative learning. In

P. M. A. Rabbit & S. Dornic (Eds.), *Attention and performance V*. New York: Academic Press, 1975.

LaBerge, D. Perceptual learning and attention. In W. K. Estes (Ed.), *Handbook of learning and cognitive processes IV: Attention and memory*. Hillsdale, N.J.: Erlbaum, 1976.

Lindsay, P. H., & Norman, D. A. *Human information processing: An introduction to psychology*. New York: Academic Press, 1977.

Maggio, E. *Psychophysiology of learning and memory*. Springfield, Ill.: Charles C Thomas, 1971.

Marteniuk, R. G. Retention characteristics of motor short-term memory cues. *Journal of Motor Behavior*, 1973, *5*, 312–317.

Marteniuk, R. G. *Information processing in motor skills*. New York: Holt, Rinehart & Winston, 1976.

Maser, J. *Efferent organization and the integration of behavior*. New York: Academic Press, 1973.

Massaro, D. *Experimental psychology and information processing*. Chicago: Rand McNally, 1975.

Massaro, D., Cohen, M. M., & Idson, W. L. Recognition masking of auditory lateralization and pitch judgments. *Journal of Acoustical Society of America*, 1976, *59*, 434–441.

Miller, G. A., Galanter, E., & Pribram, K. H. *Plans and the structure of behavior*. New York: Holt, Rinehart & Winston, 1960.

Miller, G. A. The magical number seven plus or minus two: Some limits on our capacity for processing information. *Psychological Review*, 1956, *63*, 81–96.

Morris, P. R., & Whiting, H. T. A. *Motor impairment and compensatory education*. Philadelphia: Lea & Febiger, 1971.

Nacson, J., Jaeger, M., & Gentile, A. M. Organizational processes in short-term memory. In I. D. Williams & L. M. Wankel (Eds.), *Proceedings of the Fourth Canadian Psychomotor Learning and Sports Psychology Conference*. Ottawa, Canada: Dept. of National Health & Welfare, 1973.

Neisser, U. *Cognitive psychology*. New York: Appleton-Century-Crofts, 1967.

Norman, D. A. Towards a theory of memory and attention. *Psychological Review*, 1968, *75*, 522–536.

Norman, D. A. *Memory and attention*. New York: John Wiley, 1976.

Paillard, J. The patterning of skilled movement. In J. Field (Ed.), *Handbook of physiology: Neurophysiology* (Vol. 3). Baltimore: Williams & Wilkins, 1960.

Penfield, W., & Roberts, L. *Speech and brain-mechanisms*. Princeton, N.J.: Princeton University Press, 1959.

Schmidt, R. A. A schema theory of discrete motor skill learning. *Psychological Review*, 1975, *82*, 225–260.

Schmidt, R. A. Control processes in motor skills. In J. Keogh & R. S. Hutton (Eds.), *Exercise and sport sciences reviews* (Vol. 4). Santa Barbara, Calif.: Journal Publishing Affiliates, 1976.

Shapiro, D. C. A preliminary attempt to determine the duration of a motor program. In R. W. Christina & D. M. Landers (Eds.), *Psychology of motor behavior and sport*. Champaign, Ill.: Human Kinetics, 1976.

Shiffrin, R. M. Capacity limitations in information processing, attention, and memory. In W. K. Estes (Ed.), *Handbook of learning and cognitive processes IV: Attention and Memory*. Hillsdale, N.J.: Erlbaum, 1976.

Shiffrin, R. M., & Schneider, W. Controlled and automatic human information processing:

II. Perceptual learning, automatic attending, and a general theory. *Psychological Review*, 1977, *84*, 127–190.

Simon, H. A. The information storage system called "human memory." In M. R. Rosenzweig & E. L. Bennett (Eds.), *Neural mechanisms of learning and memory*. Cambridge, Mass.: MIT Press, 1976.

Skinner, B. F. *Beyond freedom and dignity*. New York: Knopf, 1971.

Sperling, G. The information available in brief visual presentations. *Psychological Monographs*, 1960, *74*, 1–29.

Sperry, R. W. The growth of nerve circuits. *Scientific American*, 1959, *201*, 68–75.

Stelmach, G. E., Kelso, J. A. S., & Wallace, S. A. Preselection in short-term motor memory. *Journal of Experimental Psychology: Human Learning and Memory*, 1975, *1*, 745–755.

Stelmach, G. E., Kelso, J. A. S., & McCullagh, P. D. Preselection and response biasing in short-term motor memory. *Memory and Cognition*, 1976, *4*, 62–66.

Taub, E. Movement in nonhuman primates deprived of somatosensory feedback. In J. Keogh & R. S. Hutton (Eds.), *Exercise and sport sciences reviews* (Vol. 4). Santa Barbara, Calif.: Journal Publishing Affiliates, 1976.

Temple, I. G., & Williams, H. G. Rate and level of learning as functions of information-processing characteristics of the learner and the task. *Journal of Motor Behavior*, 1977, *9*, 179–192.

Thatcher, R. W., & John, E. R. *Functional neuroscience, Vol. 1: Foundations of cognitive processes*. Hillsdale, N.J.: Erlbaum, 1977.

Treisman, A. Monitoring and storage of irrelevant messages in selective attention. *Journal of Verbal Learning and Verbal Behavior*, 1964, *3*, 449–459.

Weiner, B. *Achievement motivation and attribution theory*. Morristown, N.J.: General Learning Press, 1974.

Weiner, B., Neirenberg, R., & Goldstein, M. Social learning (locus of control) versus attributional (causal stability) interpretations of expectancy of success. *Journal of Personality*, 1976, *44*, 52–68.

Weiner, B., & Sierad, J. Misattribution for failure and enhancement of achievement strivings. *Journal of Personality and Social Psychology*, 1975, *31*, 415–421.

Welford, A. T. *Fundamentals of skill*. London: Methuen, 1968.

Whiting, H. T. A. Overview of the skill learning process. *Research Quarterly*, 1972, *43*, 266–294.

Wiener, N. *The human use of human beings*. Boston: Houghton Mifflin, 1954.

Woodworth, R. S. The accuracy of voluntary movement. *Psychological Review Monograph Supplement*, 1899, *3*.

Wooldridge, D. E. *The machinery of the brain*. New York: McGraw-Hill, 1963.

7

ABILITIES AND
INDIVIDUAL DIFFERENCES

We have examined the human behavioral system in order to determine the relationship of processes and mechanisms involved in motor acts without real concern for the way systems differ. Dissimilarities among systems become more obvious when more complex, higher order behaviors are of interest. The ability to perform gross motor activities places few demands on any system. Highly skilled acts, however, reflect differential aspects of human systems, for although the learning process is somewhat similar for all people, capabilities to achieve are not. Some systems contain more constraints than others. The status of the system, then, in terms of its distinguishing characteristics, marks its potential for achievement in assorted tasks.

In order to demonstrate higher-order learning in the form of successful motor performance, the presence of a wide variety of cognitive and perceptual abilities, motor abilities, physical and sensory characteristics, personality attributes, and control mechanisms for emotions is a necessity. Every skill reflects the need for varying degrees of physical, cognitive, motor, and emotional involvement. For example, although in some cases it may appear that certain activities are performed purely physically (running the dash) or cognitively (in the form of writing sentences), in reality there is always some degree of interaction of both these processes. The human factors varying from individual to individual and yet underlying motor skill learning and performance in some way are presented in this and in the next chapter. Specific reference is made in this chapter to the existence of individual differences and, later, to the study of them. The concept of a general unifying ability, such as motor ability or athletic ability, is contrasted with the idea of the existence of many abilities and how they potentially influence success in a variety of tasks and situations.

Motor abilities usually associated with the acquisition of skill are described, as well as techniques to measure them. Following this discussion, theory and research related to the notion of individual differences are presented. Special implications for instruction are derived from an analysis of aptitude X treatment interaction (ATI) research.

181

THE EXISTENCE OF INDIVIDUAL DIFFERENCES

The easiest way to determine the fact that individuals do differ in a particular behavior or trait is to select a number of subjects randomly and administer a test. Test scores will be spread along a continuum. Yet, there is something lawful about the way these scores fall. For, if indeed all subjects are chosen in a non-biased way and there is an ample number of them, we might predict with reasonable certainty how the scores will be arranged around the average score.

Look at Figure 7-1. Individuals will be expected to cluster around the mean, or average, score, with fewer scores in the extreme. We refer to this phenomenon as the normal curve. More people will attain a score surrounding the mean score than will attain a more removed score. Higher and lower scores are proportionally dispersed along the continuum.

But there are a number of occasions in which scores are disproportionately higher or lower. Symmetry does not always occur. Skewed curves are represented by an unusually large number of scores at one or the other end of the continuum. The degree of peak of the curve is determined by the number of cases packed at the central point versus those that are more uniformly spread over a large portion of the range of scores.

Many factors contribute to the variation of scores in a particular sample of subjects. The way scores are obtained and the data-collecting instruments will certainly affect the nature and the appearance of the data. Still, variations among the scores of individuals are expected. How they vary in relation to each other will be a function of measurement, the particular sample tested, and the behavior of interest.

Learners can be differentiated in terms of traits, abilities, learning styles and

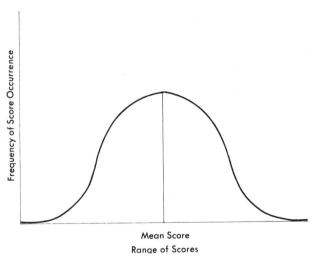

Mean Score
Range of Scores

FIGURE 7-1. The distribution of scores in the normal probability curve.

preferences, attitudes, emotions, and previous experiences related to the present situation and learning task. An analysis of how they differ in personal characteristics allows the teacher to *diagnose* and then to *prescribe* appropriate learning experiences (Levin, 1976). What personal factors are associated with success in a particular activity? Once they are known, as well as the way students in a class differ meaningfully in them, different programs of instruction can be proposed for students to maximize their potential achievement levels.

In this chapter and in the one that follows, many personal factors will be identified that contribute to differences among learners, and in turn, the realization of learning and performance potential. When teachers are sensitive to such considerations, alternative instructional approaches can be developed within a class, and special programs offered, for students with different capabilities.

ABILITIES AND SKILLS

It is not unusual to hear the terms *ability* and *skill* used quite often, many times interchangeably. Although related, they describe different behaviors. The similarities and differences between them are subtle. Explanations of these terms were presented in Chapter 2, and therefore do not need to be repeated here. As might be expected, there is much more agreement among testing specialists regarding the way to measure a particular skill or knowledge about some subject matter than there is regarding how to evaluate cognitive or psychomotor abilities. Because abilities presumably underlie potential of success in tasks and should theoretically be useful as predictors of task proficiency, an accurate assessment of abilities is quite desirable.

It should be expected, therefore, that there are many more skills than there are abilities. Skills are easy to observe and measure but the designation of abilities is more conceptual in nature. Abilities are derived by (1) general analysis and subjective appraisal or (2) statistical techniques, such as correlational and factor-analytic models. The former is a convenient but superficial approach. The latter includes the rigors of research and the application of statistics. Unfortunately, in spite of these efforts, an acceptable taxonomy of psychomotor abilities has yet to be created. A little later we will examine the current status of our knowledge on this topic.

When a number of different test scores are highly correlated, the assumption is that there is something in common among them. This underlying characteristic is termed an ability. Thus, the presence of an ability, to a high degree, increases an individual's probability to perform well in those tasks to which the ability contributes. If an accurate ability taxonomy were in existence today, prediction of task achievement from entering abilities could be a reality. However, such ideas have a way to go before practical usefulness will be realized. We must realize, in addition, that we do not know how to measure an ability in a "pure" way. What is referred to in the literature as an ability score is invariably a score registered on a specific test, or skill.

Therefore, it is difficult to answer the question: Can we improve an ability such as balance? If so, in what way? We can train someone to balance on a balance task, but can we say that we have increased balance ability in general or the ability to balance in that particular task? There is no easy answer to these questions. After you read this chapter, it will be interesting to see what you conclude.

TERMINOLOGY: MOTOR ABILITY, MOTOR FITNESS, MOTOR CAPACITY, AND MOTOR EDUCABILITY

Terms such as motor fitness, motor ability, motor capacity, and motor educability are often used interchangeably in test titles. However, their terms describe tests with different functions. Motor ability, motor fitness, motor capacity, and motor educability tests have numerous purposes and supposedly measure various aspects of human abilities and aptitudes. There are unique characteristics to tests of motor ability, motor fitness, motor capacity, and motor educability and, in some instances, a certain amount of overlap.

Motor ability presumably indicates present athletic ability. It denotes the immediate state of the individual to perform in a wide range of motor skills. A number of motor ability tests have been developed for application to both sexes at different stages in life. These tests have been proposed for classification and achievement expectancy, with the purpose of predicting an individual's possible competency in physical activities. Whether one general test can serve this broad function is debatable.

A term that has become confused with motor ability and physical fitness is *motor fitness*. Physical fitness implies the ability to perform a given task—in other words, having those physical qualities developed to the extent demanded by the task. Motor fitness refers to many of the qualities assumed to be included in physical fitness and motor ability. It is perhaps a more general term than physical fitness and, at the same time, one aspect of general motor ability.

Physical educators do not necessarily agree with the elements included in each category. To many, there is very little difference, if any, between physical fitness tests and motor fitness tests. In fact, many authors of texts in measurement in physical education include the American Alliance of Health, Physical Education, and Recreation (AAHPER) Youth Physical Fitness Test in their motor fitness chapter. Motor fitness and physical fitness tests usually contain such items as a run, sit-ups, a jump, pull-ups, and the like. Motor ability tests may include these items as well as measures of coordination.

Motor capacity is supposed to depict the maximum potential of an individual to succeed in motor skill performance. It is presumably a person's innate ability, his or her motor aptitude. Whereas a motor ability test purports to measure ultimate motor potential, a sort of "intelligence test."

The last of the related terms, *motor educability*, refers to the ease with which one learns new athletic skills. Tests so classified must incorporate novel stunts, which have not been previously practiced or learned by the performers.

Value of Tests

The worth of any test is determined by its validity—i.e., if the test measures what it purports to measure. Because of the dearth of motor capacity tests and investigations on this topic, no attempt will be made here to discuss the value of those already in existence. This is not to deny the potential impact of developments in the area, but rather to wait for more elaborate research, which might provide more concrete answers.

Tests of motor educability received the greatest amount of recognition in the 1930s. An examination of investigations concerned with motor educability tests reveals that this is but another area not well researched. Validity coefficients obtained with the Brace Test were not exceptionally high, and the criteria used have been questioned. Little work has been done with the Iowa Brace Test, and its stated function has also been attacked by numerous researchers. The Johnson Test evidently is restricted in predictive value in that high validity has been observed only through the use of tumbling stunts and track and field events as criterion measures. This might be expected, owing to the nature of the educability test. It contains stunts requiring body movements best represented by these activities.

Motor ability tests and related research have been of greater interest to physical educators than tests of and research on motor educability and motor capacity. This statement is confirmed by the greater number of publications associated with motor ability. Whether motor ability tests measure immediate athletic ability can be verified only by an examination of research results. These tests have not consistently achieved their stated purposes, that of determining present athletic ability. In general, most relationships between the motor ability tests and test of athletic competencies have been rather low and often meaningless.

Implications of Research

What, then, does the research indicate as far as the educator and trainer are concerned? First, what about the research itself? An interesting observation is that practically all the efforts in the respective area of motor ability, motor educability, and motor capacity were put forth in the late 1920s, the 1930s, and the early 1940s. One may ask why this is so. Is it felt that adequate tests for measuring skill have been constructed and well validated? Or is the trend away from viewing motor ability as something general, something that can be measured with one battery of tests? Through improved field research and intensive laboratory research, as well as sound reasoning, the emerging concept is that motor ability tests have limited value. Motor abilities in themselves are general measures, whereas task performance is specific to its peculiar nature and condition.

In many of these older studies, research techniques were used that, although sound at the time, might be questioned in the light of present knowledge in research methodology. Appropriate experimental designs and statistics are of particular concern. Second, a number of the reports lack clear and precise details on procedural operations. Finally, there have been consistent violations of terminology in the literature, with such terms as *capacity, ability, fitness,* and *educability* used interchangeably. The existence of these problems may account for many of the conflicting results obtained in the investigations. It certainly is difficult for one to arrive objectively at any definite conclusions, with regard to the respective general motor tests.

Perhaps there is such a thing as general motor ability. If there is a general factor, certainly more research is needed before doubters and disbelievers will be convinced. Much progress has been made since 1914, when Whipple wrote that many people were of the opinion that speed in tapping was the best test index of motor capacity. Other means used then to determine motor ability were hand, arm, and body steadiness tests and precision (tracing) and accuracy (aiming) tasks. There is still a long way to go.

GENERAL MOTOR ABILITY VERSUS THE NOTION OF SPECIFICITY OF ABILITIES

Do some individuals possess general abilities that allow them to succeed more easily in their undertakings when others are less favorably endowed? On the academic side, tests have been devised to predict success in college. According to Nevitt Sanford (1962) mental abilities are highly generalized—that is, there are only a few and these are basic to expected general academic achievement. Verbal and mathematical tests are significant predictors of a student's average grades in college. As far as intellectual factors are concerned, though, we know that these include reasoning, abstract thinking, memorization, creativeness, and problem solving, to name a few. IQ tests do not measure all of these qualities.

Even as there are many intellectual abilities, there are varied athletic abilities. A general mental ability test, such as an IQ test, will predict achievements in the various academic subjects fairly well. Specific tests, of course, will predict better. The general test will tend to correlate more highly with those subjects that have their matter better represented on the test. A motor ability test that purports to measure general athletic ability resembles in nature the purpose and accomplishments of a general mental test. However, in recent years, as we have seen, the so-called motor ability tests and the concept of a general motor ability have been questioned. For many years, researchers have attempted to discover general motor abilities, to isolate a few that would predict or measure general athletic achievement or ease in learning motor skills. Although their investigations have been valuable, the abundance of research attempting to find relationships between achievement in motor skills has tended to indicate the specificity of task performance. A person who performs well in one sport or in one skill will not necessarily do so in other sports or in other skills. There are many motor abilities, each applicable to certain situations. In highly refined research situations, the specificity of task performance has been well documented. Yet, we do know that the essence of most if not all learning is the positive transfer that occurs from past experiences and familiar situations to new but related experiences. The pendulum has swung back and forth: from the concept of the general compatibility of behaviors to the belief in the specificity of performance. Perhaps a compromise position will best explain what really occurs.

Research Findings

It appears that much of the research indicates that excellence in one motor ability, sport, or skill provides no assurance of accomplishment in others. The positive but low intercorrelations obtained in many investigations between motor abilities and task accomplishments support this statement. Most of the data have come from highly controlled laboratory settings.

Researchers have investigated relative success achieved when subjects perform in related movements, as well as at dissimilar motor skills. The published research from the laboratory at the University of California at Berkeley, under the direction of Franklin Henry (1961), has indicated the lack of a relationship between the speed of movement required for reaction time with that for movement time. When comparing the reaction times and movement times of 120 subjects, Henry found a correlation of 0.02. Obviously, a person could not predict achievement in one movement very well from data on the other movement. Leon Smith (1962) tested sixty male college subjects on the speed of an adductive arm movement under resting muscle and pretensed muscle conditions. Timing stations were arranged at 15°, 53°, 90°, and 105°. Small and nonsignificant correlations were obtained between the conditions at each timing station.

Since then, most research efforts have supported the idea of specific achievements of parts of the body in specified speed tasks. Lookerman and Berger (1972), for instance, tested the reaction times and movement times of subjects informed to move in any one of four directions. They concluded that the ability to react and to move was specific to the direction of the response. Recorded times were not consistently fast or slow for the subjects when directional speeds were analyzed and when hand and total body times were compared in the same direction.

Speed is not conditioned uniformly in all activities by some unitary factor or set of factors. Research findings in general tend to substantiate this proposition. For instance, Lotter (1961) timed his subjects on their ability to turn a two-handled arm crank versus the speed of the arms individually versus comparable movements of the legs. Low intercorrelations further supported a theory of motor specificity.

After administering seventeen manipulative tests, six printed tests, and twenty-three physical performance tests, Hempel and Fleishman (1955) concluded that the factors that contributed to successful gross physical task performance were not the same as those in fine motor tasks. Fleishman (1958a) found a high degree of specificity among twenty-four position (fine motor) tasks. Singer (1966) attempted to determine the relationship between throwing and kicking skills. The subjects, thirty-eight college students enrolled in required physical education classes, threw a ball at a target and kicked a ball at a target, first using preferred limbs, then nonpreferred limbs. Correlations were obtained for all of the possible limb combinations. Five of the six correlations were low, positive, and significant. However, when statistically analyzed for generality and specificity factors, great specificity was noted in the limb relationships.

It can be observed, then, that the evidence from the representative studies presented here suggests a questioning of the concept of the existence of a general motor ability. Task-to-task performance usually is related slightly, but not enough to justify predicting one's ability in many skills or sports from one test.

The notion of specificity in the psychology of learning and performance has an analogy in exercise physiology. It is becoming more and more accepted by work physiologists that training is specific to particular exercises. Consider what D. W. Edington and V. R. Edgerton (1976) have to say: "Specific energy sources within each muscle . . . respond to specific types of exercise" (p. 8). And they add that specific exercises have different nervous system requirements. Because adaptations are made within specific muscles and systems as they are used in training, it can be proposed that skilled performance in any task is partly a function of the implementation of integrated movements developed and learned especially to specific situational requirements.

The ability to perform well in many motor activities is probably based on general factors, primarily a time element (speed), strength, and coordination. Many sports require abilities related to these variables. However, performance measures of each factor vary from activity to activity; hence, speed in track is of a different nature from speed and quickness in a basketball game or on a tennis court. The balance demanded on gymnastic apparatus differs from the body balance needed when striking a ball, shooting a jumpshot, or wrestling. In other words, an athlete may demonstrate a highly refined example of balance in one sport but not in another. Evidently, one can exhibit strength, coordination, speed, and other qualities in dissimilar ways, and the relationship of tasks within a factor will depend on their degree of overlap and similarity.

The All-Around Athlete

Coaches and physical educators might be cautious in their interpretation and application of empirical evidence related to individual achievement in a number of sports. It is true that some people perform well in a variety of activities and are termed all-around athletes. However, these motor prodigies are the exception, not the rule. Success in one sport does not imply that the same situation will occur in another sport, and only when certain factors are operating will this probability increase. These underlying factors follow:

1. Experience and intensive practice in a wide range of motor skills will result in apparent ease in the acquisition of new but related skills. The person who has benefited from a childhood enriched with experiences in basic movement pat-

terns and an assortment of activities will be more favored in motor learning situations. Those past experiences and the resultant skills will serve as a foundation for the learning of new skills.

2. Genetics determines the potential of an individual in motor skill attainment. Even as heredity determines potential intelligence levels, hair color, and body size, it creates the boundaries of motor development. It should be stressed here that research, especially on intelligence, points to the possible influence of the environment and life's experiences on an individual's achievements. Furthermore, it should be realized that one has to go a long way before maximum potential is reached, whether in intellectual or motor pursuits. Thus, it may be seen that, although hereditary factors contribute to limit potential proficiency in motor acts, many of these factors can be overcome with the necessary drive and ambition.

3. Motivation is necessary for success. It is hypothesized that the athlete who has achieved success in one sport transfers this determination, motivation, and perseverance to other motor skill endeavors. The all-around athlete may very well be a highly motivated performer in general, who possesses the necessary personality characteristics for varied motor accomplishments.

4. Related sports offer a greater probability of accomplishment for the athlete. Therefore, if an athlete is proficient in a number of sports, there is a good chance that the basic skills common to all of them have been mastered.

These practical examples in sports of the nature of abilities and individual differences can be related to the final conceptual model presented in Chapter 6.

Other factors may also contribute to the relative ease a person shows in attaining success in various sports. However, there are also many reasons why an individual does not display proficiency in a number of activities. Of major concern is the unrealistic approach a coach may take in a situation involving an athlete who is superior in one sport attempting to progress in another activity in which he or she is not nearly so talented. Achievement and satisfaction may or may not come. Great success in one sport does not necessarily mean corresponding achievements will follow in other sports. To be an outstanding performer in a number of sports, even in only two, indicates an extraordinary ability.

Considerations for Performance: Specificity and Generality

So far it appears that a pretty solid case has been made in support of task specificity and the concept of many fairly independent abilities, rather than a general motor ability. We can probably rule out, at least at the present time, the concept of one unifying motor ability that is associated with proficiency in a wide variety of activities. But this is not to say that a number of general motor abilities do not operate to contribute to task success. And, to the extent that tasks are related, similar abilities will serve as contributing factors for achievement in them. There is probably a happy medium between general supports and task-specific elements to describe what motor behavior is all about.

A serious review of all the published research on the topic would lead the researcher to be disappointed if the hypothesis were in favor of general factors operating to encourage some individuals to perform well in a wide range of motor tasks while others do poorly. Nevertheless, the indirect implications of research findings and intuition suggest that general abilities, as well as specific task practice, contribute to excellence in the performance of complex skills. The presence of an ideal degree of certain task-related abilities will aid the learner in the early stages of achievement. Other abilities will be more important for higher levels of proficiency. Although genetic factors and past experiences, which contribute to the development of abilities, primarily assist the learner in the beginning stages of practice, superior skills can only be demonstrated after many hours of practice in the activity of concern. Figure 7-2 summarizes in simplified fashion the relationship between foundational abilities and specific task practice.

An expanded version of this concept is presented in Figure 7-3. More general, as well as specific, considerations are identified as they influence performance in a particular psychomotor task.

Even the ability to acquire skills at a fast rate is probably unique to each particular task. That is to say, a general learning-rate ability probably would not exist if we were to examine how people do in various activities. It is specific to each task. The inconsistency of rate-of-learning scores among individuals across a variety of tasks has been reasonably well documented for more than thirty years. Lee Cronbach (1967) thinks that it is advisable to examine instructional conditions as they interact with learning rates. He assumes that a particular instructional technique in effect helps to define the nature of the task. So when different tasks are to be mastered under the same instructional conditions, the learner is required to demonstrate a general ability to learn those tasks under the imposed condition.

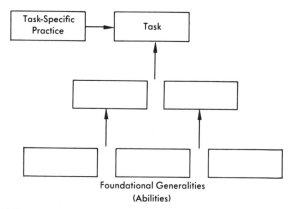

FIGURE 7-2. Abilities primarily contribute to initial task success whereas specific task practice is required in addition to the ideal presence of these abilities for highly skilled behaviors. The boxes are left blank here, because the nature of the abilities will depend on the task. For that matter, so will the number of abilities.

MOTOR LEARNING AND HUMAN PERFORMANCE

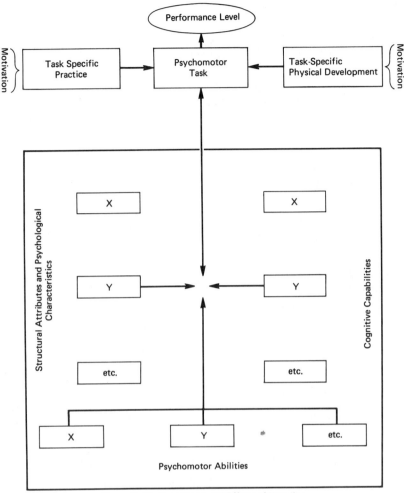

FIGURE 7-3. The interactional effect of general and specific factors on the performance of a particular psychomotor task.

The instructional method may very well dictate a person's learning rate. Further discussion on this topic will be provided toward the end of this chapter.

Expanded Issues: Specificity Versus Generality of Performance

The same kind of problem is recognized in all of these examples: (1) the relationship of a previous experience to a newly introduced one; (2) the prediction capability of a test to determine potential competency in designated activities; (3) the relationship of various performance test scores that presumably measure the same characteristic; or (4) the relationship of rate of learning scores to different tasks.

Some of these problematical areas have been discussed already, whereas others will be addressed in different sections of this book. The issue is one of generality versus specificity. Can individuals be expected to perform consistently across situations, or is each situation highly unique?

Perhaps postulates can summarize evidence and logic in regard to learning and performing expectancies in motor skills:

1. Performance in a newly introduced activity will depend on the extent and quality of previous related experiences, the presence of relevant abilities and characteristics that are developed to a desired extent, and practice or experience directly related to the activity.

(a) During the early stages of learning an activity, some learners perform better as a result of prior experiences and well-developed broad-based capabilities underlying achievement potential in that activity.

(b) Later achievement depends on the quality and extent of practice specific to the activity.

(c) The more complex the activity (considering cue availability, variations, and predictability, as well as response demands), the more homogenous the group of learners (minimal or no prior direct experiences with the activity of concern), and the more practice time available, the lower the relationship may be between the initial performance and final performance of individuals in an activity. In other words, it would be hazardous to predict terminal behaviors from beginning performance levels, the more these considerations must be recognized.

(d) Varied and enriched experiences are extremely important in early childhood to stimulate the sensory modalities, develop gross motor patterns, and develop capabilities and abilities, all of which will serve as the foundation for the later acquisition of sophisticated and refined pyschomotor skills.

2. The rate of learning activities depends on their similarity and the presence of similar motivations across activities; because both factors usually vary quite a bit, it would appear that the speed with which proficiency is shown is fairly task-specific.

3. The relationships among scores of tests that presumably measure the same "ability" have been low, but this may be due to the problems in defining what an ability is and/or the problems in measuring an ability.

(a) It is probably not possible to measure a particular motor ability purely or directly.

(b) Tests that presumably indicate an ability level probably involve, to some degree, other abilities, as well.

4. The interrelationships of the performance scores of individuals in various skills tests are generally low, as a result of such factors as (a) skill level, (b) attitude and interest, (c) testing conditions, and (d) the dissimilarity of the nature of many motor skills regarding performance demands in strategies, movement behaviors, and emotions.

5. There is no one general motor ability.

(a) Conceptually speaking, a variety of psychomotor, cognitive, and affective abilities underlie potential achievement in any activity.

(b) At the present time, no one test battery has been able adequately to explain or predict performance in a variety of motor activities.

(c) The more related a predictor test battery, in terms of behaviors measured, to a particular activity or a group of activities, the better the chance of its meaningfulness and validity.

6. Many activities require the instantaneous adaptability of behaviors to changing circumstances, and it seems that an efficient human system is one in which basic movement programs or schema have been well learned as they relate to an activity, with an allowance for performance adaptions to novel situations.

(a) It is impossible to train for every conceivable circumstance.

(b) Well-learned (semiautomatic) programs can trigger quick and accurate responses to familiar cues, but skilled adaptions are also possible to "new but related" cues, thus suggesting both specificity and a reasonably well-functioning generality capability.

7. An analysis of learning and performance, transfer possibilities, prediction potential, and the relationship among performances in activities suggests the existence of both specificity and generality combinations.

MOTOR ABILITIES

Although other classifications of abilities no doubt are involved in skilled motor performance, the motor abilities category is the one most usually associated with motor behaviors. Different approaches in formulating basic abilities have demonstrated alternative ways of thinking about them, resulting in lively debates among scholars. The consequence for the practitioner has been one of confusion. Thus:

1. An ability could be looked at as a behavioral variable with parameters defined by the particular methods used in its measurement.
2. An ability could reflect individual differences in training conditions and experiences, as well as the state of the organism as induced by the experimenter.
3. An ability could be viewed as a hypothetical construct, in which case a skill is defined as a behavioral variable, as in item 1.
4. An ability could be an artificial (observed) or constructed statistical variable, whereby a primary ability is derived from the hypothetical elements that are combined to form the ability.

Dennis Roberts (1968–69) has provided a brief but comprehensive review of the research literature dealing with abilities and learning. The relationships between abilities, learning/performance, and practice stage are complex, making it difficult to provide simple answers to trainers and teachers. He raises four major questions:

1. How do you assess a student's pattern of abilities? Strengths and weaknesses need to be assessed with one or several reliable and valid tests.
2. How do you identify, through task analysis, the abilities required to learn a task? The abilities necessary for a minimum level of performance should be specified as they relate to the task components.
3. Can deficiencies or poorly developed abilities be remediated? Abilities must be isolated and remedial activities identified and implemented in order to contribute to task achievement.
4. Are abilities differentially related to practice stages? Initial task performance may be a poor indicator of later accomplishments, because certain abilities are primary contributers to early success, an indication that screening procedures on the basis of early task performance may not be a good idea.

Perhaps the most extensive work in the area of motor abilities completed thus far by any one scholar (and his colleagues) is attributed to E. A. Fleishman. In his many publications (e.g., Fleishman, 1964), he describes the statistical techniques (correlational, factor-analytic) he used to derive both motor abilities and physical proficiency factors. From the administration of more than two hundred different psychomotor tasks (most of them oriented to the laboratory and instrumentation) to thousands of subjects, Fleishman feels that he has been able to account for performance of these tasks in terms of a small number of abilities. Those abilities are identified here:

1. Control precision: primarily involves highly controlled large muscle movements.
2. Multilimb coordination: simultaneous coordination of the movements of a number of limbs.
3. Response orientation: selection of right response (visual discrimination), irrespective of precision and coordination.
4. Reaction time: speed of response to a stimulus.
5. Rate control: continuous anticipatory motor adjustments to changing situational cues (speed, direction).
6. Speed of arm movement: speed where accuracy is not important.
7. Manual dexterity: manipulation of large objects under speed conditions.
8. Finger dexterity: manipulation of tiny objects with precision and control.
9. Arm–hand steadiness: control of movements, while motionless or in motion.
10. Wrist–finger speed: tapping activity.
11. Aiming: printed tests requiring pencil accuracy and speed.

These eleven abilities, according to Fleishman, underlie achievement in many motor tasks. Yet, it should be emphasized that most of the tasks from which these abilities have been derived have not been athletic or real-life in nature, a restriction in the interpretation and application of Fleishman's findings.

Fleishman (1964) also postulates nine physical proficiency abilities that presumably are associated with athletic and gross physical performance. The factors identified are (1) static strength, (2) dynamic strength, (3) explosive strength, (4) trunk strength, (5) extent flexibility, (6) dynamic flexibility, (7) gross body coordination, (8) multilimb coordination, and (9) stamina.

From over twenty years' work, the following interpretations of Fleishman's work can be made:

1. A particular combination of abilities can be identified that contribute to motor skill performance.
2. Changes in the combination of these abilities occur with continued practice and improvement.
3. Motor abilities become more important in task performance than nonmotor abilities with practice.
4. A task-specific factor emerges with practice.

Ability changes associated with practice and predictive possibilities will be discussed in more detail in Chapter 11 that deals with practice and training. It is sufficient here to indicate the high points of the research findings.

H. P. Bechtoldt (1970) has been extremely critical of Fleishman's work. He objects to the idea that an ability can refer to the power to perform an act, with or without training. Also, because performances are clearly specified as to situations and responses, an ability is thereby defined by a specified test procedure and scoring method. Bechtoldt raises the issue that it is conceivable for every test to define a separate ability. Conceptually speaking, of course, this should not be the case.

An ability can also be derived hypothetically, rather than defined: it is assumed or inferred from the results of factor-analytic studies or from experiments when subjects with high test scores are compared to subjects with lower test scores. Bechtoldt takes offense that Fleishman does not clearly define abilities but instead infers them. Other objections are made, including one to Fleishman's use of factor-analytic statistical techniques, which Bechtoldt claims are inappropriate for the data measured. Nevertheless, at the present time, Fleishman's work is the most prominent in the field of categorizing abilities and determining their relationship to motor skill performance. Two useful summaries of his efforts and his conclusions are recommended to the interested reader (Fleishman, 1972a, 1972b).

The recognition of those abilities required for task proficiency assists in understanding task requirements more fully. A systems anlaysis would require the identification of the hierarchical arrangement of abilities associated with achievement in a particular activity. Fleishman and Stephenson (1970), in reviewing the future plans of their taxonomy project, recommend the design and use of binary decision-flow diagrams in order to simplify decisions about ability requirements. The binary decision diagram (three tentatively described ones are illustrated in Figures 7-4 to 7-6), encourages go-no-go decisions at various steps in the task analysis. In order to be really meaningful, the flow diagrams presented here must be developed in much more detail, as admitted by Fleishman and Stephenson.

Although Fleishman and others have attempted to categorize motor abilities, there are at least four factors that seem to be of most interest to motor learning

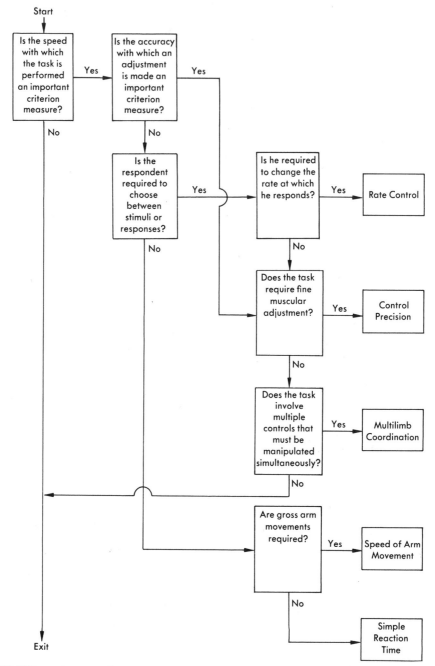

FIGURE 7-4. Tentative binary decision-flow diagrams that can be used to make decisions about the relevance of selected perceptual motor abilities. (*From Fleishman, E. A., & Stephenson, R. W. Development of a taxonomy of human performance: A review of the third year's progress. Washington, D.C.: American Institutes for Research, 1970.*)

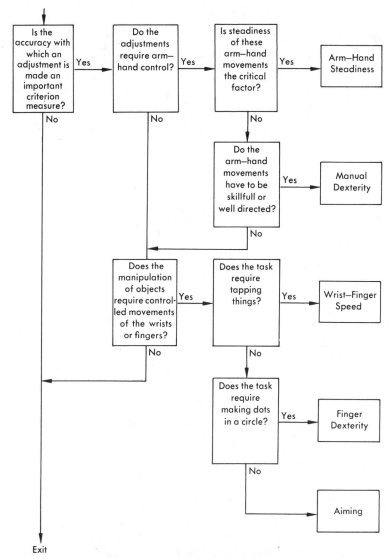

FIGURE 7-5. Tentative binary decision-flow diagrams that can be used to make decisions about the relevance of fine manipulative abilities. (*From Fleishman, E. A., & Stephenson, R. W. Development of a taxonomy of human performance: A review of the third year's progress. Washington, D.C.: American Institutes for Research, 1970.*)

researchers. Abilities have been used to determine relationships to task proficiency. They have been identified by task requirements in order to study learning phenomena, with little particular concern for the actual abilities involved. Terminologies have not been consistent in different sources, but we will identify these factors as coordination, kinesthesis, balance, and speed of movement.

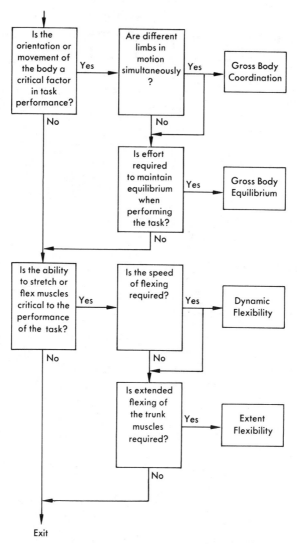

FIGURE 7-6. Tentative binary decision-flow diagrams that can be used to make decisions about the relevance of gross physical proficiencies. (*From Fleishman, E. A., & Stephenson, R. W. Development of a taxonomy of human performance: A review of the third year's progress. Washington, D.C.: American Institutes for Research, 1970.*)

The four primary research purposes, then, of tasks that are associated with these factors, would be their usage:

1. as learning tasks (novel, neutral).
2. for establishing ability norms.
3. for determining task specificity versus generality.
4. for predicting how well someone will learn and perform in a given activity.

Now let us turn to a discussion of specific abilities.

Coordination

Coordination of various parts of the body implies an ability to perform a skilled movement pattern. It is the ability to control the independent body parts involved in a complex movement pattern and to integrate these parts in a single, smooth, successful effort at achieving some goal. The skill itself primarily may involve eye–foot coorindation, an example of which is kicking a football or soccer ball; or eye–hand coordination, such as throwing an object at a target. Some sports require an overall coordination of the body: a gymnastic routine on the parallel bars requres perfect timing; a football halfback demonstrates agility and speed in movement; and swinging a golf club requires smoothness and rhythm.

Sometimes the word *coordination* is used interchangeably with *timing, skill,* or *general motor ability.* However, these words are so vague as to have no real meaning. We must always ask the question: Coordination for what? Task demands will determine those parts of the body that must be sequenced in some relationship and according to what timing arrangements.

Many laboratory tasks have been developed to measure coordinated movements (primarily eye–hand) and to predetermine success in certain fields. In industrial jobs that require manual dexterity, for example, manipulative tasks help in predicting success. An example of a widely used task utilizing arm–hand coordination (manual dexterity) is the Minnesota Rate of Manipulation Test, whereas the Crawford Small Parts Dexterity Test requires finger dexterity (see Figure 7-7).

Although evidence is fragmentary, there has been an attempt to relate predictor task performance to success in industry, dentistry, and piloting a plane. The tests have demonstrated moderately predictive values in these cases. The Complex Coordination Test, which requires stick and rudder movements in response to specific signal lights, has been reported to correlate 0.40 in predicting pilot success. The Hand-Tool Dexterity Test correlated 0.46 with the actual performance of machinists, and the Metal Filling Work sample correlated 0.53 with dentistry course grades. Obviously, the more related the task to the actual criterion, the higher the anticipated correlation. Relationships between movements required for the coordination tasks, often used by psychologists, and the coordinated movement patterns desired in sport should probably not be high because of the lack of similarity in the nature of the required responses.

Other devices are used for testing potential pilot success or probable athletic achievement. Also, they serve as a medium for viewing the effects of environmental manipulations and understanding the psychological phenomena associated with motor tasks. In physical education, coordinated movements may be demonstrated in target-accuracy skills and in the performance of various stunts. However, the laboratory environment is better for the control of the many extraneous variables that are apt to confound the field study. This is why various types of apparatus have been constructed by those interested in understanding and explaining the learning process, especially as it relates to motor skills. Unfortunately, there is

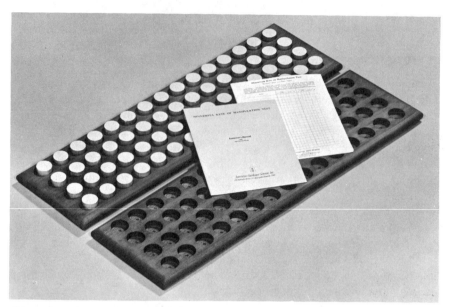

Minnesota Rate of Manipulation Test

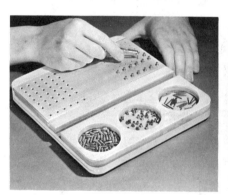 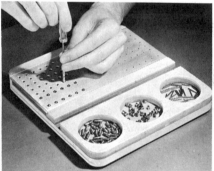

Crawford Small Parts Dexterity Test

FIGURE 7-7. The Minnesota Rate of Manipulation Test measures capacity for manipulative work. In the five tests that are administered with this equipment, the blocks are turned, moved, and placed in certain prescribed ways. This involves finger movement and hand-and-arm movement. It involves movements with the preferred hand and also with both hands simultaneously. As usage of this test has spread, it now appears that more than speed is involved in gross finger, hand, and arm movements. Also involved are gross body movements, intelligence, vision, and perseverance. (*From American Guidance Service, Inc., Minneapolis, 1966.*)

The Crawford Small Parts Dexterity Test measures fine eye-hand coordination. Part I measures dexterity in using tweezers to insert small pins in close-fitting holes in a plate and to place small collars over the protruding pins. Part II measures dexterity in placing small screws in threaded holes in a plate and screwing them down with a screwdriver until they drop through the plate into a metal dish below. (*From the Psychological Corporation, New York, 1965.*)

a danger in assuming that the learning of practical skills, those performed in daily life, is governed by the same principles as skills learned and performed in the laboratory. Arguments have been presented for and against both laboratory research and classroom or gymnasium research; but both are needed for a better understanding of the psychology of learning. Both research methods can and should complement each other and not provide fuel for debate.

Laboratory researchers concerned with coordination tasks have constructed ingenious devices for measuring coordination. One of the forerunners in attempting to uncover the factors underlying psychomotor performance success was Fleishman (1957, 1958a, 1958b). Besides employing previously used tasks in other experiments, he devised other tasks to measure the many aspects of psychomotor skill. They are basically coordinating, positioning, and speed tasks. Figure 7-8 contains a number of the apparatus that have been widely used in his investigations.

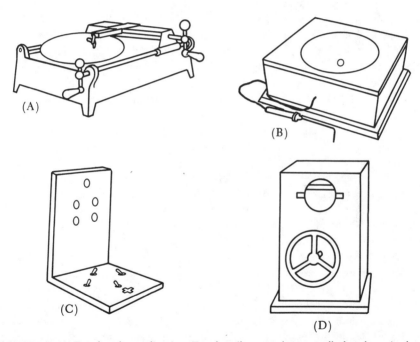

FIGURE 7-8. (A) Two-hand coordination. Two handles must be controlled and manipulated in order to keep a target follower on a target disk as the target moves unpredictably; (B) Rotary pursuit. The stylus is kept in contact with a small metallic target that is set on a revolving phonograph-type disk; (C) Response orientation. The subject manipulates one of four toggle switches as rapidly as possible in response to rapidly changing light patterns; and (D) Single-dimension pursuit. The subject makes adjustments to the wheel in order to keep the line in the window centrally located as it moves unpredictably. (*From Fleishman, E. A. Dimensional analysis of movement reactions. Journal of Experimental Psychology, 1958, 55, 438–453.*) Copyright 1958 by the American Psychological Association. Reprinted by permission.

A familiarity with the design and nature of laboratory tasks demanding motor coordination, like the pursuit rotor, will be most profitable for the person interested in reading and analyzing the literature concerning the learning of motor skills. Many deductions from the phenomena related to motor learning, transfer, retention, practice, and the like have been derived from the utilization of these tasks under manipulated environmental conditions. Differences in terminology and applications exist among research specialists and educators. For instance, whereas physical educators may have regarded only sports skills as motor tasks, psychologists include in this category all previously discussed devices and the responses required for them, as well as many others.

Balance

The ability to maintain body position, referred to as balance, is necessary for the successful performance of many gross motor skills. It is essential in those dynamic sports that require sudden changes in movement, exemplified by the tennis player who has to pursue a ball, regain balance, and then strike the ball. The wrestler, whether standing or kneeling on the mat, has to retain balance when moving toward or away from an opponent. Each sport demands a particular type of balance. In other words, an individual does not possess one general balancing ability that will lead to good balance for all tasks and under all conditions.

Standing erect under trying or even normal conditions involves an interaction of a number of neurophysiological structures, senses, and pathways. Equilibrium is obtained through the combined efforts of simple reflexes, proprioceptive information relayed to the cerebrum and cerebellum, an activation of the recticular formation, the vestibular apparatus, visual information, and voluntary movements.

The *stretch reflex* works in sustaining body posture. *Proprioceptors* in various parts of the body contribute to equilibrium: the neck proprioceptors stimulate the recticular nuclei; the head receptors for movement activate the vestibular apparatus; and proprioceptors from other parts of the body stimulate the *reticular pathways, cerebellum,* and *cerebral cortex.*

The *bony labyrinth,* which is a cavity in the temporal bone, contains the cochlear duct (concerned with hearing), the saccule, the semicircular canals, and the utricle (see Figure 7-9). The *semicircular canals* and *utricle* combined constitute the *vestibular apparatus* and are sensitive to body movement and position. The canals respond to acceleration or deceleration changes in head velocity. Head movements stimulate proprioceptors and vestibular nerves, which in turn extend to the reticular nuclei and cerebellum, producing impulses that are sent to the appropriate muscles for body equilibrium.

Vision assists in providing information about the body's position with regard to its environment. Even with destruction of the vestibular apparatus, vision can compensate and allow the person to maintain a degree of equilibrium. *Voluntary movements,* directed from a cortical center, allow us to have a conscious awareness of our body's position and to do something about it. After an observation of the environment and perception of the changing position of the body, through con-

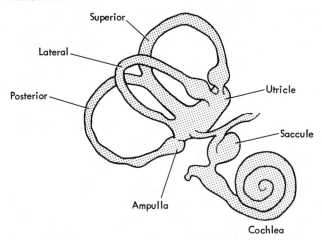

FIGURE 7-9. Bony labyrinth apparatus. The cochlea is concerned with audition. The semicircular canals, the utricle, and probably the sacule are essential for equilibration. (*From Langley, L. L., & Cheraskin, E.* Physiology of Man. *New York: Van Nostrand, 1965.*)

scious effort we can direct the necessary movement adjustments in order to maintain the desired posture.

Tests have been constructed to determine dynamic and static balancing ability. However, highly positive relationships between the two have not been obtained, as is the case when comparing the results of tests measuring dynamic and static strength. Static equilibrium requires continuous, even muscle tension, which underlies standing perfectly still, without swaying. Dynamic balance demands body orientation in off-balance situations. R. C. Travis (1945) measured static balance with an ataxiameter (which records body sway while standing) and dynamic balance by means of a stabilometer. He found no relationship between static and dynamic balance. Additional interesting findings of this study indicated that weight, not height, is an important factor in dynamic performance. Subjects with greater weight balanced better. Also, there was a small, insignificant sex difference in balancing, favoring women. Finally, balancing scores were much greater with the eyes open than closed.

The balance required for each skill varies and is evidently unique to the skill employed. There is inconclusive evidence on balance transference from task to task, task to sport, and sport to sport. The more similarity that exists between them, the more we can expect a positive influence.

An excellent example of this relationship is found in a study reported by Singer (1970). College athletes, fifteen in a group and representing basketball, baseball, football, gymnastics, and wrestling teams; water skiing experts; and nonathletes, were tested on a stabilometer apparatus. Athletic groups were compared with each other and against the nonathletes in balance performance. The nonathletes scored lowest on the task, demonstrating some balance required in respective sports carried over to the stabilometer task. More interestingly, because the stabilometer requires skill similar to the balance required by the water skiers, it is not surprising that this group attained the highest balancing performance. Gymnasts were second best, and, in fact, they and the skiers were significantly superior in achievement to most of the other groups. Evidently, although balance as an ability is demanded in a variety of athletic situations, those athletes who practice balance in skills similar to those tested on the stabilometer do better in this testing situation.

Balance tasks designed in varying degrees of complexity range from simple balance beams to stabilometers. Basically, a stabilometer requires one to balance on an unstable platform. Investigators have constructed different types of stabilometers for determining balancing ability, and each apparatus has certain advantages and disadvantages not associated with another model. A work adder has been used in conjunction with a stabilometer in certain investigations. A picture and description of this apparatus appear in Figure 7-10.

Other types of balance tasks found in the literature include rail walking (walking a narrow beam without falling off), standing on one foot for a length of time, and the Bachman ladder climb (climbing as many rungs as possible before a free-standing ladder falls).

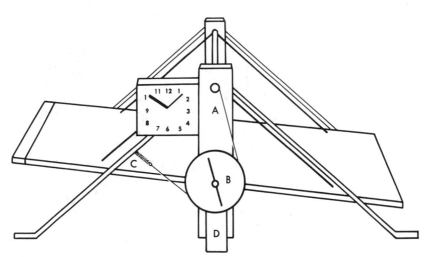

FIGURE 7-10. Stabilometer with work adder. A short cord drive lever is screwed into the protruding end of the main axle just above (A). The cord passes downward and bends over a large pulley on the back of the work-adder dial (B), terminating at a coil spring fastened to the frame just above (C). A pawl at (D) engages the milled periphery of the work-adder dial, restricting its turning to a single direction so that movement of the platform is cumulated on the dial. Various A-frame rods brace the platform and the vertical posts that rise from the base to carry the main axle. Motion of the board is measured by the work adder. (*From Bachman, J. C. Specificity vs. generality in learning and performing two large muscle motor tasks. Research Quarterly, 1961, 32, 3–11.*)

Kinesthesis

The terms *kinesthetic* and *proprioceptive* generally refer to the same sense—providing information concerning the body's position in space and the relationship of its parts. Experimental psychologists usually refer to this sense as kinesthetic; physiologists prefer the term *proprioceptive,* it having been introduced by the great physiologist Sherrington.

The confusion in the interchangeable use of the terms *proprioception* and *kinesthesis* has prompted Hopkins (1972) to address the issue. After a historical perspective of the problem, he offers four alternatives: (1) to accept the two terms as referring to the same thing; (2) to accept J. J. Gibson's interpretations—that proprioception is not a special sense but a function common to all systems, whereas kinesthesis is restricted to sensitivity of skeletal movement; (3) to use the terms *kinesthesis* when certain receptor mechanisms are activated and *proprioception* when additional mechanisms are activated; or (4) never to use the term *kinesthesis.* Hopkins favors the last proposed: to use *proprioception* exclusively.

When the special sense receptors in the muscles, tendons, and joints (called proprioceptors) are stimulated, the impulses pass through the posterior column of the spinal cord to the thalamus and finally to the somatic area of the cerebral cortex. If the posterior column is destroyed, there results a loss of sensation in limb movement and position. Coordination of the visual, vestibular, and somatic sensory receptors contributes to the body's orientation in space.

Stretch receptors of muscles alone are not responsible for kinesthesia. These receptors have not been found to provide information about joint position because they discharge over their full frequency range at any muscle length. The following receptors in the joints contain the source of kinesthetic sensations: the Ruffini receptors, which have spray-type endings and are the most common in connective tissue; the Golgi tendon organs, which are less numerous; and the Pacinian corpuscles. Whether muscle spindles (stretch receptors) that react to muscle stretch also play an important role in kinesthesis is open to question.

The importance of proprioception in contributing to proficiency in motor performance has been noted by many researchers and instructors. The "sense of feel" enables one to divert energies elsewhere, for there is a limited amount of capacity within a person to process information. For example, the beginning basketball player learning how to dribble constantly looks at the ball to see where it is. The highly skilled player doesn't have to look at the ball. Instead, vision is freed to scan the court as kinesthetic receptors provide the necessary information and control. The responsibility for dribbling is delegated to lower control centers, thereby releasing the central channel to process other information. Central and peripheral mechanisms can exert more apparent control and regulation during movement, the slower the action to be performed.

It is little wonder that researchers have attempted to develop tests to measure kinesthetic ability. We might assume that those learners who would score high on such a test would learn and perform motor skills more ably. Tests of kinesthesis

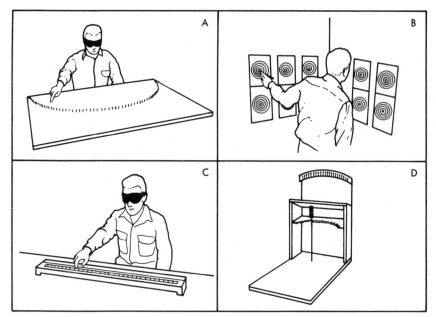

FIGURE 7-11. Tests of kinesthesis that require kinesthetic discrimination. In these tests the blindfolded subject in A must reach a certain peg or in B mark a certain target, in response to verbal instructions. In tests C and D, he reproduces certain movements with a knob or a stick control. (*From Fleishman, E. A. An analysis of positioning movements and static reactions.* Journal of Experimental Psychology, *1958, 55, 13–24.*) Copyright 1958 by the American Psychological Association. Reprinted by permission.

vary in nature and bodily involvement. Batteries of tests have been devised by a number of physical educators interested in the kinesthetic sense. M. Gladys Scott (1955) developed a twenty-eight-test battery that she administered to women college students. She noted a specificity in the function of the tests. A twenty-one-test battery was administered to thirty college men by Vernon Wiebe (1954), who also found a low correlation between the tests and deduced a lack of general kinesthetic sense. Some tests of kinesthesis are illustrated in Figure 7-11.

Many tests of kinesthesis have been static, involving positional sense. Examples of some kinesthetic tests described by Louise Roloff (1953) are the Balance Stick, Arm Raising, and Weight Shifting tests.

- *Balance stick.* A 1 x 12-inch stick is taped to the floor. The subject, with eyes closed, must balance on one foot on this stick for as long as possible.
- *Arm raising.* The subject is tested on the ability to raise each arm to the horizontal position while blindfolded. Deviations in degrees are measured with a goniometer.
- *Weight shifting.* The subject has to straddle a scale and a block of wood. With eyes open, getting the feel of running the scale up one-half one's weight in

pounds is first practiced. Then, with eyes closed, the subject attempts to do it again, and deviations are determined to the nearest half pound.

Other investigators have expressed dissatisfaction with the design of these static tests. Henry (1953) created a device that required continuing constant pressure exerted by the subject against a pad while the pressure continually changed under the influence of a cam. This dynamic test brought about an increase or decrease in muscular tension caused by the changing pressure of the cam. In two separate tasks, his twelve subjects were required to adjust to pressure changes or to perceive pressure changes.

A. T. Slater-Hammel (1957) felt that kinesthetic tests involve tactile stimulation as well as muscular force. He therefore suggested a task in which individuals had to reproduce a specific muscle contraction. With the use of muscle potentials, he measured the intensity of the muscle contraction after an initial prescribed contraction of 125 microvolts.

A means of demonstrating the effects of kinesthetic impairment has been offered by Judith Laszlo (1966). By raising the systolic blood pressure 40 millimeters mercury higher than the subject's normal reading with the use of a sphygmomanometer cuff and having the subject continually tap on a Morse key as quickly as possible, Laszlo found an expected decrease in key-tapping efficiency with a loss of kinesthetic sensation. She also tested her subjects in other ways. Once again, with the cuff on the arm and head turned away, each subject's finger was touched lightly with a Q-Tip. The finger was also manipulated up or down and the subject was asked to move it up or down. This was done regularly after the cuff was in place for ten minutes. On the average, the subjects lost their tactile sense after 19.2 minutes, their passive kinesthetic sense after 22 minutes, and their active kinesthetic sense after 22.4 minutes. The experimental methods employed in this investigation offer investigators ideas on how to study the function of kinesthesis when one learns and performs skilled movements. A complete description of the compression block technique is described by Laszlo and Bairstow (1971), which they feel is safe and useful in examining movement control in the absence of the kinesthesis. Further analysis of this technique suggests that it does not eliminate feedback in certain situations and that there is serious gamma impairment affecting fine motor control. Nevertheless, sensory restriction has provided a means for psychologists to determine sensory involvement in behavior, learning, and perception.

In summary, a variety of methods of measuring aspects of kinesthesis can be found in the literature. In a general sense, kinesthesis is believed to underlie many discriminating functions of the body required for successful motor skill performance: locomotion, perception of pressure changes, balance and body equilibrium, and overall body coordination. Its presence is thought to contribute to an individual's ability to learn as well as to perform motor skills. However, this presence must not be thought of as a general factor but rather as specific to the skill or a group of skills that requires certain movements of the body.

The reason for this conclusion is twofold: (1) correlations among tests that presumably evaluate the level of kinesthetic sense within a person are fairly low in various studies; and (2) physiological evidence indicates that the nature and extent of recruitment and use of motor units and sense receptors are fairly specialized and unique to each act. As performance level in an activity improves, there is every reason to believe that kinesthetic information is used more effectively, whether consciously or subconsciously.

Speed of Movement

Although the average person tends to look at performance speed and use certain descriptive terms in general and conflicting ways, researchers have been more precise in their analysis. It is not unusual for three people to view the same athletic activity and for one to remark about the athletes' reflexes, another about their reactions, and the third about their movement speed.

Reaction time (RT) involves an integration of the higher centers of the nervous system: perception of the stimulus (a noise, light, or the like) and the initiation of the appropriate movement. It is the elapsed interval of time from the presentation of a stimulus to the initiation of a response. A *reflex* is usually nonvolitional, involving the lower centers of the nervous system. It is an automatic response, predictable, and does not require perceptibility.

Movement time (MT) is usually viewed in research literature as the time a particular action takes to be completed after it has been initiated. *Response time* is the time it takes to complete the entire movement and includes the other times mentioned here (see Figure 7-12).

The time elapsed from the pistol shot to the sprinter's response is referred to as RT. From that point to the completion of the race, the time recorded is actually movement time. Obviously, a typical time for the track athlete includes both RT and MT. It is often taken for granted, but the initial reaction to a stimulus may be as important as running speed, especially in the short sprints. The time it takes to react to a stimulus may provide information concerning potential success or failure in the events, as is running speed in different phases of the race.

If the track athlete were standing on a shock source at the starting line, the

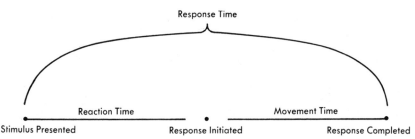

FIGURE 7-12. Relationship of reaction time, movement time, and response time.

MOTOR LEARNING AND HUMAN PERFORMANCE

time elapsed from the stimulation to the initiation of movement would be recorded as *reflex time*. Because a reflex requires neither willed movements nor judgment, it may be expected that an individual's reflex time will be faster than his or her RT.

Performance-time factors are of obvious interest to athletes and coaches. But they also have concerned researchers for many years, for different reasons. Many mental processes underlying performance have been inferred from the results of studies in which RT has been collected under various circumstances. For instance, when viewing a person as a processor of information, RT experiments have been used to provide data to suggest functions related to capacity, attention demands, decision making, and the like.

Historically, H. von Helmholtz conducted the first reaction time experiment in 1850 in order to assess nerve conduction speeds. F. C. Donders, in 1868, established three prototype simple and choice reaction-time experimental designs in order to calculate the time elapsed for certain mental operations. He identified nonoverlapping serial stages in the processing of information. By constructing basic paradigms, he was able to use a subtractive method to determine the time it took the average person to recognize or identify a stimulus or to select a response. These studies, as well as the more powerful experimental techniques devised by Saul Sternberg, are analyzed by Massaro (1975).

Sternberg (1969a, 1969b) accepted the beliefs of Donder's critics that the manipulation of a particular stage would affect the operations of another stage. Using what he termed the additive-factor method, Sternberg did not attempt to add a stage of processing in his experiments but rather to influence the amount of processing at a particular stage. By increasing the number and nature of alternatives, such as stimuli and response compatibility conditions, he demonstrated how a task can be analyzed as to the number of stages of processing involved, how a particular stage is influenced by the interactive influence of specified variables, and that the time it takes for a particular stage, such as stimulus recognition, to transpire will depend on the nature and effects of the interactive variables. Even the typical RT experiment, which appears so simple, involves a series of complicated information-processing stages, from signal detection, to recognition, to response selection, to the actual response.

Physiologists and experimental psychologists have investigated and suggested theories about other internal mechanisms activated during a response. For example, J. Botwinick and C. W. Thompson (1966) have proposed that RT be thought of as involving premotor and motor time. Premotor time includes the time elapsed from the stimulus presentation to the muscle firing, and motor time describes the point when the muscle fires to the actual response, which, in the study, was a finger lift. Results of this study indicated that premotor and reaction time are highly related; no direct relationship could be discerned between motor and reaction time.

Some researchers, interested in the characteristics of performers, have compared the RTs and the MTs of individuals to determine relationships between these factors; in other words, to see whether a person with a fast MT also has a fast RT.

Also compared in RTs and MTs have been select groups, such as athletes versus nonathletes. Some examples of devices and methods utilized in obtaining these data are shown in Figure 7-13.

The simplest method for deducing RT is to have a subject place the second finger on a button, with instructions to remove it after observing a light signal just above the button. The chronoscope is activated with the presentation of a stimulus and is terminated when the button is no longer depressed. In the choice RT method, the subject may be faced with a number of visual cues and is expected to react to one specific cue. Of course, the same is true for auditory cues. If reflex time is desired, the button may be wired for shock, and the response is a result of withdrawal from a noxious stimulus.

Henry (1961) has provided psychological reasoning as to why RT should be considered a separate factor from MT. Some individuals have suggested a common factor—speed—as underlying RT and MT. Henry postulates that separate mechanisms are involved in movement speed and in RT. Muscular forces cause speed of the limb movement, whereas reaction latency, a premovement operation of the central nervous system, determines RT. Henry and his co-researchers have consistently obtained near-zero correlations between RT and MT.

Most sports require fast responses to stimuli that vary in degree of predictability. Therefore, it is natural for physical education researchers to analyze the relationship of RT to athletic success. The abundance of evidence in the literature indicates that athletes do have faster RTs than nonathletes. For instance, E. A. Olson (1956) has compared athletes, nonathletes, and an intermediate group consisting of intramural and junior varsity players as well as participants in a recreation program. The athletes had the fastest reaction times. Other studies have produced similar results.

Furthermore, most of the RT and MT data collected in laboratory-controlled circumstances have revealed an independence of the factors; R. Groves (1973), using the racing start in swimming has produced similar results. RT was recorded from the pistol shot fired by the starter to the first discernible body movement (using film analysis). MT was recorded from that first movement until the subject's feet left the starting block. College varsity swimmers were used as subjects. The correlation between RT and MT was low, and only 5 per cent of the variance of RT was association with MT. Even in gross motor skills, as in laboratory artificial skills, RT and MT scores are apparently not related.

RT may be induced by the presentation of light, sound, or touch stimuli. (One source reports RTs in milliseconds, as follows: light 180, sound 140, and touch 140.) In a study by G. Forbes (1945), 178 subjects provided a mean reaction time of 28.26 hundredths of a second to a light stimulus and 19.19 hundredths of a second to a sound stimulus. Although a number of researchers hold the opinion that a person who reacts quickly to one stimulus will do so to another, Forbes obtained only a modest positive correlation of 0.43 between sound and light RTs. The intensity and distinctiveness of a particular stimulus, and in the case of sound, its audibility, as well, are factors that can alter reaction time. Other

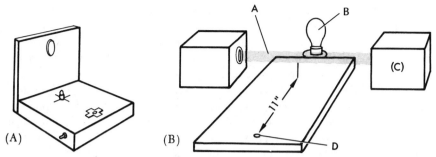

FIGURE 7-13. Tests of RT and MT. (A) Simple RT. The subject must press the button as quickly as possible when the light comes on. *(From Fleishman, E. A. A Dimensional Analysis of Motor Abilities. Journal of Experimental Psychology, 1954, 48, 437–454.)*; (B) RT and MT apparatus. At the signal of the light stimulus (B) the subject releases the reaction key (D) and attempts to move his or her hand quickly through the light beam (A) generated from the photoelectronic eye (C) at a target just behind the light beam. RT is recorded by one chronoscope that is activated on the presentation of the stimulus and broken upon the release of the key. A second chronoscope measures movement time; it is activated upon the release of the reaction key and deactivated when the hand passes through the light beam. *(From Youngen, L. A comparison of reaction and movement times of women athletes and nonathletes. Research Quarterly, 1959, 30, 349–355.)*

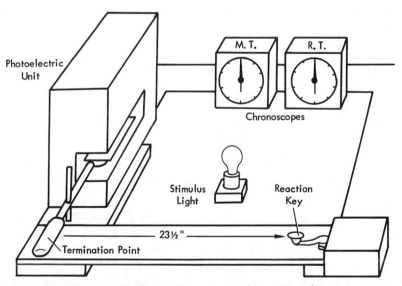

FIGURE 7-13. (continued). (C) RT and MT apparatus. The reaction chronoscope starts with the presentation of the light stimulus and stops with the release of the reaction key. The speed-of-movement chronoscope is then activated; upon contact with the terminating rod, is deactivated. *(From Hodgkins, J. Reaction time and speed of movement in males and females at various ages. Research Quarterly, 1963, 34, 335–343.)*

factors that may affect reaction time include the subject's attention, age, prior warning, fatigue, and practice.

RT, and thus performance, can be affected by numerous factors. Consider the possibility of concentrating on the movement behavior or on the stimulus. Should the competitive swimmer be tuned in to the starting gun or should attention be focused on the to-be-made starting movements? Carl McGowan (1976) has observed that the sensory set was favored for quicker reaction than the response set in a number of recent investigations. His own data have shown that stimulus intensity will make a difference in the outcome of a particular set. In other words, either set may be effective, depending on the quality of the stimulus cue.

When a person is warned of an impending event, reactions are usually quicker if the signal is presented in an optimal time frame prior to the intended action. S. M. Ross and L. E. Ross (1977) state that the optimal warning interval appears to be in the 300- to 500-milliseconds range. The signal affects the state of readiness and alertness and influences processes that occur between the stimulus and the response.

RT does not seem to be an inherent constant response to a stimulus. Rather, it varies with the existence of certain conditions:

1. RT varies according to type of stimulus (visual, auditory, tactile, olfactory, gustatory, and pain).
2. The strength and/or duration of the stimulus influences the RT.
3. Another factor influencing RT is readiness for response: whether the subject is warned before the response and the length of time before the actual stimulus presentation.
4. A very important factor is practice, as RT usually improves with increased practice.
5. Reaction time also seems to improve to a point with age in youth and then worsens during old age.
6. Choice RT lengthens when the number of stimuli presented and number of responses from which to select are increased.

THE STUDY OF INDIVIDUAL DIFFERENCES

It has been argued for some time that behavior is studied from two vantage points: (1) from experimental data, with which groups of subjects are compared and inferences made about the "average" person from cause-and-effect relationships with appropriate statistics; and (2) from descriptive data, analyzed with correlations, factor analyses, and the like, to determine normative data on certain characteristics or the way individuals are likely to differ with regard to them. The study of individual differences, of human abilities and characteristics, has generally but not exclusively fallen into the latter category.

Interestingly enough, differences among individual subjects in the same group are a nuisance to experimenters attempting to determine significant treatment effects. The more limited the spread of scores around mean, the smaller the magnitude of individual differences, the smaller the "within-group error" score. Because this score is in the denominator of the fraction in which the treatment difference score is in the numerator of statistical models, we can readily see that if individual differences can be minimized, the smaller the denominator in proportion to the numerator, the better the probability of demonstrating statistically significant effects. Differential psychologists, on the other hand, are very much concerned with individual scores. Their research has been oriented to measuring individual differences in abilities, interests, aptitudes, and personality. The relationship of factors with practice and the psychological processes that accompany learning are also in their province of study. The extensive work of Fleishman (e.g., 1972a, 1972b) has been alluded to in reference to psychomotor abilities, their measurement, and their contribution to success in various tasks. But his is one approach in this area, adhering to a changing person (abilities) model with practice. Another approach is to view tasks as changing in demands as skill is acquired.

Person and Task Models

Because the work of Fleishman has already been alluded to, let us examine M. B. Jones' method of studying individual differences. Jones has unearthed interesting patterns with correlational analyses that seem to develop with more practice. One general observation is that, with more practice trials and higher mean scores, trial variances tend to increase as well, and vice versa. Individual scores surrounding the mean usually vary more as scores improve with practice.

Jones (1972) has identified the *superdiagonal form* that emerges when correlations among practice trials are examined. The correlations between any two trials are highest when the trials compared are closer together. The more removed the trials—say, the first and last of a number of trials—the lower the correlation. Table 7-1 illustrates this point. For example, the correlation between trials 1 and 2

TABLE 7-1 Means, Standard Deviations, and Intertrial Correlations for the Two-Hand Coordination Test*

Trial	1	2	3	4	5	6	7	8	$\bar{X}$	SD
1	—	0.79	0.77	0.74	0.73	0.71	0.71	0.70	34.9	11.8
2		—	0.87	0.87	0.84	0.82	0.82	0.82	42.9	14.9
3			—	0.91	0.89	0.87	0.85	0.86	46.1	15.8
4				—	0.91	0.88	0.86	0.88	50.4	16.2
5					—	0.89	0.90	0.90	54.7	18.9
6						—	0.93	0.93	58.1	18.1
7							—	0.94	61.0	18.6
8								—	63.3	18.7

*Jones, M. B. Practice as a process of simplification. *Psychological Review*, 1962, **69**, 274–294. Copyright 1962 by the American Psychological Association. Reprinted by permission.

on the two-hand coordination test is 0.79; between trials 1 and 5 it is 0.73 and between 1 and 8 it is 0.70. Note that the variances expressed in the form of standard deviations (SD) increase, as do the mean scores, with each trial. Furthermore, each succeeding pair of trials yields a higher correlation until the process of stabilization in scores sets in.

Jones recommends that the analysis of learning center on stabilization, which is the terminal process in learning. An average score on all terminal scores (as many trials as appropriate for score stabilization to be demonstrated through statistical analysis) would constitute the subject's learning score—finished or accomplished skill. Bradley, as we saw earlier when discussing learning curves, questioned whether a final asymptote is ever reached in performance. Although he makes some valid points, it is possible, as Jones and other writers have pointed out, to select what appears to be those trials in which reasonable score stabilization occurs to be used as the learning score.

Further implications from Jones' efforts parallel those that can be made from the work of Fleishman. Initial task performance is often related to general abilities, with differences in performance primarily the result of the presence of these abilities in desired amounts. As practice proceeds, differences among performers can be ascribed to task-specific requirements. The natural consequence of this relationship is the realization that prediction of terminal proficiency from initial performance is extremely tenuous with complex tasks in which an adequate amount of practice is provided. Jones and Fleishman, in attacking the prediction problem from different research strategies, generally agree that the relationship between usual task predictors and actual performance diminishes as a function of practice. Kenneth Alvares and Charles Hulin (1972) provide an excellent review of the two approaches and attempt to resolve theoretical differences.

The superdiagonal matrix shows adjacent trials to be highly related but more distant ones to be less so, and the study of abilities as task predictors reveals poorer predictability with increased time and/or practice. Alvares and Hulin (1973) suggest that apparently different and conflicting models (e.g., Jones versus Fleishman) are really descriptions of the same underlying phenomena. In Jones's approach, fewer and fewer factors are posited to contribute to successful performance with practice. Fleishman believes that abilities contribute more or less to successful performance, depending on the status of the learner, with less of them of primary influence with increased performance level. The conflict, as Alvares and Hulin 1973) see it, is between belief in the "changing subject model" or the "changing task model." In the latter case, it is believed that the structure of the task undergoes change with practice and the acquisition of skill. The task is defined by the set of abilities necessary for performance. In the former case, it is believed that training changes the magnitude of the abilities. Alvares and Hulin suggest that the finding of decreasing correlations with more remote trials occurs because of changes in abilities rather than changes in the structure of the task.

Support for the notion of changing levels of abilities resulting from training is offered by Alvares and Hulin (1973), although in another article (1972) they do stress that both models can adequately offer post hoc explanations for the available data. Is it wiser to analyze the task according to ability requirements of a person with various ability dimensions that change with experience? In order to predict performance effectively, tests must be developed that will tap the ability requirements for termination-of-practice accomplishments, and cues and abilities most important at different stages of practice would be emphasized. Otherwise, equations must be established that predict changes in ability level. This approach, associated with the changing subject model, is a more dynamic and perhaps a potentially more fruitful area of investigation.

Intraindividual Factors

The study of intraindividual variability as related to experimental procedures and learning and performance variables provides additional insight into differential learning processes. The novice realizes that individuals will differ in performed scores at any time. However, the components of these scores deserve special consideration, for theoretical and practical purposes. Differences in scores do not necessarily reflect true score differences. Other factors that might influence performance include trial-to-trial fluctuations resulting from any one of a number of personal reasons, as well as variable errors, in the form of limitations in apparatus or weaknesses on observation. The total variability that is observed in the performances of a sample of subjects consists of true score variance (individual differences), intraindividual variance, and error variance. Individual difference scores result from all these scores.

Given that r_{ab} = the correlation between any pair of trials:

S_a^2 and S_b^2 = the observed variance of subjects' scores for any two trials
S_t^2 = true score (interindividual, individual difference variance)
S_x^2 = intraindividual variance

interindividual and intraindividual variances are computed in the following way:

$$S_x^2 = \frac{S_a^2 + S_b^2}{2} = \text{average variance for a group of subjects for a pair of trials}$$
$$S_t^2 = r_{ab} S_x^2 \quad = \text{individual difference variance.}$$

Using these formulas, Welch and Henry (1971) found that stabilometer task practice of twelve trials per day for six days yielded interindividual and intraindividual variations that decreased exponentially as a function of the amount of practice. However, they point out that there was an increase in both factors with practice in ratio of variability to mean score. In this study, individuals tended to become more alike in performance as practice increased, a finding that is not typical with complex learning tasks.

Stelmach (1969) tested subjects on a stabilometer for eight continuous minutes and recorded scores every thirty seconds. He found that true score variance (individual difference) increased slightly with practice. Intraindividual ability was relatively unaffected by continuous practice, but when performance improvement was canceled by examining relative variability, both sources of variance increased. Intraindividual variability, repeated scores on the same subjects, interpreted as consistency in motor response, was found by Albert Carron (1970) to be moderately reliable but tended to be specific to particular response components.

It has been questioned whether response inconsistency is a random or a systematic variable, or a biological phenomenon. Many researchers favor the notion of systematic influences on performance inconsistencies. A number of studies indicate that the imposed practice conditions will differentially affect inter- and intraindividual variances. For instance, Stelmach (1968) found the true score variance to decrease 49 per cent under distributed practice conditions. Intraindividual variance decreased 37 per cent with distributed practice and 11 per cent with massed practice.

A review of the recent literature on the topic of interindividual and intraindividual variance changes with practice indicates that individual differences become greater with practice, whereas intraindividual variations diminish. The study of individual differences helps us to determine the nature of inter- and intraindividual variability of performance scores. With more literature, trends in the data will become more apparent in order that generalizations can be made. Actually, differential psychology, or the analysis of individual differences, is associated with research on personal abilities and characteristics. The establishment of normative behavior and ranges of deviation has provided a means of learning more about individuals and how they may be expected to perform in certain situations. Marteniuk (1974) has written on excellent chapter on individual differences related to motor behavior that can provide more perspectives than possible here. Respect for individual differences in learning styles, motives, and other characteristics can be reflected by sensitive designs for instruction, a topic to which we will now turn.

INSTRUCTIONAL CONSIDERATIONS

If all teacher-learner situations were on a one-to-one basis, individual considerations would be maximized. Unfortunately, most training and instructional programs involve a high proportion of learners to one instructor. Principles of instruction, generally favorable to most learners in a group, can probably be identified and implemented.

Yet, it must be recognized that learners differ in many ways, notably in motivation, rate of learning, and strategies and techniques for learning. For the learning of written material, it has been possible to develop alternative and individualized learning mediums with the use of advanced technology. Students can thus work at their own speed and with personally selected materials and means of learning. It is possible to develop similar approaches to the learning of fine motor skills. But gross motor skills, to be performed with and against others, do not lend themselves so easily to self-directed and individualized learning.

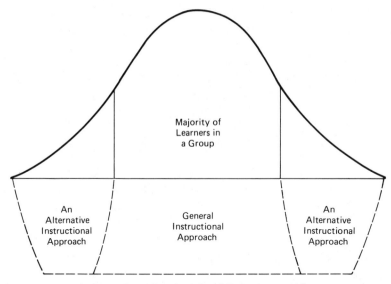

FIGURE 7-14. Considerations for different types of learners.

Although individual accommodations are more limited in the learning of gross motor activities than for written matter, sensitivity is advised for students not apparently orienting well to the general instructional technique decided on by the instructor for the group. On a probability basis, we might expect learners in general to respond acceptably to well-designed and formulated instructional programs, based on approaches consistent with scientific findings. Exceptions will be noted, as well. Figure 7-14 suggests a basic instructional approach for most students, and possible alternative approaches for small groups at either end of the continuum.

Aptitude and Instruction Interaction

A number of conditions have influenced the recognition of the important ways learners may differ from each other and what the potential outcomes are for alternative instructional approaches for them. The advancement of cognitive psychology, in contrast to behaviorism, has led to the analysis of various internal processes that operate within people. People can be categorized in the way they view and respond to learning situations.

A number of concerned citizens and educators have philosophized about the right of all students to learn and achieve. This has led to the development and evaluation of various experimental educational programs and courses. Culturally disadvantaged and handicapped children of all types have been studied. In particular courses, students with dissimilar cognitive styles or aptitudes have been instructed differentially with the intent of producing favorable outcomes for all. L. J. Cronbach and R. E. Snow (1977) have written a powerful argument recognizing that differential aptitudes can predict learning outcomes as well as often interact with alternative instructional conditions. Their position is that a particular type of method would be more appropriate for some learners.

Unfortunately, the efforts of Cronbach, Snow, and others have been directed to cognitive materials rather than motor skills. Therefore, it is through extrapolation and implication that we can assume that instruction should be adapted to learners of skills as it might be for other learning matter. No one learning condition is optimum for everyone. No one instructional model of prescription fits all people. The challenge for researchers is to determine the critical factors to consider, while instructional designers must implement and incorporate these findings into meaningful programs.

In what ways do individual differences influence instructional theory and practice? Snow (1977) has stressed persuasively that individual differences must be considered (1) in the formulation of models of learning integrated to incorporate notions of normative as well as individual expectations; (2) at the onset of a learning experience, as the initial state of the learner includes present knowledge, motivation, problem-solving abilities, personality traits, and other characteristics; and (3) as they interact with specific instructional treatments to produce certain outcomes. Snow describes other points, but these should suffice here as indicants of the primary ones.

We do not know enough about the aptitudes of learners and special treatments for them in the learning of motor skills in general, or for that matter, for specific categories of skills. There is no doubt, however, that motor learning research will progress to help answer the many questions related to this topic.

CHAPTER HIGHLIGHTS

1. Normative data are often calculated with regard to abilities, aptitudes, and learning level, but individual scores vary around the mean score; the extent of that variation is determined by the nature of the sample, the test, and the testing situation.

2. The terms *skill* and *ability* often have been used interchangeably, but they should be distinguished: skill refers to a well-defined act, but an ability is an enduring and somewhat stable trait, partially underlying success in related skills. Unfortunately, abilities are difficult to measure directly, and when they are, they become another skill test.

3. Tests that presumably assess motor ability, motor educability, and motor capacity have limited value in their stated purposes. Rather than think in terms of the existence of a general motor ability within a person, it is more profitable to expect that each person possesses different levels of a number of abilities based on genetic and experiential factors.

4. Much laboratory research, artificially contrived, has tended to support the idea of task specificity rather than task generality. Prediction of task performance from performance on another task is usually inadequate, and achievement in activities is somewhat specific to the person and the activity. There are exceptions, of course. Success in real-life endeavors is dependent on existing

abilities and capabilities brought to the learning situation, but task specific practice is required for highly skilled behaviors.

5. Psychomotor abilities have been deduced from logical reasoning or factor-analytic studies, but an acceptable taxonomy or description has yet to be developed.

6. Abilities and tasks related to coordination, kinesthesis, balance. and speed of movement (reaction time, movement time, response time) have been of the greatest concern to motor learning researchers. Tasks that primarily measure each of these factors have not correlated well with each other; i.e., test scores on coordination tasks seem to be somewhat independent of each other. It is probably impossible to tap only one ability in one test. However, many of these tasks have provided important information in regard to learning processes and have aided in the ultimate prediction in activity performances in certain cases.

7. The study of individual differences through factor-analytic and correlation approaches has given rise to two models: the changing task model, and the changing person (ability) model. Either the structure of the activity changes with practice and improvement, thereby making different demands on the learner; or the task is constant, however, and different abilities play different roles in various stages of practice.

8. Intraindividual (within subjects) and interindividual (between subjects) variations have been studied across practice trials, with differential trends in the data noted by researchers.

9. A growing body of literature in the cognitive area has been termed aptitude and instructional (treatment) interaction. Aptitudes (the learner status prior to a learning experience) and specific instructional conditions interact to produce the most beneficial outcomes. The optimum learning condition is unique from person to person. It is hoped that more research will be conducted with psychomotor skills so that abilities and capabilities can be identified and matched to pertinent learning conditions.

References

Alvares, K. M., & Hulin, C. L. Two explanations of temporal changes in ability-skill relationships: A literature review and theoretical analysis. *Human Factors*, 1972, *14*, 295–308.

Alvares, K. M., & Hulin, C. L. An experimental evaluation of a temporal decay in the prediction of performance. *Organizational Behavior and Human Performance*, 1973, *9*, 169–185.

Bechtoldt, H. G. Motor abilities in studies of motor learning. In L. Smith (Ed.), *Psychology of motor learning* (Proceedings of CIC, Symposium on Psychology of Motor Learning). Chicago: The Athletic Institute, 1970.

Botwinick, J., & Thompson, C. W. Premotor and motor components of reaction time. *Journal of Experimental Psychology*, 1966, *71*, 9–15.

Carron, A. V. Intra-task reliability and specificity of individual consistency. *Perceptual and Motor Skills*, 1970, *30*, 583–587.

Cronbach, L. J. How can instruction be adapted to individual differences? In R. M. Gagné (Ed.), *Learning and individual differences*. Columbus, Ohio: Charles E. Merrill, 1967.

Cronbach, L. J., & Snow, R. E. *Aptitudes and instructional methods: A handbook for research on interactions*. New York: Irvington, 1977.

Edington, D. W., & Edgerton, V. R. *The biology of physical activity*. Englewood Cliffs, N.J.: Prentice Hall, 1976.

Fleishman, E. A. A comparative study of aptitude patterns in unskilled and skilled psychomotor performers. *Journal of Applied Psychology*, 1957, *41*, 263–272.

Fleishman, E. A. An analysis of positioning movements and static reactions. *Journal of Experimental Psychology*, 1958, *55*, 13–24. (a)

Fleishman, E. A. Dimensional analysis of movement reactions. *Journal of Experimental Psychology*, 1958, *55*, 438–453. (b)

Fleishman, E. A. *The structure and measurement of physical fitness*. Englewood Cliffs, N.J.: Prentice-Hall, 1964.

Fleishman, E. A. On the relation between abilities, learning, and human performance. *American Psychologist*, 1972, *27*, 1017–1032. (a)

Fleishman, E. A. Structure and measurement of psychomotor abilities. In R. N. Singer (Ed.), *The psychomotor domain: Movement behavior*. Philadelphia: Lea & Febiger, 1972. (b)

Fleishman, E. A., & Hempel, W. E., Jr. Changes in factor structure of a complex psychomotor test as a function of practice. *Psychometrika*, 1954, *19*, 239–252.

Fleishman, E. A., & Stephenson, R. W. *Development of a taxonomy of human performance: A review of the third year's progress*. Washington, D.C.: American Institutes for Research, 1970.

Forbes, G. The effect of certain variables on visual and auditory reaction times. *Journal of Experimental Psychology*, 1945, *35*, 153–162.

Groves, R. Relationship of reaction time and movement time in a gross motor skill. *Perceptual and Motor Skills*, 1973, *36*, 453–454.

Hempel, W. E., Jr., & Fleishman, E. A. A factor analysis of physical proficiency and manipulative skill. *Journal of Applied Psychology*, 1955, *39*, 12–16.

Henry, F. M. Dynamic kinesthetic perception and adjustment. *Research Quarterly*, 1953, *24*, 176–187.

Henry, F. M. Reaction time-movement time correlations. *Perceptual and Motor Skills*, 1961, *12*, 63–66.

Hopkins, B. Proprioception and/or kinesthesis. *Perceptual and Motor Skills*, 1972, *34*, 431–435.

Jones, M. B. Individual differences. In R. N. Singer (Ed.), *The psychomotor domain: Movement behavior*. Philadelphia: Lea & Febiger, 1972.

Laszlo, J. I. The performance of a simple motor task with kinesthetic sense loss. *Quarterly Journal of Experimental Psychology*, 1966, *18*, 1–8.

Laszlo, J. I., & Bairstow, P. J. The compression block technique: A note on procedure. *Journal of Motor Behavior*, 1971, *3*, 313–317.

Levin, J. *Learner differences: Diagnosis and prescription*. N.Y.: Holt, Rinehart & Winston, 1977.

Loockerman, W. D., & Berger, R. A. Specificity and generality between various directions for reaction and movement times under choice stimulus conditions. *Journal of Motor Behavior*, 1972, *4*, 31–35.

Lotter, W. S. Specificity or generality of speed of systematically related movements. *Research Quarterly,* 1961, *32,* 55–62.

Marteniuk, R. G. Individual differences in motor performance and learning. In J. H. Wilmore (Ed.), *Exercise and sport sciences reviews* (Vol. 2). New York: Academic Press, 1974.

Massaro, D. W. *Experimental psychology and information processing.* Chicago: Rand McNally, 1975.

McGowan, C. The effect of motor and sensory set on reaction time and muscle electrical activity. *Research Quarterly,* 1976, *47,* 709–715.

Olson, E. A. Relationship between psychological capacities and success in college athletics. *Research Quarterly,* 1956, *27,* 79– 89.

Roberts, D. M. Abilities and learning: A brief review and discussion of empirical studies. *Journal of School Psychology,* 1968–69, *7,* 12–21.

Roloff, L. L. Kinesthesis in relation to the learning of selected motor skills. *Research Quarterly,* 1953, *24,* 210–217.

Ross, S. M., & Ross, L. E. Warning signals and alerting: Effects on differential classical conditioning. *Journal of Experimental Psychology: Human Learning and Memory,* 1977, *3,* 590–599.

Sanford, N. Higher education as a field of study. In N. Sanford (Ed.), *The American college.* New York: John Wiley, 1962.

Scott, M. G. Assessment of motor ability of college women through objective tests. *Research Quarterly,* 1955, *10,* 63–83.

Singer, R. N. Interlimb skill ability in motor skill performance. *Research Quarterly* 1966, *37,* 406–410.

Singer, R. N. Balance skill as related to athletics, sex, height, and weight. In G. S. Kenyon (Ed.), *Contemporary psychology of sport: Proceedings of the Second International Congress of Sport Psychology.* Chicago: Athletic Institute, 1970.

Slater-Hammel, A. T. Measurement of kinesthetic perception of muscular force with muscle potential changes. *Research Quarterly,* 1957, *28,* 153–159.

Smith, L. E. Influence of neuromotor program alteration on the speed of a standard arm movement. *Perceptual and Motor Skills,* 1962, *15,* 327–330.

Snow, R. E. Individual differences and instructional theory. *Educational Researcher,* 1977, *6,* 11–15.

Stelmach, G. E. Distribution of practice in individual differences and intra-variability. *Perceptual and Motor Skills,* 1968, *26,* 727–730.

Stelmach, G. E. Individual differences and intra-individual variability in motor performance under continuous-practice conditions. *Human Factors,* 1969, *11,* 201–206.

Sternberg, S. Memory-scanning: Mental processes revealed by reaction-time experiments. *American Scientist,* 1969, *57,* 421–457.

Sternberg, S. The discovery of processing stages: Extensions of Donder's method. *Acta Psychologica,* 1969, *30,* 276–315. (b)

Travis, R. C. An experimental analysis of dynamic and static equilibrium. *Journal of Experimental Psychology,* 1945, *35,* 216–234.

Wiebe, V. R. A study of tests of kinesthesis. *Research Quarterly,* 1954, *25,* 222–230.

Welch, M., & Henry, F. M. Individual differences in various parameters. *Journal of Motor Behavior,* 1971, *31,* 78–96.

8 OTHER PERSONAL FACTORS RELATED TO SKILLED PERFORMANCE

As noted in Chapter 7, abilities and capabilities differ among individual learners. The same instructional circumstances for all participants in a program do not lead typically to similar performance levels for them. In this chapter, additional factors that make up "the personal equation" will be described.

The performance of various skills may be handicapped for many reasons, among them a lack of adequate physical qualities necessary for the skilled movement. All the appropriate teaching methods and understandings of the learning process will be of little use if the performer does not have, say, enough strength or endurance to undertake the task. Specific acts require the use of and emphasis on unique qualities. Consider, if you will, physical and motor attributes, the senses, and cognitive and perceptual processes, which vary among learners and which are involved in unique ways from task to task. Emotional and motivational states differ from individual to individual and situation to situation. These individual difference variables must be understood and considered as training programs are devised.

PHYSICAL CHARACTERISTICS

Body Build

The idea of classifying a person according to physical structure is by no means new. From the days of ancient Greece when body types were classified as *phthisic habitus* (long and thin) and *apoplectic habitus* (short and thick), to the early 1920s and Kretschmer's concepts of typing, *pyknic* (squat and compact), *asthenic* (thin, anemic in appearance), and *athletic* (muscular) types, and finally including Sheldon's (Sheldon, Stevens, and Tucker, 1940) concept of *somatotyping,* various methods of body typing have been employed. Sheldon's method and the suggested modifications initiated by various researchers have become widely recognized as the most promising and accurate means of body classification.

In order to classify individuals, Sheldon designated three types: *endomorph* (round and soft body), *mesomorph* (muscular and masculine looking), and *ectomorph* (tall and thin, linearly constructed). Individuals are photographed, and then rated by judges on a 1 to 7 scale for each type, according to the degree of dominance. The somatotypes are described by three numerals, each of which contains a number ranging from 1 to 7, with 7 indicating the highest presence of certain components. The descriptive sequence of numbers refers to the components in the following order: endomorph, mesomorph, and ectomorph. Thus, a rating of 1–7–1 indicates extreme mesomorphy, 7–1–1 extreme endomorphy, and 1–1–7 extreme ectomorphy. In actuality, an individual will have certain amounts of each component and is thus not specifically one type. In all, eighty-eight different somatotypes have been recognized.

Of particular interest is the question of whether certain body types are associated with success in specific activities. For instance, Olympic athletes have been analyzed and categorized according to body structure. During the 1960 Olympics, J. M. Tanner (1964) compiled data on 137 track and field athletes; they were somatotyped and classified by event. His results indicate distinct somatotypes for the different events. For example, a somatotype of 3–6–2 was designated to the discus, shot, and hammer throwers; 2–5–3 for the sprinters; 2½–4–4 for the middle- and long-distance runners; and 2–6–2 to 2–3–6 for the high jumpers.

Present methods indicate a refinement of the original somatotyping techniques, and the usage of somatotypes is widespread. There have been attempts to determine the body types of successful athletes in various sports so as best to predict the achievement one might expect in a given sport. Although there are exceptions, research has shown some relationship of body type to given sports.

In some sports, it is important to have momentary muscular strength, and a muscular and stout build promotes successful performance for such events as weight lifting, wrestling, short-distance cycling, and throwing events. Longer-distance track events require more endurance than strength, and the combination of an efficient cardiorespiratory system with a ligher weight results in better performance times. In general, the evidence in K. Hirata's (1966) study of the Olympic Games in Tokyo appears to justify the idea that physique and constitution have an important effect on athletic performance, at least when the athletes have trained to top-level physical condition. Hirata expresses the opinion that the individual with the most adequate physique will win an event when the participants in that event have all trained hard and achieved maximal physical condition. Certainly cultural, socioeconomic, and peer influences should not be overlooked as important determiners of activity interests and success.

Investigators concerned with body builds have noted a positive relationship between mesomorphy and athletic performance and a negative correlation between endomorphy and athletic performance, greater strength and general physical fitness with mesomorphy, and better balance and flexibility with ectomorphy. An important consideration is that *although a certain body type or build may contribute to success in specific activities, it is by no means necessary.* Skill attainment is the result of many complex factors, and a limiting body structure may very well be overcome by an emphasis on other variables.

Strength

There is no doubt that, in varying degrees, strength underlies all motor performance. In an isolated sense, *strength* may be thought of as the capacity of a muscle or group of muscles to exert maximum pressure against a given resistance in a limited period of time. A weakness in any area of the body may severely limit the coordination and effort needed for the performance of a skill. Thus, a minium amount of strength is a necessity for motor skill performance. The type and location of strength necessary for performance are unique for each activity.

Muscular Endurance

The capacity of a muscle or a group of muscles to contract repeatedly against a moderate resistance reflects *muscular endurance*. The individual must maintain a moderate energy output over an extended duration of time. Whether it be muscular or cardiovascular in nature, endurance permits the individual to prolong the performance of an act. Although the constant practice of a skill promotes improvement, a degree of muscular as well as mental endurance is needed in order for the performer to be able to concentrate at length on the skill itself. Many motor skills are arduous to learn and perform, and the development of such physical qualities as strength and endurance delays fatigue, thus permitting attention to be focused for a longer period of time on the skill to be learned.

Flexibility

Flexibility is determined by the range of movement of a joint. Joint flexibility is related to the nature of the joint structure, the condition of the ligaments and fascia that surround the joint, and muscle extensibility. A flexible range of motion is needed by athletes, especially those in track and swimming.

This premise has been verified by Thomas Cureton (1951), who found above-average flexibility in the champion athletes he measured from 1946 to 1948. In one study, he found the 1936 Japanese champion Olympic swimmers to have 31 per cent greater trunk flexion than the American swimmers. In comparing twenty-one Olympic swimmers with one hundred college competitive swimmers, the Olympians proved to be superior in ankle flexion by 11 per cent and in trunk flexion by 8 per cent. Flexibility is a physical quality involved in many skilled motor patterns, and its inadequate development may well be regarded as another possible deterrent to achievement in certain sports.

Level of Physical Condition

The presence of ideal physical characteristics for performance is related to the learner's state of physical training or level of physical condition. These qualities cannot be taken for granted in gross motor activities. And, to repeat a point made in Chapter 7, training is specific to the unique demands placed on the person by the particular activity.

An intelligent and sensitive teacher would anlayze carefully the physical demands placed on learners attempting to acquire skill in an activity. Deficiencies in learners in pertinent physical characteristics should be noted and remedial programs proposed to develop any insufficient flexibility, strength, or endurance underlying potential achievement in a particular task. Remember that a person can learn a task but may not have the means to practice adequately and perform what is known! Task analysis and personality analysis will be helpful to facilitate the goals of any instructional program in which gross motor skills are to be learned. As a training regimen, much research in exercise physiology supports the idea of specificity: that training induces adaptations at the local muscle level. Recent subcellular research (McCafferty & Horvath, 1977) with regard to metabolic activity and the involvement of different muscle fiber types also supports the concept of specificity of exercise. In drawing implications for the training of athletes, McCafferty and Horvath state that exercise and athletic training must be specific in order to stress the energy sources demanded by a certain activity. The same would also hold true for nonathletes.

THE SENSES

While physical characteristics and motor abilities are always emphasized for successful motor skill performance, the senses are often taken for granted. Those remarkable sense organs have the ability to detect minor changes in stimuli. Such senses as taste and smell rarely function as part of the typical performance of motor skills. Hearing, of course, plays an important role in isolated instances, such as responding to the starting gun in an athletic event. Learners must be able to hear and understand directions, in order to tune in to verbal cues when they are given. The importance of *vision, equilibrium,* and *proprioception* to skilled performance is obvious. The range of function in the various sense organs among individuals is great, another contributing factor in the potential to learn and perform effectively.

Vision

During the initial photoelectronic process of visual activity, retinal potentials are formed. Messages, in the form of impulses, are sent by certain ganglion cells of the retina to the visual region of the occipital cortex. There is a perceptive interpretation of the information in this area. In most sports, this perceptive analysis must occur in a matter of moments if the performer is to react successfully to given stimuli, which are often unpredictable in nature. The importance of early, normal visual experience for the development of visual capacities is stressed by Robert McCleary (1970). In order to determine accurately the spatial location of objects, one must first have meaningful and integrated visual and motor experiences.

Any malfunctioning link in the human subsystems that lead to intended behavior will create noise (potential error signals) in the system. In the learning and performance of many motor skills, specific types of visual information must be received and attended to correctly. Static or dynamic visual acuity may be required of the person, depending on the nature of the activity. Obviously, dynamic visual acuity is much more demanding, especially with a moving object (e.g., a baseball) which must be attended to quickly (e.g., with a bat). G. S. D. Morris (1977), states that a ball traveling at 80 miles per hour allows .51 of a second of viewing time; 60 miles per hour = .68 of a second, and 40 miles per hour = 1.02 seconds. The velocity and direction of an object in movement must be received by the ocular apparatus and perceived in time to allow an appropriate response. Morris, recognizing the sparse literature dealing with dynamic visual acuity, suggests that this quality should be assessed in athletes who compete in sports in which projectiles move at great speeds. The information could be helpful in predicting potential success or in suggesting when activities should be directed to help improve acuity.

Many investigations in the psychological literature yield results that stress the importance of vision, in addition to tactile and kinesthetic experience, in learning skills. Evidently, even for skills that require no perception of a changing external field, vision enhances performance. Yet, the performer does not always attend to all available information, as R. B. Wilberg (1969) has shown with kinesthetic cues. However, individuals can be trained to make use of minimal visual information in given situations. In such tasks as balancing, restricted peripheral vision is apt to diminish performance. There are probably many occasions when learners need to be instructed about how to gain more information from the presence of visual cues.

A comparison of twins, one blind from birth and the other with full vision, was made by H. G. Williams and V. L. Blane (1969). Activities involving large amounts of space or powerful and fast movements of the body favored the sighted subject. Smaller space areas in which manipulation tasks occur favored the nonsighted subject. "Thus, where total body involvement was minimal and fine manipulative movements of the hands and fingers were stressed, lack of visual information seemed to have little effect. Frequently, blindness seemed to enhance the performance of such tasks, since the nonsighted individual was forced to rely upon other sources of sensory information as a basis for performing daily tasks" (p. 271). If the task permits compensation for sensory impairment, learning can occur effectively.

The relationship of visual attributes—e.g., depth perception, spatial orientation, and visual acuity—to skilled performance has been the topic of some investigations. The hypothesis tested is that the presence of high-quality visual sense apparatus is associated with greater proficiency in those tasks requiring visual scanning, spatial orientation, and target shooting. In a recent study, R. D. Beals, N. M. Mayyasi, A. E. Templeton, and W. L. Johnston (1971) tested the static and dynamic visual acuity of college varsity basketball players. Shooting records from the field and foul lines were kept for all home games. A relatively high correlation of 0.76 between field shooting accuracy and dynamic visual acuity and a moderate correlation of 0.57 between field shooting accuracy and dynamic visual acuity and a moderate correlation of 0.57 between field shooting and static visual acuity was obtained. Characteristics of vision, according to these researchers, can be used reliably to predict basket shooting accuracy. Research findings are by no means in agreement. Consider, for instance, the lack of supportive evidence by Jacquelyn Shick (1971) for any relationship between foul shooting and depth perception with female college students.

Nevertheless, more theoreticians and researchers believe that vision and visual attributes contribute heavily to the learning and performance of most complex motor skills, especially in the early stages of practice. Later as acts and situations become more familiar, kinesthesis plays an important role in successful performance. The receipt of the right cues at the right time enables the subsequent processing activities to be more appropriate.

Kinesthesis

Information concerning the kinesthetic sense seems more limited than that regarding the other senses. A leading reason for this circumstance is the great difficulty researchers have in isolating this sense for study. In spite of this problem, those receptors responsible for informing the body of its change in position, direction, acceleration, and rate of movement, as well as of the relationship of its parts in space, have been demonstrated to be necessary for the smooth movements of the skilled act. Probably this sense is appreciated most by persons having visual limitations, for it is this sense they must rely on in order to perform motor skills adequately. Nevertheless, better usage of the kinesthetic sense is associated with the performer being more skilled, and research findings appear to indicate its greater presence in those who demonstrate outstanding skill in motor activities.

Touch

Closely related to the kinesthetic sense is the tactile sense. The ability to detect changes of touch and pressure involves many of the same type of proprioceptors involved in informing the body of changes in its position. Senses that enable us to feel pain, temperature changes, touch, pressure, and the body's position in space are referred to as *somatic senses*. The receptors for pressure lie deeper in the skin and tissues than those for touch, although most of the same nerve endings serve both functions. Pressure is automatically considered a type of touch sensation. In such sports as wrestling, it is important to be able to react quickly to changes in pressure applied by an opponent.

Equilibrium

The nature of body balance and equilibrium has already been discussed from physiological and psychological viewpoints. It should be sufficient merely to reiterate the role this sense plays as a basis for voluntary movement and control. Although posture and locomotion impulses can be distributed by the spinal cord alone, refinement of these impulses under changing body and environmental conditions is the responsibility of the higher nerve centers. Equilibrium must be extremely well developed in such performers as divers, trampolinists, and gymnasts, although it is obvious that most skills require a certain degree of body equilibrium.

PERCEPTION

Limited knowledge of the structures involved in perception and in the nature of the perceptual process (or processes) has proved in the past to be a difficult obstacle for psychologists to overcome in explaining learning. Perhaps this is one of the reasons why traditional S–R theory, association theory, and reflex-arc models were widely accepted in years gone by. After Gestalt theory (which was heavily oriented toward perceptual considerations, in opposition to S–R theory) made its mark in psychology in the 1920s and 1930s, its impact gradually weakened. In recent years, new research and theories have emerged from social psychologists, experimental psychologists, clinical psychologists, and physiological psychologists, once again emphasizing the role of perception as a factor in learning, adjustment, and personality. Difficulties still arise in the definition and clarification of terminology, as may be expected in an area where so many interpretations are possible, as well as plausible.

Description and Definitions

There is no doubt that the senses underlie perception and that several senses probably interact simultaneously during the perceptual process. The old idea that perception is a passive process has met with disfavor. It is now well accepted that perception, as well as learning, is an active process. It is also evident that perception depends on the psychological and physiological characteristics of the perceiver, in addition to the stimulus.

The elementary process of sensation, or receipt of information, underlies the more complex perceptual process, or making meaning of information. The senses involved will depend on the object(s) to be perceived. Perception depends on differences between stimuli and perceptibility, or ease of discrimination, and is closely related to the magnitude of the difference between stimuli. Perception is dependent on learning and is influenced by such individual factors as personality, attitudes, emotions, experience, and expectations, in addition to environmental variables. It becomes more complex as learning becomes more complex.

Perception is usually distinguished from other processes involving thought, consciousness, and judgment. It is a form of discriminating behavior involving the overall activity of the person *immediately* following stimulation of the sense organs. It may assume overt or introspective characteristics: e.g., viewing a painting is experiential, whereas reacting to a choice RT apparatus produces observable motor activity. Perception may be defined as knowledge through the senses of the existence and properties of matter and the external world. As a continuous process, perception causes actions that, in turn, change it. A clearer distinction between sensation and perception might help us to understand these terms better. *A sensation involves the means for reception of stimuli. A perception, on the other hand, involves the means for the interpretation of stimuli.*

Some scholars have found fault with the application of the same term, *perception,* to describe an act, an event, a process, and learning. C. M. Solley and G. Murphy (1960), in their book *Development of the Perceptual World,* have attempted to clarify the generalized application of perception. They have defined an event experienced as a *percept.* Perceptual learning is a change in the status of the logically inferred perceptual state or process of an individual as a result of successive applications of the operations of a learning paradigm. The perceptual act, as they theorize it to be, involves five steps: expectancy, attending, reception and sensory reactions, trial and check, and conscious perception, or organization. Perception may be a process or a product. The process is stimulation structured and is referred to as perceiving. The product of the structural process is a percept. And finally, perception, along with such processes as memory, thinking, and imagination, composes the cognitive process. So far, perception has been discussed in a general and somewhat theoretical manner. Some specific references may help to clarify this area, such as the personal variables that affect perception.

Personal Factors in Perception

Although many people may generally perceive the same cue in the same manner if it is quite obvious, differences in perceptual processing exist as a result of a variety of personal factors. Some of these factors are related to differences in

1. perceptual style (field independent versus field dependent).
2. selective attention and set.
3. motivation.
4. previous experiences similar to the present one.
5. development and maturity.

Subjects who are considered to be field independent can distinguish figures or objects from backgrounds; field-dependent subjects cannot do this so easily. *Perceptual style (field independence-field dependence)* can be assessed with the Rod and Frame Test or the embedded figures tests. In either case, a person reacts to the tests to determine his or her *figure-ground perception.* Visual-spatial organizational characteristics are determined; this information may be helpful in distinguishing field-dependent from field-independent persons and, in turn, in predicting potential for success in particular experiences involving reactions to objects in space. George Sage (1977) suggests that "although there is little empirical support at the present time, it would appear that persons who tend to be field dependent might have more difficulty in sports in which they have to catch or hit a ball [externally paced], since they tend to be poor at distinguishing figure from ground" (p. 283).

How and what one perceives in a given situation have been shown to be affected by many personal factors. The ability to attend to, or to disregard, extraneous and irrelevant information contributes to perceptibility. Selectivity in perception reduces the number of stimuli or the amount of information surrounding the object, allowing it to be perceived more easily and quickly. *Selective attention,* the process referred to, is associated with highly skilled performance. The batter concentrates on the ball and disregards irrelevant cues. Similarly, the successful shooting of a foul shot requires attention to the feel of the ball and concentration on the rim of the basket. Possibly, any awareness of the fans and their comments, of the other players, or any feelings of nervousness will contribute to the player's ineffective performance. The athlete is faced with situation after situation where appropriate cues must be discriminated and detected and irrelevant ones excluded, many times at the spur of the moment.

Actually, the amount of sensory information yielded in any situation is more than any one person can perceive. Because there are many sensory channels, much data can potentially be presented to the individual and duplicated at one time through the medium of the senses. The performer must be set to know what to look for. This factor of set, the ability to single out objects, is necessary in all motor activity. Skill is demonstrated when there is a minimal involvement of the senses; just those needed for the distinction of cues in order that the perceptual process will work quickly and accurately. There is no doubt that the learning and performing of motor skills certainly depend, to a great extent, on perceptual abilities.

Another factor that influences perception is *motivation.* A person must have the will to perceive in order to attend to the necessary cues that influence discrimination. Motivation prepares the individual; a set or hypothesis is developed as to what to expect. This anticipation, or expectancy, permits one to attend to the meaningful stimuli. In fact, sometimes we perceive what we wish to perceive, with needs and wishes channeling the direction.

Previous experiences in the same situation with the same objects help in facilitating the perceptual process. These past experiences also promote a sense of expectancy, which in turn leads to better perception. Familiarity with stimuli in similar situations not only affects perceptual learning but learning in general, and it might be deduced at this stage of the discussion that many similarities exist between perceptual learning and motor learning.

William Epstein (1967) concludes his analysis of research in the area of perceptual learning with five propositions

1. Assumptions that are learned through everyday experience are important determinants of perception.

2. Practice, in the form of prior exposure, controlled rehearsal, or differential reinforcement of selective perceiving, can modify perception.
3. Extended exposure to conditions of conflict leads to a gradual modification of perception.
4. When visual stimulation is transformed or distorted, the perceiver adapts to the distortion.
5. A variety of perceptual functions exhibit developmental changes (p. 290).

Psychophysics

The study of sensations, their relationships within a given sense modality, and the stimuli that cause them is called psychophysics. Some authorities feel that the most precise knowledge of perceptions comes from the psychophysical field. Certain aspects of sensations have been studied more than others for their role in perception, notably, size, color, pitch, space, depth, and distance.

Problems associated with the absolute threshold and the differential threshold of people have been studied primarily but not exclusively by means of psychophysical methods (Corso, 1967). *Absolute threshold* refers to the value of a stimulus, the point at which a person will make a response, versus being nonresponsive. By example, what is the least amount of acoustic energy at a frequency of 1,000 cycles per second that would be detected by the average young adult? According to research, it would be about 5 decibel CPS (cycles per second). *Differential threshold* refers to the least amount of change in a stimulus in order for it to be recognized. We might ask the question: How many grams of weight must be added to a given amount in order for a person to recognize a difference in the weights? That question will be answered shortly.

Certain laws concerning the sense modalities have been formulated through the years. One of the most famous is the Fechner-Weber law, which describes a person's ability to distinguish between two stimuli. Weber's original law, written in 1834, stated that in order for a second stimulus to be discriminated from the first, there must be a noticeable difference between them. Increments must be in constant fractions of the original stimulus. For instance, perhaps we would have to add one gram weight to ten grams in order to observe the bare difference between two weights. If this is the case, a 20-gram weight would require two additional grams to the second stimulus in order for it to be perceived as different from the first. Consequently, a 40-gram weight necessitates the addition of 4 grams to the second stimulus; 80 grams would require 8, and so on. Fechner's law was a mathematical transposition of Weber's law. The Fechner–Weber law, which can be applied to the heavier of two weights, the longer of two lines, and the louder of two noises, has not always proved to be accurate at the extremes of a sensory continuum, but it is a generally accepted law.

The mathematical formulation for Weber's law follows:

$$\frac{\Delta I}{I} = k$$

where:

k = the constant fraction for the given type of physical energy
I = the intensity of the stimulus
ΔI = the different threshold

The constant fraction must be determined for each type of stimulus. It describes the ''just noticeable difference,'' that difference between two stimuli (two tones, two light intensities, and so on) of sufficient magnitude so that detection is possible. The differential threshold tends to approximate a constant fraction, as described by Weber's law. It has been ascertained from research findings, for example, that the ratio is 1:53 for detecting the heaviness of lifted gram weights. The ratio is 1:11 for distinguishing loudness in tones.

Figural Aftereffects

A commonly occurring phenomenon in perception is the effect that an extended experience with a particular stimulus or situation has on the individual, once it has been discontinued. When a person continually concentrates on curved lines for a period of time, and then straight ones, these straight lines appear to be curved in the opposite direction. *Figure reversals* can and have been demonstrated under a wide range of experimental conditions.

Every child has had the experience of turning in a circle a number of times and then noticing, upon stopping, a feeling that the body is turning in the opposite direction. The problem of maintaining balance after continued circular rotation confronts the ice skater attempting to master this skill. Other types of kinesthetic aftereffects are observed in other sports situations. The baseball batter swings the weighted bat in the on-deck circle in order that his regular bat will seem lighter. Thus, it is thought that the bat can be swung faster. The track athlete may practice with weighted boots in order to experience the feeling of lightness and speed once they are removed and track shoes replaced during actual competition.

A *figural aftereffect is a perceptual distortion that is produced by satiation with a particular stimulus or a combination of them.* The most pronounced effect is experienced immediately following the satiation. A kinesthetic aftereffect would be the effect of a movement experience, contrasted with, say, the visual inspection of a straight line after viewing curved lines. When B. J. Cratty and K. Duffy (1967) administered a number of movement-oriented tasks to their subjects, aftereffects of movement were found to be highly specific to the task. Aftereffect observations from task to task are not consistent. Active tasks produced more aftereffects than passive tasks.

Although some investigators have obtained results favoring an overload prior to actual performance, such as throwing a heavier baseball before throwing a regulation baseball or warming up with a weighted bat, the bulk of the research indicates that little is to be gained by this practice. Interestingly enough, subjects invariably feel they perform better following an overload routine, even though their performance does not improve more than the preoverload performance. R. Nelson has noted this phenomenon in a series of experiments. In one experiment (Nelson and Nofsinger, 1965), male students were tested for elbow flexion speed prior to and following the application of selected levels of overload. The subjects all stated that they felt faster on the postoverload test, but, in actuality, no significant differences were realized between pre- and postoverload tests. In other words, a *kinesthetic illusion* was created.

Perceived differences or distortions are generally temporary in nature, and the actual benefit to performance has yet to be objectively substantiated through experimental research. However, the reported better feeling derived from practicing with weighted objects on subsequent speed and strength performances certainly necessitates a more thorough examination of this area.

Perceptual and Motor Learning

The role of perception and its importance in motor learning and performance should now be evident. Perceptual learning has on occasion been studied separately from learning in general, but there is no doubt that although one refers to the learning of skills as motor learning, perceptual mechanisms operate prior to any skilled motor act or subsequent to that act. A person's ability to receive and distinguish among available cues in a given situation enables performance to be enacted more skillfully. The batter may have the smoothest, most ideal practice swing. But if he or she cannot concentrate and attend to the important cues when up at bat in a game and follow the ball as it comes to the plate and perceive a fastball or curve, a ball or a strike, performance cannot be effective. Perceptual activities occur in a variety of ways in any complex motor behavior, as we saw in Chapter 6.

INTELLIGENCE

Cognition consists of such higher mental processes as concept formation, problem solving, imagination, perception, decision making, and intelligence. Cognitive processes are extremely difficult to study objectively, and much of our knowledge of them has been inferred from behavior. This was shown to be the case with perception. Although we rely on the senses for the receipt of environmental information, the object ultimately perceived results from the complex involvement of many neural mechanisms and the state of the organism. Even learning, whether simple or more involved, must be measured through performance.

As was pointed out in earlier chapters, cognitive psychology has become increasingly popular. Psychologists have formulated ingenious techniques to evaluate the functioning of various cognitive operations as information is processed, leading to purposeful behavior. In this section of the book, however, we will examine research from another perspective. Rather than concern ourselves with processing factors here, we will focus on the relationships between cognitive capabilities (such as intelligence) and aspects of motor performance. In other words, achievements in the cognitive and psychomotor domains will be compared.

In most of the research on this topic, the IQ score or some other standardized measurement of intelligence has been used. Of course, intelligence can be interpreted by various behaviors, not merely by IQ score. Different types of intelligence are not all necessarily related in the same person. For a global perspective, the nature and development of cognitive abilities have been described in detail by Raymond Cattell (1971). His book offers a historical perspective as well as a contemporary way of looking at cognitive abilities, their structure and measurement. But for our purposes here, some measurement of intelligence or academic achievement will be analyzed for any relationship with achievement in motor skills.

Relationship of Intelligence to Motor Abilities and Physical Characteristics

J. P. Guilford (1959) has factor analyzed physical performance to arrive at underlying psychomotor abilities and has attempted to determine the component abilities that comprise the intellect as well as their relationships. Through the factor-analysis method, he examined data obtained from a series of intelligence tests and proposed the least common denominators, i.e., independent factors. From fifty intellectual factors, he derived five: cognitive abilities, memory, evaluative abilities, divergent thinking, and convergent thinking. He interpreted the process of cognition as including discovery and recognition abilities.

Evidently, there is a lack of agreement among psychologists in many instances of interpretation and categorization of the higher mental processes. Guilford's use of the word *intellect* might very well be interchangeable with the term *cognition,* depending on one's viewpoint. However, in this section, the concern is with intelligence tests and what they measure, and the relationship of these scores to various physical characteristics, motor abilities, and athletic success. Much research has been completed, in an attempt to determine the relationship between intellectual and physical factors.

Intelligence tests, which measure various aspects of intelligence, depending on the nature of the tests, and academic achievement scores have been utilized as a means of measuring intelligence. The most often administered and respected intelligence tests are the Revised Stanford-Binet Scales and the Wechsler Intelligence Scale, both of which yield IQs that correlate fairly well with academic achievement. These scales have been used in investigations in order to distinguish intellectual groups or relate intelligence to some other variable. The mentally retarded and the superior have been compared in physical performance; athlete and nonathlete differences in intelligence have been tested; and the relationship of motor skill success to academic achievement has been investigated.

Intelligence and Physical Status

Some researchers have been concerned with the relation of intelligence to such physical factors as height and weight and performance on strength tests. In a sense, they have attempted partially to resolve the issue of whether a sound body usually coincides with a sound mind. The theory of organismic unity, that physical and intellectual factors are interrelated in a meaningful manner, has not been supported in any convincing manner in the research literature. There is considerable doubt about the relationship of academic achievement and intelligence test scores with physical status. Early research evidence indicated that nothing more than low, positive relationships exist between physical status and mental status. Much of the present research permits the same conclusion. Exception to this has been demonstrated when mentally retarded children are compared to average and superior children in physical characteristics and motor abilities.

Intelligence and Ability to Learn Motor Skills

Some scholars have argued for a motor intelligence quotient (MQ) to depict a person's ability to learn motor skills, separate from but similar in principle to an IQ score. Others feel there is a direct relationship between such variables because the organism reacts totally to all experiences. According to the latter belief, if a student does well on an intelligence test or tests, he or she should be expected to learn motor activities more quickly and proficiently than those students who obtain lower intelligence ratings.

In E. D. Ryan's (1963) investigation, eighty college students were required to learn how to balance on a stabilometer. Academic achievement did not distinguish the subjects in their ability to learn and perform the task. K. B. Start (1964) had forty-four college students mentally practice a novel skill for five minutes on each of six days. Performance on the skill, a single leg upstart on the Olympic high bar, was then rated by four judges. When the ratings were compared to IQ scores, a meaningless r of 0.08 was obtained.

Generally, it appears that the research, although by no means in complete agreement, indicates little relationship between cognitive abilities and the ability to learn motor tasks. The sheer frustration of resolving available research evidence with common beliefs is illustrated by Philip DuBois (1965).

> Up to the present time, certain of the findings in the study of complex skills have been contradictory. Intelligence has been defined as the ability to learn, yet most of the correlations between measures of intelligence and changes resulting from training are reported to be essentially zero. One talks of the ability to learn, and yet gain in proficiency in one task is often reported to be unrelated to gains in other tasks. It is widely believed that new knowledge must be built on old, and yet many a study has come to the conclusion that those who know the most at the beginning of training profit least from instruction (p. 64).

Using factor-analytic techniques, James Duncanson (1966) indicated more optimism in being able to determine the relationship of measures of learning and measures of abilities in cognitive tasks. His conclusions, compromising between specificity and generality notions, were that

1. learning is related to abilities.
2. there are learning factors independent of the abilities measured.

3. learning in one situation is related to learning in other situations. (There is no general learning factor, but there are fewer learning factors than tasks.)

It should be emphasized that in most experiments in which intelligence was compared to motor factors, college or high school students have served as subjects. Distinctions on intelligence tests and IQs are slighter in this case than if an entire population were analyzed; the range of scores also would be much greater for an entire population. Research on preschool youngsters, elementary school children, and slightly older children tends to show greater relationships among physical, motor, and intellectual factors. Another concern is the nature of the tests employed. For instance, A. Ismail, N. Kephart, and C. C. Cowell (1963) distinguished high academic achievers from low ones on tests of coordination and static balance. Tests of speed, accuracy, and strength did not differentiate the groups. The authors were able to conclude that for boys and girls between the ages of ten and twelve, coordination items were fairly good predictors of IQ and Stanford Standard Achievement scores.

Thus far, it appears that research investigating intellectual and motor relationships has indicated higher relationships among young school-aged children than among college students. Child psychologists and others interested in growth and development have attempted to show the relationship of motor development to academic aptitude and achievement. Their work and the research of others, summarized in Chapter 10, is inconclusive in prescribing motor patterns for children as a means of promoting intellectual growth.

Athlete Versus Nonathlete in Intelligence

For many years, the popular conception of the big dumb athlete has plagued physical educators and athletes themselves. It takes only a few examples to confirm a hypothesis, especially one that is quite entrenched in the mind of the believer. Fortunately, most of the literature dispels such thoughts.

Some isolated studies do show athletes to score lower on intelligence tests than nonathletes. However, the majority of investigations have found little difference between the two groups on intelligence tests and academic achievement tests. A number of studies have even produced results favoring athletes. As far as grade-point averages are concerned, athletes do as well as, if not slightly better than, nonathletes.

Motor and Physical Characteristics of the Mentally Retarded

The "normal" population of children, from birth to college age, has been extensively investigated. For many years, the mentally retarded have been neglected. With federal encouragement and enthusiasm at the local level, much work has been recently undertaken by educators, physical educators, and psychologists in order to promote more effective learning situations for the mentally deficient child.

Evidence has been quite consistent with respect to certain points. It generally indicates a direct relationship between motor and physical factors and intellectual achievement. T. G. Thurstone (1959) undertook a comprehensive project concerned with educating the mentally handicapped. Her subjects, 559 boys and girls ranging in age from seven to fifteen years, had IQs recorded from 50 to 79. One phase of the study had to do with the acquisition and performance of gross motor skills. All the subjects were tested on such skills as (1) volleyball or soccer ball punt, for distance; (2) tennis ball or softball throw, for distance; (3) grip strength; (4) 40-yard run; (5) standing broad jump; (6) tennis ball throw, for accuracy; and (7) side stepping for fifteen seconds. The scores of the mentally retarded children were compared with those of the normal children at different ages. The scores of the normal children were consistently and significantly better on almost every test, at all age levels.

In another study, C. E. Howe (1959) formed two groups of children from six and one half to twelve years of age, equated as to age, sex, and background. A number of physical skills were tested, including a jump test, grip strength, ball throw for distance, tapping speed, balancing ability, and others. The normal children were superior to the mentally deficient on these tests. An astonishing discovery made by the author was that forty-one of the forty-three retarded children *could not balance on one foot for one minute.* This information coincides with the data obtained by Ismail et al. (1963). They had found that motor coordination and balance tasks were highly related to the intellectual achievement of normal children.

The retarded child is usually two to four years behind the normal child on performance measures. In fact, motor performance appears to be more evenly equated when comparing the mental ages of children. The pattern of learning skills—that is, developmentally—is basically the same for both normal and subnormal boys and girls. However, at a given chronological age, the retarded perform with a lesser degree of skill than normal children.

Can physical educators assist the retarded in improving their cognitive and motoric capabilities? A few studies have reported remarkable contributions of physical education programs to the total growth of subnormal children. J. N. Oliver (1958) matched two groups of mentally deficient boys. One group (the experimental group) had a ten-week course in conditioning; the other group (the control group) did not. For the experimental group, all academic subjects except arithmetic and English were replaced by physical education activities. The control group continued under their regular program. Both groups were given pre- and postphysical and mental tests. The experimental group improved significantly on both the physical and mental tests; Oliver hypothesized that the change was because of the effect of achievement and success, improved adjustment, improved physical fitness, and the effect of feeling important. The experimental group improved significantly on many physical, motor, and intelligence measures, and their IQ *improved significantly by 25 per cent!*

It might be concluded, then, that motor proficiency is directly related to intellectual ability, when groups of intellectually subnormal and normal children are compared. Children who range within the normal intelligence limits are not distinguished on motor skill measures. This point has been well brought out in an experiment by E. Asmussen and K. Heebøll-Nielson (1956). Out of 204 boys, three groups were formed, two within the normal IQ limits and one below them. They were tested on the vertical jump, strength of the leg extensors and finger flexors, and maximum expiration and inspiration force. These tests did not distinguish performers within the normal range, but did distinguish the low IQ group from the other two. The investigators concluded that there is no difference in performance as long as the IQ is above 95. Below this (their low group had an IQ average of 83) performance is lower than in normal boys.

Although it might seem reasonable to expect the intellectually gifted to do exceptionally well in motor skill performance because the retarded are below average efficiency, this is not the case. General findings indicate that a greater intellect and outstanding academic achievement are not related to physical performance.

PERSONALITY

An individual's personality, one's characteristic way of behaving, is the result of learning and experiences in life. Heredity sets limits and predisposes the person to react in certain ways to environmental events. One's actions and feelings are the result of previous experiences, and the interaction of many traits, some more modifiable than others, determines a particular uniqueness. Personality can be viewed from two vantage points. One, the effect or impact an individual has on other people usually results in an evaluation on a social basis. For instance, is he or she pleasing and popular? Besides this so-called external personality, another type may represent the *real* person. Personality, according to most experts in this area, should be defined in terms of the way a person really is, not necessarily the way that person is perceived by others. In determining an individual's personality, a difficult endeavor indeed, an indication of behavioral patterns and actions is also uncovered. When we know an individual's personality, we understand that person better. To know someone's personality, then, is to increase the potential to predict behavior in particular situations.

Traits, Situations, and Interactions

But how do we assess personality? How, in fact, can predictions be made about a person's behavior under particular circumstances? Distinct alternatives exist. The philosophical and methodological approaches taken for the study of personality sometimes provide complementary, and at other times conflicting, knowledge. Consider clinical, factor-analytical, and experimental orientations.

The clinician obtains information about clients through individual or group therapeutic situations. Through observations, dialogue, or the administration of projective tests, an analysis is made of behaviors, especially underlying contributory factors to observable behaviors. Often, subconscious problems are uncovered.

The clinician's approach is thus a personal one, probing and delving, in order to understand, explain, and help.

Personality psychologists, on the other hand, have attempted to determine the composition of personality. Social and personal orientations, need states, and traits have been identified by various theoreticians using different methodological approaches. A number of personality tests have been devised to assess the degree to which people score higher or lower than the norms established for certain traits or characteristics. Many of these tests have been established through factor-analytic methods and are found widely in the published literature and used in various research contexts.

The assumption behind these tests is that each one can describe the composites of personality and assess a profile of a person. Presumably such information will predict how a person will behave when confronted with a number of circumstances. By definition, a trait is a relatively stable characteristic within a person. Consequently, a person should behave predictably and consistently across situations, depending on the emphasis of certain traits over other ones. Trait theory dominated the thinking and methodology in personality psychology until the late 1960s. Since then, a strong movement has grown in opposition to trait theory, in which the assumptions of trait theory have been questioned.

With experimental paradigms, it has been shown that different situations can elicit behaviors from the same person. Perhaps situations need to be analyzed in order to predict how people will behave in them, instead of analyzing people and assuming that certain behaviors will be emitted across situations. Then again, a compromise between the trait approach and the situation approach (trait X situation) might be the most viable. Indeed, N. S. Endler and D. Magnusson (1976) write that empirical results support an interactional view of behavior.

Present research indicates that some people are fairly consistent in their behaviors from situation to situation; others are not. Situations interact with the dispositions of people, and behaviors are produced. A major objective is to determine patterns of behavior within individuals: e.g., consistency and inconsistency. Then, the evaluation and interpretation of personality characteristics in individuals becomes more meaningful. From a motor learning point of view, it is not usual to view the presence of certain dimensions of personality as more favorable for learning and performance. For instance, there should be an optimal level of motivation, emotion, and anxiety for each person and for each task.

The appraisal of personality traits provides some understanding about people's dispositions. However, these measures would be more informative if related to specific circumstances. They would also be more meaningful if they could be assessed in less crude ways than is presently the case.

Measurement

Because personality is viewed from diverse points of view, it is understandable that approaches to measuring it also range in many directions. Personality can be assessed from (1) interviews, (2) observations, (3) ratings, (4) projective tasks, and (5) psychological inventories. Defined aspects of personality depend on the evaluative tools used.

Interviews, observations, and ratings are quite subjective means of determining personality. Interview and observational techniques are self-explanatory; ratings are usually obtained from rating scales, in which the rater develops a number of questions or statements for measuring certain attributes and proceeds to rate the subject on each phase, not discretely, but to the degree that each pertains to the subject. Ratings may be on a 1 to 5 basis, with 1 indicating little relevance to the subject and 5 indicating extreme relevance. In any case, a scale is formulated in order that the attributes may be measured in degrees rather than absolutes.

Projective tests are used primarily as clinical tools, and they should be administered and evaluated by clinically trained psychologists. These tests contain unstructured stimulus objects, and as such, the subject is encouraged to respond freely to certain stimuli and thus reveal his or her true personality. Probably the two most popular and widely used instruments are the Rorschach ink-blot test and the Thematic Apperception Test (TAT). The Rorschach test consists of a series of cards, each containing a complex ink blot that the subject is asked to interpret orally.

Ambiguous situations concerning people are represented by the TAT pictures. The person is asked to relate orally a story concerning each picture. In all projective tests, it is hoped that there will be a personal projection into the interpretation of the stimulus objects.

The personality inventory is by far the most popular technique for obtaining information. This may be verified by merely glancing at the completed research on personality in psychology and education. Inventories usually contain questions or statements about personal feelings, attitudes, and interests and are designed to measure various aspects of personality. As such, they are easy to score (although validity measures may be questioned), permit group testing, and do not require an exceptional amount of administration time or clinical background on the part of the examiner.

The personality inventory has been criticized for a number of reasons, namely: (1) falsifications on the part of the respondent (people may answer as they think they should, rather than as they actually believe); (2) misinterpretations of the questions by different respondents; (3) the inability of some respondents to answer certain questions (not knowing oneself well enough); and (4) a lack of validity (the test items may be questionable in terms of what they are supposed to be measuring).

Nevertheless, if administered properly, many personality inventories can provide a reasonable assessment of the characteristics they purport to measure. Here are some of the more popular instruments for making personality assessments:

1. *The Minnesota Multiphasic Personality Inventory (MMPI)*. The MMPI is probably the most clinically oriented assessment and is used extensively in research. It was designed to diagnose pathological conditions, not to discriminate

individuals from a normal population; yet, it is amazing how often it is employed in the latter case (inappropriately) in published research.

2. *The Cattell 16 Personality Factor Test.* The Cattell test is another popular instrument. Through the factor-analysis method, Cattell obtained sixteen independent scales representing aspects of the personality.

3. *The California Personality Inventory (CPI).* The CPI has been designed with four variations, for four different age groups from elementary school to college.

4. *The Edward's Personal Preference Schedule (EPPS).* The EPPS is based on needs and is scored in such a way as to determine one's need to achieve, to be dominant, to affiliate, and the like. It is one of the few instruments in which the forced-choice technique is employed; that is, the respondent is faced with paired descriptions (each unrelated) of him- or herself for each question and must select the one that is most representative.

There are many other personality inventories currently in use, but those mentioned here are representative. An easy-to-read paperback, prepared by Jozef Cohen (1969), provides a reasonable discussion and analysis of the various means of appraising personality.

By our definition of personality, everything we do has an effect on us. By the same token, our behavior is determined by unique personal characteristics. The relationship of personality to motor activity is an important area of study in the psychology of sport. A number of studies have been completed on such topics as (1) differences in personalities between athletes and nonathletes, (2) differences in personalities between better and lesser athletes, (3) personality comparisons among various athletic groups, and (4) social status and athletic achievement. Personality variables, with the exception of anxiety and related emotional states, have rarely, until recent years, been the concern of motor learning researchers. Yet, it should be readily apparent that behavioral systems differ greatly in output as a result of the personality distinctions among them. Attitudes toward the learning and performing of a task, the felt need to achieve, and interest in the activity are all aspects of personality contributing to performance level.

Values and Attitudes

Our feelings toward something—our dispositions to evaluate and/or act in a particular way to certain stimuli—are learned and develop with experience and maturity, or even from tradition. These attitudes, or ways of regarding something, become more pronounced with age. They may be formed because of personal experience with an object or in a special situation, rendering favorable or unfavorable attitudes. Complete lack of personal involvement will not hinder the formation of attitudes, for tradition, culture, subculture, and familial attitude formation encourage similar thought patterns in a person. For example, there are many people who have no valid reason for disliking certain races or ethnic groups, yet they do so because of traditional biases. In this case, an attitude is a predisposition to evaluate someone or something as good or bad, as desirable or undesirable.

The importance of the many types of experiences that occur with age and influence attitudinal patterns has been demonstrated in experiments, as well as through empirical observations. Extremely young children do not display the prejudices older children do, and adulthood brings fairly well-established attitudes. With age comes a greater awareness of social expectancies and pressures and a desire to conform to the value system of a culture or subculture.

The introduction of the word *value* in the previous sentence serves to place it in the context of our discussion and to point out its relationship to an attitude. The value system of a society establishes certain standards that provide direction to an attitude and account for its persistence. Attitudes are conditioned by values, they are not inseparable. Our attitude to make a choice from a number of alternatives is mediated by personal values. Some psychologists think of values as generalized attitudes, for attitudes supposedly have fairly specific objects. Regardless of semantics, both have a place in personality formation. The sequence of events leading to a value choice may be thought to occur in the following manner:

Expression of personality → attitudes and values → motivation → choice

Attitudes and values are primarily social in nature but also represent the individualized response. In other words, although social pressure will result in a great amount of conformity, each person perceives situations differently and varies in needs, desires, values, and other characteristics. Not only will individuals react dissimilarly in situations, but the same individuals may not be consistent in their values. A person may be dominated by a single unitary value system or demonstrate inconsistent values.

An interesting topic is the relationship of established attitudes to learning. If the matter to be learned contradicts these attitudes, possibly learning and retention will be hampered. Learning, as we have seen, is not a simple conditioning process, and even our values and needs affect our perception and ultimately what we learn. This attitudinal effect on learning has been designated as *frame of reference*.

If the athlete or student does not respect the coach or teacher, or agree with what is being taught, these negative attitudes will suppress learning effectiveness. Many times, a person has a personal feeling of how a skill should be performed, and if committed in attitude, the unwillingness to accept a new learning approach will be evidenced in a lack of progress. Perhaps even more serious is the situation in which the coach or instructor is not respected as a person or seems to lack knowledge and have little teaching ability. The barrier formed between learner and teacher will be difficult to overcome and certainly will not lead to a favorable learning situation.

Need to Achieve

Various types of activities service the needs and interests of people. Interests may be thought of as attitudes we have with respect to certain objectives. Usually, attitudes refer to social or political opinions and feelings, interests to vocational or physical activity preferences. Needs are deeply rooted in biological drives and as such might be thought of as presupposing interests.

Needs determine behavior, for the body is in a state of disequilibrium when a need state is aroused. An individual's personality can be explained through needs. A person's actions are caused by an interaction of personal needs and the surrounding environmental stimuli but are modified and restricted by social sanctions. In other words, the forces within an organism provide the impetus to search for or react to various environmental objects.

It is commonly thought that needs can best be met through involvement in need-gratifying activities. For example, athletic participation helps to meet certain needs. Not only this, but the nature of the sport—e.g., team, individual, recreational body building—will dictate which needs are best met for certain people.

Successful undertakings often depend on the need to achieve. Of the many aspects of one's personality, though, need to achieve is probably not a sufficiently powerful trait to ensure proficiency. There must be an ideal proportion and interaction of the many desirable traits. The relationship of a person's motivation, or need achievement, and anxiety level on performance has been investigated by J. W. Atkinson and G. H. Litwin (1960). Evidently the two variables interact in such a way as to determine predictability of behavior.

These authors ascertained the need for achievement and test anxiety levels of their college subjects, who were to perform in a ring toss game. The students were told to stand any distance up to 15 feet from the wooden peg and attempt to toss a ring over the peg. They thought they were being measured for score, but in actuality it was their chosen distance from the peg that was recorded. Subjects high in need for achievement but low in test anxiety preferred a distance of nine to eleven feet away from the peg—of intermediate range. Those subjects who were low in need for achievement and high in anxiety level took the least number of attempts at the intermediate range; they performed primarily at the extreme distances. The other types of students selected distances somewhere between these two classified groups of subjects. In applying these findings to other types of testing situations, it appears that a high need to achieve coupled with a low test-anxiety level results in realistically high levels of aspiration and superior performance. The inhibitive effects of high anxiety on complex test performance will be discussed shortly.

EMOTIONS

Rarely is a person not emotionally involved to some extent in any activity in which he or she performs. Emotions are basically involuntary, but they can be altered under conscious direction. They determine actions, and if strong enough, emotions will initiate activity before there is involvement of the higher nervous centers. Emotions or feelings represent a wide range of states in the human organism, such as joy, sorrow, and anxiety. Not only are there many forms of emotion, but as many if not more varied causes. The athlete may be highly anxious before the event, fear competition, dread its consequences, and/or react poorly in front of spectators. Although this emotional level will have a negative effect, optimal degrees of stress and motivation will promote better performance.

Physiologically speaking, the parts of the brain involved in emotion appear to be the reticular activating system and the limbic system (parts of the thalamus, hypothalamus, and inner cortex). Pleasure and pain areas associated with the autonomic nervous system are located within the limbic system. During various emotions, glands are stimulated and homones are secreted in an attempt to recover body homeostasis (internal body equilibrium).

The word emotion means ''agitation of the feelings'' (from the French word émouvoir, ''to stir up''). Emotion may be referred to in two ways: (1) as a conscious experience or feeling, or (2) by the physiological changes that take place within the body as a result of it. Emotions are psychological and physiological responses and reactions resulting from perceived situations. Some authorities feel that emotions are a special class of motives, whereas others disagree. There is no doubt, though, that *emotions, much like motivation, may have an organizing or disorganizing effect on performance.*

Although we are born with certain basic emotional instincts, other factors later influence them. Maturation brings about the development of various emotions, although many of them can be learned and even conditioned. Both maturation and learning increase emotions in number and complexity.

Stress

Any situation or activity can be perceived to be stressful by anyone at any time. The greater the degree of perceived stress, the stronger the reaction to it, usually manifested in a heightened arousal state. Sometimes, the effects of stress are desirable, sometimes not. Nevertheless, we are continuously in situations that can be considered as potentially stressful.

What may be stressful to one person may not be so to another, and one condition may promote or be detrimental to the performances of different people. An example of this paradox is the effect of spectators on an athlete's performance. Some athletes do not perform as well in actual competition before an audience as in practice; thus, this circumstance is detrimentally stressful to them. Others are relatively unaffected and perform about the same under both practice and game conditions. Still other athletes put on a superior demonstration in front of spectators; it appears that to them this stress is beneficial.

It is commonly observed that certain situations are stressful to some people. By the same token, some situations are generally stressful to everyone. Regardless of the cause, the general state of stress is apparently physiologically reacted to in a specific pattern of internal adjustments. It is a state that disrupts the homeostasis (internal body equilibrium) of the body.

With regard to stress effects on the performance of a task at different levels of mastery, a number of researchers have found it convenient to apply Clark Hull's drive theory (briefly presented in Chapter 4). Apparently, stress encourages a person to exhibit the dominant responses of those responses that are available. In any situation, a number of alternate responses may be emitted. More complex situations and tasks create the possibility of the occurrence of alternative responses. During the early stages of learning, where incorrect response alternatives are usually dominant, stress would be predicted to be detrimental to performance. When higher levels of skill exist and correct responses are dominant, reasonable stress should benefit performance. The effects of stress will depend on the strength of the to-be-learned (correct) response, relative to other competing (incorrect) responses.

The prediction of performance under various stressful conditions is an important problem facing educators and trainers. Associated with this problem is the consideration of a general resistance factor to stress; more specifically, do individuals who react favorably to the effects of one stress do the same to a second type of stress? To answer this question, O. A. Parsons, L. Phillips, and J. E. Lane (1954) had fifty-seven industrial workers perform on the Dunlap hand-steadiness apparatus. The task required the subjects to keep a stylus from touching the side of a hole one-eighth of an inch in diameter. Stress was introduced during performance either by distraction or by informing the subjects of failure through false results and comments. No significant relationship was obtained between the two stress performance scores, therefore not substantiating the concept of a general resistance factor to stress (as induced in this experiment).

An obvious question, and a real concern in training programs, is whether procedures can be developed to prepare performers effectively for stressful conditions that might agree with real conditions. Assuming that stress of sufficient magnitude can be detrimental to performance, how can this circumstance be planned for and controlled in a reasonable way? If resistance to stress can be trained for, then it behooves the designer of training programs to build in appropriate mechanisms for this effect. In one of the few investigations on the topic, D. C. Prather, G. A. Berry, and J. M. Bermudez (1972) examined this problem, along with other related concerns. These authors concluded that it is possible to train a resistance to aversive conditions. Implications are that training programs should include moderately stressful conditions that are related to the kind that will be present in real performance situations. Transfer of training would be quite positive and desirable. Always remember that proficiency in performance depends not only on the ability to coordinate appropriate responses to cues, but also on the demand characteristics of the situation.

Research indicates that stress affects complex tasks differently from simple tasks. Stress is usually more disruptive for the learning and performing of complex tasks, whereas simple task performance either is not affected or else is facilitated under stress. Other studies suggest that if a stress is introduced early in the learning of a skill, it will be more disruptive than if introduced later. Frequently, if the skill has been learned well enough, the effects of stress will be unnoticed. In some cases, stress will improve performance with increased learning.

There is great practical importance in understanding the effects of stress on the learning and performing of motor skills. Stress may benefit, disrupt, or have no effect on a particular individual learning a specific skill. Emotional factors in general, then, are interwoven in every learning situation. Their effects will depend on the nature of the organism and the stimulus situation, which includes the to-be-learned skill and its relative difficulty, the stage of learning, and the surrounding conditions. Understanding the emotional nature of each student will enable the teacher to be more aware of possible problems. Some students may be expected to learn certain tasks with ease and others to experience great difficulty with them.

Anxiety

Anxiety refers to a tendency to perceive a situation as threatening or stressful. The reaction to stress with feelings of anxiety is a fairly common occurrence. Anxiety can be viewed as two distinct concepts, instead of one. *State anxiety* refers to how a person feels at a particular moment in response to a specific situation. *Trait anxiety* is the general disposition of individuals to respond to psychological stress. Whereas trait anxiety is relatively stable, state anxiety is considered to be a transitory emotional state (Spielberger, 1977).

Emotional distress displayed by a person prior to performance can be traced to a number of possible factors. They can be categorized according to the influence of the *situation and activity* or with regard to the *disposition of the person* in general. An understanding of the causation of anxiety should lead to the possible reduction of it, for there exists, theoretically at least, an optimal state of anxiety for each person and each task.

With regard to external factors, situations with which we are less familiar tend to induce higher anxiety levels. Tasks that are newly introduced can do the same, especially if we are asked to perform in front of others. Situational familiarity and increased learning experiences should help to diminish undesirable anxiety. Observations in the sporting world suggest that there are athletes who perform exceptionally well in practice and poorly in the actual contest. This may be attributed to insufficient experiences in the contests and the stress of competiton, responsibility to a team, and the presence of spectators. With practice in simulating the "real" event and more experiences in the "real" situations, stress will be coped with more satisfactorily and performance improved.

On the personal level, anxiety has been considered to be a general characteristic of a person, cross-situational in its manifestation, as well as specifically expressed in reaction to each circumstance. We probably are disposed to function at a generally predictable level across a variety of situations, but particular events can evoke different emotions from the same person. Also, some people are more consistent in behaviors than others. One who is highly anxious by nature in many activities may need to learn special relaxation techniques. A variety of such techniques has been developed through the years. The highly skilled performer has learned to adjust emotions appropriate to the demands of the activity. The mere possession of skills and techniques is insufficient to yield ideal performance standards. Motivational and emotional factors greatly influence the performance of what has been learned.

It has been suggested here that too much anxiety will hinder performance, and situations and people need to be analyzed for possible sources of problems. More particularly, (1) when anxiety is due to the situation, more familiarity and experiences with the situation should be provided; (2) when anxiety is due to the person, relaxation techniques should be learned.

Many researchers have been concerned with comparing the performance of more anxious versus less anxious subjects in motor skill tasks and written tests. Some researchers claim that anxiety disrupts and disorganizes behavior through a lowering of attention, concentration, and intellectual control. Supposedly there is a reduction in perceptual efficiency under anxiety. However, low levels of anxiety provide a general alerting mechanism whereby the organism can better distinguish environmental stimuli.

When comparing anxious to nonanxious subjects on performance tasks, investigators have arrived at conflicting conclusions. This circumstance may be explained partly by the method of determining the characteristics of the subjects and partly by the varying test procedures employed by the experimenters. In such investigations, the attempt has been to discover the effect of anxiety, hence drive, in learning and performance situations. No major differences between high and low anxiety subjects are expected when tasks are not overly difficult. However, on more complex tasks, studies generally show that people high in anxiety do worse than those low in anxiety. Also, those who score low on anxiety tests perform more effectively under stress (on complex tasks) than under normal conditions. This is not the case with individuals high in anxiety, who are less effective performers under stress. Even the ability to cope with stress early in learning is shown to be a function of one's anxiety state. Using a stabilometer task and electric shocks, Carron (1968) concluded that stress is detrimental to the performance of highly anxious subjects in the early stages of practice. Subjects low in anxiety were hardly affected at all.

Arousal Level and Performance

Anxiety has often been interpreted within the framework of drive theory. If anxiety has drive properties, then more anxious people should be conditioned in certain simple behaviors more easily than less anxious people. Theoretically, drive theory supports the notion that increased arousal, such as that caused by increased motivational level, results in improved performance. However, it is doubtful that this is true for all tasks. Those tasks that require energy expenditure and effort are probably best described by the predictable linear relationship between drive state and performance.

There is another theory that is often described as a rival to drive theory. Termed the inverted-U hypothesis, and favored by Rainer Martens (1971) to explain motor behavior satisfactorily, it is usually discussed in terms of arousal, or activation theory. The hypothesis predicts a nonmonotonic relationship between drive level and performance. More specifically, it is predicted that performance improves with increases in arousal, to a point. After that, increases in arousal result in increasingly poor performance. Figure 8-1 illustrates a comparison of

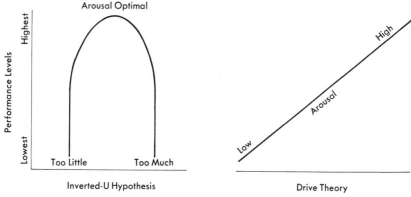

FIGURE 8-1. The inverted-U hypothesis, showing an optimal arousal level for best performance; drive theory indicating a linear relationship between performance and arousal levels.

these two models. Actually, both drive theory and the inverted-U hypothesis are plausible explainers of behavior. The inverted-U hypothesis fits tasks requiring control, finesse, and complex skillful execution, whereas drive theory seems best to describe tasks that involve effort.

Muscular tension and its relationship to motor-skill performance has been investigated by a few researchers who were interested in discovering the facilitating or detrimental effects of muscular tension on performance. Tension provides a state of arousal and a level of activation in the individual and, as such, is an aspect of emotion and motivation. The results of the research in this area have been conflicting. Perhaps this is because physical tension has been induced by different means and the learning tasks have varied.

We might speculate, however, that an optimal amount of tension, or arousal, exists within each person for each task. Charles Wood and Jack Hokanson (1965) induced different levels of muscular tension in subjects in order to determine the effects on performance of a simple intellectual task. Heart rate increased linearly with tension, which supported the idea that performance is facilitated by increasing levels of tension and that it deteriorates with further tension (see Figure 8-2). The data reflect the inverted-U hypothesis in dramatic fashion. This hypothesis has been explained and illustrated and is popularly used in the literature to associate arousal, anxiety, activation, motivation, and other related variables to performance.

Measurement of Emotions

Emotional reactions to particular situations can be observed in everyday behavior or in research laboratory under controlled conditions. Under the latter, it is possible directly or indirectly to measure physiological changes taking place in the organism. Some methods used in the research include

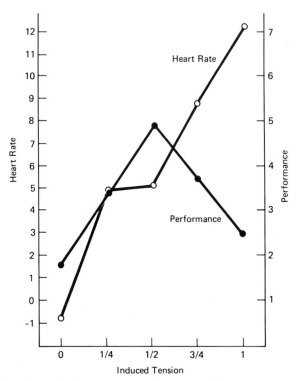

FIGURE 8-2. The relationship between mean heart rate difference scores and mean performance difference scores as a function of increasing levels of tension. (*From Wood, C. G., & Hokanson, J. E. Effects of induced tension on performance and the inverted U function. Journal of Personality and Social Psychology, 1965, 5, 501–510.*) Copyright 1965 by the American Psychological Association. Reprinted by permission.

1. *measuring respiration, blood pressure, or heart rate:* An increase is associated with an emotional state.
2. *measuring body temperature:* It may rise or fall, depending on the nature of the stimulus and its particular effect on the organism.
3. *determining amount of sweating:* It increases with the onset of stronger emotions.
4. *analyzing electrical potentials of the brain (EEG or electroencephalogram):* They become irregular during emotional conditions.
5. *evaluating galvanic skin responses or muscle action potentials:* They demonstrate greater magnitude with emotions.

Krahenbuhl (1971) used the level of catecholamine in the urine as a measure of stress reactivity. Six college tennis players were tested under basal, practice, competition-anticipation, and competition circumstances. An elevation of catecholamines is related to physical exertion as well as to various emotional states.

TABLE 8-1 The Taylor Manifest Anxiety Scale (MAS)*

Answer yes or no after each question.

1. I do not tire quickly. ____
2. I am troubled by attacks of nausea. ____
3. I believe I am no more nervous than most others. ____
4. I have very few headaches. ____
5. I work under a great deal of tension. ____
6. I cannot keep my mind on one thing. ____
7. I worry over money and business. ____
8. I frequently notice my hand shakes when I try to do something. ____
9. I blush no more often than others. ____
10. I have diarrhea once a month or more. ____
11. I worry quite a bit over possible misfortunes. ____
12. I practically never blush. ____
13. I am often afraid that I am going to blush. ____
14. I have nightmares every few nights. ____
15. My hands and feet are usually warm enough. ____
16. I sweat very easily even on cool days. ____
17. Sometimes when embarrassed, I break out in a sweat which annoys me greatly. ____
18. I hardly ever notice my heart pounding and I am seldom short of breath. ____
19. I feel hungry almost all the time. ____
20. I am very seldom troubled by constipation. ____
21. I have a great deal of stomach trouble. ____
22. I have had periods in which I lost sleep over worry. ____
23. My sleep is fitful and disturbed. ____
24. I dream frequently about things that are best kept to myself. ____
25. I am easily embarrassed. ____
26. I am more sensitive than most other people. ____
27. I frequently find myself worrying about something. ____
28. I wish I could be as happy as others seem to be. ____
29. I am usually calm and not easily upset. ____
30. I cry easily. ____
31. I feel anxiety about something or someone almost all the time. ____
32. I am happy most of the time. ____
33. It makes me nervous to have to wait. ____
34. I have periods of such great restlessness that I cannot sit long in a chair. ____
35. Sometimes I become so excited that I find it hard to get to sleep. ____
36. I have sometimes felt that difficulties were piling up so high that I could not overcome them. ____
37. I must admit that I have at times been worried beyond reason over something that really did not matter. ____
38. I have very few fears compared to my friends. ____
39. I have been afraid of things or people that I knew could not hurt me. ____
40. I certainly feel useless at times. ____
41. I find it hard to keep my mind on a task or job. ____
42. I am usually self-conscious. ____
43. I am inclined to take things hard. ____
44. I am a high-strung person. ____
45. Life is a strain for me much of the time. ____
46. At times I think I am no good at all. ____
47. I am certainly lacking in self-confidence. ____
48. I sometimes feel that I am about to go to pieces. ____
49. I shrink from facing a crisis or difficulty. ____
50. I am entirely self-confident. ____

*(From Taylor, J. A. A personality scale of manifest anxiety. *Journal of Abnormal and Social Psychology*, 1953, **48**, 285–290. Copyright 1953 by the American Psychological Association. Reprinted by permission.)

A significant difference in catecholamine levels between practice and actual competition situations appeared to show that the psychic variable more than physical activity influenced stress reactivity. No differences were noted between basal and practice conditions.

A number of self-report measures also have been developed to assess emotional reactions to stress. The Manifest Anxiety Scale (MAS) (Taylor, 1953) and other written tests have been used to determine the anxiety level of a person. The MAS is presented in Table 8-1. For many years it was one of the most popularly used tests in research undertaken in the area of anxiety. At the present time, it is being rivaled by Charles Spielberger's (1970) State-Trait Anxiety Inventory (STAI) for theoretical acceptance, in clinical usage and as a research tool. In the motor behavior area, the STAI appears to be favored. Some items from the STAI are presented in Table 8-2.

TABLE 8-2A The Trait Anxiety Test*

Directions: A number of statements which people have used to describe themselves are given below. Read each statement and then circle the appropriate number to the right of the statement to indicate how you *generally* feel.

There are no right or wrong answers. Do not spend too much time on any one statement but give the answer which seems to describe how you generally feel.	Almost Never	Sometimes	Often
21. I feel pleasant	1	2	3
22. I tire quickly	1	2	3
23. I feel like crying	1	2	3
24. I wish I could be as happy as others seem to be	1	2	3

TABLE 8-2B The State Anxiety Test*

Directions: A number of statements which people have used to describe themselves are given below. Read each statement and then circle the appropriate number to the right of the statement to indicate how you feel right now, that is, *at this moment.*

There are no right or wrong answers. Do not spend too much time on any one statement but give the answer which seems to describe your present feelings best.	Not At All	Somewhat	Moderately So	Very Much So
1. I feel calm	1	2	3	4
2. I feel secure	1	2	3	4
3. I am tense	1	2	3	4
4. I am regretful	1	2	3	4

*(From Spielberger, C. D. *The state-trait anxiety inventory.* Palo Alto, Ca.: Consulting Psychologists Press, 1970. Copyright 1970 by Charles D. Spielberger. Reprinted by special permission.)

A checklist instrument has been developed to measure perceived stress in situations; and P. D. Jacobs and J. Thornton (1970) have defended its practical significance. They found the self-report stress instrument, the Perceived Stress Index (PSI), to be sufficiently sensitive in distinguishing among groups of subjects administered different instructional sets as to forthcoming shock treatments. In an earlier publication, Jacobs and Munz (1968) presented the final fifteen-item checklist with pleasant to unpleasant words and phrases ranging along a continuum (see Table 8-3).

TABLE 8-3 Item Content, Median Intensity Values, Semi-Interquartile Ranges (Q), and Factor Loadings for the PSI items *

Item No. and Content	Median Intensity Value	Q	Factor Loading	
			I	II
6. Extremely terrified	10.72	.50	−.92*	.30
14. Scared stiff	10.04	.54	−.91*	.28
7. Fearful	9.38	.64	−.85*	.44
3. Threatened	8.74	.63	−.91*	.36
1. Distressed	8.24	.64	−.80*	.58
8. Uneasy	7.60	.65	−.75*	.60
5. Timid	7.21	.69	.95*	−.03
11. Not mattering	5.98	.32	.96*	.05
2. Unruffled	5.68	.68	.87*	−.37
10. Alright	5.12	.80	.85*	−.39
4. At ease	4.47	1.01	.75*	−.44
15. Keen	3.77	.70	.27	−.92*
13. Feeling good	2.99	.50	.38	−.91*
9. Marvelous	2.30	.64	.32	−.92*
12. Thrilled	1.97	.60	.18	−.98*

* (From Jacobs, P. D., & Munz, D. C. An index for measuring perceived stress in a college population. *The Journal of Psychology*, 1968, **70**, 9–15.) Copyright 1968 by the American Psychological Association. Reprinted by permission.

FORM

Individuals differ in the nature and extent of personal abilities and characteristics, as well as their manner of executing various motor patterns associated with complex gross motor skills. This method of expressing movement in space and time with a purpose, the way of doing something, is called form. The specific characteristics of one performer's act make it unique from others, sometimes worthy of emulation, other times best forgotten. Although form in executing skills is unique from person to person, generally accepted *good form* is usually associated with the outstanding athlete in a given sport. And yet, a definition of what good form is defies us. As such, the desirability of molding a beginner in the style of the champion is open to question; certainly reasons can be provided for and against such a practice.

Differences

Differences in form exist between performers. Either these differences are extremely slight and almost unnoticed by the untrained eye, or they are obvious to all. The following factors are associated with dissimilarities in form, or the characteristics of movement, among people: (1) skill level in the particular act or sport; (2) personality factors; (3) age; (4) the nature of the act or sport, e.g., its complexity; and (5) physical and mechanical characteristics.

Higgins (1977) has made some useful points with regard to the understanding of the organization and structure of human movement:

1. The organization of movement is reflected in the spatial and temporal components of the pattern of movement.
2. The regulatory effect of the environment is of vital importance for successful performance and is reflected in the performer's pattern of movement.
3. Each performer, for each skill, will exhibit a different pattern of movement, dependent upon morphology and the imposed cnvironmental and biomechanical constraints.
4. Level of skill for each performer and type of skill will influence the resultant pattern of movement.
5. Analysis of the interaction between the moving organism and defined constraints leads toward understanding of movement (pp. 139–142).

Simple acts can be fulfilled in a similar manner from individual to individual. Form uniqueness becomes more observable when the act becomes more detailed, when there is a series of events that constitutes a skill, or when gross motor movements are involved in the act. Participants in gross motor skills are more apt to display observable form differences.

The nature of the performer, physically, mentally, and emotionally, will decide the method used to perform. Some people are flamboyant, whereas others are introverted, and their personality may be reflected in their actions. Skill already attained in the to-be-performed act(s) distinguishes success and form. If we assume that the outstanding athlete generally displays good form, it is apparent that a beginner will not be able to duplicate performance potential as to relative skill attainment and the form in displaying it. Height, weight, body build, strength, flexibility, and other physical and motor factors usually moderate the manner in which one performs. In other words, the available means often contribute to the style of expression.

Maturation, from infancy to adolescence, often facilitates motor skill performance. Children frequently have to approximate the way a skill should be ideally performed. Desired form in skill performance is assisted by mature minds and bodies, with knowing what to do and having the available resources with which to do it.

Relevance to Success in Skill Attainment

Successful performance may be displayed through a variety of forms and techniques, but it is rare when they violate established performance principles. In other words, for a given act or sequence of skills, there is a generally accepted good form, consistent with kinesiological, physical, and psychological evidence, with variations of the ideal form. This is not to deny the possibility of success in spite of form, but rather to emphasize the probability of success and form going together.

In actuality, in most sports, the outcome is more important than the means. The relationship between some stereotyped form and success in a particular activity is probably quite low. Some activities, such as gymnastics, figure skating, and diving, are judged on skill and form. However, the baseball coach will not tamper with the batting style of a .300 hitter, even if he hits with his "foot in the bucket." The avid baseball spectator can readily picture the differences between the stances of Stan Musial and Ted Williams, yet both were great hitters. Evidently, at the point of ball contact with the bat, both men had coordinated their body parts in a similar fashion, and both hit effectively for many years.

Some people have to adjust their style because of body build and other factors. Consistent conscientious practice can overcome many limitations. The displayed form may not be aesthetic, but the effectiveness of the movement can be measured by the results. Perhaps one of the greatest problems the parent, physical educator, and coach is confronted with, is that of the youngster attempting to emulate a professional athlete, a particular idol. On the one hand, the policy is good, for great insight may be gained into the nature of the sport and the means of attaining success. However, progress may be impeded by differences in physical characteristics, age, and other factors.

It is usually a poor idea, therefore, for a beginner or even an advanced learner to attempt to copy every phase of an act or activity from someone else. The physical educator and coach should explain the reasons for the execution of a movement in a certain style and then expect and allow for individual variations. Robots do not make the best performers. Form, or information about how to move, to a certain extent, provides direction for the learner and facilitates the learning process, but probably not to the degree imagined in years past. If it is possible to designate a performer as displaying such a thing, reasonable form is to be expected for probable success in skill attainment. A thought to remember is that the ideal form for a given act is continually remodeled as new evidence is accumulated. Therefore open-mindedness and flexibility in style are necessary in order to take advantage of the research that points to a more effective means of executing acts. *The interaction between biomechanical constraints, environmental constraints, and morphological constraints determines personally appropriate form in movement,* as emphasized so well by Higgins (1977).

Aesthetic Appeal

One of the prime reasons for the demonstration of a certain form, other than that of scientific substantiation, is often merely to satisfy aesthetic appeal. Posture varies from person to person, as does the concept of what good posture actually is. Even so, form and ideal conceptual form for athletic performance also vary among individuals. Good posture implies either effective posture or pleasing-to-the-eye posture, or both, but these two conditions are not necessarily related. An individual can demonstrate physical efficiency with scoliosis, lordosis, or kyphosis.

Good form can be likened to good posture. Is the reference to effectiveness, attractiveness, or both? Each type of good form can occur independently or in conjunction with the other. Whereas in the past the saying was, "Do it because it looks good," athletes now are more concerned with their own effectiveness in the performed skills, even if it means sacrificing aesthetic appeal.

For the same reasons that a pleasing posture impresses people and may promote an inner feeling of confidence, good form in skill execution can also be advocated. Highly skilled athletes want to look good—aesthetically and skillfully—in front of spectators. A unique form, sometimes called showmanship when displayed at an extreme, helps to sell the player and the sport to the fans. As long as skill is not worsened, this practice will serve its purpose. However, it is important for the individual to realize when performance is primarily for aesthetic appeal and when performance style leads to effectiveness. Ego involvement is the basis for one, whereas science is the foundation of the other.

LIMITATIONS

A host of factors at any one given moment can contribute to variability in the output of a system. Restrictions in the design and functioning abilities of the system limit potential performance levels. The human system, like any other, depends on the quality of the component parts and their ability to interact in appropriate coordinated fashion to fulfill reasonable objectives. Defects in any system can occur, however. Some can be remedied with functions restored to full usage. Others can never be restructured. In still other cases, compensation may overcome the dampening effect of an inferior component part of the system.

Because the functioning ability of a system is weighed against the criterion of input versus output match, it is useful to identify parts of the system that may trigger noise or bias, negatively influencing performance. A quick survey of the human system would indicate that faulty working senses, perceptual distortions, learning disorders and damage to the nervous system, and physical handicaps can place a heavy toll on any expectations of quality performance.

An individual's chance at skilled behavior depends greatly on being able to accommodate or compensate for structural and functional handicaps. In many situations, adjustments can be made so that reasonable performance is demonstrated. The seriousness of a limitation and the ability to compensate and adjust will obviously be reflected in the quality of performance. As we saw with the model of motor behavior presented in Chapter 6, any kind of limitation may contribute to differences among individuals as they attempt to learn and perform skills.

Physical Handicaps

The satisfactory functioning of the musculature involved in any motor task of concern depends on the extent of any temporary or permanent damage. Temporary damage needs to be repaired, permanent damage compensated for, and poor condition remediated. A structural defect leads to a functional problem. Yet, functional problems may occur as well without structural defects. For instance, poor motor performance is noticed when appropriate muscles do not possess the needed tonus for strength; tissue elasticity is insufficient for flexibility; or cardiorespiratory functions are below par for the needed endurance to continue practicing a task.

The organic efficiency of the body can be improved on so that the person will possess the necessary physical properties to practice tasks and eventually demonstrate skilled performance. If the physical components involved in the tasks are carefully evaluated, practice can sufficiently improve them to provide the learner with the "tools" to proceed. On the other hand, temporary damage to body tissue may suggest nonparticipation in activity until healing occurs. Permanent damage to tissue requires the learner to seek out alternative methods of achieving goals. The performance may not appear smooth, but nevertheless the task may be completed in a satisfactory manner.

Sensory Handicaps

Because what comes out of the system (behavior) depends greatly on what went into it (information), the senses should not be impaired in any way that might cause input to be distorted as it is transmitted through the system. Of interest in the research has been the effect of damage to the distance receptors (visual, auditory) on learning and performing a task.

In cognitively oriented tasks, the deaf have often been found inferior to "normals." Yet, recent researchers have pointed out that the deaf were restricted and penalized in the learning strategies they could employ under the design of the experiments. At present there is a strong belief that deaf people use different strategies than hearing people and can, consequently, perform similar in many tasks if they are (1) taught to use special strategies or (2) allowed to, by removal of situational learning constraints.

Can individuals with a severe handicap in one sense modality compensate for it by developing a greater-than-average ability to use another sense modality? The question is raised often. Thare is some evidence to support the compensation notion for vision.

Larry Beutler (1970) offers data along the same line for deaf children. Deaf and hearing subjects learned three high-relief finger mazes of increasing complexity while blindfolded. The presumed verbal advantage of hearing subjects was not demonstrated in this study, in that they did not outperform the deaf on any of the tasks. In fact, the younger group of deaf children was superior to their hearing counterparts on the most difficult task. Perhaps with age these differences would not be noted, as language skill and verbal concepts are developed in the hearing children. These concepts are needed to achieve in verbal and motor tasks. At any rate, it appears as though deaf children use a different problem-solving approach on tasks when compared with hearing children.

Because individuals who possess a sense impairment are likely not to be active in vigorous activities in which that sense might have a major role, their overall physical fitness might be expected to be lower than average. Handicapped children need the opportunity to move and to stimulate physical development. In those educational programs where special planned physical activities are available to handicapped students, their development will be similar in general to the nonhandicapped. Balance ability stands out as a variable distinguishing the handicapped. As Samuel Case, Y. Dawson, J. Schartner, and D. Donaway (1973) reported, 81 per cent of the deaf subjects failed to demonstrate a particular balance task and 50 per cent of the blind failed it, but only 15 per cent of the nonhandicapped subjects could not do it. Special balance training may help to compensate for a vestibular pathology associated with the deaf or the fear of the blind if they are to accomplish in those gross motor activities that require some degree of balance.

Perceptual Handicaps

As we will see in Chapter 10, which deals with developmental factors, the quality and nature of early and timely experiences in life for all living organisms may have some bearing on adult behavior. Enriched environments and experiences, in contrast with deprived ones, stimulate the senses and in turn the perceptual processes. Coping behaviors are learned. So are problem-solving abilities. One learns to perceive relationships between objects, to determine functioning abilities of the body, and in general to make sense of the environment. A number of theories related to cognitive achievements and dependence on adequate perceptual-motor development of the child have been proposed; the leading ones are presented and discussed in Chapter 10. As far as effective performance in motor skills is concerned, perception plays a major role in making sense of cues and helping to suggest the decisions leading to the right behavior. Insufficient previous experiences or neurological impairment will impede performance in the learning of complex motor skills.

Cognitive Handicaps

The human system that is retarded mentally will typically show an inferior level of performance in a variety of motor activities when compared to those systems in the normal intellectual range. The mentally retarded will also show a greater individual variability in scores than normals. This handicap suggests that special training procedures need to be considered, such as more time, simple explanations, and sufficient breakdown of the activity into subtasks.

The problem that the mentally retarded have with learning motor skills implies the degree cognition plays in skill mastery. Following verbal or written directions, applying verbal labels to motor acts (self-verbalization), using tactics and strategies, following rules, and problem solving are activities associated with the cognitive domain of behaviors. The ideal integration of cognitive, affective, and psychomotor behaviors can only occur if all subsystems are operational at an adequate level.

Learning Disorders

Any inability to perform an activity typically performed by others within the same range of intelligence can be considered a learning disability. A learning disorder, by comparison, can be due to a host of problems:

> Learning disorder might best designate a known impairment in the nervous system. The impairment may be the result of genetic variation, biochemical irregularity, perinatal brain insult, or injury sustained by the nervous system as a result of disease, accident, sensory deprivation, nutritional deficit, or other direct influence (Frierson and Barbe, 1967, p. 4).

Brain damage may only be one of several reasons why persons do not function properly. A number of alternatives have already been presented. We will concentrate here on any injury or damage to the central nervous sytem that can occur prior to, at the time of, or after birth. Injury, infection, and the like can cause functional disturbances, as manifested by perceptual, judgmental, emotional, and response impairment. The learning process is consequently impeded.

An Overview

Chapters 7 and 8 contained an abundance of material in which many factors were discussed that may influence differences in the way persons learn and/or perform motor skills. The degree to which an ideal bodily structure, interests, and capabilities are present, the higher the probability of a successful learning experience. When the so-called ideal combination of factors is not present, compensation can occur, to a certain extent.

As we learn more about the factors that contribute to achievement in motor skills, performance level expectations can be modified when such factors are not present at an ideal level. Furthermore, instructional programs can be adjusted to take such limitations into consideration. The manner in which content is taught, skills practiced, and environments manipulated could reflect a sensitivity to learners.

Figure 8-3 summarizes the major characteristics of learners that should be considered when instructional programs are designed. Of course, it is virtually im-

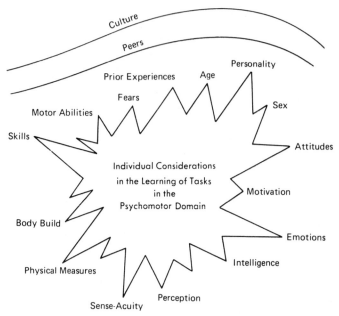

FIGURE 8-3. Factors that contribute to individual differences among learners.

possible to recognize all these individual considerations. Yet, one of the fallacies in any group learning circumstance is to treat all individuals as if they possess the same characteristics. Unless individualized instruction is the medium, group instruction will probably proceed with the establishment of procedures that will seemingly benefit most participants, with some alternatives available for those who would apparently fare better under other arrangements.

CHAPTER HIGHLIGHTS

1. Physical characteristics associated with type of body build, strength, endurance, flexibility, and level of physical condition allow the learner to execute correctly and to practice extensively the skills to be learned. Such considerations are obviously more important with gross motor activities than fine motor activities. Physical characteristics must be trained specific to the demands of the skill-learning situation if a program is to be effective.

2. The senses operate as receptacles for information, and consequently they must be in good functioning order: the output of any system depends, in part, on the appropriateness of the input. In motor learning, visual, kinesthetic, tactile, equilibrium, and even auditory cues may need to be responded to.

3. Just as individuals differ in physical characteristics and acuity of the senses, they may also utilize perceptual processes in dissimilar ways. We make meaning of information depending on its nature and availability, as well as on such personal factors as set, selective attention, perceptual style, motivation,

MOTOR LEARNING AND HUMAN PERFORMANCE

previous experiences in the same situation (familiarity), and personal development and maturity.

4. Two topics in perception that are of special interest to motor behaviorists are psychophysics and figural aftereffects. Psychophysics is the study of sense modalities and absolute and differential thresholds to stimuli. An understanding of an individual's ability to detect stimuli helps us to explain behavior better. A figural aftereffect refers to a perceptual distortion following a prolonged satiation to a particular stimulus. Its existence, in certain situations involving vision, kinesthesis, and balance, has been recognized. But improved performances due to such experiences have not been found.

5. Attempts to determine a meaningful positive relationship with intelligence or academic achievement with physical status have failed. The same finding generally holds true when intelligence and the ability to learn motor skills have been compared with subjects of normal intelligence. With more youthful learners, there is more of a tendency for some of these factors to go together. Athletes and nonathletes usually do not differ from each other in intelligence or academic achievement. Mentally retarded children, however, usually are behind normal children of similar age in physical development and level of skill in various motor activities.

6. Personality factors can contribute to more successful learning and performing circumstances. Various observational, projective, and instrumental techniques have been used to measure aspects of personality or all of it, with strengths and limitations associated with each procedure. Whereas trait theory dominated personality testing for many years, the concept of person and situation interaction is gaining increasing popularity. Some people show fairly consistent patterns of behavior across situations; others do not. Normative and situational information are helpful to understand how learners can be expected to respond to certain learning situations. Attitudes toward the learning experience and the instructor, as well as the need to achieve, are dimensions of personality to consider in any learning situation.

7. Emotional reactions, or feelings, to situations also reflect aspects of personality. Emotions, like motivation, may have an organizing or disorganizing effect on motor behaviors. Drive theory and the inverted-U hypothesis have been used to explain the relationship between anxiety level and performance. The latter model has greater popularity, but each can explain different kinds of motor behaviors more effectively.

The notion of state and trait anxiety levels helps to understand behavior better, and this concept should probably be applied to other personality variables. People with high and low levels of anxiety usually perform similarly on simple tasks; anxious individuals usually do worse with more complex tasks. Highly skilled performers must learn the mechanics of the movements, as well as how to control and use emotions appropriate for the circumstances. When too much anxiety is due to situational factors, more experiences and greater familiarity with the situation should be provided. When anxiety is due to personal factors, relaxation techniques need to be learned.

Stress can help or hinder behavior, as individuals respond to situational demands depending on their interpretations of the circumstances and skill level. As might be expected, excessive stress will be more disruptive for complex skill learning than simple task learning.

8. Form, or the expression of movement, in the performance of complex gross motor activities is an individual matter. Sometimes a standard form can aid performance and at other times hinder it. The interaction between biomechanical constraints, environmental constraints, and morphological constraints determines personally appropriate form in movement.

9. Personal limitations, such as sensory handicaps, perceptual handicaps, cognitive handicaps, and learning disorders should be recognized as possible sources of learning and performance problems. Special accommodating instructional procedures may need to be implemented.

References

Asmussen, E., & Heebøll-Nielsen, K. Physical performance and growth in children, influence of sex, age and intelligence. *Journal of Applied Physiology,* 1956, *8,* 371–380.

Atkinson, J. W., & Litwin, G. H. Achievement motive and test anxiety conceived as motive to approach success and motive to avoid failure. *Journal of Abnormal and Social Psychology,* 1960, *60,* 52–63.

Beals, R. P., Mayyasi, A. M., Templeton, A. E., & Johnston, W. L. The relationship between basketball shooting performance and certain visual attributes. *American Journal of Optometry and Archives of American Academy of Optometry,* 1971, *48,* 585–590.

Beutler, L. E. Hearing-loss effects on a procedural task sequence. *Journal of Motor Behavior,* 1970, *2,* 207–215.

Carron, A. V. Motor performance under stress. *Research Quarterly,* 1968, *39,* 463–469.

Case, S., Dawson, Y., Schartner, J., & Donaway, D. Comparison of levels of fundamental skill and cardio-respiratory fitness of blind, deaf, and non-handicapped high school age boys. *Perceptual and Motor Skills,* 1973, *36,* 1291–1294.

Cattell, R. B. *Abilities: Their structure, growth, and action.* Boston: Houghton-Mifflin, 1971.

Cohen, J. *Personality assessment.* Chicago, Ill.: Rand McNally, 1969.

Corso, J. F. *The experimental psychology of sensory behavior.* New York: Holt, Rinehart & Winston, 1967.

Cratty, B. J., & Duffy, K. Studies of movement aftereffects. *Perceptual and Motor Skills,* 1969, *29,* 843–960.

Cureton, T. K. *Physical fitness of champion athletes.* Urbana: University of Illinois Press, 1951.

DuBois, P. The design of correlational studies in training. In R. Glaser (Ed.), *Training research and education.* New York: John Wiley, 1965.

Duncanson, J. P. Learning and measured abilities. *Journal of Educational Psychology,* 1966, *57,* 220–229.

Endler, N. S., & Magnusson, D. Toward an interactional psychology of personality. *Psychological Bulletin,* 1976, *83,* 956–974.

Epstein, W. *Varieties of perceptual learning.* New York: McGraw-Hill, 1967.

Frierson, E. C., & Barbe, W. B. (Eds.). *Educating children with learning disabilities.* New York: Appleton-Century-Crofts, 1967.

Guilford, J. P. Three faces of intellect. *American Psychologist,* 1959, *14,* 469–479.

Higgins, J. R. *Human movement: An integrated approach.* St. Louis, Mo.: C. V. Mosby, 1977.

Hirata, K. Physique and age of Tokyo olympic champions. *Journal of Sports Medicine and Physical Fitness*, 1966, *6*, 207–222.

Howe, C. E. A comparison of motor skills of mentally retarded and normal children. *Exceptional Children*, 1959, *25*, 352–354.

Ismail, A., Kephart, N., & Cowell, C. C. *Utilization of motor aptitude tests in predicting academic achievement, Technical Report No. 1*. Purdue University Research Foundation, P. U. 879-64-838, 1963.

Jacobs, P. D., & Munz, D. C. An index for measuring perceived stress in a college population. *The Journal of Psychology*, 1968, *70*, 9–15.

Jacobs, P. D., & Thornton, J. Scale sensitivity of the perceived stress index. *Perceptual and Motor Skills*, 1970, *30*, 944.

Jones, M. B. Practice as a process of simplification. *Psychological Review*, 1962, *69*, 274–294.

Krahenbuhl, G. S. Stress reactivity in tennis players. *Research Quarterly*, 1971, *42*, 42–46.

Martens, R. Anxiety and motor behavior: A review. *Journal of Motor Behavior*, 1971, *3*, 151–180.

McCafferty, W. B., & Horvath, S. M. Specificity of exercise and specificity of training: A subcellular review. *Research Quarterly*, 1977, *48*, 358–371.

Morris, G. S. D. Dynamic visual acuity: Implications for the physical educator and coach. *Motor Skills: Theory Into Practice*, 1977, *2*, 15–20.

Nelson, R., & Nofsinger, M. R. Effect of overload on speed of elbow flexion and the associated aftereffects. *Research Quarterly*, 1965, *36*, 174–182.

Oliver, J. N. The effect of physical conditioning exercises and activities on the mental characteristics of educationally sub-normal boys. *British Journal of Educational Psychology*, 1958, *28*, 155–165.

Parsons, O. A., Phillips, L., & Lane, J. E. Performance on the same psychomotor task under different stressful conditions. *Journal of Psychology*, 1954, *38*, 457–466.

Prather, D. C., Berry, G. A., & Bermudez, J. M. Effect of prompting and feedback on performing during learning, stress, and transfer of a perceptual skill. *Proceedings of the 80th Annual Convention of the American Psychological Association*, 1972, *7*, 643–644.

Ryan, E. D. Relative academic achievement and stabilometer performance. *Research Quarterly*, 1963, *34*, 184–190.

Sage, G. *Introduction to motor-behavior: A neuropsychological approach*. Second edition. Reading, Mass.: Addison-Wesley, 1977.

Sheldon, W. H., Stevens, S. S., & Tucker, W. R. *The varieties of human physique*. New York: Harper & Row, 1940.

Shick, J. Relationship between depth perception and hand-eye dominance and free-throw shooting in college women. *Perceptual and Motor Skills*, 1971, *33*, 539–542.

Solley, C. M., & Murphy, G. *Development of the perceptual world*. New York: Basic Books, 1960.

Spielberger, C. D. *The state-trait anxiety inventory*. Palo Alto, Calif.: Consulting Psychologists Press, 1970.

Spielberger, C. D. State-trait anxiety and interactional psychology. In D. Magnusson & N. S. Endler (Eds.), *Personality at the crossroads: Current issues in interactional psychology*. Hillsdale, N. J.: Erlbaum, 1977.

Spielberger, C. D. *The state-trait anxiety inventory*. Palo Alto, Ca.: Consulting Psychologists Press, 1970.

Start, K. B. Intelligence and the improvement in a gross motor skill after mental practice. *British Journal of Educational Psychology*, 1964, *34*, 85.

Tanner, J. M. Physique, body composition and growth. In E. Jokl & E. Simon (Eds.), *International research in sport and physical education*. Springfield, Ill.: Charles C Thomas, 1964.

Taylor, J. A. A personality scale of manifest anxiety. *Journal of Abnormal and Social Psychology*, 1953, *48*, 285–290.

Thurstone, T. G. *An evaluation of educating mentally handicapped children in special classes and in regular classes*. Cooperative Research Project Contract Number OE-SAE-6452 of the U. S. Office of Education, The School of Education, University of North Carolina, 1959.

Wilberg, R. B. Response accuracy based upon recall from visual and kinesthetic short-term memory. *Research Quarterly*, 1969, *40*, 407–414.

Williams, H. G., & Blane, V. L. A comparison of selected behavior of identical twins, one blind from birth. *Journal of Motor Behavior*, 1969, *1*, 259–274.

Wood, C. G., & Hokanson, J. E. Effects of induced tension on performance and the inverted U function. *Journal of Personality and Social Psychology*, 1965, *5*, 501–510.

9
DEVELOPMENTAL FACTORS AND INFLUENCE ON BEHAVIOR

In an experimental sense, learning is usually measured independently of maturation. Practically speaking, though, maturation is related to behavior, and the two are inextricably interwoven. Maturation determines human potential and sets the upper limits of learning and performance.

As the youngster grows, develops, and matures, certain patterns of behavior unfold, mostly learned, but in some cases occurring in spite of a lack of experience. Researchers can measure the effects of maturation on learning and behavior when practice in or experience with certain skills is held to a minimum. Those interested in distinguishing learned acts from the natural instinctive behavior of a species have used this method. Some simple reflexes and simple acts of human babies have been identified as being independent of learning. However, it is generally conceded that the attainment of complex skills and most behavioral patterns as defined by adult standards is the result of maturation and experience.

Certain behavior is primarily influenced by learning, whereas other behavior is affected most by maturation. Educators by necessity should expect unique behavior and abilities relevant to an individual's age and maturational level. They should also understand how to teach, when to teach, and what to teach children at each level. Often a mistake is made in assuming that body size represents development and readiness to learn. *Growth* implies an increase in stature, *development* denotes increasing complexity of structure and function, and *maturation* indicates that the organism is approaching a somewhat stable structure. Behavior is more purposeful when development and maturation take place. Age is another factor that is misconstrued as representing maturity. This is why we should distinguish the chronological age from the maturational age of a child.

Throughout life, from birth to death, experiences accumulate, the body grows and changes, and individual differences in abilities and achievements are observable. Age differences, sex differences, innate abilities, personality factors, environmental experiences—all and more—interact to determine human attainment.

The readiness of the organism to learn presumes the presence of structure, functioning capabilities, and motives. Genes regulate and mediate the developmental process and serve to lay the framework for a person's potential achievement in certain endeavors at particular points in the early years of life. Body build, tendencies toward emotionality, and other characteristics are partially determined through heredity. These factors, along with rate of maturation, will favor some people and stifle others, in regard to their readiness to learn and ability to perform motor skills. Such environmental factors as conditions in the home, socioeconomic level, sociocultural surroundings, and peer associations will also influence motor development and attitudes toward participation and achievement in motor skills. As we can see, an enormous number of variables will potentially impinge on any child, interacting and influencing motor development and behavior.

Any attempt to determine the factors that influence how and what children learn will be rather general and fruitless unless consideration (Singer, 1978) is given to the following:

1. Various activities and unique demands placed on learners.
2. The development of such cognitive processes as understanding, perception, attention, memory, inference, evaluation, and deduction.
3. Neurological development.
4. The development of physical characteristics, psychomotor abilities, psychological attributes (motives, attitudes, etc.), learning capabilities, and human interactive processes (e.g. cooperation).
5. The influence of sociological, cultural peer, and familial factors.

It is not the intent in this chapter to describe how all factors interact to produce skilled behavior in children. The emphasis, instead, is on the child as an information processor, with implications for understanding and teaching. Some normative performance data will be presented as well, as will discussion on related topics.

CHRONOLOGICAL VERSUS MATURATIONAL AGE

Chronological age often misrepresents readiness skills and expectant behavior. Children, in general, seem to go through the same sequence of developmental stages but vary in their rate of progress. To post norms based on age is often a matter of convenience and practicality, and deviations should be weighed accordingly. It would be better to understand the child and his or her stage of maturational development, because early and late maturers do not display similar characteristics at the same chronological age.

Mental age, as represented by the IQ test, is, in a sense, independent of chronological age. The intelligence quotient is a ratio of the child's mental age as determined by an intelligence test over chronological age. It is possible, indeed probable, that students in a given class composed of children of the same chronological age will be widely distributed according to mental age. By the same token, children making the transition from childhood to adulthood demonstrate physical development according to their rate of maturation rather than age. Such a factor as strength is an important determiner of potential success in many motor activities, and obviously early maturers may be expected to perform more ably in sports because their physical development is accelerated.

Caution in grouping children by chronological age without concern for maturation rate is pleaded by Robert Malina (1972). It should be recognized that a child's growth status at any one time depends on (1) final adult size and (2) the rate at which the size is being attained. Any two persons may reach the same ultimate size at different speeds. In this case, the factors are independent, for at different developing ages these two persons will show dissimilar growth profiles. The factors are related, however, in that one's size at a particular age is related to maturation rate. Early maturers are larger than slower maturers of the same chronological age. Great variations among developing individuals, even those who will eventually attain similar size characteristics, is a warning to teachers in group-activity learning situations.

Numerous investigations have been completed relating motor achievement to chronological age. Reservations should be present in any application of norms to one person's scores, but there is value in comparing age and motor performance variables. This information is somewhat helpful at the first level of understanding, in order that generalizations can be made about behavior and age. Major deviations in behavioral expectations can then be examined on an individual basis, at which time other variables might be considered. A maturational average or advanced youngster at a given chronological age who is performing substandardly might be lacking in motivation, interest, and enthusiasm to learn and perform certain activities.

HEREDITY AND EXPERIENCE

When discussing motor skills, such as those involved in athletic performance, arguments are often heated as to whether the outstanding athlete is born or made. It is the old problem of nature versus nurture. What are the relative effects of genetics and experience on performance? Such descriptive phrases as "what a natural athlete" or "a born hitter" are ways of commonly referring to particular performers. Does the physical educator or coach waste time training individuals "who don't have it" and "never will have it" (whatever "it" may be)?

An examination of the problem should probably begin with the effects of heredity and environmental circumstances on intelligence, for it is the development of the cognitive processes that has been the primary concern of educators and psychologists during this century. The results of their research pave the way for understanding motor skill accomplishment. No informed person would state that what we are is caused by purely genetic factors or solely environmental experiences, but rather that the end product is formulated by the interaction of both. The problem is in determining the relative contributions each makes to one's level of attainment in a particular endeavor.

Various methods have been employed in investigations concerned with the relative effects of heredity and environment on the organism. The usual laboratory techniques with lower forms of organisms have included (1) selective breeding and (2) analysis of behavioral characteristics shown by different but ideally pure strains. Obviously these techniques are not possible with human subjects. Families may be observed in order to find the characteristics that are prevalent among members, and correlations are computed to determine the degree of relationship among members on a specific variable.

Twins have been the subject of much research. If twins are identical and raised in the same home, then differences between them are probably due to genetics. Twins who are reared apart also offer data valuable for gaining insight into the problem. Finally, a comparison of monozygotic twins (MZ) with dizygotic twins (DZ) permits further analysis of the relative effects of heredity and environment. Monozygotic twins are identical twins, originating from a single zygote and provided with identical hereditary endowments. Dizygotic twins are fraternal twins, coming from two separate zygotes, who may or may not be alike. MZ twins raised apart yield the simplest comparison data for estimating the heritability of a particular characteristic (the percentage of impact inheritance has on the characteristic relative to effect of environmental experiences on it). When the genetic constitutions (genotypes) of the subjects are controlled and are more similar, deductions on environmental effects are more easily formulated. The particular characteristic of interest, observed and measured, is referred to as a phenotype.

It is no easy matter to control the many influencing variables adequately in order to estimate environmental versus hereditary effects accurately. Therefore, results of studies must be accepted with reservation. Such findings are more suggestive than conclusive, although certain general assumptions may now be made because of accumulating evidence, as we will see.

Cognitive Processes

With intelligence, as with any other factor, environmental variables operate within the limits offered by heredity. How influential is heredity in determining intelligence? Apparently it is quite influential. The IQs of identical twins raised apart correlate higher than those of fraternal twins raised together. Environmental circumstances, to a much lesser degree than heredity, also affect intelligence, for it is noted that the IQ of one identical twin can be predicted from the IQ score of the other, with the accuracy depending on their upbringing. When the IQ correlation of twins raised in the same house is analyzed, a predictability of 80 per cent has been obtained. It is reported to be 60 per cent for identical twins raised apart. In other words, twins living apart have a greater difference in IQ scores than twins living together.

Investigators have found similar results; some show that less than 10 per cent of the IQ variance is accounted for by the environmental component, and that as much as 96 per cent of the variance is contributed by the genetic background. Jensen (1970), in summarizing the literature, noted that a comparison of MZ twins raised apart is probably the easiest way of determining the heritability of certain factors. These twins do not differ by more than seven to ten IQ points, on the average, when reared apart; they differ by about two or three points when raised in the same home. Jensen writes that twenty-four points is the largest IQ difference ever reported for a pair of identical twins raised apart, but more than 17 per cent of children, fraternal or nontwin, raised together differ by more than twenty-four points. Jensen concluded that the genes outweigh the effects of environment by 2:1 for the average person's IQ score.

Using thirty-three pairs of MZ twins and twelve pairs of DZ twins, ages thirteen to eighteen, T. R. Osborne and J. A. Gregor (1966) administered a battery of cognitive tests described as visualization, perceptual speed, and spatial orientation. The range of the heritability coefficients was from 0.15 to 0.89, indicating that specific abilities are independently inherited. That is to say, the role of genetics on task performance is different for different tasks. As might be expected, MZ twins showed higher relationships in task performances (0.46 to 0.91) than DZ twins (0.08 to 0.72). Presented in this article is an excellent review of the literature, and the degree of compatibility of various techniques for determining heritability coefficients is demonstrated.

The heredity-versus-environment issue reveals an interesting history whereby similar questions are raised, but at no time was it so volatile as in the late 1960s, with the publication of an article by Arthur Jensen (1969) in the *Harvard Education Review*. In this article and in a number of other ones, Jensen has strongly supported his stance with his own research and the interpretation of other research that heredity is by far the major factor in IQ scores. Most controversial was his claim that there are probably genetic differences of intelligence among races and that blacks have an average inherited intelligence below that of whites. Intensive debates on the point occurred on many campuses and were covered extensively by the media. Major psychology and educational research journals are still publishing articles that include data or thoughts on both sides of the issue. Because the issues cover political and racial grounds, it is not at all surprising that howls of outrage from civil rights people have been heard. Scientists also disagree about the practical interpretations of the position that heredity largely affects IQ. Data can and are being interpreted in different ways, as scholars attempt to formulate acceptable theories and determine what kinds of environmental situations and programs can produce desired behavioral changes within genetic limitations.

Although environmental factors may not have a dramatic effect on intellectual growth, they have a great influence on achievement. Extremes in environmental surroundings will have a dramatic effect on IQ scores and academic achievement in general. It should go without saying that enriched environments will promote achievement, but impoverished conditions will result in progressively poorer returns. The implication here is that although genetic factors limit potential, there is quite a distance between the operational level of an individual and personal theoretical limits. Much can be done through environmental manipulations to raise the intellectual achievement of an average or below-average youngster.

Motor Skills

Just as differences in intellectual performance may be caused by hereditary and environmental factors, these same factors operate for potential success in motor skill performance. The extent of influence is not easy to ascertain, for most of the research has been completed on mental growth. However, it should be readily apparent that it does not necessarily follow that the same amount of practice on similar skills will benefit all individuals equally. Some people will perform more effectively after a few tries, some will show skill following many practice sessions, and others may never reach the level of performance that might be termed skilled. Obviously, dissimilar capacities for performing various tasks will be due to hereditary factors and/or previous experiences.

There exists some relationship between the body build of the oustanding athlete and his or her chosen sport. To the extent that heredity might contribute to success in particular activities via physical characteristics, studies have found correlations approximating 0.50 between family physical qualities, such as height and weight (McClearn, 1964). (A statistical correlation, r, of 1.00 demonstrates a perfect relationship between variables, whereas one of 0.00 indicates no relationship.) Even anxiety level has been shown to have a firm genetic basis, and certainly the effective usage of emotions in activity can affect outcomes.

The influence of parent size on the size of offspring has been documented by R. M. Malina, A. B. Harper, and J. D. Holman (1970). Also studied were sex differences, race differences, gross motor performance, and static strength. Parent size has differential effects on the strength and motor performance of children, and those effects are more noticeable during the first few years of life than by school age. In general, however, an inconsistent trend was observed between parent size and motor performance.

Genetics will usually determine body type, and it is often witnessed that identical twins have similar body constitutions. Anatomically speaking, body structures may be influenced greatly by nonhereditary variables, such as health, nutrition, and exercise. A good example of an environmental factor exerting influence over genetic tendencies is the fact that first-generation Japanese immigrants exceed their former countrymen in height by two inches. Nutrition and diet evidently had much to do with this situation.

Q. McNemar (1933) undertook an early study to analyze the inheritance of abilities involving certain motor skills. The tests involved the use of the pursuit rotor, the whipple steadiness tester, the Miles speed drill, the Brown spool packer, and a card sorter. Forty-eight pairs of junior high school age twins were diagnosed as fraternal and forty-seven pairs were identical. The fraternals achieved higher scores than the identicals on all five tasks, but only in spools and cards did the difference achieve statistical significance. The identicals showed a higher degree of resemblance in their performance than the fratnerals.

As to actual research on the born-versus-made athlete, L. Gedda (1961) investigated the families of outstanding athletes and made comparisons of the sports practiced by twins. In this study, Gedda obtained data on genotype twins and twins with dissimilar genotypes. Among his many observations, he noted a difference between type of twin and sports participation and success. Little dissimilarity in sports participation and practice could be found between genotype twins. It was equivalent to a 6 per cent difference in the case of identical genotype twins but was 85 per cent in the case of twins with different genotypes. Evidently, twins with contrary genotypes (fraternal twins) had individual interests and differed widely in general sports practice.

Gedda interpreted his data to indicate that there is a great similarity between identical genotypes and the sports in which they participate successfully; hence, the relationship of heredity factors to activity interest and certain characteristics to athletic success. He hypothesized that sports aptitude is attributed to exogenous factors, or environmental conditions, including training, experiences, socioeconomic level, and an endogenous factor, or inherited phenotype, which refers to the transmitted characteristics necessary for skill attainment in a specific sport.

In another investigation, Gedda, Milani–Comparetti, and Brenci (1964) surveyed the athletes who participated in the 1960 Olympic Games in Rome. After accumulating data on each athlete's family, the authors formulated two indexes: an Index of Isosportivation (number of the athlete's family members participating in the same sport) and an Index of Allosportivation (number of family members practicing some other sport). Interpretation of the information allowed the following conclusion: (1) the athlete and family practiced similar activities and (2) specific physical and psychological qualities of the Olympians could be attributed to heredity. These qualities occur repeatedly in the same family and are therefore attributed to heredity and environmental influences.

It appears, then, that the capacity to perform motor skills is primarily determined by heredity. However, although achievement in intellectual pursuits and athletic endeavors will ultimately be determined by genetics, environmental experiences will do much to influence the level of achievement. Unless energies are guided in a constructive manner and abilities developed through instruction and practice, even the most favorably endowed individual will not be an outstanding performer. Certain people are born with particular potential general talents or abilities, and these permit them to excel more easily in a given area. Yet, if all success were based on hereditary components, what would be the purpose of developing a psychology of learning, of developing learning techniques and theories? Why attempt to modify behavior? Obviously, much can be done with any individual if instructed effectively, and life's experiences will either facilitate or hinder the development and acquisition of motor skills.

EARLY MOTOR DEVELOPMENT AND LEARNING

We have spent some time on the relationship of heredity and experience with development and achievement. Now it is important to analyze early motor development and the evolution of learning processes. This will be followed by a discussion of information processing and development and then one on later learning. A review of the model in Chapter 6 will help if children's learning is viewed from an information-processing perspective. Perhaps a logical starting point is Lewis Lipsitt's (1971) statement that the newborn, contrary to usual expectation, is not "inept, befuddled, bewildered, disorganized, or diffuse" (p. 18). Older concepts held that the infant was nonresponsive and could not be encouraged to learn faster than "normal" maturation would allow. Thus, the true learning potential of the infant was virtually untapped until recent years.

Lipsitt dramatically emphasizes that the human newborn is a responsive organism. A state of helplessness does not exist; enrichment environments can have a considerable influence on development. The degree to which an infant responds effectively to stimuli is usually used as an indicant of intelligence. Although there are obvious motor patterns forming that can be viewed from a motor development point of view, such responses can be regarded in their cognitive aspects. After all, the baby's perceptual and discriminating abilities, among others, are determined from the outcome of motor responses. As the sense organs and the rest of the nervous system develop, more advanced motor patterns can be displayed. The combination of maturation and enriched experiences helps to give rise to more highly differentiated and yet integrated coordinated responses. From the general behaviors related to manipulation and locomotion will come a variety of movement-oriented skills.

With the increased development of the nervous system and the musculature, as well as overall maturation, learning capabilities also increase. Performance level usually reflects *less* than what we *really* know at any given time, and learning processes have usually been developed *less* than our developmental potential allows, as we can observe in Figure 9-1.

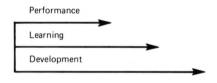

Performance

Learning

Development

FIGURE 9-1. The relationship of development, learning, and performance.

During the early portions of this century, G. Stanley Hall and later, Arnold Gesell, conceptualized a maturational hypothesis, or what Robert Gagné (1968) calls the *growth-readiness model*. It was thought that environmental factors were supportive of behavioral changes, but that, generally speaking, organisms acquired the same motor patterns in a preplanned (genetic) manner. Genetics predetermine the evolvement of behaviors, regardless of situational and learning factors. Even the Piaget approach, mentioned previously, places minimal influence for learning on a child's behavior and heavy reliance on maturational factors. The child passes through stages that are maturationally associated, although environment can facilitate or inhibit the phasing in or out of a stage. Another early description of the process of motor development was behavioristic. Behaviorism embraced concepts related to the learning of S–R associations, as we saw in Chapter 4.

Whereas Piaget relies heavily on maturational factors to explain the child's behaviors, Gagné talks in terms of the learning of prerequisite skills and behaviors, which can be related to maturation but is not of major concern. Gagné suggests that the learning of associations does not encourage the child to pass from one point to another in development. Rather, it is learning of an ordered set of capabilities. These build up in hierarchical fashion through the processes of differentiation, recall, and transfer of learning. In a simple sense, the reference is to building blocks, cumulatively adding up to more complex learned capabilities. This notion, primarily expressed by Gagné as an explanation of a child's intellectual development, has an analogy in Jerome Bruner's (1970) explanation of skill development.

Learning general and basic movements is not the same as learning skills. The latter involves far more complex processes. The structural components, dependent on maturation, must be present in the child, as well as precise practice of responses to cues under the direction of plans and strategies. As we have noted, motor behavior proceeds from primarily reflexive and generalized movement patterns to more differentiated, specialized, and integrated movments (Breckenridge & Murphy, 1969). Visual and neuromotor components are integrated in eye–hand coordination tasks. Although maturation provides the ability to control one's body and a readiness to learn, complex skills need specific rather than general practice. Maturation is important for generalized responses, but specific experiences lead to highly specialized behaviors.

Concepts and skills are built up with use. The child must continually react to environmental stimulation. Because a number of significant human characteristics develop most quickly in the first five years of life and changes in development are more difficult with age and maturation (Bloom, 1964), the implications are great for quality preschool and early school years in developing learning patterns and general achievement.

The child's readiness to learn skills will depend, in part, on the stage of development of his or her cognitive structures and processes. Teaching strategies and performance expectations should reflect a sensitivity to this development status. As I. E. Sigel and R. R. Cocking (1977) astutely observe in this regard, communication level between adult and child must be appropriate. An understanding of the way children process information would be helpful, for they process adult communications "not in terms of some objective basis but rather in terms of developmental level" (p. 101). With development, a child thinks, analyzes, and reasons more like an adult.

There is abundant information that cognitive processes can be accelerated with effective stimulation in early childhood. With little research on motor skills learning but continuing with the same rationale, it appears that a similar statement can be made about motor development processes. Of question are the long-term effects. Do early cognitive enhancement experiences make a difference in later years? What about special'motor enrichment programs? Arguments can be made in defense or attack of special early childhood programs, but the position taken here is that, within the structural and functional constraints of the organism, enriched early experiences *of all kinds* experienced in a satisfying atmosphere should increase the likelihood of beneficial long-term effects.

The potential for young children to learn complex motor skills has been shown by Ken Leithwood (1970–71). He reports the terrific gains made by four-year-olds learning standard gymnastic activities. During a period of four months, the children met for three times a week for a maximum of thirty minutes in each session. With most activities, the specially trained group made gains almost five times as great as those made by comparison groups. The experimental subjects were all able to combine tasks into their own created routines. Leithwood also scaled down gymnastic apparatus (parallel bar, horizontal bar, balance beam, trampoline), and specially trained children learned one-third more tasks. A strong possibility exists that simple activities are generally learned at the same rate for specially trained and nontrained children, in which case the maturational hypothesis would be supported. But children are ready and can effectively learn complex motor activities when involved in specific training for development.

We have already stated that learning occurs soon after birth. Many experiments with babies and other young demonstrate that conditioning can occur under appropriate situations and manipulations. But do the young learn as well as the mature organisms? At present, it appears that it is difficult to relate age and learning, for performance is determined by a host of interacting variables. Rate of acquisition and capacity affect performance but are not always found to be related to age.

In order for stimulation to be meaningful, it must not only be provided early, but *continuously* as well. Intellectually gifted children have stereotypically been stimulated early, intensively, and extensively. The gains from early intervention programs disappear shortly after termination of the programs, which is further rationale for continuity in programming, suggests Thomas Ryan (1971). It becomes clear that the young child is capable of learning a great deal, if the opportunities for learning are properly presented.

INFORMATION-PROCESSING CAPABILITIES IN DEVELOPMENT AND LEARNING

The child can be viewed an an active information processor in a *critical stage* of developing plans or programs in order to resolve situations. Although concepts associated with cybernetic and information-processing models were initially presented after World War II, it has only been in recent years that attempts have been offered to relate them to developmental processes in children in general (Farnham–Diggory, 1972) and to motor skills (Connolly, 1970, 1977) in particular.

Information-processing theorists concerned with the acquisition of skill have raised questions related to the organism's capability and capacity to receive information and attend to it, to place information in and retrieve it from memory. Processes and functions associated with perception, selective attention, decision making, short-term and long-term memory, and feedback are major factors in the learning of skill within the limited channel capacity of the individual, as we saw in Chapter 6. As a result of developmental limitations and inexperience, and their impact on these processes, special expectations and instructional procedures should be considered with children.

Similarly, motivation and motives need to be explored, Certain principles hold true across most ages, although there are unique considerations with children. Rather than deal with this topic in this chapter, the nature of motivation from different perspectives will be explored in Chapter 12.

A major consideration is that *children experience many of the same difficulties as adults when they attempt to learn a new task, although there are differences, as well.* For instance, adults have probably developed learning strategies, based on past experience, whereas children have little prior experience to draw from. As Michael Wade (1977) warns, "the child is a less elegant information-processing system than the adult" (p. 379). This is best illustrated by the child's lack of speed of response, anticipation, and timing behaviors. From a practical point, those who would assist youth in the learning of motor skills should be sensitive to the problems any beginner might have, as well as those unique to systems with developmental and experiential constraints. We are warned by C. D. Wickens (1974) that information-processing capacity does not necessarily develop as a function of age. Rather, the child learns how to use processes more effectively. Tasks and situations with similar characteristics and demands are recognized with experience and are responded to more ably as a result of experience.

And what should be analyzed here? It is somewhat hazardous, if not impossible, to discuss information-processing demands and a child's potential for handling them specific to each information-processing stage. These stages obviously interact and are interwoven in a complex fashion. Therefore, topics that have received reasonable attention in the research literature will be described here, with special reference to (1) selective attention, which is associated with input and perception; (2) goal-image formation; (3) decisions, response selection, and response execution, which are associated with central processing; and (4) feedback, the result of output or performance. Finally, neo-Piagetian theory is described briefly as a viable means to examine a child's processing capabilities in a conceptual and quantitative manner. At the outset, however, we must remember that *limits on information processing at any one of these stages interfere with effective performance output.*

Selective Attention

Attentiveness refers to the readiness of the organism at any moment to receive and process information. It should not be confused with the state of arousal or the act of concentration, although all three are somewhat related. The cognitive and affective processes associated with them need to be trained, as development occurs, if learning is to be effective.

As D. E. Berlyne (1970) discriminates by example, high arousal may result in poor sensitivity (attention) to the ever slight variations in input. He further suggests that concentration refers to attending to a wide or narrow range of impinging stimuli. Many difficulties in learning skills may be related to ineffective states of attention, concentration, and arousal. In fact, A. O. Ross (1976) points out that many learning disabilities (with cognitive materials) are due to children's problems in maintaining attention. The same is probably true with motor skills.

Much research evidence indicates that time delays in performance are predictable according to the degree of certainty or information present in the situation. Compared to an adult, the child is quite inexperienced; so much is unknown, that he or she lacks rules and, therefore, considers more eventualities. Anticipation has to be learned. Anticipation, decision making, and response integration are facilitated as external events are modified. For example, the number of cues or choices to be made can be reduced or the entire operation can be slowed down. In RT studies, children perform better when preparatory (alerting) intervals are brief and the length is predictable. The more we realize how the external environment can impede information processing and motor performance, the more teachers, coaches, and parents can reduce potential interventions.

Children are not as task oriented as adults are. They usually demonstrate inferior cue-selective attention functions as well as poorer task perseverance. As they become more skilled, they learn to respond to the minimal number of most meaningful cues in a situation. Young children, Karl Newell (1977) reminds us, fail to attend selectively to the available cues in a learning situation and also are unaware of how to do without guidance. The implications for effective teaching are obvious. The presence of an irrelevant stimulus will lengthen decision time. The child has not learned how to concentrate on only the appropriate cues. Adults even respond more effectively than children to partial cues, as they possess a faster visual processing time (Haith, Morrison, & Sheingold, 1970). A realization of the limitations of the child with regard to attention and selectivity to the pertinent cues suggests that the teacher should construct a learning environment that possesses cues relevant to the learning situation. As few cues as possible should be given to the learner. Once the learner has mastered the association and has created the appropriate strategies and programs, the next higher-level cues could be emphasized. This process would continue as the learner achieved more and more. With guidance, experience, and maturity, the developing organism learns to use perceptual and cognitive mechanisms in a specialized and precise manner.

It must be recognized, as Simon (1972) stresses, that "attention cannot be increased or diminished; it can only be relocated" (p. 15). With age, children learn to control their allocation of attention with appropriate strategies. Only the essential aspects of the task need be attended to, freeing the limited channel capacity to make quicker correct decisions. Similarly, the potential for anticipation is increased. More complex activities can be demonstrated as the system switches among available cues, especially as we consider the demands of externally paced activities. Young children (seven-year-olds) are distracted more easily than older children (ten- and thirteen-year-olds) when a secondary task is to be performed with a primary task (Birch, 1976). The ability to concentrate and not be distracted is a consideration in skills learning and apparently is developmentally related.

Developmental changes in selective attention have been described by A. D. Pick, M. D. Christy, and G. W. Frankel (1972). Children do not develop at the same rate, however. The many experiences associated with increasing age will enhance the learning of some activities and hinder others. Generally speaking, though, J. W. Hagen and G. H. Hale (1973) feel that the ability to use selective attention may or may not occur, depending on the coping strategy decided on to maximize performance. We can conclude that selective attention is an acquired skill.

With regard to generalized age considerations, Ross (1976) states that the young child seems to be "captured by one aspect of the situation" (p. 53). Visual scanning is restricted until age six. As a result of what has been termed overexclusive attention, incidental learning is low. Adaptive learning and problem solving are hindered. *Incidental learning* seems to hit a peak at ages ten to twelve, whereas afterward it decreases, when selective attention dominates. In other words, the same cue can result in a different focus of attention, depending on the age and development of the learner.

Ross (1976) explains that overexclusive attention has also been referred to as overselective attention. The characteristics of the task cause the child to respond in a predictable way to certain of its elements as a function of developmental characteristics. In incidental learning, a child perceives incidental features, as well as the most distinctive features of a stimulus. Between the ages of approximately six and eleven, many aspects of the situation can be and are attended to, as observational and perceptual capabilities increase. With age and development, the capability to selectively attend becomes pronounced. Individuals select the most relevant cues for them from the vast array available in a learning situation. They depend on past experiences. Incidental cues are attended to or disregarded as deemed necessary, resulting in a greater potential for skilled performance in more complex activities.

Overexclusive attention, which results in very fixed associations between cue and response, and incidental learning, which leads to more generalizable capabilities of handling related categories of problems, are both desirable circumstances, depending on situations and interactions.

Goal-Image Formation

Until now, the discussion has centered around information available to the learner in the task and situation. But information, in the form of instructional guidance, may also be communicated. Words, pictures, movement forms, and the like can help the learner to "get the idea" of what is supposed to be learned. The ability to identify and remember the salient features of a movement to be learned is obviously related to the facility shown in learning that movement.

How can information best be presented to enhance skill acquisition and retention? Attempts have been made to conceptualize associative learning in terms of imagery. A. Paivio (1970) proposes that adults and children differ in their use of imagery; more specifically, he proposes that children have greater difficulty in decoding from a mediator to a response than encoding from a word or picture to a symbolic mediator. The functional significance of imagery in learning and remembering at all ages is stressed by Paivio; this significance depends on the nature of the learning task and the prior experiences of the person with it.

Cues or information can be concrete or abstract, visual or verbal, in a meaningful context or in isolation. Presentation form and usefulness will depend on the developmental characteristics of the child. The capacity to use anticipatory imagery apparently makes great gains when a child is about seven or eight (Piaget & Inhelder, 1966). It also "may be the age at which the capacity for symbolic transformations—from words to images and back to words—makes a quantum leap" (Paivio, 1970, pp. 391–392). Readiness factors suggest the capabilities of children and the use of ways they may be trained to form goal images.

For instance, W. D. Rohwer (1970) suggests that attempts at imagery are more effective when verbal tabs are applied to and stored with images. Although verbal mediators may tend to confuse and to impair the performance of young children, more mature learners can intellectualize the relevant aspects of each image with words. If task components and verbal mediators will not overload a child's processing system, an instructional strategy in which visual and verbal communications are used should prove beneficial. Such simultaneous storage is more likely in older than in younger children, as is the case with imagery processes in general.

In addition, observational (imitative, modeling) learning should be considered as a facilitator in the acquisition of skill. The child who is proficient at this will, according to Hogan and Hogan (1975), "have a small but clear adaptive advantage over his peers" (p. 235). They write further that the successful child "will more readily and accurately incorporate elements of adult problem solving (i.e., culture) into his own behavioral repertoire and in this sense will be precociously skillful in dealing with the world" (pp. 235–236).

Imitation (observation, modeling) serves as the basis for most of the overt behavior of young children (Bandura, 1971; Brenner, 1974). It would be difficult to assess the extent to which skills learning depends on imitation, but one can speculate that it would be rather high. Modeling with verbalization can quickly produce new behaviors in children as well as in adults. One of the prerequisites for the successful imitation of behaviors is the accuracy of perception and what children can understand. Obviously, the ability to imitate reflects adequate physical, neurological, cognitive, and perceptual structures, the result of development and prior experience.

More mature children should benefit from an instructional strategy consisting of live or videotaped models, combined with verbalization of the skill. B. Zimmerman and T. L. Rosenthal (1974) have concluded that modeling, when accompanied by a verbal rule, produces the highest level of acquisition and generalization. In other words, the children in this condition exhibited the highest level of skill proficiency and retention and transfer of a skill when compared to other learners. A person, learning from a model, accompanied with a verbal description of the skill, would no doubt readily adapt already acquired skills in such a manner as to learn new skills rapidly.

Modeling procedures represent one format for the communication of the intended goal. Whatever means are employed, *attentiveness and concentration* need to be displayed by the learner. These are behaviors that must be acquired. They are associated with quality performance in readying the learner for the experience and in promoting quality performance during actual practice. Imagery, attentiveness, and concentration, as well as many other processes, become less consciously directed and more automatic as a learner becomes more expert at tasks. In other words, just as the skills themselves are learned, the art of concentration is also acquired.

Decisions, Response Selection, and Response Execution

The demonstration of skilled acts requires the child to emit controlled spatial and temporal patterns of movements. Skilled activity, as explained by Bruner (1970) is a "program (analogous to the way computer programs are run) specifying an objective or terminal state to be achieved, and requiring the serial ordering of a set of constituent, modular subroutines" (p. 65). From an information-processing perspective, skill is a function of input (perceptual processing), central processing (decision functions), and output (motor behaviors). Regardless of age, the organism must integrate these functions and processes in the context of a program if skilled behavior is to be observed. Any neurological and experiential limitations with regard to the peripheral and central mechanisms will potentially create some undesirable effect on the child's behaviors.

Skilled actions are developed from (1) the innate repertoire of movement patterns that interact with environmental conditions, and (2) a differentiation process that shapes gross acts into components for further use in new tasks and in new sequences. Programs are formulated that will contribute to the mastery of skilled tasks as well as to problem-solving activities. Bruner (1970) makes the startling observation that "it is difficult to say whether the tasks [that a child learns] . . . are instances of 'skill' or 'problem solving' " (p. 91). All too often, even with adults, we think of skill as symbolic of learned associations and finely tuned response mechanisms. The cognitive elements of skilled activity are either neglected or minimally acknowledged in typical analyses of skilled behavior. Recent thoughts on the child's learning of capabilities rules, plans, and strategies as underpinnings of cognitive and motor skills and, in fact, the emphasis on learning instead of maturational factors alone reflect what might have been considered revolutionary ideas ten years ago.

There is much information uncertainty in the environment of the child. This is related to selective attention abilities and the nature of the situation. Uncertainty, Sigel and Cocking (1977) observe, requires one to deal with problems on a probability basis. With experience and age, this, of course, will change. Piaget has been quoted as indicating that children between seven and eleven begin to develop a conceptual organization of stability, coherence, and logic. The quality of the experiences, prior to, during, and following this period; the type of guidance given for problem solving and the formation of skills; and the direction for effective plans of action are important considerations. The child has to learn how to use corrective processes, to detect errors in performance, and to regulate his or her behavior. With experience and information certainty comes automatically in movement. Patterns of behavior will be predictable, uniform, and less variable.

But how does the child learn to resolve information uncertainty and, in Bernstein's (1967) terms, reduce "degrees of freedom?" To Bernstein "the coordination of a movement is the process of mastering redundant degrees of freedom of the moving organ, in other words its conversion to a controllable system" (p. 127). Apparently, changes occur with regard to hierarchical control. The person learns to adjust adaptively to the environmental situations and demands. Such possibilities occur as the nervous system develops and provides the capabilities to the child, as well as through learning experiences. The net result is internal organization and reorganization of the interactive processes involved in the activity. The child produces an undifferentiated set of behaviors, learns, and goes through a gradual process of differentiated movements, which occurs through the application of reinforcements (Dickinson, 1977). At high skill levels, organization is reflected by "more flexible, expedient, and economic methods" (Bernstein, 1967, p. 127), which reduce redundant degrees of freedom.

Any analysis of skilled performance must allude to the reduction of uncertainty, the establishment of consistent appropriate behavior, and the role of control processes associated with attention, memory, and decision making. Various instructional techniques can be employed to improve short-term memory (STM) and performance. For example, it has been noted that verbal rehearsal and prompting can improve task recall with children at the six-to-seven year age level. Children appear not to have the ability for and do not use self-prompting and self-correcting procedures. Training programs should be devised to improve these skills because young children do not perform well on tasks requiring verbal mediations. Instructional strategies can be improved when teaching young children to use active rehearsal, to tackle changing task demands, and to develop STM functions (Belmont & Butterfield, 1971). These investigators call for the formulation and usage of mnemonic processes in children. Certainly, STM is improved in part when certain cues are attended to and others are ignored. In a thought-provoking paper, Chi (1976) questioned the often-accepted belief that STM storage increases with age, and that rate of information loss from STM varies with age. Instead, Chi identified four central processes, or acquired strategies, that are differentially applied by children and adults. Rehearsal, naming, grouping, and recoding strategies are used to the advantage of adults, but children show deficits in these processing strategies, as well as in processing speed. Presumably, they improve with age through cumulative learning.

When the child advances in age, on the average to five years, increasing control is demonstrated over actual movements, thought, and mediation processes. Highly skilled performance is related to the individual's ability to regulate it voluntarily. Apparently, a child can transfer behavioral control from overt verbalization (guidance) to self-verbalization (thought) over task execution. Even infants at two or younger can show some voluntary inhibition of performance. With age and appropriate experiences, skilled performances reflect the ability to use inhibitory control to regulate actions matching corresponding images and ideas. Wozniak (1972) recognizes the importance of the emerging abilities to self-regulate and control; he writes:

> "Verbal regulation" or the transfer of the control of a child's behavior from stimuli external to the child (e.g., commands of an adult) to stimuli internal to the child (e.g., verbal planning) is a prerequisite for higher cognitive functioning. A child's success, therefore, in a wide variety of behaviors (e.g., control of attention, conscious recall, concept formation, problem solving, etc.) depends specifically upon the occurrence of this transfer (p. 13).

Not only does the child learn to transfer control over personal actions, but the repertoire of responses also increases considerably; the ability to apply verbal labels to movements increases, and directions can be more detailed and lengthier because of the developing information-processing abilities. Attention, perception, imagery, and other abilities are developed corresponding to the increased maturity and quality experiences of the organism in approach of adolescence. Such personal qualities are prerequisites for the skilled execution of complex motor skills (Singer, 1973).

Furthermore, as Singer indicates, positive transfer probably occurs more easily during youthful years than advanced years. Previous learnings affect subsequent learnings to the degree that they are related. This effect may be favorable or unfavorable. At older ages it becomes increasingly difficult to reorganize patterned behavioral responses. More established and practiced routines impede possibilities for modification and change. A child has fewer competing, and, for that matter, well-learned responses that might interfere with new learnings.

Programs are formulated in children as well as in adults that contain the logic to deal with specified and restricted conditions, as well as unpredictable, sudden, and novel circumstances. Cognitions in the form of rules, strategies, plans, and the formation of schema are closely allied to the production of skilled movement. The developing child emits skilled behavior as a function of the sophistication of cognitions, response repertoire, and the resources of the physical system. Children learn the probability of events from past experiences. With certainty and a feeling of control over one's responses to the environment, programs of action are issued with great speed and confidence. Strategies assist the child in delivering appropriate behaviors in situations in which unpredictable and rapid changes may occur. Strategies are associated with particular motor sequences, to be matched with a particular set of cues.

Previously, the discussion on selective attention indicated the limitations in the way children use their attentional processes. Considerations for the potential to parallel process or to quickly serial process information seem to favor adults over children. As such input functions improve with age, the simultaneous release of responses (output) likely does so, too. C. D. Wickens (1974) suggests that

> if children are thus more single channel than adults in processing input information, it is reasonable to conclude that they are likewise less capable of dividing attention between two simultaneous responses . . . (p. 752).

In summary, a child's performance in skills depends on the ability to create a plan to accomplish a goal, with images and programs that contain a serial set of flexible actions that are appropriate for familiar and novel settings. Adaptive behavior is often overlooked; yet it is an extremely important feature of skilled performance required in externally paced activities. Such behavior requires a quick but accurate analysis of tasks and situations and the ability to respond accordingly.

Feedback

Proficiency at skills occurs when the child is capable of achieving predetermined goals, and when ongoing or subsequent behaviors are modified through the effective use of internalized or externally provided feedback. Feedback is information provided to the learner about the nature of his or her performance or the results of the performance. When a discrepancy exists between output and input, a corrective mechanism must be initiated.

Various sensory modalities exclusively, or more often in redundant overlapping fashion, offer such information about the nature of performance as well as the results of the performance. Visual feedback, to be useful, must be attended to correctly and perhaps quickly. Auditory feedback has the same requirements, with the necessity for the communication level between teacher and young learner to be on the same wavelength. Feedback from proprioceptive sense receptors is effective if the learner understands what to feel in terms of direction and extent of movement and spatial and temporal patterns of energy.

Thus, feedback from self or external sources must be processed purposefully, efficiently, and effectively. Many scholars have stated that mature human beings process information better than children, and these results have been confirmed. The mere availability of feedback is not the answer to improved performance in children's learning. The type, form, timing, and receptivity to it must be considered. For example, K. M. Newell (1977) tested children from four different grades in school and demonstrated that the optimum precision level of externally provided feedback for motor learning varies as a direct function of age.

Reinforcement and feedback may have similar or distinctive qualities. If we consider for a moment their commonalities, then Dickinson's (1977) point is of interest here: "the evidence concerning maturation shows incontrovertibly that some motor behaviors are not susceptible to the effects of reinforcement until a particular stage of development is reached" (p. 71). With maturation, the repertoire of potential behavior is increased, as is the number of past experiences with reinforcers. Similarly, the child learns when and how to use the sources of feedback available as a function of previous experiences and current cues and directions.

One example of the interaction of the type of externally supplied feedback with age and the effects on motor performance will be described here. B. Mitchell and J. R. Thomas (1977) studied seven- and ten-year-old boys, and three groups were formed in each age category to receive no feedback, general feedback, or precise feedback. The seven-year-olds made adequate use of general feedback with the more complex task and were more consistent in their performances than when not receiving feedback. More precise feedback was not beneficial. More consistent performance was attained with the ten-year-olds with more precise rather than general feedback. Mitchell and Thomas reason that precise feedback required the detailed integration of error information too detailed to be meaningful for the seven-year-olds in the more difficult task. They discuss their results within a neo-Piagetian framework, and we will turn to this theory next.

Neo-Piagetian Theory

Piagetian theory has influentially impacted on the thinking of scholars and the actions of practitioners. His theory has been criticized in some quarters as being based on observations rather than "hard" data. It is somewhat vague and descriptive, meant to account for sequential stages of development but not the functional mechanisms that underlie learning. Neo-Piagetian theory (Case, 1972a, 1972b; Pascual-Leone, 1970, 1976) is a derivation of Piagetian concepts and an attempt to quantify Piaget's observed developmental sequence of cognitive behaviors within an information-processing framework.

A detailed presentation of neo-Piagetian theory is not possible here; hence, only its salient concepts will be identified. One essential construct is *mental space* (M-space), which is a central computing space geared to handle and process information. As a child develops, structural M-space and functional M-space need to be considered in order to predict behavior. Structural M-space (M_s-space) refers to the number and repertoire of schemes or units of information a child can attend to or integrate in a single act at one time. It is represented by a numerical value and is associated with each of Piaget's developmental stages.

The child's functional M-space (M_f-space) indicates his or her tendency to use available structural M-space. At any age, children demonstrate differences in learning and performance, perhaps attributable to discrepancies between M_f-space and M_s-space. Differences in the cognitive styles of children can be indicative of noncongruence between these two parameters. Theoretically, structural space is the same among children of the same age, but functional space varies as a result of previous experiences and learning.

Another essential construct of neo-Piagetian theory besides mental space is *schemes*. Three types have been identified: figurative, operative, and executive. Figurative schemes are facts or perceptual configurations familiar to the child, somewhat analogous to how much he or she knows. Operative schemes are rules or transformations that the child can apply to one set of figurative schemes. They help to generate new configurations of schemes, similar in principle to how much the child knows how to synthesize and elaborate. Executive schemes monitor, control, and coordinate sequences of specific operative and figurative schemes. They reveal higher-order strategies to "put it all together" to produce goal-oriented behaviors.

These propositions are in the beginning phases of formulation and analysis as they relate to the quantitative explanation and prediction of children's learning. Applications to motor development are even more recent but nevertheless vigorous and intense (e.g., Tudor, 1975). These efforts show much promise in studying children, development, information processing, and motor behavior.

For instance, P. R. Bender (1976) administered a linear positioning task to three groups of children, ages six, eight, and ten. An age-related linear increase in processing ability was found, as expected. What is even more interesting, children determined to be high mental-space processors at one age level performed as well or better than the low mental-space processors at the next age level. Furthermore, high mental-space processors performed better than low mental-space processors of a similar age. Evidently, instructional design should be ideally matched.

Similar findings were obtained by Thomas and Bender (1977) between and within six- and eight-year-olds, and with two different curve linear positioning tasks. Gerson and Thomas (1977) found differences in performance between high and low processors in the five- to six-year age bracket. In addition, schema theory was combined with neo-Piagetian theory to explain performance, and it was concluded that the combination of the two theories was profitable in this respect.

Many questions remain unanswered, as attempts are made to wed theory, research, and practical concerns. Do capacities for learning continue to grow until age fifteen or sixteen, as neo-Piagetian theories suggest, or are they somewhat complete by age five or six, as proposed by Chi (1976)? There is little doubt that experiences lead to a greater capability to tackle problems and to resolve situational uncertainties. But is the structural system "ready" and "completed" at a young age, waiting for the development of attentional, learning, and memory strategies and processes? We must wait for more evidence on this question. Nonetheless, neo-Piagetian theory provides the conceptual direction to study the information processing of children at different ages and with different capabilities. More traditional information-processing models, referred to earlier, have provided a path for thinking and research in other directions. The recency of the publications referred to throughout this section suggests the excitement and fervor these days in studying children's behaviors in the context of information-processing models.

From a practical teaching standpoint, John Salmela (1976) suggests diagnosis of learner problems with regard to input, central processing, output, and the like. Problems at any one point can be detrimental to the total system and the way it can potentially behave. From another framework, neo-Piagetian theory has led to the analysis of processing capabilities (such as field dependency or field independency) of children of similar or different ages and to the predicted impact on learning and performance. All these considerations point to a greater sensitivity to the learner and learning problems and to accommodating learners with appropriate instructions and expectations.

LATER LEARNING AND MOTOR PERFORMANCE

Motor behavior in infancy and early childhood has been discussed already and need not be treated here. School-age children display characteristics of skilled movements in their play; the nature of their play is such that, with increasing age, more complex skills and diverse sports are mastered and demonstrated. Two widely used methods for obtaining performance data relevant to age are the *longitudinal* and *cross-sectional* approaches. Subjects at each age are sampled under the *cross-sectional* approach, whereas the same individuals are followed for a length of time with the longitudinal method. Both research methods contribute to our knowledge of growth and development, although the longitudinal technique usually is more time-consuming and contains more administrative problems than the cross-sectional method. However, the longitudinal study more accurately describes the changes that take place within individuals in succeeding years. Famous early longitudinal studies include Lewis Terman's follow-up of genius youngsters to adulthood and Harold Jones's observations at Berkeley of strength changes during the adolescent period. The longitudinal study permits an analysis of the growth process and does not conceal unusual occurrences, such as growth spurts.

When normative motor skills performance data are collected, without any prior special learning or treatment conditions, one can expect performance to be directly related to age during the developmental period. As a general rule, performance increases with age throughout childhood. Running, throwing, jumping, balance, agility, stroking, and catching skills in primary grade children have been found to be greater at each age level. M. Humphries and A. H. Shephard (1959) trained their subjects, from four to ten years of age, in a reversed task of the Toronto Complex Coordinator. These investigators noted that the level of performance was positively related to age and that all age levels constantly improved with training. Extending the analysis of age to performance in later ages, improvement increments are noticed to a certain time in life, depending on the skill. It should go without saying that individuals learn and improve in performance up to varying ages, and any evidence presented here is based on average performance.

Four hundred and eighty female subjects with ages ranging from six to eighty-four had their reaction times taken by Jean Hodgkins (1962). It was discovered that reactions improved from childhood to nineteen years, remained constant from ninteen to twenty-six, and decreased afterward. Similar results were obtained in another study by Hodgkins in which she tested both the reaction time and movement time of males and females. Figure 9-2 illustrates her findings.

Slowness of behavior is characteristic of older age and may be caused by many factors. Some evidence suggests the process of aging in the nervous system as being a leading cause. Some studies show a 10 to 20 per cent slowing of reac-

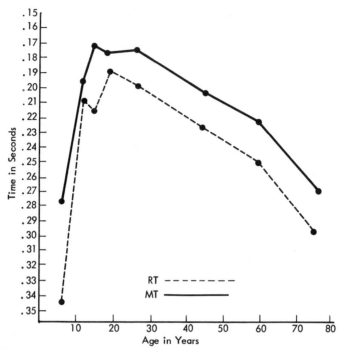

FIGURE 9-2. RT and MT changes as a function of age. (*From Hodgkins, J. Reaction time and speed of movement in males and females at various ages.* Research Quarterly, *1963, 34, 335–343.*)

tion times between twenty- and sixty-year-olds. However, the actual time difference may be as little as 0.02 of a second, which, practically speaking, is not much.

Some researchers have found conflicting results using different tasks to measure a similar variable. For instance, Cron and Pronko (1957) tested balance by having their subjects walk on a balance board, whereas Bachman (1961, 1966) used the stabilometer and vertical ladder climb. In the former study, 501 children were represented, spanning in age from four to fifteen. Balance ability improved with age, then leveled off, and declined in the twelve- to fifteen-year-old group. The girls were superior in the four- to eight-year bracket, but the boys exceeded the girls in the eight- to fifteen-year range. In the first study by Bachman, the subjects were from six to twenty-six years of age, and in the second investigation, they aged from twenty-six to fifty. In both tasks and in both studies, it was generally found that learning was not related to sex or age.

Talland (1962) tested three groups of men; members of group 1 were in their early twenties; of group 2, between forty and sixty-three; and of group 3, between seventy-seven and eighty-nine. There were eighteen subjects in each group. The tasks they performed were (1) continuous working of a manual counter, (2) moving beads with a tweezer, and (3) selecting beads of one hue from a mixed stock

MOTOR LEARNING AND HUMAN PERFORMANCE

and moving them with a tweezer. Significant differences were found between each group in favor of each preceding younger group. The results suggest that even the simplest motor skill declines in speed with age, even though it involves little exertion or coordination of movement.

It appears that athletic skills are continually developed to a high degree of proficiency, especially in the first two decades of life. Individuals may continue to improve in skill attainment throughout a good portion of life, depending on the nature of the skill and the training habits and personality of the performer. Many top athletes in baseball, football, and a host of other sports appear to reach their prime in their middle and late twenties.

A picture of Olympic champions raises serious questions about whether we justifiably can indicate a given age for optimal athletic performance. Ernst Jokl (1964) has presented age and sport data from the 1952 Olympic Games in Helsinki. The swimming participants had the lowest mean age: twenty-one and a half. Boxers, cyclists, short-distance runners, hurdlers, and jumpers were on the average under twenty-five. As to the running events of over 1,500 meters, an average increase in age was noted as the distance increased. Those who participated in the decathalon, free-style wrestling, long-distance running events, and weight lifting were between twenty-five and thirty, on the average. The ages of the male Olympians were from thirteen to sixty-six, and a number of middle-aged men were observed to give excellent performances.

Data from the 1964 Olympics substantiated Jokl's earlier findings. Hirata (1966) categorized Olympic athletes by age and event. Much of his data indicates that those events in which a performer relies primarily on muscular strength are represented by more youthful athletes. Those events requiring more refined skill and technique are accomplished later in life. Swimming, for example, which does not demand so much technical ability, was represented by the youngest athletes. Male swimmers averaged approximately twenty years of age, whereas performers in such technical sports as gymnastics and wrestling were in the middle and late twenties. Some other mean ages, representing the male Olympians of various sports, were found to be as follows:

Sport	Age
Volleyball	26.2
Basketball	25.3
Foil fencing	27.5
Track: 100-meter	24.5
marathon	28.3
Cycling	24.0
Weight lifting	27.2
Soccer	24.9

Although it would appear as if certain ages are more desirable for successful sports participation, there was a wide range of ages for the Olympic champions, as was the case in the 1952 Olympics. The male Olympians ranged from fifteen to fifty-four years in age, whereas the ages of the female Olympians went from thirteen to thirty-five years.

It is evident then, that, through ability and hard training, a person can demonstrate superior skills at earlier and later ages than ever before. Perhaps one of the reasons why drop-offs in performance are noted in early adulthood is because of incentive loss. Additional responsibilities, new values, and even boredom from practice repetition may contribute to a decline in performance with age. High levels of skill, once attained, are not easily forgotten. Most highly skilled activities demand a well-conditioned body, but once strength, endurance, and speed deteriorate, coordination also falls. Certain sports, with constant practice and the maintenance of good body condition, allow successful participation until a person is in the fifties and even sixties.

James Birren (1964) writes that industrial studies indicate that there is little change in worker performance up to the ages of sixty and sixty-five. Performance in typical industrial tasks should be little influenced by physiological changes except where time limitations are present, i.e., when a task must be performed in some time context. An older person may be limited in performing a number of tasks in a short period of time or over a long period where fatigue sets in. Older persons generally demonstrate poorer performance on complex and difficult tasks.

Athletic competition is usually more demanding. Reductions in such capacities as strength, sense acuity, and reaction time are more apparent in their relative effects. In those sports where the response is self-pacing—e.g., archery, bowling, and golf—high skill achievement can be more easily attained. Also, when the older person has a long time to anticipate or preview the stimulus conditions, there is a better chance for success. Certainly this is the case in noncompetitive sports. Finally, the quality and quantity of the cues present in the situation will determine task performance.

Summarizing the research literature, it has been shown that

1. reaction time is longer in older people.
2. older people need more time to finish complex tasks.
3. older people process information more slowly.
4. older people tend to pay attention to irrelevant information and, on occasion, even warning signals do not measurably affect performance.
5. strength decreases after the mid-twenties.

Learning is not only associated with maturation, for it can continue throughout life. Changes with age in ability to learn are usually small up to sixty. Learning difficulty may be attributed to perception, motivation, set, attention, and the physiological state of the organism. Nevertheless, it is harder to teach an adult because of the complexity and maturity of the organism. A structured past and movements that have to be unlearned lead to learning difficulty. Motor abilities are more general in childhood, and with advancing age and varied experiences they become more specific. Differences in age and learning methods have been examined by Henry and Nelson (1956). Ten-year-olds were characterized by their ability to learn with less task specificity than fifteen-year-olds. The initial level of skill rather than ability to learn was important in the older group in ultimate task performance.

Thus, it can be seen that age groups can be characterized by unique learning abilities, developed capacities, attitudes and interests, maturational levels, and physiological development. Specific sports and tasks differ in the optimal age a human should have for highest skill attainment. Even within a given activity, a wide range of age levels may be represented by successful performers.

CHAPTER HIGHLIGHTS

1. In the research literature as well as in everyday experiences, performance comparisons are made among children. These comparisons are usually referenced according to chronological age, in spite of the fact that behavioral expectations according to maturational status might be more meaningful and useful.

2. Techniques to determine the relative influence of situational experience and genetic factors have demonstrated the interactive effect of both. Studies of twins have provided the most relevant data. Although the capacity to learn and perform skills is primarily determined by heredity, personal experiences will do much to influence level of achievement in various endeavors. We never come close to realizing our true potential.

3. A child's capabilities to learn motor skills are great, but special considerations should be given to the nature of the learning task and the demands placed on the developing organism. Abilities, physical structure, cognitions, and psychological variables are associated with the potentiality to practice appropriately, to learn, and to perform at a high level of proficiency.

4. Young children are at a disadvantage in learning skills, as compared to more mature individuals, but a consideration of certain factors can lead to more fruitful learning outcomes with motor skills. A child is limited in information-processing capabilities. Distraction occurs easily and attention span is poor. Gross movements precede fine movements. Need to achieve is apparent, and failure results in frustration, loss of motivation, and little desire to continue the experience.

5. Children's learning can be improved if learning activities involve more gross muscle movements, simplified actions, and minimal cues to which to respond. For instance, a two-year-old learning to catch a ball should experience a large ball before a small one. Soft throws to a predictable location allow the child to concentrate on fewer alternative cues. Verbal cues by an outsider should be simple and limited. One or two of the most relevant to the child's developmental level should be emphasized. Too many cues are confusing. Experiences should be enjoyable and successful. With success, increased difficulty in the activity is appropriate; with failures, reversal to more simplified activity is a necessity. Children learn rules in the activity and expectations when certain situations and stimuli are present. Anticipation improves, as will skill.

6. The child's limited channel capacity to process information dictates a concern for the quality, quantity, and speed at which cues are presented. Although it is true that for certain behavior adults and children will perform equally poorly, the reasons may be to some extent similar and to some extent dissimilar. The development of skill undergoes similar processes for the child as well as the adult. Yet, differences in neurological organization and maturation, previous experiences, and motivation suggest different operational factors.

7. Each child should be analyzed carefully for information-processing capabilities (from input through central process to output stages), or general considerations at a particular age should be made, in order to gain a more realistic understanding of a child's potential for learning and performing those activities that have different information loads and demands. Instructional procedures also should reflect these considerations.

8. Learning activities should be modified to accommodate the stage of a child's development, or the child should be provided with special instruction that might aid the processing of information, from perception and selective attention, to STM, to decision making, to response integration, to feedback.

9. A child learning a new activity can be considered on occasion to possess many of the same problems as the beginning adult learner, and yet there are differences primarily associated with the cumulative learning effect, which favors the adult. Children appear to develop an information-processing capacity similar to that of adults, but the effective use of this capacity must be learned, to free it in terms of selective attention, anticipation, and decision-making and response execution possibilities.

10. The formation of the appropriate goal image depends on behaviors associated with imagery, symbolic transformations, verbal labeling, and modeling; such capabilities are related to age, experiential, and instructional variables.

11. Practice and experiences breed situational and activity familiarity, reduce uncertainty, and promote a hierarchical level of control over generated movements that deliver them quickly, accurately, and adaptively.

12. Feedback during and after performance, response produced or provided from an external source, is an important corrective source of input, and the type of delivery and potential for effective usage must be considered relevant to performance expectations and instructional design.

13. Cognitive structures and processes play a far greater role in the production of skilled movement than realized in past years. Neo-Piagetian theory has been influential in recent years in providing a framework for the study of the information-processing capabilities of children.

14. Performance data matched according to chronological age point to improved performance until the age range of twenty to thirty, after which it usually declines. Considerations must be made for type of task and demands placed on the learner, information-processing changes with age, and other phenomena.

References

Bachman, J. C. Motor learning and performance as related to age and sex in two measures of balance coordination. *Research Quarterly,* 1961, *32,* 123–137.

Bachman, J. C. Influence of age and sex on the amount and rate of learning two motor tasks. *Research Quarterly,* 1966, *37,* 176–186.

Bandura, A. *Social learning theory.* Morristown, N. J.: General Learning Press, 1971.

Belmont, J. M., & Butterfield, E. C. What the development of short-term memory is. *Human Development,* 1971, *14,* 236–248.

Bender, P. R. *A developmental explanation of motor behavior: A neo-Piagetian interpretation.* Unpublished doctoral dissertation, Florida State University, 1976.

Berlyne, D. E. Attention as a problem in behavior theory. In D. I. Motofsky (Ed.), *Attention: Contemporary theory and analysis.* New York: Appleton-Century-Crofts, 1970.

Bernstein, N. *The coordination and regulation of movements.* New York: Pergamon Press, 1967.

Birch, L. L. Age trends in children's time-sharing performance. *Journal of Experimental Child Psychology,* 1976, *22,* 331–345.

Birren, J. E. *The psychology of aging.* Englewood Cliffs, N. J.: Prentice-Hall, 1964.

Bloom, B. S. *Stability and change in human characteristics.* N. Y.: John Wiley, 1964.

Breckenridge, M. E., & Murphy, M. N. *Growth and development of the young child.* Philadelphia: W. B. Saunders, 1969.

Brenner, C. *An elementary textbook of psychoanalysis.* Garden City, N.Y.: Doubleday-Anchor, 1974.

Bruner, J. S. The growth and structure of skill. In K. J. Connolly (Ed.), *Mechanisms of motor skill development.* New York: Academic Press, 1970.

Burt, C. Quantitative genetics in psychology. *The British Journal of Mathematical and Statistical Psychology,* 1971, *24,* 1–21.

Case, R. Learning and development: A neo-Piagetian interpretation. *Human Development,* 1972, *15,* 339–358. (a)

Case, R. Validation of a neo-Piagetian mental capacity construct. *Journal of Experimental Child Psychology,* 1972, *14,* 287–302. (b)

Chi, M. T. H. Short-term memory limitations in children: Capacity or processing deficits? *Attention and Cognition,* 1976, *4,* 559–572.

Connolly, D. J. (Ed.). *Mechanisms of motor skill development.* New York: Academic Press, 1970.

Connolly, K. The nature of motor skill development. *Journal of Human Movement Studies,* 1977, *3,* 128–143.

Cron, G. W., & Pronko, N. H. Development of the sense of balance in school children. *Journal of Educational Research,* 1957, *51,* 458–464.

Dickinson, J. *A behavioral analysis of sport.* Princeton, N. J.: Princeton Book Co., 1977.

Eaves, L. J. The genetic analysis of continuous vairation: A comparison of experimental designs applicable to human data: II. Estimation of heritability and comparison of environmental components. *The British Journal of Mathematical and Statistical Psychology,* 1970, *23,* 189.

Farnham-Diggory, S. (Ed.). *Information processing in children.* New York: Academic Press, 1972.

Gagné, R. M. Contributions of learning to human development. *Psychological Review,* 1968, *75,* 177–191.

Gedda, L. Sports and genetics, a study on twins (351 pairs). *Health and fitness in the modern world.* Chicago: The Athletic Institute, 1961.

Gedda, L., Milani-Comparetti, M., & Brenci, G. A preliminary report on research made during the games of the XVIIth Olympiad, Rome, 1960. In E. Jokl & E. Simon (Eds.), *International research in sport and physical education.* Springfield, Ill.: Charles C Thomas, 1964.

Gerson, R. F., & Thomas, J. R. Schema theory and practice variability within a neo-Piagetian framework. *Journal of Motor Behavior,* 1977, *9,* 127–134.

Hagen, J. W., & Hale, G. H. The development of attention in children. In A. D. Pick (Ed.), *Minnesota symposium on child psychology* (Vol. 7). Minneapolis: University of Minnesota Press, 1973.

Haith, M. M., Morrison, F. J., & Sheingold, K. Tachistoscopic recognition of geometric forms by children and adults. *Psychonomic Science,* 1970, *19,* 345–347.

Henry, F. M., & Nelson, G. A. Age differences and interrelationships between skill and learning in gross motor performance of ten- and fifteen-year-old boys. *Research Quarterly,* 1956, *27,* 162–175.

Hirata, K. Physique and age of Tokyo Olympic champions. *Journal of Sports Medicine and Physical Fitness,* 1966, *6,* 207–222.

Hodgkins, J. Influence of age on the speed of reaction and movement in females. *Journal of Gerontology,* 1962, *17,* 385–389.

Hogan, J. C., & Hogan, R. Organization of early skilled action: Some comments. *Child Development,* 1975, *46,* 233–236.

Humphries, M., & Shephard, A. H. Age and training in the development of a perceptual-motor skill. *Perceptual Motor Skills,* 1959, *9,* 3–11.

Jensen, A. R. How much can we boost IQ and scholastic achievement? *Harvard Educational Review,* 1969, *39,* 1–123.

Jensen, A. R. The heritability of intelligence. *Engineering and Science,* 1970, *33,* 1–4. (a)

Jensen, A. R. IQs of identical twins reared apart. *Behavior Genetics,* 1970, *1,* 133–146. (b)

Jensen, A. R. Note on why genetic correlations are not squared. *Psychological Bulletin,* 1971, *75,* 223–224.

Jokl, E. *Medical sociology and cultural anthropology of sport and physical education.* Springfield, Ill.: Charles C Thomas, 1964.

Leithwood, K. A. Early childhood motor learning. *Early Childhood Education,* 1970–71, *5,* 7–20.

Lipsitt, L. Infant learning: The blooming, buzzing, confusion revisited. In M. E. Meyer (Ed.), *Early learning, the second Western symposium on learning.* Bellingham: Western Washington State College, 1971.

Malina, R. M. Anthropology, growth, and physical education. In R. N. Singer, D. R. Lamb, R. M. Malina, & S. Kleinman (Eds.), *Physical education: An interdisciplinary approach.* New York: Macmillan, 1972.

Malina, R. M., Harper, A. B., & Holman, J. D. Growth status and performance relative to parental size. *Research Quarterly,* 1970, *41,* 503–509.

McClearn, G. E. Genetics and behavior development. In M. L. Hoffman & L. W. Hoffman (Eds.), *Review of Child Development Research.* New York: Russell Sage Foundation, 1964.

McNemar, Q. Twin resemblances in motor skills and the effect of practice theron. *Journal of Genetic Psychology,* 1933, *42,* 70–99.

Mitchell, B., & Thomas, J. R. *Developmental trends in motor performance of boys related to precision of knowledge of results.* Paper presented at the Southern District Meetings of the American Alliance for Health, Physical Education, and Recreation, Atlanta, February 1977.

Newell, K. M. *Knowledge of results and children's motor learning*. Paper presented at the North American Society for the Psychology of Sport and Physical Activity Conference, Austin, Texas, May 1976.

Newell, K. M. *Motor control: Developmental issues*. Paper presented at the National College Physical Education Association for Men—National Association of Physical Education for College Women Conference, Orlando, Florida, January 1977.

Osborne, T. R., & Gregor, J. A. The heritability of visualization, perceptual speed and spatial orientation. *Perceptual and Motor Skills*, 1966, *23*, 379–390.

Paivio, A. On the functional significance of imagery. *Psychological Bulletin*, 1970, *73*, 385–392.

Pascual-Leone, J. A mathematical model for the transition rule in Piaget's developmental stages. *Acta Psychologica*, 1970, *32*, 301–345.

Pascual-Leone, J. Metasubjective problems of constructive cognition: Forms of knowing and their psychological mechanism. *Canadian Psychological Review*, 1976, *17*, 110–125.

Piaget, J., & Inhelder, B. *L'image mentale chez l'enfant*. Paris: Preses Universitaires de France, 1966.

Pick, A. D., Christy, M. D., & Frankel, G. W. A developmental study of visual selective attention. *Journal of Experimental Child Psychology*, 1972, *14*, 165–175.

Rohwer, W. D. Images and pictures in children's learning: Research results and educational implications. *Psychological Belletin*, 1970, *73*, 393–403.

Ross, A. O. *Psychological aspects of learning disabilities and reading disorders*. New York: McGraw-Hill, 1976.

Ryan, T. J. Poverty and early education in Canada. *Interchange*, 1971, *2*, 1–11. (Published by the Ontario Institute for Studies in Education.)

Salmela, J. H. A human information processing approach of the child and skill. In J. G. Albinson & G. M. Andrew (Eds.), *Child in sport and physical activity*. Baltimore: University Park Press, 1976.

Sigel, I. E., & Cocking, R. R. *Cognitive development from childhood to adolescence: A constructivist perspective*. New York: Holt, Rinehart & Winston, 1977.

Simon, H. A. On the development of the processor. In S. Farnham-Diggory (Ed.), *Information processing in children*. New York: Academic Press, 1972.

Singer, R. N. Motor learning as a function of age and sex. In L. G. Rarick (Ed.), *Physical activity: Human growth and development*. New York: Academic Press, 1973.

Singer, R. N. *Readiness to learn skills applied to motor skill acquisition*. In R. A. Magill, M. J. Ash, & F. L. Smoll (Eds.), *Children and youth in sport: A contemporary anthology*. Urbana, Ill.: Human Kinetics, 1978.

Talland, G. A. The effect of age on speed of simple manual skills. *Journal of General Psychology*, 1962, *10*, 67–76.

Thomas, J. R., & Bender, P. R. A developmental explanation for children's motor behavior: A neo-Piagetian interpretation. *Journal of Motor Behavior*, 1977, *9*, 81–93.

Tudor, J. I. Age differences in integration of components of a motor task. *Perceptual and Motor Skills*, 1975, *41*, 211–215.

Wade, M. G. Developmental motor learning. In J. Keogh & R. S. Hutton (Eds.), *Exercise and sport sciences reviews* (Vol. 4). Santa Barbara, Ca.: Journal Publishing Affiliates, 1977.

Wickens, C. D. Temporal limits of human processing: A developmental study. *Psychological Bulletin*, 1974, *81*, 739–755.

Wozniak, R. H. Verbal regulation of motor behavior: Soviet research and non-Soviet replications. *Human Development*, 1972, *15*, 13–57.

Zimmerman, B., & Rosenthal, T. L. Observational learning of rule-governed behavior by children. *Psychological Bulletin*, 1974, *81*, 29–42.

10 ADDITIONAL DEVELOPMENTAL CONSIDERATIONS

In Chapter 9, the emphasis was primarily on the learning characteristics of the developing human organism, from birth to maturity. We now turn to some additional considerations. The analysis of the behavior of lower forms of organisms has provided us with an understanding of the notion of critical learning periods, a topic that will be treated in this chapter only. Often it is difficult, if not impossible, to study certain aspects of behavior directly in humans. The control needed to detect the existence of certain phenomena through the ability to manipulate specified conditions directly can best be done with subhumans. This has been the case with studying critical behavioral periods. However, as we will see, the ease—or, for that matter, the credibility—of applying these findings to humans may be difficult and tenuous. The question is whether critical periods exist in all living things or are species-specific and behavior-specific.

Yet, of great interest to everyone is that period in the development of a child in which certain skills should be introduced. When is this age of readiness? Do critical, or even optimal, periods exist for humans? Athletes train earlier and more intensively than was the case years ago. But we really know very little about the influence of this practice on the acquisition of skill, how it influences tendencies to persevere at or to maintain involvement, and perhaps most importantly, its psychological impact on the developing child.

Another area full of controversy is the relationship of special perceptual motor training programs oriented to young children to enhance cognitive development and academic achievement. The association of cognitive and motor attributes was discussed in Chapter 9 in a different context. With that material as background, and the introduction of the material in this chapter, it will be of interest to see how you interpret the proposed validity of the various perceptual motor training programs as to claimed or potential outcomes.

Also included in this chapter is an introduction to some tests that have been formulated to assess motor development. Such tests can be used to determine "normal" characteristics of children, as well as deviations that might be the result of inadequate experiences in motor activities or neurological disorders. In addition, sex differences in motor performance will be presented, as well as an attempt to determine any differences in learning potential or learning style (preferences for approaches to learning and activities themselves). Finally, the nature of body, or self-, concept will be explored. Can success in motor activity improve one's personal concept and in turn lead to a more generalized feeling of confidence? Will this experience in turn lead to a desire to undertake other activities to achieve a reasonable degree of accomplishment in them? This topic as well as the others included in this chapter have created much controversy, primarily because of a lack of conclusive research and the existence of popular opinions.

CRITICAL LEARNING PERIODS

One of the most fascinating concepts in psychology is that of critical learning periods. It is based on the notion that certain periods during growth and development are optimal for affecting behavior and promoting learning. This phenomenon has been observed in a number of species, although it is more apparent in infrahumans. In fact, most research accumulated on animals and birds has indicated specific periods crucial for the development of certain behavior. Types of experiences and the periods in which they are encountered by the organism may have a critical bearing on future behavior. Critical periods, as applied to human learning, refer to the crucial periods in which an attempt needs to be made to acquire fundamental and complex skills. The critical period for any specific sort of learning is that time when maximum sensory, motor, motivational, and psychological capacities are present. The natural questions that relate to the concept of critical learning periods are (1) Will intensive and extensive training at a relatively early age result in superior achievements later in life? (2) What is the critical age, and is it unique for each activity? (3) Will deprivation of certain motor experiences ever be compensated for? (4) Will deprivation result in producing inferior performances in activities in subsequent years?

A critical period for the learning of certain tasks or development of behavioral patterns can be determined by (1) sense or experience deprivation, (2) introduction to the experience, or (3) environmental enrichment at a given time in life. Humans and animals have been subjected to all three conditions by researchers intent on discovering these periods. In order to determine the best time for learning, it is necessary first to examine the normal learning progress from birth to later childhood. More complicated behaviors are demonstrated with increased development of the nervous system. Earliest activity is primarily reflex in nature. Doctors can usually detect unusual neurological activity and disturbances if the baby exhibits certain involuntary movements or lacks others. Through examination of numerous babies, doctors have come to expect the presence of specific types of activity with progressing age. After approximately six months of life, many of the innate reflexes are replaced by purposeful responses.

Anna Espenschade has undertaken much research in children's motor devel-

MOTOR LEARNING AND HUMAN PERFORMANCE

opment; she and Helen Eckert (1967) have presented an excellent summary of the research in this area. They point out that early behavior patterns are generally consistent from infant to infant, but developmental rates differ widely. This may be because of heredity and/or environmental deprivation or enrichment.

A baby should receive the opportunity to explore and practice: to reach for toys, to walk, to roll over, to pull the body upward. Throughout life, more complex skills will be built on a foundation of simple movements. With experience and maturity, the child will learn how to perform gross motor patterns and eventually fine motor skills. Genetic factors will influence performance potential, but there is much untapped potential in everyone. Meaningful experiences help to close the gap between existing capabilities and what can be achieved. Within limitations, preadolescent children are able to perform in a wide range of sports, especially those based on running, throwing, and jumping skills. These skills are developed to an adequate degree in most children by reason of frequent opportunities for participation in activities requiring these movements. It should be emphasized that *movement mastery,* the ability to coordinate motor patterns into a highly skilled act, *is learned.* Skilled movements do not occur as a result of the maturation process.

The impact of early experiences on later behavior and development has been explained through the popular *stage* approach. Previously, it was thought that periods of expectant transition occurred as a result of increments in age. At present, many psychologists believe that children do not go through the same experiences according to their chronological age, but rather, through similar stages of development that emerge in children at different points in time. Some will progress through certain stages more quickly or slowly than others. When one stage has been achieved, the child progresses to the next stage. Figure 10-1 illustrates the dissimilarity between the chronological age approach and the stage approach.

The works of a few outstanding psychologists have helped to substantiate the stage approach in child development. Sigmund Freud made child psychology an appealing area of study in the beginning of this century and emphasized the im-

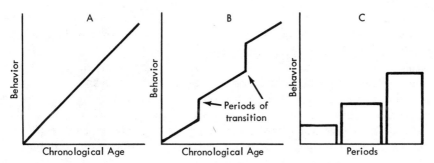

FIGURE 10-1. Illustrations A and B represent the traditional concept of behavior expectancies according to chronological age. Illustration C discounts the importance of age and emphasizes the stage approach: children progress from one stage of behavior to another, irrespective of age.

ADDITIONAL DEVELOPMENTAL CONSIDERATIONS

297

pact of early sequential experiences on later behavior. He attempted to explain adult neuroses through inadequate resolutions of certain sensitive periods in childhood. D. O. Hebb depicted stage evolvement through a neuropsychological approach to learning and behavior. One of the persons most influential on our understanding of child development is Jean Piaget, and he has written extensively on the formal or specific stages that all children experience in a predictable manner. Finally, J. P. Scott (1968) has completed a considerable amount of work on critical learning periods in animals.

Freud, reports Lucy Freeman (1965), felt that specific types of drives become prevalent in the human during progressive stages in life. If the needs of these drives are not met during specific periods, then the individual will show some type of distress as an adult. Apparently these drives appear only at certain maturational stages, and their satisfaction cannot be met before then. Thus, the relationship here seems to be not between the earliness of experience and attainment, but rather between timeliness of experience and attainment, which, in Freud's theory results in a well-adjusted individual. If this type of process plays a role in mental and psychological development, then it seems quite possible that an identical process functions in the attainment of physical skills.

Piaget (1952) has presented a stage approach to learning in children. The child undergoes sequential stages, during which specific types of learning unfold. The child may start out with unsolicited gross motor responses, then begin to perceive and respond to stimuli, and so on, until a conceptual stage of understanding abstract terms is reached. The stages seem based on maturational and experiential factors. The learning accomplished appears to depend on the particular learning stage attained. The understanding of abstract and conceptual terms for instance, will not occur unless the child is maturationally and experientially prepared. Piaget has proposed a series of hierarchical critical periods for the human infant.

Lower Forms of Organisms

Supposedly, if an animal or human is exposed to a given experience at a particular critical period or stage, it has a greater effect on adult behavior than if the experience occurs at an earlier or a later period. Unfortunately because of the difficulty in investigating this point of view, research on humans is lacking, thus permitting very few generalizations. However, as is the case in so many experimental areas, animal research has paved the way for implications in human behavior as well as for procedures that may be used in human research.

Infrahuman research points to the fact that behavior development not only is dependent on heredity, maturation, and practice, but also is related to perceptual learning experiences in infancy. The findings of many studies demonstrate that, after certain times in life, an organism cannot perform a particular behavior if it has not been subjected to specific stimuli or experiences. F. A. Beach and J. Jaynes (1954) refer to numerous experiments that lend support to the critical period concept. Their article is an excellent one for both reference and evidence, as it summarizes the major works on early experience and later behavior. The areas of study touched on follow here:

1. *Sensory discrimination and perception.* A lack of early visual stimulation results in an inability to respond to visual cues later in life. However, with the higher species, usually these defective responses are not permanent and disappear with experience. There are more pronounced effects with rabbits, pigeons, and fish.
2. *Touch and proprioception.* Studies on chimpanzees, who had their feet and hands bandaged in childhood, have demonstrated that these animals show abnormal behavior when the restrictions are removed.
3. *Feeding behavior.* In studying the pecking behavior of chicks, those who were spoon-fed in the dark for two weeks never did learn how to peck.
4. *Hoarding.* If rats are deprived of food in infancy (first fifteen days), afterward there is a tendency for them to hoard. Also, the deprived rats eat faster in adulthood.
5. *Social behavior.* Birds and chicks raised in isolation have shown later antisocial behavior.

Konrad Lorenz (1970) has demonstrated a phenomenon termed *imprinting*. Imprinting refers to the first stimulus that evokes an instinctive reaction and becomes the only stimulus that will cause this reaction. It takes place in a critical stage of life and is irreversible throughout life. In a sense, it is a primitive form of learning. Geese that have been exposed to humans in childhood but never to adult geese tend later to stay near humans rather than geese. Certain species, after being brought up with humans, never can react normally to their own kind. In imprinting, a duckling within the first two or three days of life becomes attached to almost any object or organism that is introduced at this time. This behavior continues throughout life, with the bird following the imprinting object even in the presence of its own species. Thus, the bird does not recognize its own kind and will not respond normally to them. Lorenz's work has been duplicated with other organisms as well.

Personal and social behaviors, as explained through critical periods, have been of particular interest to investigators. Young rats that have been stimulated (handled) learn more quickly, are less timorous, and are more vigorous. When rats are brought up surrounded by many playthings, as compared to a barren environment, their performance on learning tasks is better. R. J. Rivizza and A. C. Herschberger (1966) raised some rats in an inhibited environment and allowed another group of rats to climb. As adults, the rats allowed freedom of exploration were more active in exploration tasks, showed superior performance on an intelligence test, and were less emotional in a novel situation.

The study of the development of social attachments in dogs as a function of critical learning periods has led to interesting speculations about human behaviors (see, for example, Scott, 1969). Furthermore, even the development of tendencies to persevere at tasks, to show ideal motivational levels, depends on early learning experiences, and successes and failures. Motivation in tasks undertaken later in life will be increased if successful experiences are had early in life. Scott reports that it is extremely hard to remotivate a puppy that has failed repeatedly.

Humans

The irreversible characteristics of poor or limited experiences on the undesirable later behaviors of subhumans is well documented. We have just examined some of the convincing evidence. The evidence with humans is far less supportive with regard to the notion that a child will not be able to remediate at a later date nonquality early experiences. For instance, when Hopi Indian infants were studied, who, as dictated by their culture practices, were bound to a cradleboard with little movement allowed or encouraged during the first year of life, they were found to be no slower in beginning to walk than those babies who were not restrained (Dennis, 1940). Many current popular concepts dealing with the development of intelligence and academic aptitudes suggest the wonderful ability of the human to be able to make up early deficiencies. Apparently, we are far more adaptable than nonhumans. We can compensate for shortcomings. Many critical behavioral periods, which exist for a very brief period in subhumans, apparently are quite lengthy in humans. Perhaps, as H. P. Mussen, J. Conger, and J. Kagan (1969) suggest, the whole of infancy is a critical period. These thoughts bring hope to situations where despair might otherwise be present. They should, however, not be construed as supportive of nonenriching and limited experiences for the child. It is more likely than not that the child who has encountered meaningful experiences appropriate for his or her maturational level will demonstrate more advanced behavior with more ease in later periods.

According to Scott (1969), there are three kinds of critical learning periods: (1) optimal periods for learning; (2) infantile stimulation; and (3) formation of basic social relationships. Infantile (human or otherwise) stimulation, in the form of large amounts of perceptual experience, leads to better learners later on than if the organisms are deprived of such experience. As development occurs, learning capacities change. When dealing with young children, we obviously are not concerned with complex sport and skill learning. Rather, we are concerned with basic movements and patterns that are performed as if by habit. Habits formed early in life persist into adult life and are resistant to change. It is therefore necessary that these learned movements be desirable, for the acquisition of one habit may prevent the learning of others. What is learned at a particular time may interfere with later learning. In the words of Scott, "organization hampers reorganization."

There is need to be concerned not only with what the child does experience, but also with what he does not. Warren Johnson (1964) repeats the statement Luria made at the 1959 World Health Organization seminar in Milan, Italy: "Sometimes, if a single link of training is missed, if a certain state in the development of the necessary operation is not properly worked up, the entire process of further development becomes retarded. . . ."

What motor skills, then, should be taught to children, and when? Myrtle McGraw's (1935) famous twin study indicated that learning varies for each motor activity; each activity has its own optimum period for rapid and skillful learning. Jimmy was the control twin and was raised in typical fashion. Johnny was the experimental twin and received special training to increase his neuromuscular development; he demonstrated an ability to acquire many skills at an early age. This study helped to refute the concept that an infant is unresponsive to practice because of an immature nervous system, a concept espoused by leading child psychologists such as Gesell.

McGraw attempted to discover the period when a child would profit by a particular experience or practice. Johnny was stimulated daily, whereas Jimmy was provided with a few toys and experienced a routine environment. At about one year of age, Johnny was directed in various motor activities usually experienced by children later in life, e.g., riding a tricycle, swimming and diving, roller skating, jumping from heights, and sliding. Jimmy received intensive practice and instruction in the same activities for two and a half months when he was twenty-two months old. When Johnny was less than a year old, he could swim the length of a seven-foot tank while supported by a strap. He swam the distance without support at 411 days, performed a dive into the tank at 422 days, and when 467 days old, dove off a five-foot board into a lake.

After Jimmy's training period, the two boys were compared in performance. In swimming and diving behavior, Johnny demonstrated superior talents and better attitudes, which were attributed to his extensive swimming experience. As to skating, Johnny had the advantage because of his earlier training. He was adjusted to falling, a problem that Jimmy had difficulty in overcoming. It would seem that the best time to learn skating occurs when the baby is learning to walk, for he is gaining control of equilibrium factors. Johnny also demonstrated a more coordinated jump from heights, having overcome fear at the early age at which he had had related experiences. These activities were learned better because of their earlier introduction. Some activities were not facilitated by earlier practice—for example, walking. Both boys demonstrated approximately similar patterns, despite the extra practice Johnny received. Other activities appeared to be disrupted because unskillful habits were formed. McGraw suggests that not only was Johnny not benefited by his earlier experience with the tricycle, but, in fact, these experiences actually hindered him. Jimmy practiced less on this skill, and the delay in his exposure to the tricycle proved to be more economical to learning.

McGraw (1939) retested the boys at school age. The skills were demonstrated in varying patterns in their tendency to be retained or forgotten. For example, Johnny and Jimmy were about equal in tricycling and in roller skating. However, although both boys demonstrated no loss of skill in tricycling after the long layoff, it appeared as if the skating skill had undergone deterioration. Nevertheless, *Johnny generally displayed greater motor coordination and daring in physical performance.* The retention of specific skills, according to McGraw, depends on whether performance was composed of well-integrated movements. Poorly developed skills are not retained to a high degree.

The McGraw investigation allows other general assumptions. *There is no one critical period, no one chronological age for all skills, as periods differ for each behavior pattern.* In fact, the critical period is not determined by chronological age; rather, it is based on the maturational status of the nervous system for a given activity and evidently may extend for quite a long period for the acquisition of many skills. As long as the organism grows, so do the powers of restoration and compensation. Unless there is an unduly long deprivation period (a time when the child does not have any experience with the skill in question), he or she can usually be brought to approximate the achievement level of another child who has begun practice earlier. (Jimmy did approximately match Johnny's skill level in the various activities after the intensive training period, but it should be remembered that Johnny demonstrated better overall motor coordination.) Finally, because the twins were normal and about equal in intelligence test scores, exercise in special motor activities did not appear to accelerate intellectual functions. The important role that perceptual-motor experiences have in contributing to potential intellectual achievements is not to be denied, though. This particular study merely indicates that additional motor activity will not improve on normal intelligence.

Empirical evidence indicates that young children can learn much more than they are given credit for. Investigations on outstanding athletes show that usually they began learning their specialties at early ages and have undergone continuous intensive training. In McGraw's study, Johnny could swim seven feet (with one breath) at one year of age. Children, in general, are learning sports traditionally associated with adulthood, such as golf, bowling, and tennis, earlier in their lives than has been the case with preceding generations. If, as Jerome Bruner (1963) suggests, *any subject can be taught in a legitimate way to be of value to the child at any stage of development,* the implications are great for physical educators. Although Bruner's thoughts in general lie more in the cognitive domain with the great issues, principles, and values of society, his concepts also can be applied to the learning of motor skills. Certainly, physical education offers experiences that most children are receptive to, i.e., a child usually does not have to be forced into participating in games and play. It is up to the creative teacher to present the material in a meaningful way, by understanding the developmental stages of childhood.

Motor skills can be taught in a modified way to a child once reasonable control of the body has been achieved. However, the desirability of encroaching on the maturing process, of teaching particular activities to children who are too young to comprehend and respond to them adequately, is questionable. *Successful skill attainment at maturity is not dependent on the earliness of instruction, but rather on its timeliness.*

Scott (1968) feels that one answer to the problem of how to enhance the maximum development of motor skills in young children is to permit a great amount of freedom of movement. Confinement does not permit the experience necessary for developing motor capacities. Capacities attained reflect maturational level and practice. It is often found that children raised in orphanages have poorer motor capacities than those raised by their parents, perhaps because of less enriching and more constricted environments. The same is true when comparisons are made between upper- and lower-class children. In lower-class homes, children are often less controlled and confined; they demonstrate high degrees of motor development. Scott (1968) says:

> It is desirable to give a child contact with a variety of physical objects which can be manipulated or climbed. This encourages the development of general motor skills that can be applied later to the learning of more complicated tasks. The results at boths ages are more satisfactory than those obtained by trying to teach complex physical skills directly at an early age. Most children are not able to perform activities requiring good coordination of the whole body much before the ages of seven or eight, and introducing them too early in such activities only results in unskillful performance or failure (p. 123).

Research on critical learning periods permits only generalizations from animal research to human behavior. It does not, at this time, tell us the optimal time in life at which to learn, say, basketball, golf, or archery. It does call attention to the theoretical impact of the proposition that there are critical periods in life for the learning of everything. It remains for researchers to investigate this area further, to determine the stage of approximate age of readiness for specific motor skill experience.

It appears, however, that the concept of critical learning periods is slightly different for humans and infrahumans. In infrahuman studies, critical learning periods are considered to be points in time at which either a behavior is learned or it probably will never be learned. For humans, on the other hand, the phrase *critical learning periods* seems to be more correctly substituted with the phrase *optimal learning periods*. This is the time when the minimal abilities necessary to learn a skill are present in the learner. Before this period, one is unable to learn the skill, and after it, certain aging or interfering factors might impair the learning. As long as prerequisite abilities and skills are present, the learner should be able to master more complex activities. If they are not attained, they must be acquired before proceeding further.

To summarize, humans display remarkable plasticity in their nervous systems. Such is not the case with lower forms of organisms. We adapt, adjust, and modify behaviors at different developmental stages in life. Yet the importance of experiences early in life cannot be denied. Infants are not at the mercy of their environments. They can respond, react, and develop to their capabilities if they are stimulated appropriately.

It would appear that the foundational blocks for later in life learning are formed early in life. Gross movement patterns, developed in the early years, lead to the refinement of movement associated with skilled behaviors. Consequently, the child who has learned how to throw smoothly, to kick, to run, to balance, and the like will probably be favored in later years in attempting to master more complex tasks.

After the first six or eight years of life, perhaps nothing that we ever learn is completely new. Everything is related somehow to what has been learned before. As we approach maturity, our nervous system develops, allowing us to perform more complex activities. Many tasks require a greater precision, or perhaps a difference in timing, of movements than was the case in earlier years. More encouragement should be given to children to explore, move, problem solve, and, in general, to develop these foundations for movement. In turn, children develop foundational capacities to acquire more complex motor skills.

The readiness to learn activities can be interpreted in two ways: attitudinally or developmentally. From an attitudinal point of view, learning is much more productive when the child is mentally and emotionally set for the experience. Favorable disposition toward an activity may be brought to the situation by the child or else induced by the creative teacher. Environmental settings, if manipulated appropriately, and instructional and communication styles, if warmly received, can do much to shape the attitudinal process.

From a developmental point of view, one can easily observe that activities cannot be learned unless children are at the appropriate stage of development. The teacher is then left with an alternative: wait until the child is ready to master the activity or attempt to modify the activity so that it will be experienced at a level compatible with the developmental state of the child. Teachers should try to understand the developmental level of the child and, in turn, modify experiences so that they can be meaningfully engaged in at given stages of development. If children are constantly faced with failure they will attempt to avoid the activity. They need to be challenged and yet have the feeling of success. The happy blend of these "feelings" can best be attained when activities are suitably presented to children with consideration of their stage of development.

SPECIAL TRAINING PROGRAMS

A child begins elementary school and displays poor readiness skills. It may appear that the child has low intellectual potential, brain damage, or mental retardation. Can anything be done to remedy the situation?

Obvious solutions include reading therapy, special training in intellectual skills, or allowing nature to take its course. A more practical approach would be to assess the determinants of the child's problems and to proceed from there. Causes of problems associated with a low level of readiness for achievement in school may be genetic factors, brain injury, or inadequate environmental experiences. Barring extreme cases in the first two categories, research evidence indicates the possibilities and limitations in attempting to overcome intellectual difficulties through a corrective program. Basically, this program includes the introduction and practice of certain basic motor patterns.

Evidence for the low correlation between motor skill achievement and intelligence in adults and older school-aged children is recognized. What of the relationship in infancy and early childhood? Statements by pioneer researchers, educators, and psychologists concur on the concept of a general maturational trend early in life. That is to say, "things seem to go together" at this time. Reasonably strong relationships exist among various maturational and behavioral characteristics of the young child. As age increases, these associations lessen. Performance tasks that were general and gross become more specific and complex. Nonetheless, if a child proceeds through progressive development stages, success in one may depend on successes in the previous ones. We must pause and speculate about the ramifications of such a notion.

Crudely put, perhaps, the stages are

1. physical (reflexive, simple).
2. motor (more purposeful).
3. perceptual-motor (more complex).
4. cognitive (various forms of intelligence).
5. conceptual (abstract thinking).

Rationale would have it that a child with problems at the cognitive stage perhaps had difficulties in the perceptual-motor stage. Remedial activities are needed that will serve as preparation for the more advanced stage. With this kind of reasoning, a number of so-called perceptual-motor training programs came into being in the 1960s. They often differed in emphasis and mode of operation, but a commonality was in the belief that cognitive learning disorders can be remediated through special programs that emphasize body awareness, multisensory stimulation, and a variety of movement experiences. A large number of these programs are in operation throughout the United States, often as preschool experiences for the culturally and socioeconomically disadvantaged. Many have been supported by huge federal grants in the hope of preventing later learning problems or remediating existing ones.

Although special training programs are typically perceptual-motor or sensorimotor oriented, with the hope of assisting the intellectual qualities of the child, it is of interest to note the lack of literature on programs specially designed for youngsters to develop their movement patterns for later-in-life highly skilled movements. McGraw, as reported earlier, made a stab at this problem when she trained the twin Johnny at specific motor skills to determine effects in subsequent years on performance in these same skills. Perhaps a few reasons can be offered for the relative nonexistence of special skill training programs.

For one thing, our culture places a heavy emphasis on the mastery of intellectual tasks. Although we are noted as a country of great athletes and athletic teams and we support them well through attendance and finances, actual participation in and mastery of athletic and recreational skills—the effective use of the body in the attainment of skill and selffulfillment through movement—are virtually underplayed in value relative to so-called intellectual attainments. The successful person is thought to be the wise one—the doctor, lawyer, or businessman. Children are encouraged to elevate their social prestige and their economic status by striving for such professional positions. Skill mastery has a lower prestige rating.

Also, a controversy exists over the desirability of specially training young children in skills associated with athletics. Is the child ready to learn these skills and to compete? To what degree will personality be enhanced or harmed through involvement in special programs? On top of this, to what degree should programs be structured for specific skill learnings versus spontaneous, open-structured, creative activities? We do know that children can learn skills to a much greater extent than was once believed. As to the long-term benefits and disadvantages of special skill training programs, we can only speculate.

Yet, as we mature and grow older, the effective use of our body in activities that require skilled motor patterns is rewarding. Mechanical skills, recreational activities, various occupational endeavors, and athletic events make perceptual-motor demands on the individual. What with more leisure time and interests in recreational pursuits, the ability to express oneself through skilled movement is quite an advantage. It is true that high degrees of proficiency result from prior general learning experiences that relate to the task at hand, as well as to task-specific practice. Precise spatially and temporally timed movements can only be acquired from extensive quality practice and experience. The general perceptual-motor abilities developed in childhood will contribute to later possible success in more complex activities. Throwing, jumping, and striking movements are similar in many skills. Many so-called new activities usually merely require a modification or restructuring in already existing routines or response patterns. Thus, the argument can be made for programs of special instruction, as well as for unstructured programs that encourage general skill development in an enjoyable atmosphere, corresponding to the child's maturational level and readiness.

Development of the ability to move has long been the major concern of the coach and the physical educator. The relationship between this movement ability and later development of motor skills and physical fitness is justification enough for the inclusion of movement in the young child's learning experiences.

During the past few decades, this interest in movement has spread beyond the realms of physical education into such fields as developmental psychology, neurology, educational psychology, and remedial reading. With this diffusion of movement into other areas, recognition of the existence of a relationship between movement and cognitive development has occurred. The majority of the work that has been done in this area has generally been associated with attempts to overcome learning disabilities, particularly in the area of reading.

Although a paucity of research literature exists on special skill-training programs, such is not the case with perceptual-motor training programs geared to enhance the general learning abilities of the child. Perceptual-motor programs have been approached from many different angles; thus there exists a variety of theories based on various aspects of perceptual-motor development. Carl Delacato (1966) joined with Glenn and Robert Doman to establish a theory based on neurological organization. The late Newell Kephart, also a prominent leader in the perceptual motor area, based his theory on the perceptual and integrative processes that result from having had vast experience in the motor area. Other leaders in this field, G. Getman and Marianne Frostig, have worked in the direction of visual perceptual training. The program developed by Ray Barsch is referred to as a "movigenics" curriculum.

Perceptual-motor training programs are more individualized in nature than physical education programs, which tend to be group oriented. Typically, an awareness of sensory skills is established and activities are geared to the developmental level of the child. James Fleming (1972) states that the common variables of all the perceptual-motor programs proposed appear to be

1. the use of gross motor activities or physical exercises incorporating awareness of the necessary body movements.
2. the use of structured activities organized in planned programmed procedures.
3. training to improve basic sensory skills (visual, auditory, and tactile), as well as motor skills.
4. the relative importance and emphasis that is placed on these programs in relation to academic learning and/or gains.

Differences within the various perceptual motor programs appear to stem from

1. the theoretical models on which [researchers] base their programs.
2. the areas of major emphasis in remediation.
3. the claims linked to the specific programs and procedures on personal development (pp. 251–252).

Let us examine some of the programs. In the book *Success Through Play,* and in subsequent books, Kephart (Radler & Kephart, 1960) emphasized the importance of visual development in intellectual development, which in turn depends on simple motor skills. Poor motor coordination results in decelerated intellectual growth. According to Kephart, coordination is composed of (1) laterality— the sense of one's symmetry, of leftness and rightness; and (2) directionality—laterality projected into space, which is obtained through and experienced in motor skills. An inability to perform or realize laterality and directionality must be overcome if the child is to be successful in school. And, indeed, Kephart recommends various movement patterns that can be learned and practiced by youngsters needing a corrective program.

Kephart clarified his thoughts at the annual convention of the American Alliance for Health, Physical Education and Recreation, held in Chicago in 1966. He offered the proposition that systematic motor exploration is the basis for all learning, because motor activity is information gathering. Ultimately, we may be teaching motor activity through physical education in order to promote reading. Kephart stated that 15 to 20 per cent of all children suffer from learning disorders; they have difficulty in learning. Children need generalized motor experiences; they need to explore, in order to have the background necessary for later success in school work. These motor generalizations include

1. *balance and posture:* The child must know where gravity is, as well as comprehend direction.
2. *propulsion and receipt:* The child should be able to move both body and objects away and toward something.

3. *locomotion:* Locomotion refers to body movement through space, overcoming obstacles, and changing pace. Locomotive generalizations go on unconsciously so that the child can explore.
4. *contact and manipulation:* The child's relationship with objects is determined by such abilities as reaching, grasping, and releasing.

Because of the importance attached to motor generalizations in intellectual development, natural questions arise. Are professional athletes more highly intelligent individuals? Kephart states that this is not necessarily so, as they may have dropped out at one of the developmental levels above motor skill accomplishment. Athletes have the potential for high intellectual attainment, but only if they have successfully gone through all the development levels during childhood. He calls for more emphasis on the developmental aspects of sports and less on the competitive and social aspects. What about high degrees of skills in many motor performances? This is not necessary, but, instead, what is desired is a minimum ability in a wide range of activities. Overconcentration on one skill is not as effective as varied motor experiences in contributing to the cognitive processes.

Just as Godfrey and Kephart (1969) suggest that low achievers in school lack basic readiness (motor) skills that can be made up if they are taught, Delacato expresses similar thoughts. In a series of articles and books, culminating in *Neurological Organization and Reading,* Delacato (1966) favors a concept of neurological organization. It is used to explain deficits in readiness and to show how a child develops physically and neurologically in his early years and, ultimately, intellectually. Neurological organization describes the process of control over activities that begins at the level of the spinal cord and medulla at birth, then goes to the pons, to the midbrain, and finally to the cortex. This organization terminates when the child is approximately six to eight years of age. In other words, the neurological development process is complete at that time.

Delacato has tested children on various tasks to see whether they have progressed normally from one state to the next. For example, cortical-level control is measured by the child's ability to perform cross-pattern walking and visual pursuit. A failure on a test at any control level indicates that the neurological organization is incomplete, with potential detrimental effects in reading ability. Reading problems are thus created before a child enters the school; the school merely points them out. The most important element for successful reading endeavors is cortical hemispheric dominance, or one-sidedness. Lack of complete and constant laterality results in reading and language problems. (Compare this view with Kephart's.) From his observations, Delacato concludes that 60 to 80 per cent of the superior readers are completely one-sided. Preventive or corrective measures include mastering general motor patterns, such as homolateral crawling at the lowest stage, and creeping, walking, and walking in cross-patterns at later stages.

A number of studies, on the other hand, have not found any difference in reading ability between established and nonestablished laterality groups. R. J. Capobianco (1967), for example, administered five tests of handedness and four tests of eye dominance to subjects with special learning disabilities. The test scores were correlated with reading ability measures. Results indicated that lateral dominance did not facilitate reading achievement; in fact, incomplete dominance, in certain cases, resulted in better reading performance.

Research that questions the Delacato theory was conducted by Melvin Robbins (1966). Delacato had made several claims concerning the educational benefits of his theory when used with children. Robbins questioned three of those assertions in his study of 126 children from three second-grade classes. Class I continued with its normal curriculum, class II continued with its normal curriculum but was subjected to a program consistent with the Delacato theory in addition to its regular activities, and class III was given a general program of activities now known to be correlated with reading achievement. A pre- and posttest were given in the areas of arithmetic, general intelligence, laterality, reading, and creeping. Robbins made the following conclusions:

1. The data did not support the relationships between neurological organization and reading achievement.
2. The addition of Delacato's program did not enhance the reading and lateral development of these children.

Robbins, based on these conclusions and literature he reviewed, advised against acceptance of Delacato's work until more scientifically based research could be conducted concerning the validity of the theory.

A year later, Robbins joined with Gene Glass (Glass & Robbins, 1967) to examine the Delacato theory further. They presented a brief overview of Delacato's theory in an attempt to determine the validity of the theory. Fifteen studies were critiqued, and a great deal of inconsistency, as well as lack of objectivity, was reported in the Delacato studies and studies that supported the Delacato theory. The authors concluded that the research done by Delacato and his supporters contained major faults in design and analysis and, if validity of the theory is to be found, studies must be designed without bias and be conducted in a scientific manner.

Kephart's theory is more acceptable and seems to be based more on fact than Delacato's. Kephart's theory was endorsed by the Reading Research Foundation in 1970 and has achieved widespread support more recently, although there is research evidence to contradict the supposed benefits of the program.

Barsch (1967) also feels that movement efficiency is a fundamental principle underlining human development. His theory of movigenics is based on the development of movement patterns and the relationship of those patterns to learning efficiency. The child must learn to move within spaces. If this movement efficiency is developed completely, then learning will not be impaired. The development of this efficiency depends on fifteen fundamental units that are placed under three separate headings. The first of these headings is Postural-Transport Orientation. Within this area of development of movement efficiency, Barsch has placed: (1) muscular strength, (2) dynamic balance, (3) body awareness, (4) spatial awareness, and (5) temporal awareness.

The second heading, Percepto-Cognitive Modes, deals with reception and expression within the child and encompasses the information-receiving gustatory, olfactory, tactual, kinesthetic, auditory, and visual modes. The final heading, Degrees of Freedom, includes the qualities that allow the child to achieve range, amplitude, and broadness with behavior. These qualities are bilaterality, rhythm, flexibility, and motor planning. Barsch (1967) writes that

> All fifteen components are simultaneously active and developing from birth throughout life. The human performer is at all times a composite of relative efficiencies and inefficiencies of all components. Each component provides its own emphasis in contribution to the total in a hierarchial pattern from infancy. As they have been listed in order, we hold that order to be chronologic. The first to receive emphasis is muscular strength and the last to be emphasized is motor planning. Each provides a foundation for the emergence of the subsequent components and each subsequent one continues to enhance and enrich those that have gone before. All are interrelated and interdependent (p. 83).

Throughout this progressive order of emphasis, Barsch looks at the physical phenomenon of each component, as well as the cognitive aspect of the development. Thus, he views the individual as learning to move in space through the dual physical and cognitive aspects of these fifteen components of movement.

Frostig (1971) has developed a perceptual training program geared specifically to vision. Her theory deals with visual perception and the remediation of visual perception and assimilation, with some attention to certain motor responses. Frostig has based her program on the sensorimotor training of the child. This training includes four groups of sensorimotor skills that the child must develop. The first two groups are termed *awareness;* in these groups the infant becomes aware of its environment and the outside world and gains awareness of the self. The third group of skills is comprised of the motor skills, in which the child learns to turn over, sit, stand, kneel, crawl, walk, and so on. The final group of skills includes those necessary to the child for the manipulation of objects. All of the skills within each group must be incorporated into a sensorimotor training program to ensure the total development of the child.

Based on the idea of these four necessary groups of sensorimotor skills, Frostig evaluates the child to determine dysfunctions in the skills and then prescribes a movement education program that will enhance the development of those skills, thus improving movement function. She utilizes the Frostig Sensorimotor and Movement Skills Checklist in each evaluation. Children who are admitted to the Marianne Frostig Center of Educational Therapy are prescribed remedial programs on the basis of their evaluation on this checklist.

General Analysis

In general, research that concretely supports any of the programs is sparse. It almost appears that for every positive report, a negative report can be found in regard to any of the proposed programs. Perhaps one of the more careful analyses of the research data and theory surrounding perceptual motor programs has been offered by Cratty (1970). He, as well as Seefeldt (1974), illustrates the frailities upon which these programs are based and, indeed, both the weaknesses in the research and the lack of research support for the various programs.

One idea that has evolved with the emergence of the perceptual motor training theories is the premise that the slow learner or underachiever need no longer be sent to the back of the room to color or play with blocks. Through perceptual training, the underachiever has been brought into the limelight of education and an increasing amount of research, study, and work is being expended in order to help this child. Perceptual motor training programs are far from being a panacea for educational difficulties, but they do afford the learner a new and different medium for learning as well as a break in the regular day-to-day curriculum.

There is evidence that perceptual motor training can enhance achievement in deficient and mentally retarded children. To what degree there is something inherent in these programs to cause beneficial results or to what degree these results are associated with psychosocial factors, such as parent, teacher, and learning enthusiasm in the possibility of curing the deficiency, remains to be seen. Special attention and love may contribute much to achievement, although one might argue that the important concern is the outcome, not necessarily what causes it.

MOTOR DEVELOPMENT TESTS

Many of the perceptual motor training programs suggest assessment techniques for determining the motoric development level of the child. Such tests can reveal where the learner stands in reference to normative data. They might also imply remedial work that needs to be accomplished.

For instance, the Purdue Perceptual Motor Survey allows the examination of a number of behaviors that presumably undergird academic skills (Roach & Kephart, 1966). They are as follows:

1. Walking board: Forward
2. Walking board: Backward
3. Walking board: Sidewise
4. Jumping
5. Identification of body parts
6. Imitation of movements
7. Obstacle course
8. Chalkboard: Circle
9. Chalkboard: Double circle
10. Chalkboard: Lines, lateral
11. Chalkboard: Lines, vertical
12. Kraus-Weber (items 4 and 5)
13. Angels-in-the-snow
14. Ocular pursuits: Both eyes, lateral

15. Ocular pursuits: Both eyes, vertical
16. Ocular pursuits: Both eyes, diagonal
17. Ocular pursuits: Both eyes, rotary
18. Ocular pursuits: Right eye, lateral
19. Ocular pursuits: Right eye, vertical
20. Ocular pursuits: Right eye, diagonal
21. Ocular pursuits: Right eye, rotary
22. Ocular pursuits: Left eye, lateral
23. Ocular pursuits: Left eye, vertical
24. Ocular pursuits: Left eye, diagonal
25. Ocular pursuits: Left eye, rotary
26. Developmental drawing: Form
27. Developmental drawing: Organization
28. Rhythmic writing: Rhythm
29. Rhythmic writing: Reproduction
30. Rhythmic writing: Orientation

Roach and Kephart state that the survey is geared to detect errors in perceptual motor development. Performance scores on the test can suggest areas for remediation. One admitted restriction in the survey is that it was developed with only second-, third-, and fourth-graders in mind.

Keith Kershner and Russell Dusewicz (1970) have attempted to modify the original Oseretsky Tests of Motor Development. Referred to as the KDK–Oseretsky Tests, they presumably measure

1. general static coordination.
2. general dynamic coordination.
3. dyamic manual coordination.
4. simultaneous voluntary movement.
5. speed.

Time is shortened greatly in the administration of this abbreviated test, which can provide descriptive and normative information about motor development. Diagnostic purposes can be served as well. The Osertsky test items are large-muscle activities, often novel in nature.

From another perspective, J. L. Schulman, C. Buist, J. C. Kaspar, D. Child, and E. Fackler (1969) developed a battery of fine motor tasks that are to assess speed of fine motor functioning of children aged three to eight. Presumably, the tests are most helpful in the study of brain-injured children. The tasks that comprise the test are:

Pegs: The score is the length of time required to place the six pegs into the square-hole pegboard from the Cattell Infant Intelligence Scale. This is done for both the preferred and nonpreferred hand.

Picks: The score is the number of seconds required to place fifteen toothpicks into a styrofoam ball 2½ inches in diameter. This is done for both the preferred and nonpreferred hands.

Beads: The score is the number of seconds required to string ten beads one half inch in diameter.

Taps: The number of seconds required for S to tap sixty times on a laboratory blood cell counter. This is also done for each hand. These tasks generate a total of seven measures (p. 244).

From the data collected in the study, it was concluded that the age and time required for task completion were related in a negatively accelerated manner. Speed, as an exponential function of age, is plotted in Figure 10-2. Sex was not a factor in performance. Children with impaired intellectual functioning performed more poorly on the motor tasks than the standardized population.

The literature is replete with tests that claim to measure general motor ability, specific motor abilities, developmental abilities, brain dysfunctioning, cognitive achievement predictable from motor test scores, and the like. An excellent survey of tests that are supposed to assess motor impairment, along with research findings, is presented by Morris and Whiting (1971). But in spite of the existence of so many tests with so many stated purposes, in reality their practical value, ex-

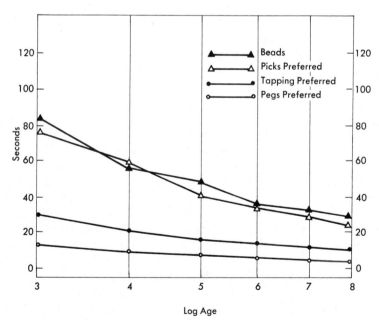

FIGURE 10-2. Speed with preferred hand × log age. Reprinted with permission of authors and publisher. *(From: Schulman, J. L., Buist, C., Kaspar, J. C., Child, D., & Fackler, E. An objective test of speed of fine motor function.* Perceptual and Motor Skills, *1969, 29, 243–255.)*

cept in extreme cases, has yet to be determined. Conflict exists between theory and the stated functions of certain tests. Further confusion appears when generalization of the usefulness of some tests goes beyond the data presented. As developmental indices of emerging perceptual motor patterns, normative information, and potential clinical usage, a number of tests serve useful purposes. But care should be exercised in score interpretation and student evaluation. Diagnostic and remedial possibilities can only be realized when it is clearly understood what test scores really measure. And, it goes without saying, the validity and reliability of any score, and the care with which testing is administered will influence performance outcomes and, in turn, evaluation.

SEX DIFFERENCES AND PERFORMANCE

In the past, sex differences in motor performance became more apparent with increasing age. Young boys and girls, it was felt, could compete in similar activities with satisfaction until they approached adolescence. During this period, motor skills related to the dominant form of play of each sex presumably distinguished the two sexes. From adolescence to adulthood, it was found that boys continually advanced in motor performance, girls improved very slightly or even worsened, and the gap in performance between the sexes widened. Why this occurred and indeed, if it actually should, is open to conjecture.

As we examine data that follow, we must keep in mind the years in which they were reported. Sex differences in gross motor performance are diminishing due to changes in socio-cultural factors, and their influence on the attitudes and motivations of young girls and women to become involved in such endeavors as sport.

The female infant is distinguished from the male by her earlier maturation and more advanced motor development, which permits her to demonstrate a higher level of proficiency in movement-oriented behaviors. Yet, males tend to participate in more vigorous activity. Because of greater strength and muscular development, the average male child, at the age of two and a half and beyond, performs better than the female in a great variety of gross motor activities. Throwing patterns are superior for boys than girls at age five; at ages five to seven and nine to eleven, research shows that boys perform better in tests of running, jumping, catching, striking, and kicking. Numerous studies in which normative data have been collected on boys and girls at school age indicate the superiority of boys to girls in gross motor activities. An excellent summary of sex differences in motor development and of motor tasks, abilities, and various cognitive processes has been presented by J. E. Garai and A. Scheinfeld (1968).

An analysis of the research literature on sex differences in simple perceptual-motor tasks has led D. M. Broverman, E. L. Klaiber, Y. Kobayashi, and W. Vogel (1968) to conclude that young girls and women exceed their male counterparts in tasks of fine manual dexterity. Furthermore, females perform better than males in the perceptual motor behaviors associated with speech and reading, as well as in small-muscle, simple perceptual motor activities that require speed, repetition, and skill. More specifically, Broverman et al. (1968) indicate behaviors in which one sex is superior to the other.

The behaviors in which females are superior to males seem to have the following attributes:

1. The behaviors appear to be based mainly upon past experience or learning, as opposed to problem solving of novel or difficult tasks. Thus, color naming, talking, reading, etc., are based upon extensive previous experience.
2. As a result of extensive prior practice, the behaviors appear to involve minimal mediation by higher cognitive processes. Sensory thresholds represent an extreme of this attribute; but other more obviously learned behaviors such as typing, color naming, or conditioning are termed skilled or well-acquired as they move toward reflexive automatic responses.
3. The behaviors typically involve fine coordinations of small muscles with perceptual and attentional processes, such as in typing or reading, rather than coordination of large muscle movements, as in athletics.
4. Finally, the behaviors are evaluated in terms of the speed and accuracy of repetitive responses, as in color naming, rather than in terms of production of new responses or "insight," as in maze solutions (p. 28).

The behaviors in which males are superior to females seem to be characterized by the following:

1. The behaviors involve an inhibition or delay of initial response tendencies to obvious stimulus attributes in favor of responses to less obvious stimulus attributes, as in the Embedded Figures Test.
2. The behaviors seem to involve extensive mediation of higher processes, as opposed to automatic or reflexive stimulus-response connections.
3. Finally, the behaviors are evaluated in terms of the production of solutions to novel tasks or situations, such as assembling parts of a puzzle or object, as opposed to speed or accuracy of repetitive responses (p. 28).

Broverman et al. have determined an inverse relationship between the physiological processes associated in the simple perceptual motor abilities and those involved in inhibitory restructuring tasks. Perceptual restructuring tasks often call for the identification of stimuli patterns from more complex patterns in which they are embedded. Another example is a widely used experimental task, the Rod and Frame Test, in which the subject, while in a darkened room, must adjust a luminescent rod from a tilted luminescent frame. Differences in performance in the two categories of tasks (simple perceptual motor and restructuring), according to Broverman et al., represent the balance between adrenergic and cholinergic neural processes. Androgens and estrogens influence activation and inhibition processes, thus helping to explain sex differences in the performances of the type of tasks examed by Broverman et al.

One of the more complete research projects having to do with the interaction of age and sex on performance was completed by C. E. Noble, B. L. Baker, and T. A. Jones (1964). A Discrimination Reaction Time apparatus was used that required the subject to snap one of four toggle switches in response to changing light stimulus patterns. A total of six hundred subjects took part in the study, ranging in age from eight to eighty-seven. Twenty males and twenty females were placed in each of fifteen experimental groups, according to age. It can be observed that the expected performance curves were obtained—i.e., peak performance for both groups was attained at approximately the late teens and early twenties and worsened with advancing age. These data coincide very nicely with those reported by Hodgkins (see Figure 9-12).

It is interesting to compare performance differences at the various ages. With the exception of the ten- to thirteen-year age bracket and the seventy-one-to eighty-seven-year age bracket, males displayed a general superiority over females in response speed. The two sexes performed similarly until the age of sixteen, when the females leveled off in performance and show decrements with increasing age. Males continued to improve until the early twenties, and then they too underwent declining performance.

The following measures were recorded by Singer (1969) for third- and sixth-grade children: height, grip strength of the dominant and non-dominant hands, elbow flexion and elbow extension strength, hip flexion and hip extension strength, dynamic balance, ball-throwing accuracy, speed of hand-arm movement, eye-hand coordination, stimulus discrimination and hand speed, perceptual ability, academic achievement, and intelligence. Figure 10-3 includes all the measures taken on the four groups, converted to standard scores from raw.

It can be concluded that sixth-grade boys had, in general, the most favorable recorded measures, followed by sixth-grade girls, third-grade boys, and third-grade girls.

In most gross physical and motor measures, both boys and girls compare favorably, with boys holding a slight edge until approximately the age of twelve or thirteen. Body size and strength have much to do with athletic accomplishments. During adolescence, boys generally grow larger and demonstrate a greater magnitude of strength, and as these differences between sexes become more apparent, so do motor performances. Jones (1949) followed the strength development of boys and girls over a period of time. Figure 10-4 presents a comparison between boys and girls, from age eleven through seventeen, in right- and left-hand grip strengths. The girls begin trailing off at about fifteen years of age, whereas the boys are still increasing with great rapidity at the age of seventeen. Differences in strength, although in favor of the boys at eleven, become more noticeable at thirteen, and continue to widen at each succeeding age.

In summary, generally it can be stated that boys typically increase in performance until the late teens, whereas girls decline in performance in the early teens. There are exceptions, of course. The relative performances of boys and girls at comparative ages may be attributed to many factors. One of the more prominent variables is the influence of social approval, which, of course, is culturally determined. For many years, boys have been encouraged to develop athletic prowess, whereas girls have been told to act feminine, to avoid most sports and vigorous activities. With a lack of incentive, performance levels naturally decline.

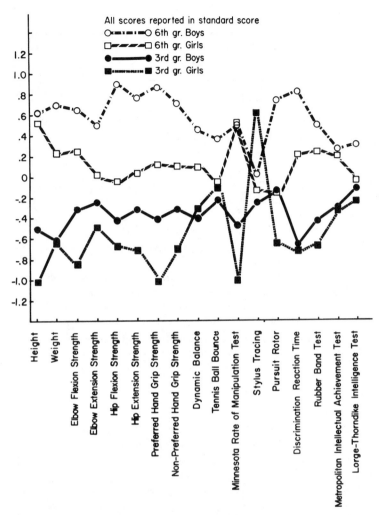

FIGURE 10-3. Comparison of four groups of children on various physical, perceptual motor, and intellectual abilities. (*From Singer, Robert N. Physical characteristics, perceptual motor, and intelligence differences between third- and sixth-grade children.* Research Quarterly, *1969, 40, 803–811.*)

Although much information on the nature of sex differences indicates the superiority of males over females in most gross motor activities, this does not necessarily mean any differences in learning abilities or rates between the sexes. Some possible reasons for performance dissimilarities have been offered. Physiological differences also provide the male with a more favorable apparatus (body build, strength, and so on) to exceed performances of females in a number of activities. A fair conclusion from the evidence is that males and females learn motor tasks in a similar way and at a similar rate. Differences in actual performances may be the

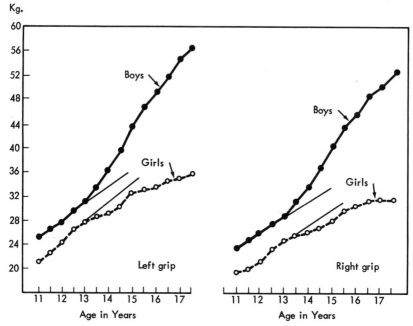

FIGURE 10-4. Comparison of right- and left-hand grip strength of boys and girls from the ages 11 through 17. *(From Jones, H. E. Motor performance and growth (Vol. 1) Berkeley: University of California, University of California Publications in Child Development, 1949.)*

result of previous learnings and transfer possibilities, structural differences, motivational differences, and, most obviously, sociocultural factors.

In fact, if a greater field of vision is related to more highly skilled performance in certain tasks, it is of interest to note that Albert Burg (1968) found that females consistently demonstrated slightly higher visual fields than men at just about all ages (see Figure 10-5). Eye fields peak at a later age for the females than for the males. As might be expected, and being consistent with data on other personal abilities, visual field, after the early twenties, decline with age for both sexes.

More factual evidence offered by Hirata (1966) indicates the relationship of achievements in various athletic endeavors with sex and age. Using the 1964 Olympic champion athletes as subjects, he found the mean age of the male champions to be twenty-six years, whereas the female champions were twenty-three years in age, on the average. Most of the male champions were in the twenty-to-thirty age group, whereas the majority of female champions were located in the seventeen-to-twenty-five age bracket. Hirata concludes that the males's motor and physical development are completed later than the female's and is maintained for a longer time. However, other factors as well, perhaps social and physical in nature,

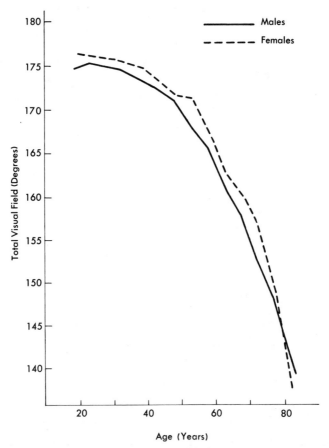

FIGURE 10-5. The relationship of age, sex, and field of vision. (*From Burg, A. Lateral visual field as related to age and sex.* Journal of Applied Psychology, *1968, 52, 10–15.*) Copyright 1968 by the American Psychological Association. Reprinted by permission.

may account for some of the difference in peak performance years between the sexes.

From a physiological point of view, various differences between the sexes usually favor the male in athletic performance, but not to the extent once supposed. With social encouragement, girls and women are displaying remarkable skills in a wide range of activities. Jokl et al. (1964) observed that "the time-honored statement that women are invariably the weaker sex no longer holds true as an unqualified assertion" (p. 691). Constant hard drilling and training result in outstanding athletic performance, regardless of sex. Examine the following selected contemporary data in swimming as to record times to support this point:

Event*	Year Difference
100-meter freestyle: Women: 1976—Ender—55.65 Men: 1952—Scholes—57.4	(24 years)
400-meter freestyle: Women: 1976—Thumer—4:09.89 Men: 1964—Schollander—4:12.2	(12 years)
1500-meter freestyle: Women: 1974—Turrall—16:33.94 Men: 1968—Burton—16:38.9	(6 years)
200-meter breaststroke: Women: 1976—Koshevaia—2:33.55 Men: 1960—Mulliken—2:37.4	(16 years)
200-meter butterfly: Women: 1976—Kother—2:11.22 Men: 1960—Troy—2:12.8	(16 years)
100-meter backstroke: Women: 1976—Richter—1:01.51 Men: 1960—Thiele—1:01.9	(16 years)

*The English Channel swim record is held by a woman, Tina Bischoff, who swam it in nine hours and three minutes in 1976. The best male performance is that of Barry Watson, who swam it in nine hours and thirty-five minutes, in 1964.

BODY IMAGE

The child develops many characteristics in the early formative years that will be fairly well established, although modifiable, in subsequent years. Self-image, the appearance of oneself, is one of those characteristics. Other terms often used along with *self-image* are *body image, self-concept* and *body awareness*. They all refer to the impressions one has of his or her body, impressions that develop in the course of time, with perceptual sensitivity, experiences, and the like. In turn, an individual's self-image may very well be associated with activity involvement and possible success.

A review of the literature by Morris and Whiting (1971) reveals that body image, or concept, is associated with a variety of expressions, such as

1. the ability to make body movements appropriate to the demands of the environment.
2. bodily sensations.
3. imagination—mental imagery that is not purely representational.
4. ego development.
5. affective development.
6. cognitive development.

7. development of body boundaries.
8. kinesthetic sensitivity.

Regardless of the usage and interpretation of *body image,* the development of an ideal body image is the result of a personal interpretation of one's actions and appearance, as well as environmental feedback. It begins, according to perceptual theorists, with a child's differentiation between self and environment, of body and field. The awareness of the body's potential and limitations, in general and in relation to particular circumstances, is an expected process. Faulty development can lead to personality and learning disorders, according to many psychologists and special educators. Furthermore, fundamental to some perceptual motor training programs to remediate learning disorders is the child's mastery of body awareness. Laterality (awareness of two sides of the body), sensory dominance (perferential use of one of the eyes, hands, or feet), and directionality (movement in space to a correct location) are aspects of body awareness thought to be important factors in a developing child.

In fact, Harriet Williams (1973) suggests three foundational components in the development of the image one has of oneself: (1) a sensorimotor component; (2) a conceptual component; and (3) a feeling, or opinion, component. Body awareness first begins for the child through feedback received from personal activities. The senses provide input, which helps the child to learn more about his or her being. With development, the child learns to verbalize and conceptualize about the self, personal experiences, and personal environment. At the same time, body attitudes are developed. A variety of experiences in which the child learns to perceive and accept reality promotes a more accurate body image. Personally rewarding experiences in which the child learns to perceive and accept reality promotes a more accurate body image. Personally rewarding experiences as an outgrowth of sensitive and quality child-rearing practices lead to a body image that is satisfying to the child.

The relationship between one's self-image, personality factors, activity interest and proficiency, body build, and other variables has not been clearly established. Positive but low associations have often been reported in the literature. Yet, the effects of a sensorimotor training program on the body image of mentally retarded children were quite beneficial, report Maloney and Payne (1970). When compared to control subjects, the sensorimotor trained subjects showed better body image scores immediately after the two-month training session, as well as eight months later. Assuming the value of a high body image, apparently, special body awareness programs can produce desirable changes, at least in the mentally retarded.

To what degree a generalized feeling of confidence can be developed within a child as a result of successful and rewarding experiences in some motoric activity is difficult to assess. As might be expected, it is an extremely arduous task to isolate and control variables to determine these effects. Consequently, research is lacking that might enable us to make conclusive statements at this time. However, many psychologists would probably agree that every child needs to be successful at some undertaking. Subjective wisdom suggests that this experience should be personally rewarding enough to facilitate attempts at other undertakings.

CHAPTER HIGHLIGHTS

1. Critical learning periods refer to that crucial time in the development of an organism when the ideal intermix of sensory, motor, psychological (maturational), and motivational factors is present for the learning of a specified behavior. Presumably, an experience introduced before that time will be a waste, and afterward it might not be as effective. Behaviors have been identified as specific to certain species of organisms with regard to the existence of critical learning periods. With humans, it appears that these might be optimal times for the introduction of certain behaviors, but that humans are highly plastic as compared to subhumans and can compensate later in many ways for limited earlier experiences. But timeliness, not earliness, is apparently the most important variable with humans. Critical learning periods for the learning of specific skills have not as yet been identified in humans.

2. A variety of perceptual motor training programs have been formulated to enhance cognitive development and, in turn, achievement in academic matters. The premise is that poor intellectual performance may be the result of prior inadequate perceptual and motor development. A remedial program would presumably overcome academic deficits for a number of children. These programs have received wide endorsement in some areas, rejection in others. Some programs have gained greater acceptance than others. Because of methodological problems in the research that are difficult to overcome, it is hard to evaluate cases in which positive conclusions are reported. Improvements in academic learning may be the result of side benefits of perceptual motor programs, rather than the improvement of learning capabilities in general.

3. Motor development tests provide normative data on various performance tasks that can be useful in learner diagnosis for learning disabilities or the lack of previous quality motor learning experiences.

4. Differences between the sexes in gross and fine motor performances have been noted in the research for years. Many of them are disappearing with changes in cultural values toward a female's participation in motor activities, especially of the vigorous, large-muscle kind. Differences may also be due to physiological, biochemical, and hormonal distinctions. However, the evidence does not clearly point to differences in learning abilities or rates between the sexes.

5. Body image, self-image, or self-concept, describes the feelings one has about oneself. It is thought that a greater positive image reflects more confidence and, in turn, contributes to success in a particular undertaking. Whether experiences that contribute to this ideal state in turn help a person to participate and achieve in other undertakings is not known from the research, although the concept is supported by many educators and psychologists.

References

Barsch, R. H. *Achieving perceptual-motor efficiency: Special child publications* (Vol. 1). Seattle: Seattle Sequin School, Inc., 1967.

Beach, F. A., & Jaynes, J. Effects of early experiences upon the behavior of animals *Psychological Bulletin*, 1954, *51*, 239–263.

Broverman, D. M., Klaiber, E. L., Kobayashi, Y., & Vogel, W. Role of activation and inhibition in sex differences in cognitive abilities. *Psychological Review*, 1968, *75*, 23–50.

Bruner, J. S. *The process of education.* Cambridge, Mass.: Harvard University Press, 1963.

Burg, A. Lateral visual field as related to age and sex. *Journal of Applied Psychology*, 1968, *52*, 10–15.

Capobianco, R. J. Ocular-manual laterality and reading achievement in children with special learning disabilities. *American Educational Research Journal*, 1967, *4*, 133–138.

Delacato, C. H. *Neurological organization and reading.* Springfield, Ill.: Charles C Thomas, 1966.

Dennis, W. The effect of cradling practices upon the onset of walking in Hopi children. *Journal of Genetic Psychology*, 1940, *56*, 77–86.

Espenschade, A. S., & Eckert, H. M. *Motor development.* Columbus, Ohio: Charles E. Merrill, 1967.

Fleming, J. W. Perceptual-motor programs. In R. N. Singer (Ed.), *The psychomotor domain: Movement behavior.* Philadelphia: Lea & Febiger, 1972.

Freeman, L. *Why people act that way.* New York: Thomas Y. Crowell, 1965.

Frostig, M. Program for sensory-motor development at the Marianne Frostig Center of Educational Therapy. *Foundations and practices in perceptual motor learning: A quest for understanding.* Washington, D. C.: American Association for Health, Physical Education, and Recreation, 1971.

Garai, J. E., & Scheinfeld, A. Sex differences in mental and behavioral traits. *Genetic Psychological Monographs*, 1968, *77*, 169–299.

Glass, G. V., & Robbins, M. P. A critique of experiments on the role of neurological organization in reading performance. *Reading Research Quarterly*, 1967, *3*, 5–51.

Godfrey, B. B., & Kephart, N. C. *Movement patterns and motor education.* New York: Appleton-Century-Crofts, 1969.

Hirata, K. Physique and age of Tokyo Olympic champions. *Journal of Sports Medicine and Physical Fitness*, 1966, *6*, 207–222.

Johnson, W. R. Critical periods, body image and movement competency in childhood. *Symposium on Integrated Development*, Purdue University, 1964.

Jokl, E., Karvonen, M., Kihlberg, J., Koekela, A., & Noro, L. Olympic survey (Helsinki, 1952). In E. Jokl & E. Simon (Eds.), *International Research in sport and physical education.* Springfield, Ill.: Charles C Thomas, 1964.

Jones, H. E. Motor performance and growth. Berkeley: University of California publications in child development, 1949.

Kershner, K. M., & Dusewicz, A. R. KDK-Oseretsky tests of motor development. *Perceptual and Motor Skills*, 1970, *30*, 202.

Lorenz, K. *Studies in animal and human behavior* (Vol. 1). (R. Martin, Trans.). Cambridge, Mass.: Harvard University Press, 1970.

Maloney, M. P., & Payne, L. E. Note on the stability of changes in body image due to sensory-motor training. *American Journal of Mental Deficiency,* 1970, *74,* 708.

McGraw, M. B. *Growth: A study of Johnny and Jimmy.* New York: Appleton-Century-Crofts, 1935.

McGraw, M. B. Later development of children specially trained during infancy: Johnny and Jimmy at school age. *Child Development,* 1939, *10,* 1–19.

Morris, P. R., & Whiting, H. T. A. *Motor impairment and compensatory education.* Philadelphia: Lea & Febiger, 1971.

Mussen, H. P., Conger, J. J., & Kagan, J. *Child development and personality.* New York: Harper & Row, 1969.

Noble, C. E., Baker, B. L., & Jones, T. A. Age and sex parameters in psychomotor learning. *Perceptual and Motor Skills,* 1964, *19,* 935–945.

Piaget, J. *The origins of intelligence in children* (M. Cook, Trans.). New York: International Universities Press, 1952.

Radler, D. H., & Kephart, N. C. *Success through play.* New York: Harper & Row, 1960.

Ravizza, R. J., & Herschberger, A. C. The effect of prolonged motor restriction upon later behavior of the rat. *The Psychological Record,* 1966, *16,* 73–80.

Roach, E., & Kephart, N. C. *The Purdue perceptual-motor survey.* Columbus, Ohio: Charles E. Merrill, 1966.

Robbins, M. P. A study of the validity of Delacato's theory of neurological organization. *Exceptional Children,* 1966, *32,* 517–523.

Schulman, J. L., Buist, C., Kasper, J. C., Child, D., & Fackler, E. An objective test of speed of fine motor function. *Perceptual and Motor Skills,* 1969, *29,* 243–255.

Scott, J. P. *Early experience and the organization of behavior.* Belmont, Calif.: Wadsworth, 1968.

Scott, J. P. A time to learn. *Psychology Today,* 1969, *2,* 47–48, 66–67.

Seefeldt, V. Perceptual-motor programs. In J. H. Wilmore (Ed.) *Exercise and sport sciences reviews* (Vol. 2). New York: Academic Press, 1974.

Singer, R. N. Physical characteristic, perceptual-motor, and intelligence differences between third- and sixth-grade children. *Research Quarterly,* 1969, *40,* 803–811.

Williams, H. G. Perceptual-motor development in children. In C. B. Corbin (Ed.), *A textbook of motor development.* Dubuque, Iowa: William C. Brown, 1973.

11 INSTRUCTIONAL AND TRAINING PROCEDURES: PREPRACTICE CONSIDERATIONS

Individuals possess unique qualities and specific characteristics as a result of inheritance, enabling some people to have greater potential than others for success with a particular motor skill. However, actual skill attainment does not depend only on genetic factors. Qualitative and quantitative environmental experiences will promote learning and ultimately determine performance levels.

Recognition of individual differences requires allowance for the fact that all people will not benefit in the same way from the same practice techniques and methods of instruction. This does not mean, though, that we proceed in a haphazard way in attempting to attain skill. Research has cleared the way for a better understanding of the learning process, with the result that certain concepts and procedures may be applied with confidence to many learners in a variety of learning situations. Learning, Benjamin Bloom (1976) believes, is the function of (1) those behaviors or competencies a student brings to a situation; (2) motivation; and (3) the quality of the instruction. Certainly, a competent instructor should be able to influence a student's motivation and to instruct effectively.

In this and the next two chapters, we will be concerned with pre-, in-, and post-practice conditions and considerations. Figure 11-1 indicates the relationship between these factors and those from an information-processing framework, as well as simplified expressions in the form of personal activities. Discussions on

FIGURE 11-1. Practice considerations with regard to information-processing terminology and personal activities.

Practice Considerations	Information Processing Dimensions	Personal Activities
prepractice	preprocessing	readiness
during practice	processing	doing
post practice	reprocessing	doing again

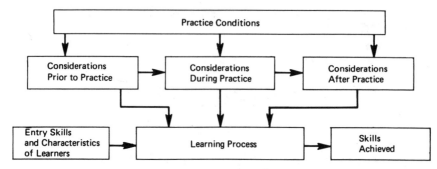

FIGURE 11-2. Considerations for the achievement of skill in motor learning. (*Adapted from Singer, R. N. The learning systems approach and instruction in psychomotor activities. Motor Skills: Theory Into Practice, 1977, 1, 113–122.* (a))

the topics associated with each of these three major headings follow nicely in some cases in the chapters but are arranged more arbitrarily in other cases.

The management of practice, for oneself or others, requires a great deal of planning if benefits are to be reaped as quickly as possible. An understanding of the learning process and how to manipulate practice conditions is of obvious value. Performance level achieved is a function of the quality and extent of practice undertaken by the learner; three facets of practice can be identified, as can be seen in Figure 11-2.

Figure 11-2 contains the framework for the guidelines of the content of Chapters 11 through 13 and emphasizes the potential role of instruction in the different phases of learning, from the readiness state of the learner to ongoing practice conditions to considerations for transfer and retention.

In this particular chapter, our thoughts will be directed to the preparatory state of the learner and the learning environment. The learner must be in an ideal state of readiness and the situation prepared appropriately in order for learning potential to be realized. Consequently, factors associated with the learner's orientation to the learning activity, communication between instructors and learners, and the learning environment will be discussed. In addition, special programs designed to enhance learning through the establishment of the learner's readiness and willingness to perform will be described briefly and analyzed.

THE LEARNER'S PREPARATORY STATE

The learner brings feelings, expectations, ideas, and previously developed competencies to the learning situation. Beginners usually need to be guided in their orientation to the activity, whereas the more highly skilled have typically learned how to prepare themselves for additional learning and performance.

Goals and Intentions

An approach to instruction should begin with some type of implicit or explicit statement about what one wants to teach. It is quite common to talk about what is going to be taught rather than to talk about what the students are going to learn. Too often we say that our instruction is in fifth-grade mathematics or sophomore biology. Mathematics and biology are really content domains and do not reflect what the student learns or is able to do as a result of having received that instruction. The statement merely reflects that the teacher will somehow convey information related to those topics.

Goal identification can be applied to any unit of instruction, whether it be for a full year of instructional activity or simply for one class hour. The learners need to know what is expected in order to get the idea and to practice in a purposeful manner. The terminology, or the way in which the goal is stated, can be very critical to success in the later application of the systems approach model. More specifically stated goals and intentions increase the likelihood that students will fulfill them. No matter what means are used, written material, observation, verbal description, or others, the student can be goal-oriented only if the goals are understood. An image of the desired response must be created.

Where instructional strategies such as problem solving are advocated and students are led into the act of discovery, goals and objectives need not be specified. Much depends on what the teacher is attempting to achieve regarding the desirability of one strategy over another. Specific skill expectancies require specific explanations. If a number of behaviors of a given type are acceptable, then goal direction need not be so explicit. If an acquisition of the techniques involved in a learning process—e.g., problem solving—is important, the product, in the form of specific behaviors, becomes secondary to the experience of a process that will be applicable to other situations. What particular behaviors or tendencies to behave are hoped to be affected from the forthcoming learning experiences?

Task Meaningfulness

Tasks that are more meaningful to the learner elevate motivation and consequently are learned more effectively. Meaningfulness can be interpreted in two ways, according to David Ausubel (1968) with regard to the (1) nature of the material, or (2) function of the learner.

For instance, some tasks are "logical"; they are not contrived or artificial. A list of nonsense syllables really is meaningless; a poem contains a meaningful content. The property of the learning task is determined against a criterion of logical meaningfulness.

Another way to analyze an activity is according to its meaningfulness to the learner. The learner's cognitive structure of prior experiences and knowledge must be adequate for the task if it is to be interpreted as meaningful. How is it perceived regarding the importance of demonstrating achievement? Will proficiency fulfill personal goals? Does it make any difference to the learner whatsoever if success occurs with the task? In either case, whether task meaningfulness is analyzed according to acceptable interpretations in a society or on an individual and personal basis, a greater interest and perseverance will generally be noted in performance, as will longer-lasting learning affects. Instructional procedures encouraging favorable attitudes to the learning activity will help to make it more appealing, interesting, or challenging.

Often an activity is conceived by the instructor as meaningful for the learner; the assumption is that the learner holds the same values and perceptions as the instructor. Unfortunately, such is not always the case. This possible discrepancy between learner and instructor could result in frustration and insufficient motivation for the occurrence of adequate skill acquisition. Furthermore, the learning of meaningful material is not the same thing as meaningful learning. Meaningful learning occurs when practice conditions are set ideally for a learner who is in the appropriate dispositional state to learn.

Intent and Purpose

Practice is beneficial when it is purposeful. If the learner has the intention of improving and of attaining a goal, more than likely, performance increments will be observed on succeeding trials. Thus, both the instructor and student are obligated: the instructor to set the goals, arrange the practice format, and provide motivation, the student to follow the lead. Of course, if the task to be learned is meaningful to the student, there is less of a problem in creating interest to promote learning.

Merely going routinely through an act is a pure waste of time. It is not untypical for students in programs or classes to demonstrate the same low levels of skill at the termination of a unit as at the beginning. Although many reasons may be cited for this unfortunate circumstance, certainly one is a lack of purpose and direction. Many physical limitations can be overcome if the individual desires to improve in performance through practice. The reasons for wanting to develop a motor skill are varied, ranging from pure enjoyment in skilled performance to fulfilling some occupational or recreational goal or for attention or for some material reward. Some reasons are better than others (who is to decide?) but the fact remains that any purpose is better than none at all, and performance will be contingent on intent to better oneself.

Developmental and Psychological Readiness

Effective training procedures must be sensitive to the learner's state of readiness. Readiness refers to the learner's (1) developmental stage and maturational abilities to cope with the learning activities, or (2) predisposition at the time of instruction for favorable response to the instruction and the tasks. Both considerations of readiness need to be recognized if instruction is to proceed in a meaningful manner.

In Chapter 9 and 10, devoted to developmental factors, importance of maturational readiness for skill learning was stressed. We need not go into this topic again. It is merely reemphasized here. However, the learner's psychological state of preparedness to heed relevant cues, concentrate on task demands, and practice conscientiously is often taken for granted. Meaningful practice depends to a great extent on the learner's state of readiness. Although this condition may be present for personal reasons, there are many occasions on which the instructor must use methods to elevate learner readiness. In many ways, readiness is related to motivational state. If the learner is optimally motivated, we can assume the existence of optimal preparation to practice appropriately.

Emotional Readiness

Motivations and emotions need to be operating in the ideal manner for the person, preparatory to the experience of learning an activity or performing in it. Each person should possess an ideal state of readiness for each activity. Too much anxiety or too little concern, for example, may interfere with performance and learning, for different reasons. (See Chapter 8 for a discussion on the U-shaped hypothesis in this regard.) Although it is true that many learners are placed in situations in which they would rather not be, and must be motivated to practice, others are too highly motivated and need to be taught to relax more. Discussion on various relaxation programs will appear at the end of this chapter. Suffice it to say here that emotional readiness should be recognized and controlled by the learner, or else guided by an external source, such as the instructor. Relaxed concentration, as Tim Gallwey (1974) describes it, is an ideal dispositional state in which to begin any learning experience.

Motivation: Task Selection

Motivation operates in a variety of ways. It has just been pointed out how important an ideal motivational state is in preparation for performance. But motivation also works to promote continuance in and perseverance at practice in an activity. It is also the reason why we select one activity over another in which to participate. Preference for an activity is indicative of motivation, and when a great many choices are present, one selection truly represents a meaningful endeavor. Task meaningfulness, either for intrinsic (personally gratifying) or extrinsic (materialistically rewarding) reasons, increases the probability of its selection among alternatives, in order to gain in experience and in performance.

Attention and Set

On a number of occasions, especially with the more experienced and more mature, it may not be necessary for the teacher to employ special means of directing the learner's attention to the behaviors to be learned. But inexperienced and young students typically require special consideration with regard to the condition that gains and maintains their attention.

Attention is associated with interest and motivation. It also implies the capability to discriminate among available stimuli, to select appropriate stimuli to which a response is expected. When students are taught to hit a softball, they have to consciously direct their attention to the task through their own efforts or those of the teacher. High attention levels are important at the introductory point to the task, as well as during all stages of the experience. One of the prerequisite conditions for learning is that the learner be in a state of preparedness, alertness, and attentiveness. Receptivity to directions and concepts can be translated into effective behaviors. Various techniques have been suggested to direct the learner's attention (if it is not being demonstrated under his or her own powers) to a task. Whatever strategy is selected, once the learner is attentive, the acquisition of specified behaviors is more apt to be demonstrated.

Anticipatory Timing Behavior

In those tasks that are externally paced and in which events can occur suddenly, anticipation helps to prepare a person for the expected or the unexpected. Planning ahead and being prepared to respond in a certain way will aid in the reaction to events that occur with regularity and with a high degree of predictability. When one realizes that an event will occur, but without certainty in terms of its form, location, or timing, readiness to make an adaptable and accommodating response facilitates performance.

Assuming the possible predictability of an event, how does one obtain the pattern information from memory in order to use it effectively, as a rule prior to the occurrence of the event? How can a person judge the time interval before an event in order to anticipate correctly? Somehow, cues are self-generated for the purpose of time keeping. As R. W. Christina (1976) points out, one mechanism that has been hypothesized to function in the accurate anticipatory timing of movement responses is proprioception. Two viewpoints have been proposed in regard to proprioception used for this purpose: (1) the proprioceptive trace hypothesis, and (2) the proprioceptive input hypothesis.

The trace hypothesis accounts for perceptual anticipation, with the assumption that movements can become associated with traces of proprioceptive stimuli aftereffects. With practice, appropriate aftereffects can elicit the next correct movement sequence. In the input hypothesis, it is proposed "that incoming proprioceptive feedback, produced by movement made during the interval preceding the occurrence of a stimulus event, is the means by which a subject judges the duration of the interval so as to accurately anticipate the stimulus occurrence" (Christina, 1976, p. 193). The evidence is not sufficient to rule in favor of either hypothesis. However, evidence does exist (e.g., Schmidt & Christina, 1969) that proprioceptive feedback is a mediator in tasks requiring precise anticipation and timing.

Level of Expectation (Aspiration)

Before performing a skill, we typically formulate hypotheses about our chance for success. Success itself is relative and depends on what a person will accept as achievement. Some people would consider themselves successful if they shot golf in the 90s; other people attain this feeling when they score in the 70s. The setting of a goal is termed *the level of expectation* or *aspiration*. Past experiences in similar situations, resulting in successes or failures, affect this level. In turn, the immediate level for a given task may very well determine its outcome, as will be noted a little later in this section of the chapter.

An individual's level of expectation for a given task reflects an optimism, or lack of it, when faced with the challenge. It denotes an attitude toward the task. It also indicates a level of reality—whether the goal is consistent with prior success, actual present achievement, and ability. Finally, it can be used to improve performance. If the level of aspiration is set high enough, it acts as an incentive, something for which to strive. For each person there may be different levels of aspiration, depending on interpretation of the term. It may mean a level hoped for, expected, or minimally accepted. In other words, a level of aspiration can indicate the discrepancy between previous performance and expected performance; between wished for and previous performance; or between personally acceptable and previous performance.

It is unrealistic for a person to have a large discrepancy between estimated performance and actual performance. When the performance level is far below the expectation level, the result is consistent personal failure. When the situation is reversed, there is a better chance of success. Therefore, it can be seen that success and failure can be determined in relation to the level of aspiration. An unhealthy situation occurs when too many successes or failures are experienced by an individual; hence, it is desirable to have an approximate relationship between hoped-for and actual performance.

Persons try harder in a competitive situation when there is a greater degree of uncertainty concerning goal attainment. With regard to achievement motivation, J. W. Atkinson (1957) feels that individuals in whom the achievement motive toward success is relatively strong should and will prefer intermediate-risk tasks, whereas those in whom the motive to avoid failure is relatively strong should and will avoid intermediate-risk tasks. These findings have been contradicted by Edwin Locke (1966), who has observed a linear relationship between intentions and actual level of performance. The higher level of intended achievement resulted in high levels of performance.

Locke and Bryan (1966) verified these findings. These experimenters utilized the Complex Coordination Apparatus, where red and green lights are arranged to form an H on the display. The subject has to move controls (foot pedals and a hand stick) to match lights with those lights that are illuminated. When the match is right, a new stimulus pattern occurs, and this continues until all thirteen patterns have been presented in sequence. It was found that performance goals in-

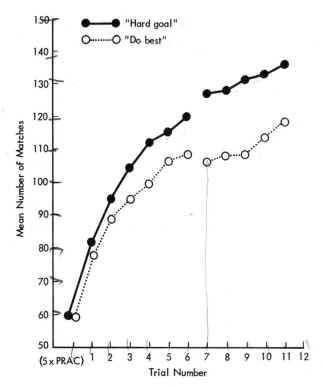

FIGURE 11-3. A comparison of two groups in performance on a complex motor task. One group had high standards and a difficult goal, the other group was merely told, "Do your best." The Hard Goal group was significantly better than the Do-Best group. (*From Locke, E. A., & Bryan, J. F. Cognitive aspects of psychomotor performance: The effects of performance goals on level of performance.* Journal of Applied Psychology, *1966, 50, 286–291.*) Copyright 1966 by the American Psychological Association. Reprinted by permission.

fluence the level of performance. The subjects with specific but high goals did better on the task than those who were told just to do their best (see Figure 11-3). Implications from these results can be applied to teaching methods. Having students set precise high, but attainable, goals may be more effective as a learning technique than haphazard methods of motivation.

Certain statements concerning level of aspiration appear to be warranted. Research findings by Irvin Child and John Whiting (1949) and other investigators are in agreement:

1. Success lends to a raising of the aspirational level.
2. The greater the success, the greater the probability of a rise in the level.
3. Level of performance is influenced more by success than failure, and the effect of success is more predictably stable (more upward shifts are noted after success than downward shifts after failure).

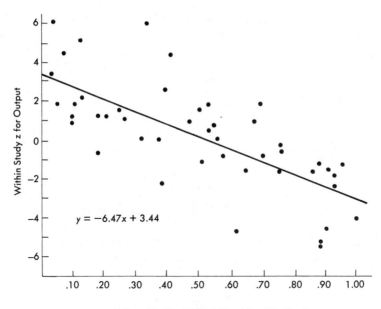

Mean Empirical Probability of Reaching Goal

FIGURE 11-4. Goal difficulty is a function of the number of trials in which subjects attempting to achieve a particular goal actually perform higher than it. Performance level is expressed in terms of the Within Study z-score (converted raw score to a standard score) for performance for a particular goal. Each point represents a particular group (a particular goal) in a particular study; it indicates the probability of the subjects in that group reaching their mean output in relation to the other goal groups in that study. (*From Locke, E. A. Toward a theory of task motivation and incentives.* Organizational Behavior and Human Performance, *1968, 3, 157–189.*)

Locke (1968) has summarized the literature on consciously set goals and intentions and task performance. It can be observed in Figure 11-4 that the harder the goal, the higher the level of performance. These data reflect the combined results of twelve investigations on the topic. It is true that subjects with very hard goals reached them less often than subjects with very easy goals. Yet, the hard-goal subjects consistently outperformed the easy-goal subjects.

In theorizing about events that lead from a particular situation to action, Locke proposes the following schema (1968, p. 184):

> Environmental   Goal-setting
> Event → Cognition → Evaluation → Intention → Performance
> (e.g., incentive)

Goals and intentions can be manipulated by others. Instructions are commonly deployed and will be especially valuable if the performer accepts them and, indeed, possesses the capabilities demanded for the task. Providing evaluations (e.g., knowledge of the results of performance) or competition may suggest specific standards to the performer. The benefit of these conditions is contingent on the desire of the person to use performance knowledge to compete against his or her own score or the score of others. Various rewards and incentives (money, praise, and so on) may motivate a person generally to perform better, but much depands on the value to one of such rewards.

To conclude, expectation levels continually change with repeated experience with a task and will be dissimilar from task to task. The skill level of the learner, as well as a desire to improve, as demonstrated by high but attainable goals, describes important considerations in the learning process. However, high expectations in and of themselves do not necessarily lead to better performances. Some learners deliberately set expectations that are unrealistically high for themselves so that they can fail with pride. Others set expectations so low that failure is minimized, and performance changes are slight, if at all.

We should also remember the self-prophecy concept. If we think of failing (low expectation level), the probability for failure is indeed increased. Thoughts on performing well lead to improved probabilities of performing well.

Situational Generalizability (Transfer Possibilities)

Learners often panic in learning situations when they think they are learning something completely new to them. Yet, much present learning is associated in some way with previously experienced encounters. When learners understand this relationship, confidence and progress should be improved. More complex movements can be simplified to show relationships to previously experienced movements. Initial task learning should be facilitated when the past is bridged to the present, when learning experiences are related to each other.

Intended Outcomes

Practice conditions should be directed toward the intended outcomes of practice. This point can be emphasized easily as we consider the differences between self-paced and externally paced skills. In a self-paced activity, such as golf, response consistency in one movement is the desired outcome, and the golf swing can be practiced repeatedly to achieve what some might call an automated state. Externally paced activities, such as handball, require adaptive behaviors to changing situational contexts. Variable behaviors need to be practiced, to improve transfer potential from practice conditions to test conditions.

Experimentally, H. D. McCracken and G. E. Stelmach's (1977) data support this idea. Two groups of subjects were formed to learn a task that involved moving a slide along a trackway between two points as near to 200 milliseconds as they could. One group was trained with four different lengths to move the slide. The other group trained on only one movement length. After three hundred trials, both groups were tested on a new movement length for transfer effects. The variable group transferred more effectively to the new task. This finding suggests that practice variability increases transfer potential to a previously nontrained motor response that is related to some previous experience. Schmidt (1977) emphasizes that these and other data support schema theory (see Chapter 5) and the role of variability in practice.

Warm-up

So far we have discussed psychological means of readying oneself for a learning activity. But there are physical ways as well, and the most familiar one is the warm-up. Athletes often prepare themselves for an athletic contest by engaging in certain preevent rituals. Such activities are usually referred to as a *warm-up*. They take the form of exercises or specific practice in the skills that will be required in the contest. Presumably, they prepare and prime the athlete for competition, enhancing performance. We are all familiar with the concept of *warm-up* in this sense, for there are many practical examples of such activities.

A number of research articles have been published in this area, and a review and analysis lead to surprising conclusions. The data by no means confirm the value of a variety of warm-up procedures in promoting more effective performance; nor, for that matter, is there a clear indication that athletic injuries are minimized by this practice, although common sense suggests that this would occur. However, it does seem that, if warm-up activities are to be of benefit, they should be directly related to the tasks that ultimately will be performed. Furthermore, they will probably be more beneficial for those skills that require a great deal of precision, timing, and coordination—especially if there has been a long layoff from the last experience to the present event. It is extremely difficult to ascertain where the psychological aspects of these procedures outweigh the ''real'' benefits. In other words, if we think something will help our performance, performance output may be increased accordingly.

Warm-up has been of interest not only to those involved in practical situations, but also to scholars concerned with psychological learning and retention theory. The term *warm-up decrement (WUD)* was coined many years ago to describe poorer performance after a layoff, even when it was as little as a few minutes. It might be thought of as a loss in retention as a function of time, and therefore *warm-up* practice trials may have value in

1. activating or elevating, or reducing or diminishing, the level of arousal necessary for task performance.
2. reducing the performance decrement that occurs over time.
3. increasing the set of the performer, which therefore reinstates the appropriate task adjustments and readiness to perform (postural set).
4. promoting any combination of the above.

Warming up does not always increase the arousal state of the individual, for in some instances it decreases it and allows the performer to settle down to the task at hand. Furthermore, WUD is associated with a disappearing decrement in performance dependent upon the need to warm up for the task. It has been found to be different from the process of forgetting; the decrement is not simply due to a loss of habit strength. Interestingly enough, certain intervening or preliminary tasks do not always reduce WUD. Many of them increase WUD, in contrast to a rest period. The learning versus performance effects of WUD are confusing, but there is no evidence that it is a condition of practice that affects learning, only that it affects performance.

Schmidt (1972) presents an excellent overview of the literature and theory related to WUD. The more interested reader will want to examine his material and the relevant sources that bear on the different points of view offered to explain WUD.

ORIENTING THE LEARNER TO THE GOAL

Communication is the means by which the instructor conveys the intent of the outcome of the learning experience. Even if no instructor is involved, the learner observes others, reads descriptions, views films, or analyzes illustrations in order to "get the idea." Various techniques, from instructor-directed to self-managed, have and always will be used; however, their relative effectiveness is extremely hard to ascertain.

The quality of the informational medium, the nature of the task, and the characteristics of each learner interact in a complex manner. And so, we must conclude that mode-of-information presentation can be more or less effective in transmitting the idea of what is to be accomplished in the motor learning situation. With more complex motor tasks, it does appear that observation of a live or filmed model should be very beneficial. In many cases, combinations of modes of information presentation may be useful.

Communicative techniques between the instructor and learner that can impose situational modifications fall into three categories: visual, verbal, and kinesthetic. The visual area encompasses modeling procedures whereby the student "gets the picture" of what is expected in performance standards. Direct observation of expert performances, films, illustrations, and television are some possibilities. The visual area also involves cueing or prompting techniques prior to or during performance, as well as knowledge of results information (e.g., videotape) to be used as a performance regulatory mechanism. The verbal area includes words or sounds that might help the learner to understand task expectations, to cue, or to supplement feedback information about performance. The kinesthetic area includes physically guiding or manipulating the learner in difficult learning periods.

Verbal and Written Directions

It is most uncommon to discover an organized instructional or training situation where verbal directions, comments, and cues are not issued by the instructor prior to, during, and following the practice of motor tasks. Words or sounds may

(1) continually provide *instruction* and direction, (2) only be used as a *pretraining* technique for transfer value, (3) *prompt* the learner to respond to certain cues at specified moments, and (4) offer *correctional* advice following performance.

The latter two examples are found to some degree in many training programs, although the larger the ratio of learners to instructor the less likely prompting and advice will be present. Without much in the way of research to refer to, circumstantial evidence would seem to encourage verbal cueing techniques in initial learning phases of a skill until internal timing capabilities can take over. Continuous tasks in which events occur requiring immediate responses could be verbally prompted for a while. One particular act that contains a series of movements could be cued at various positioning points. As with any form of assistance, however, such information should be removed from the learning situation as soon as possible, before the person becomes too dependent on it.

Instructions for task learning can be presented orally or in written form. We cannot assume, however, that all types of instruction will be equally beneficial to all learners. Consideration must be given to

1. the ability of the learner to understand and relate verbal concepts to appropriate movement patterns. (Special problems exist with learners who are young, are less intelligent, or have communication handicaps because of being raised in a different society, culture, or ethnic tradition.)
2. the meaningfulness of the directions (quality, length, and detail) as related to the particular task and learner.
3. the need for simplicity, explicitness, or detailed directions.

Some individuals respond better to certain modes of instruction than others. Drawing from this premise, certain people will learn faster than others from verbal comments on their motor activity. At the present time, beginners as a group seem to benefit less than advanced learners from extensively detailed verbal directions. Young children have less patience than mature learners and need to be immersed in activity. With respect to the nature of the task, a more complex task would probably require greater explanation and more teacher direction, but not necessarily at the beginning states of learning.

In fact, when verbal training is offered only at the beginning of a task, it is the simple task, not the complex one, that will be most positively affected. William Battig (1956) found verbal pretraining to facilitate performance on simpler motor tasks, but no benefit was shown from this pretraining on complex tasks. The subjects were tested on a finger-positioning apparatus. The degree of transfer from verbal pretraining decreased as a function of the complexity of the task. The more important actual performance is, as with difficult motor tasks, the less value verbal pertraining seems to have.

Verbal or written instructions can at best partially take the place of actual motor skill practice, especially on skills containing a certain degree of challenge. Descriptions and ideas are one thing, experience another. The body must actively respond, and the kinesthetic receptors must be stimulated, if a high skill level is to be reached on complex motor tasks. Furthermore, verbal training that precedes motor training must be of sufficient quantity and quality in order to transfer favorably to motor skill performance. This condition becomes evident in reviewing K. E. Baker and R. C. Wylie's (1950) experiment. Before practicing on a discrimination problem involving matching the correct switch to a light stimulus, their subjects received verbal training and memorized by the oral paired-associates method. The group that had eight verbal training trials did not show evidence of significant transfer to motor performance when time or the number of errors were used as measurements. However, the twenty-four verbal training trials brought about a significant transfer effect on both these measurements.

Actually, the things we usually learn are mediated by words. In the beginning stage of learning a task, the individual has to learn instructions to know how and what to perform. Not only are there words from external sources (instructors, teachers, and coaches), but there are words spoken to oneself during activity. This latter theoretical state has been termed *verbal mediation*. It also has been referred to as conceptualization, ideation, thought processing, or implicit speech.

The ability, then, to succeed in motor performance may very well be related to a certain extent to being able to apply external and internal words to motor acts. Sometimes, however, the verbal mediation process interferes with skilled performance. Consider, for example, the performer who thinks too much and gets confused, resulting in a delayed reaction to a given situation. This is especially detrimental in an athletic contest, where players have to respond immediately to unpredictable openings and occurrences.

Instruction can be informational, directional, and motivational. Its effectiveness, therefore, depends on the timeliness, nature, and appropriateness for the learner. Instruction and cueing might occur more often where emphasis is on the demonstration of one correct behavior. Where the process of problem solving and discovery is desired, external verbal cues and aids should be minimal. Another consideration is the total time allotted to practice: more specifically, how much of it should be actual practice and how much should be devoted to instructions. Participants in most movement-oriented tasks are anxious to participate actively. They need sufficient direction, but not to the point where their channel capacity is overloaded and the information is dysfunctional; nor do they need direction to the extent that they become bored and frustrated. An optimal relationship between instruction and actual practice probably exists for any task.

Evidently, an optimal amount of instruction was received in the study reported by Dorothy Davies (1945). Figure 11-5 illustrates the effects of tuition and a lack of it on learning archery skills. One group received regular and systematic instruction; the other had none. An interesting sidelight in this study was that brighter students, as measured by a mental ability test, tended to profit more from the instruction than the duller students. If the task to be learned is relatively easy, instructional material and cues will help the individual in the beginning to proceed on the right track. With practice on this type of task, further assistance from an outsider is usually unnecessary. Later in practice, the guidance will probably be

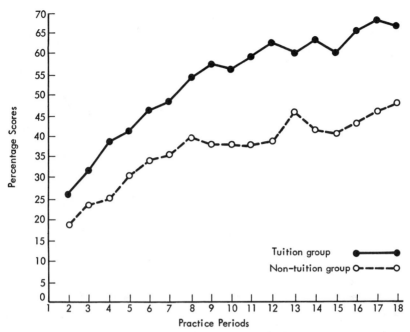

FIGURE 11-5. Daily average percentage scores for two archery groups. (*From Davies, D. R. The effect of tuition upon the process of learning a complex skill.* Journal of Educational Psychology, *1945, 36, 352–365.*)

remedial. Specific detail about the task and learner performance will lead to the highest proficiency levels.

Further support for instruction in learning a motor task is offered by Parker and Fleishman (1961). Detailed task analysis helped a group of college ROTC students to perform a tracking task better than two other groups (see Figure 11-6). Group I received no formal training other than a brief description of the task, performance expectations, and an achievement score after each trial. Group II was administered what Parker and Fleishman termed a "commonsense" program, including explanation, guidance, assistance, and critiques of performance. Group III's training program was similar to that of group II, except that special ability demands of the task were used to develop special training procedures. Figure 11-6 illustrates that group III's overall performance was superior to that of group II, whose performance was higher than that of group I.

Learning Strategies and Rules

The typical motor skills training and instructional program is conceived of as teaching specific responses to designated cues. There is a heavy emphasis on repetition of movements. If only the practiced task is of concern, this procedure is quite acceptable. Yet, it does appear that the long-term expectations of many pro-

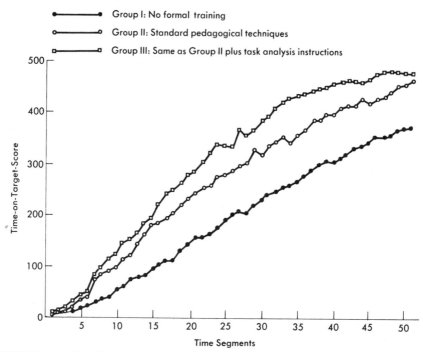

FIGURE 11-6. The effects of instruction in the training process. (*From Parker, J. F., & Fleishman, E. A. Use of analytical information concerning task requirements to increase the effectiveness of skill training.* Journal of Applied Psychology, *1961, 45, 295–302.*) Copyright 1961 by the American Psychological Association. Reprinted by permission.

grams is to enhance the probability of the learner being able to apply knowledge and skills to new and related situational demands. It is hoped that positive transfer will occur.

Cognitive involvement, in the form of learning how to formulate rules and strategies for achievement in presently introduced tasks, will no doubt enhance the probability of successfully meeting future-related activities. The learner should realize how to analyze tasks. Prerequisite and component tasks build up to complex task mastery. Identifying subtasks, learning how to do them, and eventually putting them all together constitutes a strong portion of ultiment achievement. Identifying errors, or debugging the system, is equally important. Remedial adjustments appropriately follow error identification.

New learnings must continually be related to old learnings. Establishing task relationships instead of learning subtasks in isolation will probably be an effective training medium for long-range goals, especially when it appears that the learner is expected to confront a variety of situations, not merely the situational tasks practiced in formal programs. Time limitations in training programs often do not permit experiences in the variety of tasks and situations related to the overall activity. Therefore, the importance of selecting the most appropriate learning tasks, seeing the relationships of tasks to each other, applying correct strategies

MOTOR LEARNING AND HUMAN PERFORMANCE

and rules to newly introduced ones, and rectifying errors through problem solving are apparent.

Discovery training is effective for transfer and retention if adequate time is allotted for such processes to be developed and if students are successful. Success in discovery is related to effectiveness in discovery; e.g., the more rules discovered, the more value in the training (Anthony, 1973). This should be translated into a better capability to use the problem-solving approach in new situations (Worthen, 1968).

One objective of any program should be the development of self-learning techniques (Singer & Gerson, 1977). Extra cue and instructor dependency must be minimized. The availability of an external source of instruction and assistance becomes limited once a training program is terminated. The individual may be "on his or her own" or will receive limited guidance. The learner who can analyze tasks and self-prescribe procedures to enable their accomplishment is obviously at an advantage. The role of cognition—e.g., analysis, judgment, and problem solving—should never be underestimated in the learning of motor tasks. Beyond mere recognition of this fact, practice sessions should reflect and encourage the cognitive aspects of motor performance.

R. C. Craig (1969), after reviewing the cognitive literature dealing with discovery and guided learning, concluded, "What is most probable, of course, is that no simple strategy will be generally useful under all conditions" (p. 505). True, no one strategy is consistently appropriate. But conditions and parameters can be specified, and a strategy suggested for a particular purpose (Singer, 1977(b)).

1. If the purpose of learning a skill is only for the highest level of performance in that skill, then a guided and prompted method of learning would seem to be the appropriate choice, especially if there is concern for economy in training time.
2. If the purpose of the learning situation is to lead to the application of what has been learned for transfer to other related skills and situations, it would seem that some form of discovery, problem-solving, or trial-and-error strategy should be employed.
3. Self-paced, closed-loop tasks should be learned primarily through a guided technique, for response consistency.
4. Externally paced, open-loop tasks should be learned primarily through a discovery technique for familiarity with diverse situations and response adaptions.
5. The later learning situation should be considered and might determine what the prior learning method should be; e.g., if subsequent experiences are going to occur with the availability of prompts and guides, then it would seem to be a waste of time and effort to conduct the initial learning experience under a discovery method (p. 493).

R. E. Mayer (1975) has addressed the problem of learning outcomes as influenced by what is received by the learner as well as the personal established set. He contrasts learning with an emphasis on algorithms versus learning ideas and concepts as to their effects on learning outcomes. The first, he concludes, results in a narrow assimilative set; the latter, in a broad assimilative set. Mayer summarizes by saying:

When the goal of learning is meaningful understanding which allows transformation to novel situations and which supports further learning, the conditions of learning are reception of the to-be-learned material, existence of memory of related previous experiences, and activation of a broad assimilative set that will be integrated with incoming information. When the goal of instruction is quick, efficient performance on specific tasks, less attention may be paid to the latter two conditions; i.e., a narrow assimilative set based on only a small portion of previous experience is required (p. 539).

The conclusions could very well fit the benefits of discovery learning, problem solving (resulting in a broad assimilative set), and guided or prompted learning (resulting in a narrow assimilative set).

Principles of the Mechanics of Performance

From a theoretical point of view, it makes good sense to believe that if the individual understands the mechanics of the intended movement, performance will be facilitated. The ability to succeed in complex gross motor skills depends many times on both the intended and unintentional application of biomechanical principles. Intentional usage of scientifically accepted movement patterns would seem to be a desirable objective. It is reasoned that the knowledge of mechanical principles will assist the learner in gaining quicker insight into the mastery of a given gross motor task.

Unfortunately, this "sound reasoning" of transfer has not been upheld consistently enough in experiments to gain acceptance. On the positive side, Dorothy Mohr and Mildred Barrett (1962) found that the learning of mechanical principles applied to physical activity is an effective teaching technique. In their study, an experimental group of women learned mechanical principles associated with swim strokes; the other group did not. After fourteen weeks, the experimental group improved more than the control in all strokes except the elementary backstroke.

One of the earliest studies on the problem of principle transference to a motor task was reported by C. H. Judd (1908). The task involved was dart tossing at an underwater target. One group of subjects received no theoretical training, they just practiced, whereas the other group was given theoretical explanations and practice. Although no difference between groups was found with twelve inches of water, a change to four inches favored the experimental group. These subjects evidently applied the theory in this transfer situation.

In an interesting study of principle transference to an assembly task, G. O. Johnson (1963) compared the performances of experimental and control groups of normal and retarded children. With eighteen subjects in each of the four groups, the two experimental groups were instructed in a principle to facilitate performance on the motor task. Both experimental groups were superior to both control groups when they were timed on their rate of assembling ten items. The unusual finding was that the performance of the retarded experimental group was significantly better than that of the intellectually normal control group.

Some sample experiments obtaining contrary results follow. Frances Colville (1957) attempted to determine the effect of knowledge of three mechanical principles on the learning of a number of motor skills. Two groups of college women were formed, one of which spent their time learning and practicing the skills, the other learning mechanical principles, as well as having skill practice. The results indicated that (1) instruction in mechanical principles did not promote the initial learning of a motor skill any more than did an equal amount of time spent in skill practice; and (2) such knowledge did not facilitate subsequent learning, as evidenced when similar or more complicated skills were learned, even though the same principles were applicable.

Reasons for the contradictory evidence in this area may very well be partially explained by methodological differences in experiments. Consider the following major discrepancy in two groups of studies utilizing a specialized training consideration:

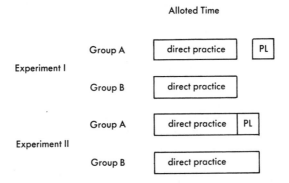

The allotment of time to direct practice in relation to principle learning (PL) differs between groups in both hypothetical experiments. Both groups receive the same amount of direct practice on a task in experiment I, with one group receiving additional time for the learning of performance principles. In Experiment II, PL is built into the direct practice time; consequently, that group will have less time in direct practice than the other group. All things being equal, we might expect the design in Experiment I to favor Group A and the design in Experiment II to favor Group B or neither group.

Wayne Sorenson (1966), an industrial researcher, was interested in the importance of a knowledge of mechanical principles for on-the-job success of mechanical repairmen. He reported that the better mechanics appeared to rely on mechanical intuition and experience rather than on formally taught principles (e.g., physics, mechanics, electricity, etc.)

Perhaps the safest statement, in view of the conflicting research results, is that some individuals will prosper more, some less, when time is devoted to learning mechanical principles, especially when this time is taken away from potential physical participation. On the more optimistic side, there is some evidence to suggest that the mastery of learning principles aids in the future discovery of new principles and, in turn, the solution of new problems (as was pointed out before).

The context in which the principles are learned and insight into how they are to be applied in given situations are conditions to be considered if such knowledge is to be beneficial to motor performance. Unfortunately, educators sometimes talk too much and expect learners to know many things in which they have no interest.

Demonstrations: The Modeling Effect

Visual guidance can be provided for the learner by allowing him or her to view expert performance. This is a procedure usually advocated and practiced by many instructors. It allows the beginner to visualize what the desired act looks like and supplies the ideal goal to which to strive. Merely watching others perform a task one does not expect to have to do results in more effective learning, a phenomenon termed incidental learning.

We know that children learn by modeling the behaviors of adults and other children. Adults can learn by observing the behaviors of other adults. As a learning condition, observation-demonstration techniques on the part of the teacher inform the students about what is expected of them. They provide the learners with direction, an understanding of where they are headed. There is a variety of ways of directing the goals of the learner, including the use of written material, illustrations, verbal descriptions, and observation of live or filmed "expert" performances.

Certainly one of the most fundamental and often used means by which new behaviors are acquired is through modeling procedures. The teacher or student who can perform an act with proficiency can be modeled by the learners. Indeed, Albert Bandura (1969), a leading exponent of principles of behavior modification, especially through modeling procedures, indicates that

> One can acquire intricate response patterns merely by observing the performances of appropriate models; emotional responses can be conditioned observationally by witnessing affective reactions of others undergoing painful or pleasurable experiences; fearful and avoidant behavior can be extinguished vicariously through observation of modeled approach behavior toward feared objects without any adverse consequences accruing to the performer; inhibitions can be induced by witnessing the behavior of others being punished; and, finally, the expression of well-learned responses can be enhanced and socially regulated through the actions of influential models (p. 118).

Bandura indicates that if the modeling behavior is to be effective, the observer must be attentive to the modeled behavior, must retain the modeled sequence of behavior, must have the physical capacity to perform the task, must have the motivation to model, and must be reinforced for modeling. In addition, the model must exhibit adequate cues for the observer (Landers, 1975).

There are many ways in which modeling, or observational learning, occurs. Donna Landers (1978) has made some practical suggestions on the basis of research findings. She suggests that (1) the learner must attend to the demonstration; (2) the model must convey the optimal information that can be processed by the learner; (3) repeated demonstrations are better than a single one, especially within the context of the observer's practice; and (4) filmed demonstrations can be equally effective as live demonstrations.

The use of the demonstration approach according to describable criteria will enhance the ease with which students learn skills. Landers shows her optimism for the approach, as compared to other means of orienting the learner, when she writes "It is a well-accepted fact that more information can be conveyed through a simple demonstration than through any other form of communication" (p. 65).

Visual Aids

Visual aids, in various forms, have been experimentally investigated for their worth in promoting motor learning. They are represented by motion pictures, videotape recorders, force-time graphs, loopfilms, pictured representation of the task, slides, and the use of the tachistoscope. These aids demonstrate ideal performance (at regular or slow speeds), performance of the subject on the skill, or simple images or pictures of the task. The value of visual aids lies in their ability to allow the learner to view the task and critically analyze the task setting and body movements involved in skilled movements. This function is especially important if we stop to consider that the problem in executing most motor skills rests not with demands placed on the motor capacity of an individual, but rather in overcoming stimulus complexity in order to react with appropriate movements to particular environmental cues.

Whereas films are primarily used for modeling purposes—that is, providing an image of reference performance standards and helping to shape learner goals (see Figure 11-7)—videotape can be used to provide a feedback function. The individual can immediately see how he or she performed. This information can be valuable in modifying the next attempt. These aids have much intuitive appeal, but surprisingly, research evidence gives only a slightly favorable indication of their value in motor learning situations. Many studies have indicated no differences in final skill proficiency between groups trained with or without these visual aids.

One may propose several reasons for the finding of no significant performance differences among groups compared in a visual aid study. Films may be of poor quality, so the learner may not be able to integrate the visual information into effective movement patterns. Criterion performance tests between groups may not be too reliable or valid. In other words, they may not be refined enough to distinguish among subjects. The duration of the film exposure or the training session itself might be of insufficient magnitude. In a few studies a problem may be associated with the use of inappropriate statistical techniques. Also, insufficient control of contaminating extraneous variables may lead to performance scores so variable that it is virtually impossible to detect performance differences between groups of subjects.

These and other attacks on the research methodology in which visual aids have been used allow us to suspect the data when the value of these aids is not

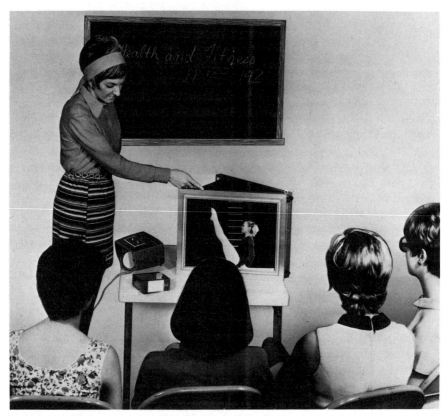

FIGURE 11-7. The super 8 projector can be used to display model performance, thereby helping the learner to understand the goals of the activity. (*With permission from the Athletic Institute; 200 Castlewood Drive, North Palm Beach, Florida 33408.*)

demonstrated. Nevertheless, popular thinking and a reasonable rationale exist for the use of films as instructional aids.

The value of the videotape recorder (instant replay) is its capability to provide immediate visual feedback to the performer. Although research data are inconclusive in confirming its role in instruction, it is widely used in sports activities for performers of all skill levels. Especially in individual sports, such as golf, skiing, bowling, tennis, and swimming, the videotape (VTR) is becoming more a part of instructional programs. We need not be reminded of how often instant replays in football, basketball, baseball, and hockey matches are shown on television. This viewing encourages a more penetrating analysis of strategy and performance. It also gives the television viewer who has missed the action (perhaps because of an urgent trip to the kitchen for a beer) another opportunity.

Typical of the studies that did not find any benefits from the use of videotape to develop sports skills are those reported by Kenneth Penman (1969) and I. S. H.

MOTOR LEARNING AND HUMAN PERFORMANCE

Gasson (1967). Penman used beginning tumbling skills and Gasson dealt with badminton skills. In both studies, two groups were formed. Only the experimental group received videotape exposure in the training procedures. No differences in performance between the groups were noted on tests administered at the end of the duration of the studies.

Patricia Del Rey (1971) made an attempt to refine the experimental methodology with regard to performance criterion variables and task classification as related to training with or without VTR. A lunging task was made open or closed (see Chapter 1), and the dependent variables were latency, accuracy, and form. Performance in the open modification of the task for form and latency was apparently aided with videotape. VTR with the closed version of the task led to higher accuracy scores. More detailed and sophisticated investigations such as this one are needed in order to begin to answer questions regarding the value of VTR. Parameters need to be defined clearly, variables controlled, and performance measures made valid and appropriate for the circumstance.

Preliminary training on visual representations of complex motor acts may help to provide greater insight into these acts. At least in one experiment, arranged by Gagné and Foster (1949), this was found to be the case. Subjects, before learning a discrimination reaction time task, were presented with a paper-and-pencil representation of the task. This procedure was found to be effective in skill acquisition, and more premotor practice resulted in better motor performance.

Constrained Approaches

In order to encourage a greater awareness of the physical movement involved in certain acts, a *manual manipulation* technique is employed by teachers on occasion. The student relaxes while being guided through a series of movement patterns. Presumably, this practice serves to activate the receptors associated with the task and provides the learner with the desired movement experience. The manual guidance procedure is based on common sense and not on conclusive affirmative experimental findings when used with the normal learners. Katherine Ludgate (1924) did find that manual assistance while learning a stylus maze helped subjects to learn faster. The manual manipulation approach is used quite often and effectively with children who have learning disabilities, however.

In recent years, and with the use of movement reproduction tasks, a research paradigm has been developed to compare the effectiveness of voluntary (preselected) or constrained movements on the potential to reproduce these movements. Voluntary movements are made by subjects to a particular location or for some distance. Blindfolded subjects are requested to reproduce the movements. Constrained subjects have their movements terminated by an imposed stop. Most researchers (e.g., Gerson, 1978; Stelmach, et al., 1975) have reported the superiority of preselected movements over constrained movements in location or distance cue reproduction.

This type of experiment contains some analogous features to the instructional situation in which learners are encouraged to make their own movements to achieve a goal or are constrained in some way. Although the experimental subjects are not manipulated to a particular goal, they are not provided with freedom of movement, either.

When the preselection effect has been observed, it has been attributed to better cue-encoding and retrieval strategies associated with that movement. Kelso (1977) has suggested that the underlying contributing process is more specifically, a corollary discharge or a superior motor image. If indeed such processes are more active in voluntary and noncontrolled movement, these arguments could be somewhat persuasive against the use of any type of teacher-controlled situations, such as in the use of manual manipulation.

In fact, Kelso has designed two experiments in which active and passive (manually manipulated) movements were analyzed for accuracy in positioning under conditions in which the intended goal was preselected, subject defined vs. constrained, or experimenter defined. In both experiments, active preselection led to better performance than any other combination. Kelso (1977) has speculated that "the information provided by selection and execution processes results in a more accurate representation of the movement" (p. 43).

Image Formation

The ultimate goal of any of these communication approaches is to help the learner internalize a goal image. Once an internalized representation of the movement has been made, probabilities increase for the actual production of that movement. It is difficult to say which technique or combination of techniques is more effective. Two major considerations in this regard are (1) the feeling of the approach—the quality of the means of communication; and (2) the nature of the learner.

In the latter case, an individual's preference in being introduced to the skill to be learned may vary. Differences in cognitive styles and preferences may suggest that some students favor one approach, others another approach. We might consider the use of combinations. Redundancy of information may be complementary in aiding the learner to understand how a complex act is to be performed. In other circumstances, it may lead to information overload and confusion. As we can see, there is no easy answer here.

To repeat, the primary consideration is to use what appears to be the best way to introduce a skill to learners in general and those with unique preferences, with the intent of helping them to create images of the act. The strength of the image does not ensure acceptable performance, but it is a step in the right direction. In the verbal learning literature, it is well established that individuals who mediate or construe an image better, who develop better visual representations or "mental pictures," are superior in learning to those who are less effective in this endeavor (Klatzky, 1975). How to induce better visual representation of movement expectations is certainly a challenge to instructional designers.

CONSIDERING LEARNER ABILITIES

When designing instruction, it is imperative to consider abilities that are related for success in particular motor skills. Task analysis suggests those abilities that would appear to be most important at different stages of learning. Instruction could be planned to accommodate this relationship, to emphasize the use of abilities at the appropriate time. We will analyze the research in this area, as well as the possibility of predicting ultimate achievement on the basis of initial performance levels of the learner.

Abilities and Learning

Many abilities contribute potentially to the successful execution of a complex task. These abilities change in relative importance to task proficiency. Some are associated with achievement at later stages.

The results of an investigation by Fleishman and Hempel (1954) provided early dramatic support of the idea of a change in factor (ability) patterns with practice. The Complex Coordination Test appeared to be more complex (in terms of the number of significantly important factors) in the initial phase of practice and less complex with the continuation of practice. Through the factor-analysis method, higher loadings on more factors were obtained at the beginning of practice. There were seven significant factors in the initial stages of practice but only three in the final stages. Beside this discovery, different abilities were found to be important during the various stages of practice.

Fleishman and Hempel conclude that it is quite conceivable that the abilities contributing to individual differences in earlier stages of skill attainment may be quite different from those contributing to more advanced and terminal levels of proficiency. This study lends further warning about the problems in predicting final achievement from early success; those abilities needed for success are called on in varying degrees, depending on the stage in practice. Also, teacher and learner should be aware of the desirability of emphasizing different factors as practice progresses. Figure 11-8 illustrates the data.

Fleishman (1957) offered further evidence in another investigation. He studied the abilities involved in early and late stages of proficiency. His subjects were tested on six motor tasks, including the Complex Coordination Test, pursuit rotor, and discrimination RT test. As training continued, he found a changing of abilities that contributed to proficiency on these tasks: the level of importance of some abilities increased, others decreased. For instance, the discrimination reaction time task measures spatial orientation and response orientation early in practice, but speed of arm movement is important later. Fleishman attempted to isolate and predict the factors necessary to high levels of skill on these complex motor tasks and found that the factors were not the same as those abilities emphasized early in training.

Although it seems reasonable to accept the hypothesis of different ability

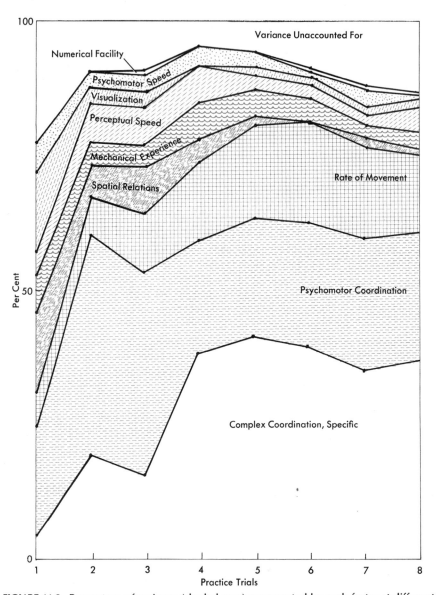

Numerical Facility

Psychomotor Speed

Visualization

Perceptual Speed

Mechanical Experience

Spatial Relations

Variance Unaccounted For

Rate of Movement

Psychomotor Coordination

Complex Coordination, Specific

Per Cent

100

50

0

1   2   3   4   5   6   7   8

Practice Trials

FIGURE 11-8. Percentage of variance (shaded area) represented by each factor at different stages of practice on the Complex Coordination Test. (*From Fleishman, E. A., & Hempel, W. E. Changes in factor structure of a complex psychomotor test as a function of practice.* Psychometrika, *1954, 19, 239–252.*)

requirements at different stages of practice and to acknowledge the implications for practice settings, almost all studies citing such findings have been executed with laboratory apparatus tests as the criterion learning tasks. In one of the few investigations in which a real-life skill was analyzed, an exception was reported.

Dickinson (1969) attempted to determine the relationship between kinesthetic sensitivity and distance perception with the task of aiming a shuttlecock with a badminton racket. Male and female subjects were novices in the sport of badminton. The aiming task consisted of striking the shuttlecock over the net into target areas, with each subject given five sets of twenty attempts.

Overall, kinesthetic sensitivity correlated 0.49 with aiming performance, whereas distance perception only correlated 0.20 against this criterion. Furthermore, a contradiction was indicated, as compared to other research data, in that kinesthetic sensitivity correlated at a constant level with both initial learning and postlearning performances. This would refute the concept of the change in relative importance of abilities at different stages of practice. Keeping these findings in mind, let us review data from Fleishman and Rich (1963) which are indeed supportive of the hypotheses originally presented.

In contrast to Dickinson's findings, it appears that visual cues are extremely important in the acquisition of skill in psychomotor tasks. Kinesthetic cues evidently are of secondary importance in these tasks, whereas in more complex motor skills, e.g., athletic skills, they seem to be more meaningful. Much depends on how and when abilities are measured during skill acquisition. It is possible that

TABLE 11-1 Performance During Ten Trials on the Two-Hand Coordination Apparatus With Respect to Obtained Correlations Between Kinesthetic Sensitivity and the Criterion and Spatial-Visual Orientation and the Criterion. [As practice continues, the correlations of Two-Hand Coordination (THC) decrease with the spatial ability measure and increase with the kinesthetic sensitivity measure.]

THC Trial	Orientation Aerial	Kinesthetic Sensitivity
1	.36**	.03
2	.28*	.19
3	.22*	.15
4	.19	.15
5	.08	.10
6	.07	.09
7	.09	.23*
8	−.05	.28*
9	−.02	.38**
10	.01	.40**

*$p < .05$, one-tailed.
**$p < .01$, one-tailed.

(From Fleishman, E. A., & Rich. S. Role of kinesthetic and spatial-visual abilities in perceptual-motor learning. *Journal of Experimental Psychology*, 1963, **66**, 6–11.)

different cues are more important at various learning stages, for there is strong evidence that exteroceptive (visual) feedback and spatial orientation ability are related to early achievement in perceptual motor tasks. Later, at higher skill levels, proprioceptive (kinesthetic) feedback and kinesthetic sensitivity ability are most important. Table 11-1 includes the data obtained by Fleishman and Rich and indicates the relationships between these two abilities in performance on a motor task.

Forty subjects received ten blocks of four trials each on the Two-Hand Coordination Test (THC). They were pretested on a kinesthetic sensitivity measure, the ability to judge the difference between lifted gram weights, and a spatial-visual measure, through the United States Air Force Aerial Orientation Test. An analysis of the data showed the spatial measure to be significantly related to performance on the Two-Hand Coordination Test only early in practice. The kinesthetic measure was significantly related to THC performance only late in learning. It does appear that individual differences in sensitivity to kinesthetic cues may determine *higher* skill levels. Other interesting results of this study point to the fact that both kinesthetic sensitivity and spatial orientation are necessary to overall performance on the task, as together they correlated 0.73 with the THC.

Assuming the validity of these suggestive findings and the possible universality of the generalizations, the implications are strong for instructional guidelines. Task analysis and ability demands should be undertaken. Specific cueing and practice on those abilities related to practice at a certain stage of skill mastery would be most beneficial.

Prediction of Success

Owing to the unique nature of individuals and their previous experiences, performers will vary in their rate of skill acquisition. With any given task, some people appear to be faster learners than others. The value of practice, especially over an extended length of time, is obviously more beneficial to those learners who demonstrate initial difficulty with the problem at hand. The necessity of practice of long enough duration has been established from research findings pointing to the fact that one cannot usually predict ultimate achievement from initial progress. Researchers such as M. Welch (1963) and E. Trussell (1965) have demonstrated that sufficient data, collected over approximately one-half the intended duration of the practice days, are needed to reflect final levels of attainment adequately.

However, there are evidently at least some tasks in which later proficiency is directly related to early proficiency, Jack Adams' data (1957), acquired from performance on a discrimination RT test, nicely illustrate this point (see Figure 11-9). Ten groups of subjects were stratified into deciles on the basis of their first trial scores. They were given 160 trials, and although some individuals shifted status with practice, the groups maintained their relative positions throughout the experiment. The reader can observe the unique asymptote for each group, and it does not appear as if the groups would converge toward a common level. All groups

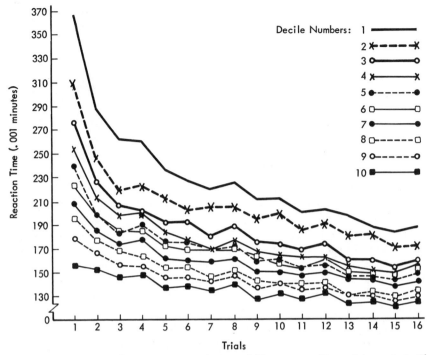

FIGURE 11-9. Mean performance curves for ten ability groups. (*From Adams, J. A. The relationship between certain measures of ability and the acquisition of a psychomotor criterion response. Journal of General Psychology, 1957, 56, 121–134.*) Reprinted by permission.

showed improvement with practice, and as might be expected, more improvement was noted with the low-ability subjects than the high-ability subjects.

There is good reason to believe, though, that the relationship between initial and final status is quite low on more complex tasks. Variations in the performance levels between learners throughout practice may be the result of the relative ease of gaining insight into the problem; the transferability of related learned skills to the task at hand, which might be of special advantage in the early stages of practice; and various psychological, physiological, intellectual, and emotional adjustments that have to be made. Whatever the cause, initial individual differences will exist, as will later differences; apparently, however, they are not related in complex motor skill learning. Hence, practice will benefit individuals in dissimilar ways and they will show varying rates of progress.

To summarize, then, predictions of final accomplishments from initial scores become more difficult to make if (1) the task is complex, (2) ample practice time for all is allotted, and (3) the group is relatively homogeneous to start with.

A final point should be made with regard to increasing the precision of predicting ultimate task proficiency. As J. R. Hinrichs (1970) emphasizes, on the basis of his data, prediction is enhanced when the reference or predictor tasks closely resemble the task itself. Also, predictor tasks are more successful when they attempt to be specifically related to later stages of performance than when they are measures of more generalizable abilities.

CONSIDERING SITUATIONAL ARRANGEMENTS

Intelligent modifications in the environment imposed by external sources can hasten insights into learning tasks, enrich the learning experience, and ultimately produce quality performance. But in some cases, the environment is "given"; that is, the individual will have to cope with existing elements in the real performance situation. Therefore, the instructor must carefully analyze the situation to determine the desirability of rearranging it, of adding certain cues and aids for the benefit of the learners.

Learning situations can be natural, untampered with by external sources. Or they can be modified for the convenience of the learner, considering the complexity of task, the skill level of the learner, and the apparent need to simplify the display to expedite the learning process.

Manipulations can lead to more effective cueing devices, enriched and additional information, and augmented feedback. Modifications for such purposes can be introduced in timely ways but also must be removed gradually as performance improves and is to be demonstrated in the natural display setting. The design of an environment compatible with task demands and learner capabilities is a real challenge. Displays can emphasize visual, tactile and proprioceptive, or auditory sensory modalities. Abilities related to these modalities may change in import as skill is acquired. The availability of aids and cues is another consideration. Any modification of situations should be made in accordance with scientific evidence and the unique dimensions of the learning tasks.

Most complex activities deserve special consideration, as simpler tasks can probably be handled without any modifications in the learning environment. Let us turn to possible ways in which a tampered-with display can be of benefit to the learner.

Performance changes, for better or worse, may be due to training techniques or changes in equipment. It should be pointed out that when equipment is changed, training procedures should be modified accordingly. Aided learning situations and special training devices are used to simplify tasks and to encourage early and frequent correct responses, with the hope that such practice will effectively transfer to "real" tasks and "real" situations. So, in essence, whenever we refer to manipulated practice tasks and situations, *transfer of training* is at the heart of the matter.

Furthermore, situational aiding and special training equipment hold implications for *mediated* instruction. In the traditional sense, the term *media* refers to the use of hardware and software equipment to aid the learning process. What with the current educational emphasis on technology and individualized instruction, a variety of media have been experimented with and implemented in instructional settings. Although certain contrived conditions may be expected to assist the average learner in skill acquisition, a respect for individual differences suggests a sensitivity to altering and adjusting instructional settings in particular cases.

Richard Burns (1971) writes that "individualized instruction is a system which tailor-makes learning in terms of learner needs and characteristics" (p. 55). After learner diagnosis, a variety of instructional materials, aids, and experiences should be made available. Training should be as individualized as possible. Technological advancements, systems designs, and behavioral change principles help to facilitate the rate and quality of skill acquisition for groups and individuals.

Every instructor differs not only in respect to communication and planning, but also in methods of implementing and enriching particular experiences. Although some adhere to routinized training procedures, others look to supplemental materials and methods. Traditional procedures can be altered in many ways. Some of these approaches to motor learning are presented here, along with an evaluation of their worth, as indicated by research.

Visual Cues

Of all the ways to alter the learning situation, visual cues and changes in structures that produce visual stimuli helpful to the learner are most often experimented with in training situations. Visually aided environments can be especially beneficial to the learner at early stages of learning. It is interesting to analyze just how visual stimuli facilitate or hamper the learning process. With a newly introduced skill, the learner typically attends to too many stimuli and has to learn to be more selective. This will occur with experience and expert guidance. Too many visual stimuli can be distracting, and, in fact, perhaps very few are necessary in the beginning stages of learning certain skills. Gymnastics, diving, and stunts on a trampoline necessitate vision for equilibrium, balance, and safety. And, of course, for many activities, vision provides a knowledge of results (e.g., basketball shooting, archery, tennis, and the like), enabling the individual to know when to compensate for inaccurate responses.

Artificial visual cues are used either as an initial learning technique, to be disregarded later, or as a continual performance aid. Although research is scattered and inconclusive on the value of these techniques, it does appear that many of them are of value in fulfilling certain objectives. Theoretically analyzing the problem, specific and precise visual cues are easier to attend to than general and vague ones. Furthermore, nearer cues should be easier to aim for than those more removed. However, not all learners will benefit equally from identical cues in the same task.

The necessity of visual cues for adequate motor performance can be analyzed in investigations in which reduced visual cues are presented to subjects. In many continuous tasks, it is assumed that a complete visual tracking of objects is important for successful responses. "Keep your eye on the ball" is an often-used expression associated with various sports activities. But is it really imperative that the ball (or some other object) be viewed until the moment of contact?

Some research evidence indicates that as visual cues diminish, so does performance. The ability to catch objects is directly related to the availability of light and visual cues; there is a need for sufficient time to preview the object prior to responding. Yet, there are exceptions. A ball need not be watched all the time for effective catching if flight patterns can be accurately predicted. In other words, the length of time ball flight patterns need to be scanned depends on the information available to the person in the situation and his skill level. H. T. A. Whiting, E. B. Gill, and J. M. Stephenson (1970) have shown a longer time period for scanning is necessary when the task is relatively unpredictable. With variable flight patterns and a dark room in which a ball to be caught was illuminated for 0.10, 0.15, 0.20, 0.25, 0.30, or 0.40 of a second from moment of release to the point of being caught, longer viewing time led to more successful catching (see Figure 11-10).

Whiting et al. discuss the possible existence of a perceptual moment, a critical time period for viewing an object in order that the central processing mechanism can function properly. A perceptual moment may be in the range of 0.05 to 0.20 of a second. Once the visual stimulation is initiated there must be an adjusted period of time to assimilate this conformation. The concept of a perceptual moment was not supported by the data in the Whiting et al. experiment, although subject variability and other rationales were offered for the lack of supportive data. It does seem that sufficient time for the registration of the stimulus and use of it for making acceptable responses is part of the process associated with skilled performance.

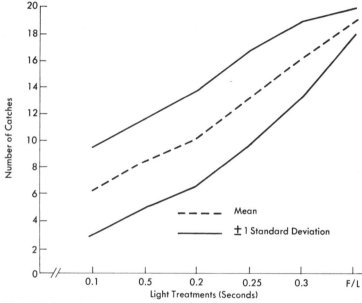

FIGURE 11-10. Performance curve—combined means of all subjects. (From Whiting, H. T. A., Gill, E. B., & Stephenson, J. M. Critical time intervals for taking in flight information in a ball-catching task. Ergonomics, 1970, 13, 265–272.)

Norman Gordon (1969) has contrasted two types of events in terms of their functional properties when visual displays are altered. There are those, called input, that provide the subject with cues about where and when to react. Others are derived from the subject's own activities and inappropriate responses and are termed feedback. It is hoped that any cues added to a situation will assist the learner in making appropriate adjustments and adaptations. Gordon's research efforts have led him to question the advisability of aiding displays. Presumably, such a circumstance facilitates early performance in a task but in the process encourages display dependency and discourages the learner from paying attention to feedback.

Early achievement in aided displays may occur because task demands are diminished and learner strategies are altered. The individual may learn less from such a situation, for less is demanded of him. Gordon has reported high performances in the early phase of practice in aided displays but poorer performance when attempting a transfer, or reference, task. We might speculate that if aided displays are constructed, be they visual, verbal, or tactual, their potential value must be considered in the context of (1) the length of time in use, (2) the nature of the cues, (3) the type of task being learned, and (4) the ultimate (true) task to be mastered.

Aided displays will probably benefit tasks that are response oriented, such as self-paced tasks, in which fixed patterns of responses are desirable. Externally paced tasks make the kinds of demands on the performer that suggest the value of learning (1) from one's mistakes, (2) a variety of acceptable responses, and (3) effective coping strategies. To be of any value, supplementary situational cues should be temporary and deployed where task complexity suggests a need for learner guidance. An effective training procedure might be the gradual elimination of additional cues as the learner gains enough skill to cope with the true task. The usual practice reflects a dichotomy of procedures: from an aided display situation to an unaided situation. A gradual reduction in assistance and guidance could be preferable in those cases where cues are deemed appropriate in only the early learning stages.

Verbal Cues and Guidance

Verbal cues and prompts prior to and during performance can help learners to be ready, to anticipate, and, consequently, to perform the right movements at the right time. Guidance during and after an act can provide reinforcement as well as important information to the learner.

The heavily guided or directed approach to learning has been supported by such learning theorists as Skinner, Gagné, and Ausubel. This method places stringent controls on the learner through the use of commands, prompts, or cues. There is little opportunity for the learner to explore and to learn alternatives through error-correction procedures. Skinner (1968) advocates a form of instruction that prompts the student's every response, while leading him or her in a logical way to achieve desired behaviors. He describes discovery learning, in contrast, as a sink-or-swim method that evades the school's responsibility for instruction.

Gagné (1977) has presented one of the most comprehensive models for guided learning. He suggests that prerequisites for learning are connected in a hierarchical fashion. Learning is described as a step-by-step approach through the hierarchy of prerequisites until the desired learning behavior is obtained. Effective instruction, to Gagné, requires the careful sequencing of learning tasks. He suggests that learners should be prompted or guided in their attempts to respond correctly, and he minimizes the need for independent discovery.

Macrae and Holding (1965a, 1965b, 1966) have indicated that guided learning procedures can be highly successful. In their first study, restriction techniques and forced-response techniques of guided learning were compared by using a manual positioning task. Both techniques were found to be successful, with the technique that most resembled the task form being the most effective. The effectiveness of guided learning across trials was investigated in the second study. It was found that the effect of guidance on learning diminished as the number of learning trials increased. For example, n number of trials of guidance is not n times as effective as one guided trial. Different instructional strategies were used in the third study and applied to the learning of a serial tracking task with a reversed relationship between the stimulus lights and control lever. It was generalized from the results of this study that guidance becomes more effective as task complexity is increased.

Guided learning usually leads to more rapid and better learning on the primary task of interest than does nonguided learning. This is true with various experimental procedural differences, dependent measures, and tasks.

It would appear that in those activities that require fixed responses to fixed cues, heavily guided learning is the most expedient method to achieve goals. If costs and availability of prompting and feedback sources are of consequence, these must be weighed against the potential payoffs.

However, for those activities that ultimately make varied and often unpredictable demands on the person, sufficient experience in an assortment of environments is in order. Practice may be guided at first to some degree for the learning of basic skills. But strategies and tactics need to be developed, as well, to troubleshoot, adapt, and adjust to the potential future demand characteristics of the situations in which the activity will be performed.

Background Music

Although music may serve as a stimulator, motivator, or relaxer, its exact benefit in motor skill attainment and motor performance has not been determined. Melodies are piped into department stores and supermarkets in order to relax the customers and encourage purchases. Investigations have been made to determine the effects of music in general, as well as different tempos and tones, on sales. The dentist uses music to relax patients and take their minds off the impending pain. Industrial workers have been observed to increase their output when motivated by music.

Because of the success tuneful and rhythmic melodies have had in these areas, it might be hypothesized that similar benefits would be derived in motor learning and performance. It is felt that lively tempos encourage more vigorous practice efforts; slow, soft music relaxes individuals who are tense; and highly rhythmic music facilitates rhythmic and coordinated movements desired in an act. Some coaches and physical educators provide music as a background for the performance of skills, with these objectives in mind. The difficulty in controlling experimental variables in determining the effects of auditory aids—hence the lack of research—permits little more than speculation. In one of the few studies done on this problem, Evelyn Dillon (1952) reported that her intermediate swimming students taught with music in the background achieved better form and speed than those swimmers taught without music.

Operating under the assumption that more repetitive, monotonous tasks would perhaps be more positively affected by the sound of music, R. I. Newman, D. L. Hunt, and F. Rhodes (1966) undertook a project to test this hypothesis. Workers in a skateboard factory heard four different types of music played on four different days; no music was played on the fifth day. No difference in output was noted as a result of the type of music played or even the absence of music. It appears that, in routine tasks, tasks in which the performers do not need a high degree of skill, music is not beneficial to performance.

However, other studies in vigilance situations have indicated that background music improved performance. Industrial productivity has been shown to improve with background music in a variety of settings (Fox, 1971). Although it is true that research is virtually nonexistent on the effects of music on learning, performance increments may be due to increased arousal and attention. Job performance and background music are currently being analyzed under the concepts of arousal theory.

From another perspective, M. H. Anshel and D. Marisi (1978) examined the effects on synchronized and asynchronized movement to music on the ability to endure a physical task. Endurance was significantly better when movement was rhythmically coordinated with a musical stimulus. The mere presence of background music (asynchronized) did not yield any better results than a no-music condition.

In summarizing the research on the effects of music in vigilance, athletic, and industrial situations, Luigi Lucaccini and Leonard Kreit (1972) have noted a lack of methodological precision as well as an atheoretical framework. The evidence, according to them, is too weak to support traditional and commonly held beliefs regarding the efficacy of music, although a few studies report findings that do support these beliefs.

Kinesthetic Aids

The role of the kinesthetic sense in skilled movement has been discussed throughout the book. A sensitivity to and awareness of body and limb position in movement is naturally an asset to performance. Can the kinesthetic sense be sharpened by means other than traditional practice?

An obvious method of attempting to accentuate this sense is to perform the desired act with the eyes closed (if it is a type of activity that can be practiced this way). Concentration is then on the movement rather than its outcome, such as projectile accuracy or distance. Environmental stimuli above and beyond response cues no longer serve as distractions. The eyes-closed or blindfold method of early skill learning has yet to be truly tested as a means of promoting learning. Therefore, at the present time, we must speculate on its effectiveness.

Let us examine the golf swing as an example. One of the greatest problems for the beginning golfer is concentrating on the swing and feeling the movement rather than worrying about how far the ball has gone. A few instructors believe in blindfolding beginners so that this kinesthetic sense can be developed. Indeed, in one study, it was reported early in this century that blindfolded golfers demonstrated greater ultimate proficiency than golfers taught using full vision.

A possible manner of activating and sensitizing more proprioceptors is through the use of heavier or lighter equipment. A measurement of transfer of skill would indicate the more desirable procedure. Projectiles of varying weights were thrown by subjects in a study conducted by G. H. Egstrom, G. A. Logan, and E. L. Wallis (1960). Greater transfer was demonstrated from a light ball to a heavy ball then vice versa, and the authors reasoned that the lighter ball sharpened the sensitivity of the receptors and the feedback mechanism. Edward Wright's (1966) experiment neither supported nor rejected this conclusion. Young children were tested on physical fitness items and sports skills, and although his results were inconclusive, Wright's evidence suggests that, if the children have limited strength, motor skills may be learned faster with light-weight equipment.

Does a player develop a greater sensitivity in shooting a basketball when practicing with a larger ball? Weighed baseball bats for warm-up swings and weighted shoes for practice runs and jumps are intended to increase speed, power, and velocity during competition. In these and related cases, the research is much too scanty to analyze the effectiveness of such practice procedures. Franklin Lindeburg and Jack Hewitt (1965) had varsity and junior varsity basketball players practice with a regulation basketball and a larger basketball. On the tests administered, no difference between groups was observed on foul shots, dribbling ability, and lay-up speed skill. There was a significant difference on the passing test in favor of the group that had practiced with the smaller basketball. Unfortunately, the authors did not test the transference of accuracy from the larger to the regulation basketball.

In motor performance, when too much kinesthetic information is withheld, the consequences can be severe. The relative importance of kinesthetic, verbal, visual, and auditory cues in the learning situation will depend on the skill in question and the skill level of the individual. All may provide necessary feedback messages, although in many cases they overlap, and duplication occurs between the senses and their information. The skilled performer is one who has learned to respond to specific cues and emphasize particular sensory modes at different stages of proficient movement patterns.

Comparison of Cues

One way of comparing cue effectiveness is in relation to the stage of practice of the learner. As indicated earlier in this book, we might expect a person to be more dependent on display characteristics (e.g., visual input) early in training. This is especially true with nonpredictable events. Later, reliance might be on proprioceptive (response-produced) cues. This rationale is derived from the numerous studies in which Edwin Fleishman has been involved, demonstrating the differential relationship of visual and kinesthetic abilities to task achievement at different stages of practice. Furthermore, an individual might be expected to be more cue dependent at first and more selective at proficient levels of performance.

Assuming that cognition (understanding the nature of the task, learning strategies for task mastery, etc.) plays an important role early in practice (see the Fitts–Posner model in Chapter 5), an investigation by D. Trumbo, L. Ulrich, and M. E. Noble (1965) attempted to clarify the role of verbal and cognitive processes in skill acquisition. Examined were the three levels of effects of display cues and verbal pretraining on tracking performance. It was expected and found that display-specific cues and verbal pretraining were more beneficial early rather than late in learning. However, this effect was not additive. Apparently, the redundancy and irrelevancy of some cues suggest the careful planning of aiding displays. Because retention performance was not affected by display specificity or pretraining, it remains for other research to reveal the function of other cue combinations in retention in contrast to initial stages of practice.

Nevertheless, redundant information can facilitate performance in certain cases, such as with reaction times. Irving Biederman and Stephen Checkosky (1970) present data that demonstrate this fact. The value of redundant and relevant cues, according to these researchers, lies in a person's ability to process information in a parallel fashion rather than serially. If serial processing occurs, reaction time should be longer. If parallel processing occurs, it should be shorter. The later occurrence with reaction data is explained theoretically in the framework of the parallel information-processing model.

Of course, in many situations, sensory information may be discrepant and therefore pose a conflict for the learner. If an information conflict exists between two sense modalities, how is it resolved? In an investigation by Pick, Warren, and Hay (1969) discrepancies between proprioception and audition, vision and audition, and vision and proprioception were analyzed. The researchers felt that different processes are involved when conflicting information must be resolved. With regard to sense modality comparisons, it was reported that proprioceptive and auditory judgments were biased strongly by vision, as were auditory judgments by proprioception. The dominance of vision over touch had been convincingly expressed earlier by Irvin Rock and Charles Harris (1967). They concluded that "the sense of touch does not educate vision; vision is totally dominant over touch" (p. 96). When conflicting information is present in a situation, visual information determines perception. This point of view has been altered to some degree by Kelso, Cook, Olson, and Epstein (1975); they have demonstrated that the allocation of attention determines situational dominance. In turn, the dominance influences the locus of adaptation. In other words, if attention is directed deliberately to proprioception among alternative sensory information available, then the proprioceptive modality will dominate.

Further implications of the dominance of vision over proprioception are noted by Timothy Jordan (1972), who suggests that the demands of visual input for attention by the brain tend to result in longer response times. In his study, blindfolded practice on a fencing skill, the disengage and lunge, which was simulated with a blade–deflection laboratory apparatus, resulted in faster response times than sighted practice. If, as Jordan states, "one is inclined to rely upon what one sees, rather than upon what one feels," he may also be correct in his observation that "in skills where kinesthetic or proprioceptive cues are considered important, this can perhaps be a hindrance to the learning of an optimal response" (pp. 536–537). Jordan's study supports the notion that blindfold practice in the early stages of skill learning, where *events are predictable,* produces best results as far as speed in movement is concerned. When visual cues are restricted, attention is more easily focused on proprioceptive feedback, resulting in faster responses. Further evidence is suggested in favor of the idea that the visual and kinesthetic systems may involve different information–processing mechanisms. In a recent review of the literature, M. I. Posner, M. J. Nissen, and R. Klein (1976) have stated that

> It seems that when information about an event is available from vision *and* from audition or proprioception, and when the visual information is adequate for responding, attention is directed to vision. In conditions in which vision does not provide adequate information, visual bias no longer prevails (p. 168).

Cues may be presented during a performance (coincident) or terminal to it (noncoincident). Laurence Karlin and Rudolph Mortimer (1963) demonstrated the superiority of a noncoincident verbal cue over coincident visual and auditory cues during training and for a transfer task. Visual and auditory augmented information stressed the acceptable target area of the task. A score at the end of each trial provided to the subject was the verbal cue. It could be, as the researchers suggest, that augmenting cues affect transfer best when they function as incentives and in defining performance standards.

When cues are tampered with and removed in a systematic way, results are somewhat predictable. Standard practice is usually most effective, and the relative import of sensory cues can be deduced from the following example reports. In a comprehensive experiment, William Battig (1954) compared performances on the Complex Coordination Test when kinesthetic, verbal, and visual cues were eliminated or emphasized. Six groups of subjects were formed, with all subjects tested on the same task on the first and tenth trials but practiced under different conditions during the middle eight sessions. Standard practice afforded the best results. The sequence of cue importance, after standard practice, was determined to benefit skill acquisition as follows: visual, kinesthetic, and, lastly, verbal.

Similar results were obtained in Dennis Holding's (1959) investigation. On a tracking task, normally trained and guided groups demonstrated little dissimilarity at the early stages of learning. The guidance group subjects gripped the control knobs, got the feel of the machine tracking itself, and finally had to track themselves. Also noted in the study was that full guidance was better than visual guidance; visual guidance was superior to kinesthetic guidance; and kinesthetic guidance did not yield a significant improvement in performance. The great success of the guidance group indicates the necessary occurrence of correct responses. Holding argues that knowledge of results is not necessary to learning, but the correct movements are, although KR is a means of correcting a response. Knowledge of results is synonymous with error feedback (to many psychologists), but there is no error to feed back if the performance is perfect.

For many tasks, conventional practice is not only sufficient but, from the evidence, often more beneficial than singling out and emphasizing either visual, verbal, or kinesthetic cues. As a final reminder, probably the best advice is to consider the nature of each task and to emphasize equally all sensory cues if the task so demands. Specific cue emphasis should be offered in such cases when one has to react to complex stimuli, execute a complex motor act, or compensate for a weakness in performance.

Training and Simulation Devices

For various reasons, industrialists, military personnel, and educators have turned to artificial equipment and devices for assistance in facilitating the learning of motor skills. The term *artificial* as used here simply implies that those devices are made especially for training purposes, to simulate to a certain extent the actual performance conditions or, perhaps, to prepare the individual for the actual task via audiovisual or tactile and kinesthetic cues. Technically speaking, we could distinguish these aids by categorizing them as trainers or simulators, although the dichotomy is not always obvious.

A trainer is some aid used to promote the learning of a task in the early stages. It could be a film, pictures, or a specially constructed piece of equipment. A simulator, on the other hand, is usually a device that more nearly approximates task conditions. It is realistic and provides the performer with concentrated practice when he is at that point of developing a high level of proficiency.

Certain tasks permit more favorable usage and, indeed, require more frequent usage of these devices if learning efficiency is the desired objective. Consider, for instance, industrial, military, and automobile tasks. The cost of training personnel, as well as the inconvenience of activating complex machinery, helped to inspire the development of simulators and trainers. Also, there is an element of danger in some tasks, such as piloting a plane. Finally, it is not practical to train a large number of people on tasks that require extreme proficiency on expensive equipment. Because of these factors, various types of aids are used instead of direct practice for the learning of complex motor skills.

Although fake cockpits and automobile controls have been devised for simulating practice flying a plane or driving a car, most athletic skills do not require the use of such costly and complex equipment. The best practice is afforded by on-the-job tasks or game situations. This is not always practical or possible, although it is certainly more reasonable to expect in educational situations than on military installations or in highly technical industrial work. But, even in education today, where teachers are faced with a greater ratio of students than ever before, training devices have certain advantages over traditional teaching procedures.

These aids allow students to practice skills that otherwise might be impossible to learn under the equipment and facility limitations faced by many institutions. Thanks to the initiative of some physical educators, golf can be taught with a certain degree of effectiveness in the gymnasium with the use of plastic or taped balls. These balls do not travel far and are safer than regulation golf balls. The absence of a golf course does not inhibit the teaching of basic golf skills. Similar measures are currently being made so that such sports as water skiing and snow skiing can be simulated in the pool and gymnasium. Although these efforts are probably not as effective as learning the skills under actual conditions, they serve a definite purpose.

The aids also alleviate the situation where there are too many students for the instructor to provide individual instruction. Devices that approximate real conditions provide each learner with an immediate knowledge of results and of performance status and facilitate learning progress. Ball-throwing machines in tennis and baseball are examples of pieces of apparatus that allow individuals to concentrate on hitting techniques. The machine for tennis tosses a ball at a preset speed and a server apparatus suspends a ball and releases it when contact is made. Both devices eliminate many of the complex factors involved in stroking and serving (see Figures 11-11 and 11-12). W. H. Solley and S. Borders (1965) were interested in determining the effectiveness of the Ball-Boy machine in promoting the learning of tennis skills. After comparing control and experimental groups, the investigators concluded that the machine was very effective. They recommended the procedure of using traditional teaching methods first, followed by the use of the Ball-Boy machine.

The Golf-O-Tron is an example of a type of equipment invented to facilitate golf learning. This highly technical instrument simulates a golf course and playing conditions and allows the individual to play a round of golf without stepping on a course. Edward Chui (1965) taught two groups to use the 7 iron and then tested transfer skill to the 4 iron. One group was instructed in the conventional method and the other learned with the assistance of the Golf-O-Tron. Positive transfer effects were noted for both groups, with no significant differences between them.

Flotation devices are used in swimming to overcome fear of the water, as well as to facilitate the learning of swimming skills. Although there has been very little scientific experimental work to analyze the effectiveness of flotation devices

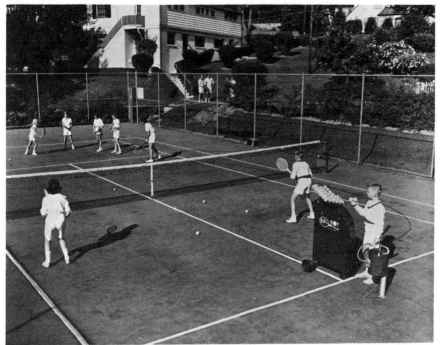

FIGURE 11-11. The automatic tennis ball machine in operation. (*With permission from the Ball-Boy Company, Inc.; 26 Milburn St.; Bronxville, N.Y.*)

as teaching devices, Richard Kaye (1965) has reported that a group of college beginning swimmers, using a waist-type flotation device, was able to swim further at the end of his experiment than a group taught without it.

These examples indicate the type of training aids currently being introduced and evaluated in physical education and sport. Audiovisual materials have already been discussed in this chapter; the value of viewing ideal performance or one's self performing should not be minimized. A final point to be considered with the use of trainers and simulators, and certainly not the least, is their value as motivators. Novel and different methods of instruction serve to elevate motivation. The anticipation, excitement, and challenge of learning under novel conditions can very well be reflected by increased performance scores.

Overload Training

A fairly common practice in the sports world is the use of overload training. Weighted shoes or weights on golf clubs or bats may have psychological value (the placebo effect?), but there is no reason why learning or performance should be facilitated. This point has been alluded to earlier in other sections of the book. Overload training will improve physical characteristics that might contribute to increased performance potential.

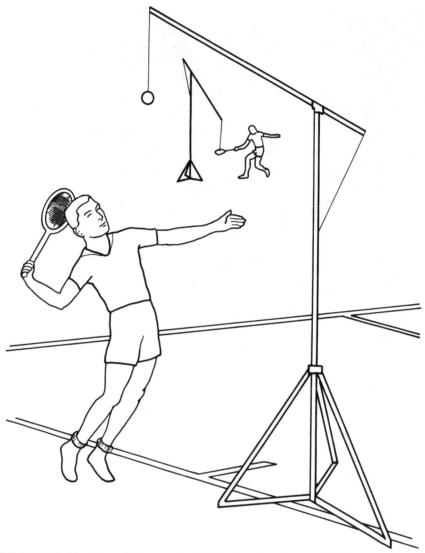

FIGURE 11-12. The Server. This apparatus holds a tennis ball at any height; at contact, the ball is released for a completely normal flight. The Server minimizes some of the complexities of the serve by eliminating the toss. (*With permission from the Ball-Boy Company, Inc.; 26 Milburn St.; Bronxville, N.Y.*)

But the learning of skills is most effective when the learning experiences are such that the same motor units and movement patterns will be activated and trained in the way required under testing conditions. When weighted training occurs, the person has to adjust his or her response timing mechanisms. After it is completed, another readjustment must occur.

SOME PSYCHOLOGICAL ERGOGENIC AIDS

Ergogenic aids have been defined by William Morgan (1972), as "substances and phenomena which elevate performance above normal expectations" (p. xi). This interpretation is broad enough to include many things. A typical understanding of the term *ergogenic aid* is negative, in a sense—that is, work output is enhanced by the intake of illegitimate or immoral substances.

Certain aids, be they changes in environment or substances or strategies directly applied to the human system, may induce an appropriate intermix of physiological and psychological variables, resulting in elevated performance. Unfortunately, in most cases, it is exceptionally hard to determine where such factors combine to produce beneficial results or the psychological component dominates the scene. For instance, many performers will do better *if they think they should.* A preevent steak meal may lead to a greater-than-expected performance in a football game simply because the players think that steak is nutritious and will enhance their athletic capabilities in the contest. Yet, there is little, if any, physiological justification for this.

Classic examples of intake ergogenic aids used in sport are pure oxygen, drugs, vitamins, hormones, special diets, and special beverages. Do these categories of substances benefit performance? There is some supporting evidence for this. For instance, oxygen can be an effective ergogenic aid when used in certain ways and for certain purposes. Oxygen inhalation is effective immediately before an event if the exertion is maximal and the duration is short. It is also effective during strenuous exercise to minimize fatigue effects, but to administer it during activity is usually not practical. Similarly, the stimulating effect of amphetamines (pep pills) on body activity has been documented with some qualifications (Cole, 1970).

Many food fads are overemphasized; their value, if any, must be more psychological than anything else because they are usually not supported by a sound nutritional base. Mineral and vitamin supplements, wheat germ oil, quick energy foods, high-protein diets, and the like, have been discussed by Ellington Darden and Harold Schendel (1972). Conflicts in assumed values and scientific findings are shown. Yet, it is indeed possible that a substance such as wheat germ oil might produce greater work output simply because the athlete thinks that it should.

Other possible ergogenic aids include *placebos,* substances or situations that should not have a beneficial effect on performance but work because one is convinced of their effectiveness. They will be discussed shortly. Hypnosis is an ergogenic procedural variable operating on the human system, and it too will be reviewed subsequently. Either contrived or natural environments can yield ergogenic effects. Warm-up, which has already been discussed, has psychological implications and a possible placebo effect where it relates to performance.

The problems involved in the use of a number of ergogenic aids (e.g., drugs, oxygen) become compounded when considered in a moral framework. Should they be recommended for use even though segments of society oppose them? Should an ergogenic aid with no known "real" value but that operates through its placebo effect in elevating performance outcomes be introduced in training programs? Is this a violation of ethical conduct? These types of questions are beyond the scope of this section of the chapter but deserve the attention of interested and informed parties.

Placebos

Areas such as psychiatry, medicine, and psychology are replete with examples revealing the power of placebos, which have no pharmacological effect. The placebo effect refers to an individual's reaction in a particular situation to some nonindependent variable (e.g., medication) as a function of personal expectations and beliefs interacting with procedures and someone else's expectations. When subjects are convinced of their value, placebos tend to elicit behaviors in an expected and often desirable direction.

Experimentation with drugs has shown that placebos can duplicate both positive and negative effects of active substances. For example, if a patient believes that a pill will reduce pain, such effects will be reported, even though the pill was a placebo. The placebo is administered as if it is the real thing, but it really has no value. H. K. Beecher (1969) indicated that saline solutions used as a pain killer in a battlefield situation when morphine was expected showed 90 per cent the effectiveness of morphine in reducing pain. In a hospital situation, saline solution was 70 per cent as effective as morphine. Thus, changes in feelings or behaviors must be attributed to the psychological properties of the substance.

The value of placebos in motor behavior situations is by and large inferred from research in other fields. Their potential influence on the learning and performance of motor tasks is unclear. In one of the few articles dealing with physical performance and an administered placebo substance, David Pomeranz and Leonard Krasner (1969) reported findings in the expected direction. A placebo salve said to be of proved merit in relieving muscle fatigue was given to subjects who were sustaining a hand grip on a dynamometer. Less decrease in grip strength on a number of trials was found with the application of the salve.

But the placebo situation need not only be limited to substances taken into a person's system. If any treatment effect is potentially analogous to a placebo situation, then other factors can be included here. Warm-up could be the treatment. In certain cases it may very well operate like a placebo. As we mentioned earlier, a person may perform better following warm-up; however, is this change caused by body chemistry or primarily psychological factors? If it is thought that warm-up is an aid to performance, expectations may be fulfilled. The placebo effect arouses a person's expectancy level; it alters attitudes toward the particular circumstance.

Environmental modifications can produce a placebo effect. A popular term associated with this situation is the Hawthorne effect. This term evolved from a series of studies undertaken a number of years ago (Roethlisberger and Dickson, 1939) in an industrial situation in which the workers interpreted changes in their working conditions as favorable to their performance. Beginning in 1927 and continuing for twelve years, the effects of such manipulated factors as office illumination and temperature, wage rate, work-rest periods, and the like on the productivity of six female subjects were examined. Even when usually perceived unfavorable conditions were present, production rate remained the same or increased. The workers may have interpreted such changes as a personal interest in them, thus inspiring greater work output.

Dale Hanson (1967) has shown the influence of the Hawthorne effect on the performance of selected physical activities. To summarize: (1) a group of subjects provided with a placebo after six weeks of no physical practice improved nineteen curls (a popular exercise) from the pretest to the posttest; and (2) a placebo group compared to a control demonstrated better performance in bench-stepping endurance.

Robert Rosenthal has repeatedly warned about the experimenter- and teacher-expectancy effect and its subtle influence on the direction of the outcome of an experiment or student performances in a classroom. Rosenthal (1970) summarized 103 studies on the topic and concluded that, in two-thirds of the research, subjects as well as experimenters gave or obtained responses in the direction of the experimenter's expectancy. Of the studies reviewed, nine dealt with animal learning, ten with human abilities, six with laboratory interviews, and sixty-four with person perception.

In one of the few real-life motor activity studies, John Burnham (1968) divided camper nonswimmers into a "chosen" group and a "nonchosen" group. Fifty per cent of each sex and age group was designated as chosen, that is, a test battery presumably predicted these children psychologically ready to learn to swim. The staff counselors were given the list of names. Based on the criterion of the number of Red Cross beginner swimmer tests passed, the experimenter's bias effect was shown. The chosen group performed significantly better than the controls.

Yet, merely administering placebos or creating placebo environments does not always produce better performance scores. Performers have to be naive and susceptible. Perhaps present motivation needs to be low for the effect to operate. If not, incentives in addition to the normal practice and testing environment might tend to be ineffective. The beneficial psychological effects of a placebo are not ubiquitous across varied tasks and dissimilar situations (e.g., Singer, Llewellyn, & Darden, 1973). Placebo effects are evidently not universal in different tasks and situations. Motor learning situations need to be investigated in more depth before more conclusive statements can be made. For many motor tasks, assuming they are nonrepetitive and reasonably challenging, sufficient performer motivation may be present.

Nonetheless, the placebo effect, the Hawthorne effect, and the experimenter and instructor expectation effect are intriguing areas of study. It is recognized that a person may perform as perceptions lead to expectations. Encouragement has a better probability of elevating performance, discouragement inhibiting it. The more a person wants to believe that performance can be improved by some substance or environment, the more this feeling is apt to be realized.

Hypnosis

There is an increasingly accepted feeling that a hypnotic state can lead to more powerful feats. Some professional baseball players have credited hypnotism with their improved performances, and indeed, there are examples of hypnotists working with professional baseball teams. Yet, in summarizing an abundance of literature, Morgan (1972) concluded that "a review of the experimental literature does not justify the view that performance in the hypnotic or posthypnotic states will necessarily surpass performance in the motivated waking state" (p. 193).

One of the serious confounding problems in the experiments dealing with hypnosis and motor performance is suggestion and actual state. It is not easy to determine a person's hypnotic state following hypnotic treatment. Many procedural contaminants, often resisting desirable control, make it difficult to undertake research on this topic. Similarly, interpretations of findings are equally distressing. Equivocal conclusions, which indicate the difficulty in making practical implications, are found in the literature.

Hypnosis has been studied in athletic events, with the learning of motor tasks, with work, strength, endurance output, reaction time, and the like. Example experiments by J. Arnold (1971) and I. Albert and M. H. Williams (1975) provide little support for hypnosis as a facilitator of learning or endurance. Arnold used a mirror-tracing and a ball-bouncing task to determine whether hypnosis could improve the learning of those tasks. Albert and Williams tested subjects for endurance with a bicycle ergometer. However, Albert and Williams did note that endurance was decreased with a posthypnotic suggestion of fatigue.

Relaxation Programs

Because the adequate performance of complex motor behaviors under stressful conditions requires the person to be in an ideal state of arousal, and because this is a problem for many individuals, it is understandable why many anxiety-reducing programs have become increasingly popular. Actually, the pressures of a highly paced society have caused emotional problems for many people. Programs to reduce anxiety and tension have caught the eye of those who train athletes and military personnel, as well as industrialists, businessmen, professionals, and others.

Regardless of the orientation and the techniques, one of the general purposes of what might be termed relaxation programs is to help people become less tense and anxious and more able to perform adequately. Although proponents endorse each program enthusiastically, limited "hard" data are available regarding the effectiveness of the programs across many kinds of situations and people. Thus, it may be that biofeedback, progressive relaxation, autogenic training, anxiety reduction, and meditative techniques are useful for some individuals in certain instances, but they should not be considered a panacea for all.

In *biofeedback training,* the individual learns to identify indicants of his or her personal emotional state through the use of feedback information from various devices. Training is supposed to help people help themselves to quiet their internal state. The principal response measures, as indicated by Bruno (1977), are (1) the electroencephalogram (EEG), which measures brain waves; (2) the electrocardiogram (EKG), which assesses pulse rate and other circulatory parameters; (3) the electromyogram (EMG), which is an indicator of muscle tension; (4) the galvanic skin response (GSR), which is associated with emotional responses; and (5) skin temperature.

In *meditation,* the idea is to free one's mind of stress by concentrating thought and feeling on inner space. Concentration might be on a particular word or image. A state of complete relaxation is reported by those who gain the ability to meditate, as are increased energies to undertake impending tasks.

In *anxiety reduction programs,* people learn to relax muscle groups. Afterward, the learners internally identify situations that normally arouse anxiety in them and attempt to produce deep relaxation in those situations. In other programs, students are told to focus on those factors that seem to cause heightened anxiety within them. They learn to cope with and to counter them. Irrational anxiety is thereby reduced.

In *progressive relaxation programs,* a particular muscle group is tensed deliberately, then relaxed. This procedure occurs throughout the body. R. M. Nideffer and C. W. Deckner (1970) report a case study with a shot putter that indicates the benefits of a progressive relaxation program on competitive performance.

It should be emphasized that a certain degree of stress facilitates performance and is a normal occurrence prior to a meaningful experience. Obviously, the attempt should be to match each person's temperament with the type of activity to be performed. Where anxiety levels are beyond the desirable range, a particular relaxation program may be helpful in enhancing learning and/or performance.

CHAPTER HIGHLIGHTS

1. A number of considerations were identified with regard to the learner's preparatory state to learn. Obviously, the more the learner is predisposed to learn, the greater the presence of an ideal receptive state, and the increased probability of favorable learning outcomes.

Meaningful goals and intentions are important prerequisites, as are purposes. The meaningfulness of the task, especially as perceived by the learner, serves as a source of motivation. Developmental readiness, the possession of ideal personal qualities to tackle impending responsibilities, must be present to match task demands. Psychological readiness implies the appropriate presence of set and motivation to learn. Emotions must be matched to the task demands, as an ideal emotional level enhances learning and performance.

Motivation for task preference over other alternatives leads to desired prerequisite conditions. Similarly, attention and set must be oriented to situational demands, to focus on key features and the most important and relevant contextual information. Expectation levels must be such that they are reasonably high, specific, and attainable. Because they are based on previous successes and failures, a reasonable amount of previous personal success must be realized to establish expectations.

Transfer of previously learned related skills and information will be more likely to occur when relationships between the past and present are understood. Every effort should be made to communicate similarities to facilitate present learning. Learners should be prepared to practice in the contextual arrangements that more likely resemble testing conditions. Finally, warm-up to refamiliarize learners with the situation is necessary after lay-offs. It helps to reorient the learner to situational demands and accommodating responses.

2. There are many ways to communicate the idea of the nature of the material or the skill to be learned. Various approaches are available: verbal and written directions, visual forms (live models or filmed demonstrations), and, on occasion, the manipulation of passive limbs and body. On occasion, learning rules or strategies, or principles of performance, are taught, with the hope that they will lead to greater insight, understanding, and learning of the content to be introduced. The communication of an act intended to be learned is effective when it stimulates the formation of an internalized image of the to-be-produced act. Obviously, the quality of the instructional approach and the receptivity of the student will have a great deal to do with understanding and performance.

3. Initial learner status is often proposed to be related to later accomplishments. But this is only true in relatively simple tasks, in which achievement can be reached rather quickly. More complex activities require the primary involvement of different abilities at different stages of learning. The learners' use of their developed abilities, individual rates of learning, motives, and other factors taken together help us to realize the hazards in attempting to predict terminal achievement in difficult tasks on the basis of initial performance.

4. Learning situations can be arranged to suit the needs and abilities of the learners. Various cues and aids can modify the environment, to prompt and guide the individual. Visual, verbal, and kinesthetic cues, or aids, have been found to be useful on occasion. They help to simplify learning by reducing information uncertainty and movement complexity. They should be used judiciously and removed as soon as possible, to minimize learner dependency. Trainers, or simulators, resemble the actual testing conditions and permit people to maintain skill or to acquire additional skill. Trainers reduce task complexity, but they should not be depended on for too long.

5. Finally, some kinds of programs have been termed ergogenic, which means that they should benefit impending activity. Actually, some have a reasonable scientific basis, others are bounded to logic, and all are usually controversial as to proposed merit.

In the case of a placebo, its influence on behavior is well-established. An inert substance or contrived situation can affect psychological disposition and behavior, if the person believes in it. The value of hypnosis in motor learning and performance seems to be rather limited, on the basis of current research findings. Relaxation programs, including meditation, biofeedback, progressive relaxation exercises, and anxiety-reduction techniques may also have value; however, much depends on individual receptivity for a particular program, personal problems (e.g., anxiety level), and task and situational demands. The appropriate emotional-motivational level in preparing to learn contributes to a more meaningful learning experience.

References

Adams, J. The relationship between certain measures of ability and the acquisition of a psychomotor criterion response. *Journal of General Psychology,* 1957, *56,* 121–134.

Albert, I., & Williams, M. H. Effects of post-hypnotic suggestions on muscular endurance. *Perceptual and Motor Skills,* 1975, *40,* 131–139.

Anshel, M. H., & Marisi, D. Effect of music and rhythm on physical performance. *Research Quarterly,* 1978, *49,* 109–113.

Anthony, W. S. Learning to discover rules by discovery. *Journal of Educational Psychology,* 1973, *64,* 325–328.

Arnold, J. Effects of hypnosis on the learning of two selected motor skills. *Research Quarterly,* 1971, *42,* 1–6.

Atkinson, J. W. Motivational determinants of risk-taking behavior. *Psychology Review,* 1957, *64,* 359–372.

Ausubel, D. P. *Educational psychology: A cognitive view.* New York: Holt, Rinehart & Winston, 1968.

Baker, K. E., & Wylie, R. C. Transfer of verbal training to a motor task. *Journal of Experimental Psychology,* 1950, *40,* 632–638.

Bandura, A. *Principles of behavior modification.* New York: Holt, Rinehart & Winston, 1969.

Battig, W. F. The effect of kinesthetic, verbal, and visual cues on the acquisition of a lever-positioning skill. *Journal of Experimental Psychology,* 1954, *47,* 371–380.

Battig, W. F. Transfer from verbal pretraining to motor performance as a function of motor task complexity. *Journal of Experimental Psychology,* 1956, *51,* 371–378.

Beecher, H. K. Measurement of subjective responses: Quantitative effects of drugs. In R. Rosenthal & R. Rosnow (Eds.), *Artifact in behavior research.* New York: Academic Press, 1969.

Biederman, I., & Checkosky, S. F. Processing redundant information. *Journal of Experimental Psychology,* 1970, *83,* 486–490.

Bloom, B. J. *Human characteristics and school learning.* New York: McGraw-Hill, 1976.

Bruno, F. J. *Human adjustment and personal growth: Seven pathways.* New York: John Wiley, 1977.

Burnham, J. R. Effect of experimenter's expectancies on children's ability to learn to swim. Unpublished master's thesis, Purdue University, 1968.

Burns, R. Methods for individualizing instruction. *Educational Technology,* 1971, *11,* 55–56.

Child, I. L., & Whiting, J. W. Determinants of level of aspiration: Evidence from everyday life. *Journal of Abnormal Social Psychology,* 1949, *44,* 303–314.

Christina, R. W. Proprioception as a basis of anticipatory timing behavior. In G. E. Stelmach (Ed.), *Motor control: Issues and trends.* New York: Academic Press, 1976.

Chui, E. F. A study of golf-o-tron utilization as a teaching aid in relation to improvement and transfer. *Research Quarterly,* 1965, *36,* 147–152.

Cole, S. O. Experimental effects of amphetamine: Supplementary report. *Perceptual and Motor Skills,* 1970, *31,* 223–332.

Colville, F. H. The learning of motor skills as influenced by knowledge of mechanic principles. *Journal of Educational Psychology*, 1957, *48*, 321–327.

Craig, R. C. Recent research on discovery. *Educational Leadership*, 1969, *26*, 501–505.

Darden, E., & Schendel, H. E. Food fads in athletic training. *Clinical Medicine*, 1972, *79*, 31–34.

Davies, D. R. The effect of tuition upon the process of learning a complex skill. *Journal of Educational Psychology*, 1945, *36*, 352–365.

Davis, R. H., Alexander, L. T., & Yelon, S. L. *Learning systems design*. New York: McGraw-Hill, 1974.

Del Rey, P. The effects of video-tape feedback on form, accuracy, and latency in an open and closed environment. *Journal of Motor Behavior*, 1971, *3*, 281–287.

Dickinson, J. The role of two factors in a gross motor aiming task. *British Journal of Psychology*, 1969, *60*, 465–470.

Dillon, E. K. A study of the use of music as an aid in teaching swimming. *Research Quarterly*, 1952, *23*, 1–8.

Egstrom, G. H., Logan, G. A., & Wallis, E. L. Acquisition of throwing skill involving projectiles of varying weights. *Research Quarterly*, 1960, *31*, 420–425.

Fleishman, E. A. A comparative study of the aptitude patterns in skilled and unskilled psychomotor performers. *Journal of Applied Psychology*, 1957, *41*, 263–272.

Fleishman, E. A., & Hempel, W. E., Jr. Changes in factor structure of a complex psychomotor test as a function of practice. *Psychometrika*, 1954, *19*, 239–252.

Fleishman, E. A., & Rich, S. Role of kinesthetic and spatial-visual abilities in perceptual-motor learning. *Journal of Experimental Psychology*, 1963, *66*, 6–11.

Fox, J. G. Background music and industrial efficiency: A review. *Applied Ergonomics*, 1971, *2*, 70–73.

Gagné, R. M. *Psychological principles in system development*. New York: Holt, Rinehart & Winston, 1966.

Gagné, R. M. *The conditions of learning* (3rd ed.). New York: Holt, Rinehart & Winston, 1977.

Gagné, R. M., & Briggs, L. J. Principles of instructional design. New York: Holt, Rinehart & Winston, 1974.

Gagné, R. M., & Foster, H. Transfer to a motor skill from practice on a pictured representation. *Journal of Experimental Psychology*, 1949, *39*, 342–354.

Gallwey, W. T. *The inner game of tennis*. New York: Random House, 1974.

Gasson, I. S. H. *An experiment to determine the possible advantages of utilizing instant television for university instruction in badminton classes*. Unpublished master's thesis, University of Washington, 1967.

Gerson, R. F. *The influence of cognitive motivational factors on the reproduction, learning, and performance of preselected and constrained movements*. Unpublished doctoral dissertation, Florida State University, 1978.

Gordon, N. B. Varied input stimuli and motor learning. *Journal of Motor Behavior*, 1969, *1*, 149–161.

Hanson, D. L. Influence of the Hawthorne effect upon physical education research. *Research Quarterly*, 1967, *38*, 723–724.

Hinrichs, J. R. Ability correlates in learning a psychomotor task. *Journal of Applied Psychology*, 1970, *54*, 56–64.

Holding, D. H. Guidance in pursuit tracking. *Journal of Experimental Psychology*, 1959, *57*, 362–366.

Johnson, G. O. Generalization (transfer of a principle) in comparative studies of some learning characteristics in mentally retarded and normal children of the same mental age. In S. A. Kirk & B. B. Weiner (Eds.), *Behavioral research on exceptional children*. Washington, D.C.: National Education Association, The Council for Exceptional Children, 1963.

Jordon, T. C. Characteristics of visual and proprioceptive response times in the learning of a motor skill. *Quarterly Journal of Experimental Psychology*, 1972, *24*, 536–543.

Judd, C. H. The relations of special training to general intelligence. *Educational Review*, 1908, *36*, 28–42.

Karlin, L., & Mortimer, R. G. Effect of verbal, visual, and auditory augmenting cues on learning a complex motor skill. *Journal of Experimental Psychology*, 1963, *65*, 75–79.

Kaye, R. A. The use of a waist-type flotation device as an adjunct in teaching beginning swimming skills. *Research Quarterly*, 1965, *36*, 164–167.

Kelso, J. A. S. Planning and efferent components in the coding of movement. *Journal of Motor Behavior*, 1977, *9*, 33–47.

Kelso, J. A. S., Cook, E., Olson, M. E., & Epstein, W. Allocation of attention and the locus of adaptation to displaced vision. *Journal of Experimental Psychology: Human Perception and Performance*, 1975, *1*, 237–245.

Klatzky, T. L. *Human memory: Structures and processes*. San Francisco: W. H. Freeman, 1975.

Landers, D. M. Observational learning of a motor skill, temporal spacing of demonstration, and audience presence. In D. Harris & R. Christina (Eds.), *Psychology of sport and motor behavior*. University Park: Pennsylvania State University, 1975.

Landers, D. M. How, when, and where to use demonstrations: Suggestions for practitioners. *Journal of Physical Education and Recreation*, 1978, *49*, 65–67.

Lindeburg, F. A., & Hewitt, J. E. Effect of an oversized basketball on shooting ability and ball handling. *Research Quarterly*, 1965, *36*, 164–167.

Locke, E. A. The relationship of intentions to level of performance. *Journal of Applied Psychology*, 1966, *50*, 60–66.

Locke, E. A. Toward a theory of task motivation and incentives. *Organizational Behavior and Human Performance*, 1968, *3*, 157–189.

Locke, E. A., & Bryan, J. F. Cognitive aspects of psychomotor performance: The effects of performance goals on level of performance. *Journal of Applied Psychology*, 1966, *50*, 286–291.

Lucaccini, L. F., & Kreit, L. H. Music. In W. P. Morgan (Ed.), *Ergogenic aids in muscular performance*. New York: Academic Press, 1972.

Ludgate, K. E. The effects of manual guidance upon maze learning. *Psychological Monographs*, 1924, *33*, 1–65.

Macrae, A. W., & Holding, D. H. Guided practice in direct and reversed serial tracking. *Ergonomics*, 1965, *8*, 487–492. (a)

Macrae, A. W., & Holding, D. H. Method and task in motor guidance. *Ergonomics*, 1965, *8*, 315–320. (b)

Macrae, A. W., & Holding, D. H. Rate and force of guidance in perceptual motor tasks with reversal or random spatial correspondence. *Ergonomics*, 1966, *9*, 289–296.

Mayer, R. E. Information processing variables in learning to solve problems. *Review of Educational Research*, 1975, *45*, 525–541.

McCracken, H. D., & Stelmach, G. E. A test of schema theory of discrete motor learning. *Journal of Motor Behavior*, 1977, *9*, 193–201.

Mohr, D. R., & Barrett, M. E. Effect of knowledge of mechanical principles in learning to perform intermediate swim skills. *Research Quarterly*, 1962, *33*, 574–580.

Morgan, W. P. (Ed.). *Ergogenic aids and muscular performance*. New York: Academic Press, 1972.

Mosston, M. *Teaching physical education*. Columbus, Ohio: Charles E. Merrill, 1966.

Newman, R. I., Hunt, D. L., & Rhodes, F. Effects of music on employee attitude and productivity in a skateboard factory. *Journal of Applied Psychology*, 1966, *50*, 493–496.

Nideffer, R. M., & Deckner, C. W. A case study of improved athletic performance following use of relaxation procedures. *Perceptual and Motor Skills*, 1970, *30*, 821–822.

Parker, J. F., Jr., & Fleishman, E. A. Use of analytical information concerning task requirements to increase the effectiveness of skill training. *Journal of Applied Psychology*, 1961, *45*, 295–302.

Penman, K. Relative effectiveness of teaching tumbling with and without an instant replay videotape recorder. *Perceptual and Motor Skills*, 1969, *29*, 45–46.

Pick, H. L., Jr., Warren, D. H., & Hay, J. C. Sensory conflict in judgments of spatial direction. *Perception and Psychophysics*, 1969, *6*, 203–205.

Pomeranz, D. M., & Krasner, L. Effect of placebo in a simple motor response *Perceptual and Motor Skills*, 1969, *28*, 15–18.

Posner, M. I., Nissen, M. J., & Klein, R. Visual dominance: An information-processing account of its origins and significance. *Psychological Review*, 1976, *83*, 157–171.

Rock, I., & Harris, C. S. Vision and touch. *Scientific American*, 1967, *216*, 96–104.

Roethlisberger, F. J., & Dickson, W. J. *Management and the worker*. Cambridge, Mass.: Harvard University Press, 1939.

Rosenthal, R. Teacher expectation and pupil learning. In Association for Supervision and Curriculum Development (Ed.), *The unstudied curriculum: Its impact on children*. Washington, D.C.: National Education Association, 1970.

Schmidt, R. A. Experimental psychology. In R. N. Singer (Ed.), *The psychomotor domain: Movement behavior*. Philadelphia: Lea & Febiger, 1972.

Schmidt, R. A. Schema theory: Implications for movement education. *Motor Skills: Theory into Practice*, 1977, *2*, 36–48.

Schmidt, R. A., & Christina, R. W. Proprioception as a mediator in the timing of motor responses. *Journal of Experimental Psychology*, 1969, *81*, 303–307.

Singer, R. N. The learning systems approach and instruction in psychomotor activities. *Motor Skills: Theory into Practice*, 1977, *1*, 113–122. (a)

Singer, R. N. To err or not to err: A question for the instruction of psychomotor skills. *Review of Educational Research*, 1977, *47*, 479–498. (b)

Singer, R. N., & Dick, W. *Teaching physical education: A systems approach*. Boston: Houghton Mifflin, 1974.

Singer, R. N., & Gerson, R. F. *A conceptual orientation to the study of motor behavior*. Paper presented at the Seminar on Learning Strategies: Measures and Modules, Carmel, Calif., December 1977.

Singer, R. N., Llewellyn, J., & Darden, E. Placebo and competitive placebo effects on motor skill. *Research Quarterly*, 1973, *44*, 51–58.

Skinner, B. F. *The technology of teaching*. New York: Appleton-Century-Crofts, 1968.

Solley, W. H., & Borders, S. Relative effects of two methods of teaching the forehand drive in tennis. *Research Quarterly*, 1965, *36*, 120–122.

Sorenson, W. W. Test of mechanical principles as a suppressor variable for the prediction of effectiveness of a mechanical repair job. *Journal of Applied Psychology,* 1966, *50,* 348–352.

Stelmach, G. E., Kelso, J. A. S., & Wallace, S. A. Preselection in short-term motor memory. *Journal of Experimental Psychology: Human Learning and Memory,* 1975, *1,* 745–755.

Trumbo, D., Ulrich, L., & Noble, M. E. Verbal coding and display coding in the acquisition and retention of tracking skill. *Journal of Applied Psychology,* 1965, *49,* 368–375.

Trussell, E. Prediction of success in a motor skill on the basis of early learning achievement. *Research Quarterly,* 1965, *36,* 342–347.

Welch, M. Prediction of motor skill attainment from early learning. *Perceptual and Motor Skills,* 1963, *17,* 263–266.

Whiting, H. T. A., Gill, E. B., & Stephenson, J. M. Critical time intervals for taking in flight information in a ball-catching task. *Ergonomics,* 1970, *13,* 265–272.

Worthen, B. R. Discovery and expository task presentation in elementary mathematics. *Journal of Educational Psychology, Monograph Supplement,* 1968, *59,* 1–13.

Wright, E. J. *Effects of light and heavy equipment on the acquisition of sports-type skills by young children.* Paper presented at the annual American Association of Health, Physical Education, Recreation Convention, Chicago, 1966.

12 INSTRUCTIONAL AND TRAINING PROCEDURES: DURING PRACTICE CONSIDERATIONS

Once the learner is oriented, or prepared, to learn, the instructor must plan for practice conditions that will best lead to the most favorable results. Many alternatives are available. Decisions among alternatives are not easy to make.

In this chapter, there will be an attempt to identify and analyze a number of practice considerations, as well as to suggest some alternatives for particular kinds of activities. Such major topics as motivation, attention, and instructional design will be addressed. Each will be developed to a reasonable degree, as there are many subtopics and issues of major concern to those who are responsible for manipulating learning environments. As we will see, many of the areas have been explored quite extensively, in an attempt to resolve such questions as whether practice should proceed under whole or part conditions, with emphasis on the speed or accuracy of the movement, according to massed or distributed schedules, and with formal guidance or under problem-solving conditions. Any decisions made should follow a consideration of the research in the psychology of learning and in instructional design, as apparently appropriate for the learning of behaviors associated with a particular content or specialization (see Figure 12-1).

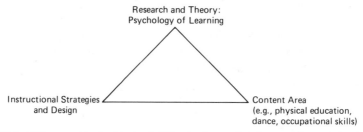

FIGURE 12-1. With regard to the kinds of skill to be learned, science and research related to the psychology of learning and instructional design should be considered, as the optimal conditions for learning are established by the instructor.

If all teacher-learner situations were on a one-to-one basis, individual considerations would be maximized. Unfortunately, most training and instructional programs involve a high proportion of learners to one instructor. Principles of instruction, generally favorable to most learners in a group, can probably be identified and implemented.

Yet, it must be recognized that learners differ in many ways, notably in motivation, rate of learning, and the strategies and techniques that will be used to learn skills. For the learning of written material, it has been possible to develop alternative and individualized learning mediums with the use of advanced technology. Students can thereby work at their own speed and with personally selected materials and means of learning. It is possible to develop similar approaches for the learning of fine motor skills. But gross motor skills, to be performed with and against others, do not lend themselves so easily to self-directed and individualized learning.

Although individual accommodations are more limited in the learning of gross motor activities than in the learning of written matter, sensitivity is advised for students not apparently orienting well to the general instructional technique decided on by the instructor for the group. On a probability basis, we might expect learners in general to respond acceptably to well-designed and formulated instructional programs, based on approaches consistent with scientific findings. Exceptions will be noted, however.

Although it is not practical to expect that every student can be treated on an individual basis, it is important to recognize that past accumulated knowledge and experiences bring different people together with different capabilities and learning approaches to the same activity. What to do about it depends on many practical considerations, most too obvious to mention here.

INSTRUCTIONAL DESIGN

Systems approaches to instruction and training are prominent in contemporary literature. They suggest organized and systematic ways of scientifically creating learning environments that most efficiently and productively lead to favorable results. One of the first sources calling the attention of educators to this approach was published by Gagné (1962). Many resources were developed in subsequent years.

The attempt has been to incorporate learning research and theory into models that are of practical value to the instructor. Learning need not proceed in a haphazard way. Although we are concerned here primarily with the identification of learning phenomena and a summary of research findings, those readers who are interested in ''putting it all together'' in a systematic way for more meaningful instruction will want to familiarize themselves with systems approaches and the science of instruction, instructional design. Many recently published books, primarily in the area of educational psychology, provide a good background for those who want to utilize systems models in their instruction (Davis, Alexander, &

Yelon, 1974), or at least understand the nature of instructional design further (Gagné & Briggs, 1974).

A variety of instructional and training strategies exists. A preference might be dictated by situational constraints and individual differences. In the latter case, it is thought that students with dissimilar attributes, interests, and capabilities might benefit from alternative strategies. Entry characteristics of the students would be matched to the task demands and expected learning outcomes, thereby suggesting appropriate instructional procedures.

The point is that learning research might suggest the most favorable conditions for the average student. Yet, a systematic and sensitive analysis of any situation in which a number of students are involved leads to a realization of individual differences and ways of coping with them. The book by Singer and Dick (1974) contains content expressly for physical educators and promotes the use of systems approaches to enhance instruction for all students.

There is no one way to teach. Some instructional methods are better than others, and a method's effectiveness may very well depend on the teacher and the task, as well as the learner. To limit and direct all instructors to one procedure would be erroneous; certainly we do not attempt to require every baseball batter to stand and swing in exactly the same way! General principles should not be violated, but there is latitude for individual variation and initiative. A comparison of teaching techniques indicates that some are more beneficial than others to a particular learner. Some help to fulfill specified goals better than others. Because of the complexity of the problem and the many operating and interacting variables, however, it should be apparent why conclusive evidence in favor of certain approaches is somewhat lacking.

All instructors must make certain judgments before a class or session begins. These judgments involve various dimensions of the class situation, and, in a sense, reflect an individual's teaching style. Muska Mosston (1966) categorizes preclass decisions in the following order:

1. Selection and apportionment of subject matter, e.g., time allotted for practice.
2. Quantity of an activity, e.g., consideration for individual differences.
3. Quality of performance, e.g., measurement standards.
4. Teacher involvement, e.g., to what extent and how.
5. Student involvement, e.g., to what extent and how.

Although Mosston is concerned with these variables primarily as they relate to teaching styles, there are other questions. In what manner should new material be presented to students? How should the student be guided during the practice of skills? Should learning be designed for social situations or for each learner as an entity? These questions are a few that may be raised as instructional materials and procedures are developed.

At this point, we will examine ways in which instructors communicate their intentions to learners and design practice conditions. We have dealt with prepractice considerations, with what happens prior to the learner's actual initiation of physical or motoric practice. Now we will analyze conditions during practice.

PRACTICE CONDITIONS

Practice Quality

For the majority of motor skills, and under certain conditions, learning progresses with an increased number of practice trials. It is foolish to expect skilled performance at the onset, although there is no doubt that some individuals learn faster and are endowed more favorably than others for the task at hand. However, practice, as a rule, is a necessary prerequisite for learning skills.

Unfortunately, there is more to learning than mere practice, for *practice alone does not make perfect*. Practice must be accompanied by such conditions as the performer's awareness of direction or goal, attained results and, in general, by motivation, or the desire to improve. Repetition of an act may result in no performance increments and even in an inferior performance. The first situation (no increments) can occur if the conditions mentioned earlier in this paragraph are not present. The latter (inferior performance) will be manifested under these conditions or when the participant practices incorrectly and with erroneous goals. Thus, we can only assume the positive effect of practice on learning and performance when other desirable factors are operating in conjunction with practice, factors that often are taken for granted. (It might also be mentioned here that some learning theorists believe that learning takes place in one trial and that further trials only enhance performance. However, this is a theoretical argument and does not concern us in this chapter.)

It is important to remember that practice may perpetuate error as well as eliminate error and improve skill. Attempts should be made to recognize and improve the environmental conditions surrounding the practice and, in turn, the participant's learning and performance.

Amount of Practice

Of natural concern is the question of how much practice is necessary for a skill to be really learned. Where is that point of diminishing returns, that point when further practice will be wasted? Much depends on the criterion for skill attainment. Is the foul shot in basketball learned when the student can score one throw, five out of five, ten in a row, or twenty consecutive shots?

In the psychological literature, the criterion of success is usually one perfect trial or match. A trial may consist of learning ten nonsense syllables, tracing a maze, and the like. Any practice after the one-trial achievement, then, would be additional, and is termed *overlearning*. Researchers have investigated the effects of practice over and beyond the point when criterion learning has occurred and have invariably come to the same conclusion: overlearning results in better retention than regular learning of the material learned.

It is felt that continuous motor tasks are retained better than discrete ones. It may be that there are more opportunities to make gains in habit strength in continuous tasks. Absolute retention is increased with overlearning, but relative retention is associated with proportionately fewer gains with overlearning. That is to say, any amount of overlearning will lead to better retention, but proportional increases in overlearning do not lead to proportional gains in retention.

It is no secret that motor skills—for example, bicycle riding, ball throwing, and typing—are retained for a much longer period of time than many of the so-called intellectual or verbal skills. When one is asked to recall from childhood the skills involved in bicycling or to remember the lines of a poem, much greater performance is typically demonstrated with the motor skill. One explanation of this is that motor skills are usually overpracticed. How much time is spent playing baseball and learning the swing, in contrast with learning prose material? For the average youngster, the answer is obvious.

However, overlearning is beneficial to a point, after which there are diminishing returns. In laboratory studies, 50 per cent overlearning is advantageous, but practice beyond this does not afford a proportional gain for the extended effort. Although 100 per cent overlearning results in a better performance yield than 50 per cent overlearning, the gains are not very worthwhile in terms of economy of the practice time.

Overlearning is associated with drill, but how much is necessary in learning motor skills? The lack of research on motor skills, especially practical ones, necessitates a cautious application of the overlearning principle. Perhaps too much drill occurs in typical situations: not only may this drill reach the point of diminishing returns, but it even may be detrimental because it (1) takes time away from other learning; (2) is boring to the learner; and (3) actually does not serve in improving skill retention significantly.

Sufficient practice to establish learning permanence is required for future success. But perhaps, instead of the number of repetitious trials providing greater motor skill retention, the answer lies in the nature of the interpolated activity. From the time a skill is learned until it is to be demonstrated again, a few years later perhaps, a minimum number of competing responses has occurred. Most motor skills are somewhat unique. Not too many other learned skills will interfere with the originally learned skill. Therefore, it can be reasoned that motor skills can be retained with less practice, proportionally, than is associated with verbal learning.

The reply, therefore, to the question of how much practice is necessary is a difficult one that can be made only after deciding on one of two possibilities. What is the object of the practice: immediate success or later retention? For many skills, reasonable achievement comes after not too many practice sessions. If the goal is immediate successful performance and there is no concern for the future, then the time spent on learning can be more limited. If, however, later performance is an important consideration, then evidently more practice, hence more overlearning, will be beneficial in determining the length of time the tasks are to be retained as well as the amount of skill that will be displayed at that time of recall.

From Situational to Personal Control

The learner, as pointed out by P. M. Fitts and M. I. Posner (1967), seems to proceed from an overwhelmingly conscious state, with overattentiveness to many external sources of information, to a self-reliant state, where control over the situation is much more internalized. Obviously, practice conditions should be such as to encourage this transitional process. Proper introduction and reduction of guidance and cues would be of great benefit.

The guidance and control of movement can be viewed from another point of view as well. It appears, as Mary Smyth (1977) suggests, that the closed-loop theory proposed by Adams (see Chapter 5) predicts that dependence on visual feedback is greater after a large amount of practice; however, motor program theorists such as Steven Keele (also see Chapter 5) indicate that response-produced feedback should become less important for movement control, as skilled movement is preprogrammed. Smyth's evidence favored the motor program model. The less learners have to depend on feedback, the better they should be able to perform. This is true whether it is given from another person or derived from the performer's own movement.

There is always the problem, also, of discrepant feedback information. If visual and kinesthetic information conflict and vision dominates (as has been reported frequently in the literature), more feedback dependency can have deleterious effects on performance. The relationship of the feedback modalities, as explained by Smyth, along with the negative effects she found in learning, was attributed to visual dominance over the feedback sources available to the learner. With less peripheral control and more central control, thereby reducing feedback dependency, the person is able to demonstrate more highly skilled performance.

LEVEL OF SKILL

In most situations, learners possess a wide range of developed skills and potential abilities for achievement. The magnitude of the range will depend on whether the students are grouped at random or there is an attempt at homogeneity. It is often convenient to categorize students learning an activity as beginners, intermediates, or advanced. This classification is arbitrary, for individuals fall in a continuum on the range of skill development. Recognizing differences in achieved level of skill allows the educator or trainer to proceed in a more effective manner, for each level requires special learning considerations.

General Considerations at Different Levels

Certain learning principles apply to the acquisition of motor skills, regardless of skill level. One of the major purposes of this book is to relate the general considerations for all learners. However, the status of the individual in skill achievement in a particular activity necessitates specific allowances and unique considerations. As might be expected, teaching techniques should be modified from the beginning to the advanced stages of an individual's motor skill development.

The beginner, the person learning a specific skill for the first time, poses problems to the instructor unlike those confronted with a highly skilled performer. Unfortunately, the beginner is often neglected, for it is much more rewarding to direct the progress of individuals who are highly skilled, coordinated, and motivated. Each novice requires individual attention, although in many cases this might be impractical. What general procedures, then, may be followed to promote learning in a group of beginners?

First, beginners must *understand the goal* that they will be attempting to achieve. If it is to swim the side-stroke the length of the pool, they should observe a demonstration of this stroke in its entirety. They will then become aware of what is to be expected, of how the parts of the body are coordinated for this skill and, generally, what lies ahead of them. The old adage of quickly involving the learner in the activity for best results may be effective in elevating motivation or performing general movements but may not really be of much advantage in skill acquisition if performance goals are uncertain. Assuming the maturity of the organism, a clear picture of behavioral expectancies should be developed.

Second, beginners appear to *benefit most from activity;* thus, verbal instruction should be kept to a minimum. Naturally, with increased age and maturity, there is less impatience and perhaps a greater mental capacity on the part of the students, enabling them to benefit from verbal instruction. However, the generally accepted rule with beginners is to allow the actual physical activity to dominate the early lessons (assuming an understanding of goals).

Third, this activity may be initiated by the performer or directed from *external sources,* such as the teacher manipulating a particular body area in order for the novice to get the feel of the desired movement. At the early stage of skill attainment, there is the unresolved question of introducing the mechanical and physiological principles related to the skill performance, as well as the merit of using the problem-solving approach, of directing the students to attempt to determine the why's and the how's in their quest for skill mastery. Visual aids, in the form of movies, slides, and pictures are possible supplementary material. The methods and means of instruction to be utilized will depend on the background, nature, and ideas of the teacher. There is no one set method of instruction. The point here, though, is that *physical activity should be emphasized in the early stages of motor learning.* This is especially true with young children.

The physical experience allows additional methods of instruction to be more meaningful. Attention to detail can then be provided in verbal instruction. Specifics can only be attended to when the general aspects of an activity have been mastered. One of the greatest mistakes a teacher can make with beginners is to spend too much time on details and talking too much.

The results of an investigation by S. Renshaw and D. K. Postle (1928) will serve to reinforce the concept of the importance of motor activity for beginners. These researchers formed three groups, all of whom learned a pursuit rotor task.

Group I received very brief demonstrations and instruction, group II had additional instructional, and group III observed a simple demonstration with detailed instructions. Groups I and II performed similarly on the task; group III demonstrated the poorest performance. In this case, greater verbal instructions had the effect of impeding the acquisition of manipulatory skill. As Renshaw and Postle reason, progress in some motor skills may be inhibited where language (verbal habits) cannot substitute for direct sensory stimuli afforded by the task. The study is aptly and humorously concluded with the statement that the pursuit rotor is operated by the hands, not the voice box.

A learner will probably fare better in a newly introduced skill if the teacher attempts to *build on skills familiar and already known* to the learner. Resemblances of already learned skills to those to be learned, if pointed out, promote faster learning. At least one leading tennis authority believes that it is quite difficult to teach anyone to hit the tennis serve if he or she cannot throw a ball overhand. Similarly, if students cannot swing their arms freely at the shoulder, parallel to the ground, learning forehand and backhand groundstrokes will be impeded.

Such simple motor skills as throwing, catching, pivoting, and the like must be accomplished before reasonable tennis proficiency can be expected. The tennis stroke is then likened to some familiar skill, as exemplified by singing a baseball bat. The acquisition of new skills would be more fun, and a faster process as well, if these rules were followed.

Consideration should be given to the length of the practice sessions. For most beginners, *frequent, short, spaced practice periods* are preferable to extended practice periods. Novice learners are more prone to a loss of interest and a lack of attention when they have to overcome the hurdles of learning something completely new. The acquisition of skill can be a stubborn process, especially without the presence of desireable practice conditions.

The beginner demonstrates symptoms of *tightness and wasted energy*. As skill is acquired, efficiency in movement is observed. At first, it is as if the parts of the body are working independently; however, later performance is characterized by minimal and only necessary coordinated movement patterns. Neurologically, control of unlearned or poorly learned skills is at the cerebral level, but this area has less of a role in the performance of advanced learners. The cerebellum is more active in the later situation. It is as if the beginner has to attend to so many cues (many unnecessary) that performance suffers. With experience and instruction, the person learns what to respond to, how to respond effectively, and how to direct thought processes during motor performance.

New skills should be taught in such a way that the *learner performs in practice the way one is expected to in the actual situation*. Slow-motion practice or emphasis on one factor when several are equally important to the successful performance of an act only makes for additional learning and relearning problems. If speed and accuracy are required, both should be practiced simultaneously. One can learn to shoot a stationary jump shot in basketball, but in actual competition the player is usually on the move before shooting. Simulating gamelike skills in practice affords a better chance of success in the contest.

Many students have trouble learning gross motor skills because of a lack of experience with *basic movement patterns* in childhood. Ease in learning new skills will depend to a large extent on these many varied previous experiences. There are indications that even in later years familiarization with simple motor patterns facilitates the learning of more complex skills, e.g., those involved in sports. It is rare that new tasks require the learning of new motor skills. Basic, simple movements—those that are performed in childhood include running, throwing, kicking, and jumping—underlie all sports. It is the means of organizing these patterns that differs from skill to skill and sport to sport. Therefore, learners who have not had the opportunity to play and develop the simple motor skills associated with childhood are handicapped in later, more complex undertakings.

Beginners should not be required to display the same ideal form for a specific skill. The important thing in the initial stages of learning is achievement and satisfaction, and casting a mold restricts the opportunity. Emphasis on particular desired styles can take place later as skill progresses.

The advanced learner, the one who demonstrates a high level of achievement in a skill or group of skills, may be approached in a different manner from the beginner. More time can be spent with the critical details of performance. Verbal instruction is more meaningful and, in general, the advanced are able to concentrate for a longer period of time on the task at hand. Practice sessions can be more intensive and extensive.

A highly skilled person usually achieves status because of motivation, among other variables. Incentive will probably be less of a problem with this performer than the beginner. As a standard rule, though, we all like to perform in activities in which we can demonstrate achievement. A beginner usually lacks confidence in the activity, the advanced learner typically does not. All in all, teaching students who fall along the continuum of skill achievement presents general and special problems. Emphasis in instructional methods and considerations changes as skill progresses.

Early Versus Late Learners

Frequently, early progress in skill attainment is misleading in predicting ultimate success. Some individuals demonstrate better performance than others in the early stages of learning, almost as if they gain quicker insight into the problem at hand. Various factors may be attributed to individual differences in early skill achievement, but one conclusion appears justified: early success does not indicate later achievement, in a reliable manner.

Marya Welch (1963) had her subjects perform a ladder climbing test (to go as high as possible before toppling). They were tested on six different days, with each test consisting of ten trials. Welch concluded that general skill attainment prediction is poor unless an estimation of learning ability extends over at least half of the practice days. Fleishman and Hempel (1954) demonstrated that different factors are emphasized with increased practice and learning. Hence, beginning success depends on certain factors and later achievement reflects the utilization of other factors. In other words, it would be quite difficult to predict end performance from beginning level of skill because variables differ in importance in each particular stage of learning.

Ella Trussell (1965) required forty college women students to learn a ball-juggling task. She found that the learning scores were not significantly related to initial scores and that the best predictability of final performance was obtained during the first 60 per cent of practice. Implications from the evidence are that people learn at varying rates of speed and that some may be handicapped if a particular unit or skill to be learned is covered too quickly. Everyone has an optimal learning rate, and unfortunately, in mass learning situations such as those found in many classes and programs, it is hard to consider individual differences. However, an awareness of this problem will at least allow the teacher to determine what is best for the group and where possible to adjust for extremes in fast and slow learners.

Further analysis of various parameters surrounding individual differences in learning is offered by Welch and Henry (1971). Using a stabilometer task and sixty undergraduate college women, some conclusions were that final prediction from initial scores over several days was not effective unless nearly 95 per cent of the potential learning had been accomplished. In this particular study, which confirms the findings of the studies of Welch and of Trussell, this point was reached after approximately 50 per cent of the total practice. In addition, rate of learning was not correlated with amount of learning. This finding has been well documented in the literature and is opposed to the popular belief in the high relationship of these factors to each other.

MOTIVATION

In any situation, at any time, and with any individual, performance is likely to fluctuate. Even outstanding athletes who have attained a high proficiency in certain skills do not always perform consistently at a particular skill level, although they are more likely to than beginners or intermediates. Variability in response can be caused by external factors. For the basketball player, the basketball, the court, the basket, the gymnasium, the spectators—all of which may vary from location to location—are sources of potential alterations in performance to which adjustments must be made.

Apart from environmental sources, internal variables such as physiological and psychological drives and needs contribute to levels of performance. So do thoughts, expectations, and appraisals of situations, as well as feelings about oneself. Many other sources of potential influence on behavior can be identified, in addition. Indeed, the study of motivation underlies the answer to the question: Why does a person behave in a certain way? For the instructor, problems include getting students to learn and perform according to their potential and helping them to maintain interests and to persevere at activities, or at least attempt "new" experiences. Variability in performance, therefore, is not only due to situational differences, but to differences in personal motives, expectations, attitudes, and reactions to activities and situations.

Interpretations and Explanations

To interpret motivation is extremely hazardous, considering (1) the potential effects of motivation, and (2) the various approaches available for the study of motivation. In the first instance, motivational forces are responsible for the selection of and participation in a particular activity over other possible alternatives at any moment. They influence the decision to persevere and practice at it for an extended period of time, perhaps even under demanding conditions. As such, they enhance learning potential. They even impact on the quality of and effort in performance. In other words, more and better practice, leading to improved learning and excellence in actual performance, is a by-product of the effects of motivational factors. In summary, motivation is responsible for:

1. selection of and preference for an activity.
2. persistence at the activity (duration of training).
3. intensity and vigor of performance (effort).
4. adequacy of performance relative to standards.

It can be seen that motivation played a part in a person's history and subsequently influences any particular performance with regard to any tasks. In sport, behaviors must be considered during the preseason, the actual competitive season, the preevent interval, and the actual competitive event. Motivational processes need to operate in dissimilar forms for the different purposes of each situation. For instance, *more* motivation leads to selection, persistence, and effort behavior, but more motivation may not be appropriate for skilled performance. The nature and demands of the activity may suggest the need for motivation to be elevated or lessened. In this latter regard, *optimal* motivational levels need to be considered relative to the nature of each individual and each activity, as we will see shortly.

As to the approaches to the analysis and interpretation of motivation, the gamut ranges from the clinician's subjective perspective to the experimentalist's contrived and controlled means of observation. As Walter Kolesnik (1978) indicates in his summary of approaches, insights into motivation come from psychoanalysis, social psychology, behaviorism, cognitive psychology, and humanism:

1. Psychoanalysis: Subconscious motivation, personality factors, psychic energies, understanding the nature of the person.
2. Social psychology: Social consciousness and concerns, sociopolitical impact on personal behavior, socialization (competition and cooperation).

3. Behaviorism: External control and regulation of behavior, reinforcement, drive reduction, contingency management (behaviors shaped by reinforcers).
4. Cognitive psychology: perceptions, expectations, attitudes, interpretations of behaviors (attributions), locus of control, the role of mental processes, achievement motives.
5. Humanism: Self-fulfillment, self-determination, purposeful behavior (satisfying needs and attaining goals), self-actualization.

These perspectives provide a feeling for the complexity of motivational processes and the variety of personal and situational factors that can influence them. Motivation is usually thought of as goal-directed behavior, an urge to push toward some goal. Actually, motivation is a concept invented to describe the psychological state of the person as it is affected by various influences. Perhaps all behavior is motivated (by something), although it is not always easy to isolate specific motivational variables.

There are at least four variables that will affect action or goal-directed behavior. A person's behavioral tendency toward and in activities will be determined, according to David Birch and Joseph Veroff (1966) by

1. availability: situational and historical factors, ability to become familiarized with the situation
2. expectancy: past association and immediate perceptions
3. incentives: extrinsic consequences of actions (positive or negative, degree and magnitude)
4. motives: intrinsic cause of action (strength depends on experience with a general class of incentives representing a particular consequence) (p. 6)

The type, quality, and orientation of action will depend on (1) the characteristics of the person and (2) the characteristics of the immediate situation.

Motives and *incentives* are terms often used interchangeably and, in fact, they have much in common. An incentive is an object or condition that satisfies a motive and removes it, but a person can be motivated without an incentive. Also, incentives may be present but appeal to no particular motive. Incentives can be used effectively to guide the learner to specified goals. Because they are distinguished and interpreted differently, depending on age, sex, socioeconomic class, abilities, and the like, care is necessary if they are to be of benefit.

Recently, Martin Maehr (1974) suggested new directions for the study of motivation. He would place behavioral patterns, which prompt motivational inferences, in a taxonomy. The three categories of behavioral patterns are change in direction (choice), persistence (in spite of or under failure), and performance level variations. When viewed in this manner, motivation can mean several different things, as was indicated previously. The theory of achievement motivation, formulated by D. C. McClelland (1972) and to be discussed shortly, is modified by Maehr to consider differences in cultures and resultant effects on personal needs to achieve.

Any of the three categories of behaviors can be examined in the following way: Behavioral manifestations of motivation can occur when the social learning experiences in a given culture influence the personality (predisposition to react in a predictable way) of an individual. Motivational patterns also can be developed as a result of experiences in situations that affect such behavior, regardless of individual personalities. A third possibility is that, depending on the situation, motivational behavior will be affected by personality predispositions, which in turn, are influenced by social learning.

A basic argument in Maehr's work is that the concept of need to achieve, or nAch, as expressed by McClelland, is not a generalized trait within a person. A ghetto youngster may score low on the nAch test and still reveal extremely motivated behaviors in athletic endeavors. Thus, achievement tests often reflect the behaviors associated with a particular culture to those of another culture. The previous situations experienced by a person will strongly influence present motivational behaviors (persistence, choice, and performance patterns). The parameters of these situations assume many forms. The individual is probably influenced by:

1. social guidelines (social systems, norm comparisons).
2. social expectancies (fulfilling prophecies).
3. social values (adhering to guidelines).
4. locus of control (individual control versus external control in situations).
5. interpersonal variables (quality feedback, social competition versus self-competition).
6. task dimensions (difficulty, appeal, relevance).

Motivation is dynamically portrayed by Maehr as influenced by societal, experiential, and personal factors. Although it often is convenient to isolate individuals and incentives or environmental intrusions to examine behavior, thereby deducing information about motivation, such an approach is limited in its ability truly to describe effects on and properties of motivation. The person, as a system, is influenced by the immediate situation (or system confines), as well as the present social and cultural system. We will expand on these issues shortly.

Effects on Learning and Performance

Motivation affects both learning and performance. When people are unmotivated, they do not practice or will not practice well, resulting in little if any learning. But then, again, the degree of arousal (motivation) present in an individual prior to and during the performance of a task will influence its execution and outcome. The following formula is derived:

$$\text{Performance} = \text{Motivation} \times \text{Capabilities}$$

$$
\begin{array}{lll}
\text{(behavior in} & \text{(attitudes,} & \text{(genetics,} \\
\text{a situation)} & = \text{feelings,} & \times \text{past experiences,} \\
& \text{expectancies)} & \text{learning)}
\end{array}
$$

In this formula we can observe that a person's actual performance depends on relevant hereditary characteristics that serve to predispose one for achievement in a particular endeavor. Heredity sets the boundaries, or the framework, of the human system. Yet, there is always room for improvement. Practice, quality practice, that is, allows the individual to more truly realize potential. Previous experiences influence the development of skills, abilities, knowledge, and tactics that might be related to the present task.

But excellence in performance is also a function of affective behaviors. These include attitudes, feelings, arousal level, and expectations. Such affective behaviors need to be developed as appropriate for the task. The training of a person with regard to these psychological variables, along with the training that promotes organic efficiency, physical development, knowledge and strategies, and specialized skills, will result in the degree of excellence observed in the performance of a motor activity.

Interactional Factors

A myriad of factors interplays dynamically to influence the ultimate achievement of someone in a special activity. To put it simply, personal characteristics, situational variables, and task dimensions interact to suggest the optimal motivation to be imposed and/or generated (see Figure 12-2).

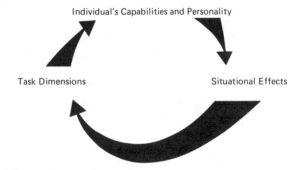

Individual's Capabilities and Personality

Task Dimensions

Situational Effects

FIGURE 12-2. The interactive, dynamic processes affecting performance.

The demand characteristics of any activity suggest ideal arousal states. Situational or environmental factors surrounding the to-be-performed event will contain cues with arousal properties. In athletics, the presence of spectators, the words of the coach, the contest conditions, and other variables are associated with potential arousal dynamics. Owing to the nature of individual differences in personality, each athlete may react differently to particular situational factors and the nature of the activity. Anxiety level, resistance to specific stressors, and perception of locus of control (internal versus external) are good examples of personal characteristics that will bear on performance outcomes. They, too, must be considered in relation to motivation. Let us first examine in more detail differences in the characteristics of tasks and implications for motivational states.

MOTOR LEARNING AND HUMAN PERFORMANCE

Optimal Level and Task Considerations

Motivational effects depend not only on environmental manipulations and the individual's personality, but on the nature of the task itself. If the motivational level can be held constant, it is observed that the relative simplicity or complexity of the skill to be learned will determine the ease with which it is learned. For instance, it is generally assumed that high or low motivation has the same effect on the performance of simple acts or skills. High motivation will, in addition, aid in perseverance at a task.

However, the level of motivation will affect the performance of a complex skill. Evidence indicates that more difficult tasks require lower motivation, for high motivation has been found to impede skill acquisition in these tasks. Highest performance is attained by subjects with intermediate motivation (drive); as tasks increase in complexity, subjects with less drive do better. The *Yerkes–Dodson law* describes the phenomenon: there is an *optimal level of motivation for the level of task difficulty.* Although somewhat exaggerated, Figures 12-3 and 12-4 illustrate some possible effects of varying degrees of motivation.

FIGURE 12-3. Level of motivation, related to the difficulty level of activity.

Highest	High Motivation	Moderate
Most Simple	Fairly Complex Skill Act	Most Complex

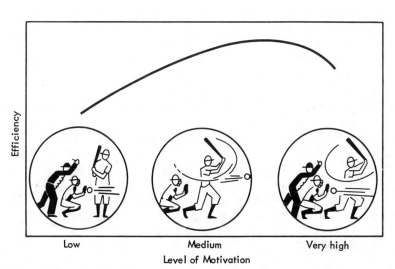

FIGURE 12-4. A schematic representation of the relationship between level of motivation and efficiency of behavior. At low and high levels of motivation the result is the same, a strike-out, but the behavior of the batter is quite different. (*From* Psychology, *Revised Edition, by Wickens, D. D. and Meyer, D. R. Copyright © 1955, 1961 by Holt, Rinehart and Winston, Inc. Reprinted by permission of Holt, Rinehart and Winston, Inc.*)

With regard to task structure and the ideal degree of motivation, we have touched on the contrasting effects of motivation on simple and difficult tasks. In sport we may contrast, for convenience, activities that are vigorous and that involve explosive power, strength, and endurance with those that require control, precision, timing, and high degrees of coordination. The first category of activities would probably benefit from the presence of the highest levels of motivation. In these cases, the act can be performed mechanically and subconsciously, and effort, as reflected by motivation, may determine final performance. The second category of activities suggests the controlled use of motivation. A reasonable degree needs to be present for arousal and cue attention, discrimination, and selection purposes. Response adequacy will also be reflected by this state. But too much motivation, either internally produced or externally imposed, will most likely hinder the control processes underlying skilled maneuvers.

Four dimensions of motor activities may be considered in regard to motivation (Singer, 1977): complexity, physical demands, appeal, and meaningfulness. A task analysis is important for realizing the potential impact on a person's attitudinal and arousal state, including any influence an instructor might attempt to exert in the situation.

Complexity. As was indicated before, task complexity is related to the degree of motivation appropriate for optimizing performance potential. Events placing relatively few cognitive, perceptual, and finely coordinated movement demands on a person require the highest level of arousal and vice-versa. The discussion in an earlier chapter on emotions and drive theory versus the inverted-U hypothesis related to performance expectations is pertinent here. The same conclusions could be reached with motivations compared with emotions. Self-generated or regulated arousal, compatible with the activity, reflects the learning of emotional discharge appropriate for skilled performance.

Physical Demands. More "pure" physical tasks require the highest degrees of arousal. Strength, speed, endurance, or explosive power is generated best under such conditions.

Appeal. Unique and interesting activities can help to generate enthusiasm and motivation. By varying the structure of the practice session, the attitude of the students for the tasks to be learned/performed will also be modified, resulting in better performances.

Relevance and Meaningfulness. The more meaningful practice routines are perceived to be by the learner, in helping to contribute to personal goals, the greater the motivation to perform well and to sustain practice in the activity. Even though specified practice activities are known by the instructor to be appropriate and necessary, the student must be convinced, as well (an example of the involvement of cognitive and affective processes).

Personal Variables

Individuals differ in many dimensions with regard to personal motives and their influence on behavior. We will identify a number of them here. They serve as a reminder of the particular considerations that must be given to individuals.

First of all, there are *under, over, and expected achievers.* If you recall, it has been stated that performance is a function of capability level and motivation, as associated with (1) persistent and quality prior practice in the activity, and (2) feelings and an arousal state associated with present performance in the activity. True levels of capability are not realized if the current motivational state is inappropriate to meet the challenges of the activity. An underachiever, a person who performs worse in the ultimate performance test than expected from previous practice, is probably unable to activate or control the arousal mechanisms to a desirable degree. In other words, the perceived stress of the performance test results in an inability of the person to cope with it effectively.

By the same token, the overachiever, the individual who produces more than expected on the ultimate performance test, may be demonstrating a reversed arousal state. Consistent performance between practice sessions and the final test imply consistent motivational responses to each.

Academic achievement is often evaluated in the form of a written or an oral test. Many students feel that their test scores and course grades do not truly reflect the information mastered by them over a period of time. These students are no doubt poor test takers; that is, they have an inability to cope emotionally with testing.

Second, we must mention here, as was discussed in the previous chapter, the relevance of *level of aspiration or expectation* to performance level. The situation is evaluated, expectations produced, and performance output influenced accordingly. Previous successes and failures in direct or related experiences, present evaluations in terms of probabilities of achievement, and realistic or unrealistic approaches influence aspiration levels. In turn, goal level affects performance yield.

Third, people differ in *need to achieve,* which is influenced by many factors. The degree of felt need to accomplish is not a generalized trait but is specific to each activity and situation. The need to achieve in a particular activity reflects the motivational strength of that activity and its interaction with a person's personality characteristics. In turn, the level of this need influences risk-taking behavior, the sustenance of practice, and momentary performance.

Fourth, differences in *need for social approval* are manifested. Activity performance and achievement are related to sociocultural factors, and perceived social expectations bear upon motivation and behavior.

Fifth, let us consider *need to avoid failure or to avoid success.* Both of these types of needs are anxiety producing; both are associated with motivation and performance. Fear of failure can produce improved skills, but it also limits risk taking and best potential for success in activities with characteristics associated with altering intended behaviors in unexpected situations. Fear of success limits achievement, for it is possible to reject the prestige and accompanying responsibilities that might accrue with elevated skilled performance, especially in team or group activities.

Sixth, what of the *level of anxiety* felt toward the particular activity? The essentials of Clark Hull's drive theory describe the relation of the task to the performer in the following way: If the correct response is dominant over incorrect responses (typical in a simple task), increased motivation or anxiety should facilitate performance. In a complex learning situation, there are usually a number of competing incorrect responses that are more dominant than the sole correct response. Performance is predicted as poorer in this case in highly motivated subjects. Figure 12-5 illustrates the data obtained in an investigation testing the theory. The subjects were children who were placed in extreme groups as a result of their scores on the Taylor Scale of Manifest Anxiety, which is a measure of one aspect of motivation. Their task was to learn a light-button motor task that requires trial-and-error learning in attempting to find the correct button that turns off each light. As can be viewed in Figure 12-5, the subjects low in anxiety were superior to the subjects high in anxiety, thus substantiating evidence accumulated on adult subjects and further supporting Hull's theory. The more highly anxious person will learn and perform better if less motivated, and the less anxious individual will do better if motivated to a higher degree. If an induced motivation level is too emotionally stressful, learning and performance will be inhibited.

Seventh, the continual undertaking of activities will depend on the *future*

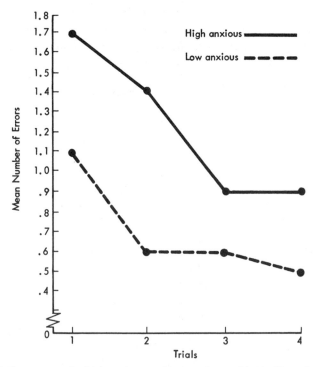

FIGURE 12-5. Error curves for high anxious and low anxious subjects. (*From Palermo, D. S., Castaneda, A., & McCandless, B. R. The relationship of anxiety in children to performance in a complex learning task.* Child Development, *1956, 27, 333–337.*) Reprinted with permission of the authors and The Society for Research in Child Development, Inc.

MOTOR LEARNING AND HUMAN PERFORMANCE

orientation, or goals, of a person. Being oriented to distant accomplishments is encouragement to practice those activities perceived as leading to the realization of those accomplishments.

Eighth, individuals may perceive their chances of success as depending on *internal or external factors,* or *locus of control.* Persons possessing an internal locus of control feel that their accomplishments are influenced through personal efforts. They believe that they are masters of their own fate, so to speak. People with an external locus of control perceive the situation as having chance outcomes. Performance will be influenced by luck, situational factors, and other variables external to their efforts and abilities. It would appear that the degree of motivation associated with overcoming fate or energizing perceived capabilities might differ, with an internal locus of control being the more advantageous of the two.

Ninth, *extrinsic and intrinsic sources* of motivation might influence behavior differentially. It is possible to be primarily motivated to practice and achieve for reasons associated with materialistic goals (e.g., praise, prestige, money) or personal satisfaction and self-realization. Rewards are incentives to perform and produce. Similarly, self-fulfillment is an inspiration to participate and accomplish. Extrinsic and intrinsic forms of motivation probably operate together in many situations, with one the more dominant of the two. In other words, a person may find experience of and achievement in an activity to be personally rewarding, as well as socially and monetarily beneficial. It is also possible for external sources of motivation to lead to internal sources, where rewards encourage one toward task selection and an increasing number of goal-directed activities; then the experience of satisfaction and fulfillment occurs, is repeated, and dominates the wish to participate and succeed. It appears as though intrinsic rather than extrinsic forms of motivation encourage greater persistence at an activity and may in the long run lead to better performances in many endeavors.

Tenth, a person's *concept* of himself or herself, the extent to which contentment and confidence are exhibited, will depend on a variety of personal experiences. A positive valence toward oneself provides a necessary impetus toward action. Such feelings will probably be represented by the level of aspiration decided on prior to performance. The personality structure of the individual, experiences and successful performances, and the reaction of others directed toward him or her, will be most influential in the development of self-image. Continual criticism and rejection can keep the sensitive person with tremendous potential from realizing this potential and cause that person to be classified as an underachiever.

As we can see, many personal factors can operate to influence motivation and, in turn, achievement potential and its realization. What can be done about those factors? A number of recomendations can be offered to resolve potential problems. After we highlight some of the orientations in psychology in regard to motivational considerations, this section of the book will be concluded with suggestions for using motivational techniques to the advantage of learners. A word of caution is in order, however. Approaches to motivational techniques depend not only on convincing research evidence, but also intuitive appeal, a sort of philosophy of human nature and what might work to promote performance/learning in situations. From the discussion so far, perhaps you have already formed opinions on to how to modify situations and influence learners and their behaviors.

Behavioristic Approaches (Reinforcements and Rewards)

A behavioristic approach toward motivation is associated with situational control over the learner, as with the deployment of positive or negative reinforcers. These are objects, events, or situations that increase the likelihood of the occurrence of some particular act. The nature of reinforcement will be discussed in Chapter 13, in which postpractice factors are analyzed. For now, we will focus on the effectiveness of rewards in directing behavior in a certain direction. Rewards are traditional examples of positive reinforcers. It should be pointed out, however, that many behavioristic techniques have been used in investigations and in real life, including threats, praise, punishment, immediate knowledge of results, varying amounts of rewards, and the introduction of prompts, cues, bells, buzzers, sounds, and music during performance. All of these techniques have been shown to improve performance. To the contrary, many have been questioned regarding their widespread use and possible deleterious side effects, as will be shown shortly, when we deal with intrinsic motivation.

Merely introducing a buzzer or bell at certain intervals of performance may elicit a greater work output. Data from the military tasks of tracking and pursuit, in which boredom from task monotony sets in, indicate the importance of novel stimuli interspersed during practice. If a motor skill is repeatedly performed, motivation, which might normally lessen, will probably increase with the introduction of various stimuli throughout a practice session.

Sometimes, experimenters do not find that various induced motivational factors influence performance. This may be because the subjects are already operating at a high level of drive on the task. Therefore, additional inducements will be ineffective. Many motor skills are by their very nature interesting and challenging to the learners. In such cases, additional incentives are unnecessary. In fact, extra imposed motivational techniques may impede performance in certain activities.

Employment of verbal instructions or inducements is one of the most widely used motivational techniques. Research evidence does indicate that this method helps in learning written materials, and there is some evidence to support the idea that it is also beneficial to motor performance.

Fleishman (1958) provides interesting data on the relationship between ability levels and motivation. Four hundred subjects were trained on the Complex Coordination Test, on which a subject must make appropriate stick and rudder control adjustments in response to successively presented patterns of visual signals. All of Fleishman's subjects were given five one-minute trials and then divided in two groups, one of which received continual verbal encouragement during certain rest periods between the remaining fifteen trials. In analyzing the data, Fleishman identified high-and-low-ability groups, based on scores made on the initial trials, and compared them under motivating and nonmotivating conditions.

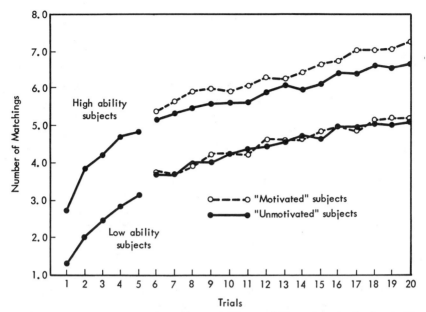

FIGURE 12-6. Acquisition curves for subjects of different ability and motivation levels. (*From Fleishman, E. A. A relationship between incentive motivation and ability level in psychomotor performance. Journal of Experimental Psychology, 1958. 56, 78–81.*) Copyright 1958 by the American Psychological Association. Reprinted by permission.

It was found that each group improved at about the same rate and in the same fashion. However, in the high-ability subjects, there was a significant difference in favor of the motivated group over the unmotivated group. The performance curves are presented in Figure 12-6. Environmental factors usually do not strongly affect the performance of skills that are well learned. There is a general stability in performance, despite different situations. However, personal observation and empirical evidence points to the fact that it is possible for the performance levels of the skilled to rise or fall when certain factors are present.

It is more likely, though, that, during the acquisition-of-skill stage, the effect of varying motivational conditions will be more noticeable. Before routines become well established and responses somewhat conditioned, environmental variations act as temporary depressants or facilitators to performance.

Varying the amount of reward appears to produce a change of performance in favor of the reward with the greatest magnitude. Studies on verbal materials have repeatedly demonstrated this occurrence. The same results appear in measuring short-term retention, for Weiner and Walker (1966) found that a greater strength of motivation during learning led to less forgetting. Four different incentives were used: 1-cent reward, 5-cent reward, shock for no recall, and withheld motivation. This investigation concerned the selecting of consonants for various colored slides, but it is inviting to speculate on the effect of similar incentives on motor performance. Assuming little or no inner drive of the learner, the instructor would have to turn to the most extreme motivating conditions in order to hasten skill acquisition. Once again, it is necessary to realize that individuals are not all motivated in the same manner by a particular form of motivation. Some respond better when they are yelled at and incited; others need inspiration as provided through different approaches. A grade, a position in the class or on the team, punishment, a note to the parents—these and many other techniques are specifically appropriate for a certain kind of person. Most ideal would be an in-depth analysis of the performer's personality and nature, so that the most appropriate motivational method, if needed, could be applied without subjecting an entire group to the same condition.

Coaches are often guilty of approaching all their athletes in the same way. One type of coach continually yells at the players to "fire them up." Unfortunately, some individuals will respond in a negative way when they are constantly under dramatic vocal fire. On the other hand, a mild-mannered coach who offers only praise when deserved and sympathy where warranted may be guilty of neglecting those athletes who need to be inspired vigorously. Anyone responsible for directing the motor learning process must understand and apply the appropriate motivational technique at the right time, one that is compatible with the demands of the task. Other approaches toward motivation, such as humanism and cognitive psychology, seem to address personal factors more than behavioristic programs.

Humanistic Approaches (Self-fulfillment)

In contrast to behavioristic control over behavior and imposed goals on students, humanists advocate ways and means of encouraging students to become more inner-directed and self-determined. Such leaders in psychology as Abraham Maslow, Carl Rogers, Gordon Allport, and Arthur Coombs have called for a greater insight into individual needs, hopes, feelings, and how students channel their energies toward self-actualization.

Such needs as affiliation, self-esteem, approval, independence, and self-preservation have been identified and analyzed. At the core is self-concept. It acts to cause present behavior and is the result of past experiences. Humanists believe in helping people to develop themselves with respect to various needs. Their concepts are associated with the new directions in cognitive psychology and the importance placed on intrinsic motivation.

Approaches in Cognitive Psychology (Attributions and Expectations)

As contrasted with the environmental control orientation of the behaviorist and the personalized self-attitudinal concepts of the humanist, motivational forces and factors are viewed somewhat differently by cognitive psychologists. According to cognitive motivational theory, our perceptions and mental processes, as they are used to interpret situations, outcomes of situations, and expectancies in situations, will have a great impact on behavior.

In Chapter 11, we dealt with aspiration, or performance expectancy level, and its influence on achievement. How one expects to do in a particular situation (reasonably high, specific, but attainable goals) will usually result in better performance, a reflection of individual control over motivation. Expectations are of central concern to cognitive psychologists. So are interpretations of the causes of behavior.

Such causative factors have been termed attributions. To what do we attribute the way we performed in an activity? The notion of locus of control (the feeling of being controlled by the situation and/or others, or the feeling of being in control over circumstances) has obvious implications for interpretations about how and why behaviors are expressed. Furthermore, attribution theory, initiated by F. Heider (1958) and advanced by Weiner (1974), has reflected an attempt to analyze the scope and impact of the factors people attribute to their performance to explain and predict behavior. These will be discussed in more detail in Chapter 13.

One of the basic tenets of cognitive motivational theory is the belief that students need to learn to be independent, in control, and confident and, in general, assume a sense of responsibility for personal actions. The position is more readily clarified in contrast to behavioristic approaches, in which behavior is to be shaped by rewards, or events external to the person, with little consideration for individual differences in expectations, attributions, perceptions, and attitudes. This discussion leads logically to an overview of the nature of achievement motivation concepts and programs, as a practical outgrowth of efforts in the area of cognitive psychology.

Achievement Motivation: Concepts and Programs

For believers in the development and maintenance of intrinsic motives, achievement motivation programs are particularly appealing. In contrast, the use and benefits of rewards, reinforcements, and behavior modification programs will be explored more fully in Chapter 13.

The need to be competent, to achieve, underlies the potential for success. Concepts and research on the need to achieve motive have been pioneered and developed through the years by psychologists David McClelland and John Atkinson. Characteristics of high achievers and low achievers indicate fundamental differences; various achievement motivation programs (e.g., Kolb, 1965) have been developed on the basis of these data. Many low achievers have the potential to accomplish, but due to personal and situational factors, do not. Extrinsic factors (rewards) and intrinsic factors (fulfillment) have been applied to influence behavioral change, although intrinsic ones are emphasized in achievement motivation programs.

Personal Characteristics of High Achievers. Individuals who have a high need to achieve usually (1) demonstrate an extremely high persistence at activities; (2) demonstrate exceptional quality in performance; (3) complete activities at a high rate; (4) are task-rather than person-oriented; (5) take reasonable risks and enjoy stress; (6) like to take personal responsibility for actions; and (7) like to have knowledge of the results of the activity in which they are involved (to judge capabilities in order to develop them further).

A recognition of these characteristics associated with a high need to achieve is important. Learners can be analyzed in order to determine the presence of such attributes and attempts can be made to develop them if they are not present in some students. It is apparent in education that the traditional approach of merely placing individuals into instructional programs is insufficient for assuming reasonable improvement. The same has been found to be true in industry and business. Productivity does not necessarily improve because procedures and policies are dictated. There are ways in which motives can be improved in order that work output and personal development can occur in a more desirable manner. Some of the key characteristics of an effective program that might be used to improve the achievement motive in those who are not well motivated have been identified.

Achievement Training. When trying to change performance and practice inclinations, instructors might first explore ways to *influence cognitive and affective behaviors.* Students like to be aware of the reasons why they should change their behaviors. Intellectualizing the experiences and attempting to modify attitudes seems to be a better approach than merely dictating training procedures. If learners are going to be involved in the program, they naturally will want to know what the program will do for them—that is, why they should be involved in it. It is through an interactive process that a rationale can be developed, ideas exchanged, understandings improved, and attitudes changed.

Somehow, *responsibility for performance* must be borne by the *participant-student* rather than the leader-teacher. Personal decision making and a perceived personal control over the situation will lead to a greater commitment. Once an understanding has been reached of the value of a particular program, procedures can then be agreed on to select the number of goals and how they can be attained. Some of the major principles, with regard to improving the achievement motive, follow:

1. Discussions between teacher and student, or coach and athlete, should be held about the *purposes* of a particular program. Communication channels should be open and conducive to an exchange of ideas. The goal is to increase understanding and to modify attitudes.
2. Working together, the participant and leader should set *specific, high, but attainable goals* in the program, under the guidance of the leader. Goals should be long term as well as short term, with the short-term goals providing the enabling activities in order to attain long-term goals. The participant knows that he or she has a role in the decision-making process and establishes personal goals.
3. *Procedures* to achieve the goals should be explored. As the student identifies the means to be used to achieve goals, the teacher can help determine whether the program can realistically help the person achieve the goals. In case there is incongruity between the program and the goals, either the goals should be low-

ered or the program intensified. Once again, this occurs through a mutual process of exploration and decision making.

4. Once the program has been determined, personal *records of progress* should be maintained. These are good for motivational purposes. They should be used for self-comparisons primarily, rather than comparisons against others.

5. Wherever possible, feelings of *self-confidence* and *self-image* should be enhanced. Much depends on the relationship of the teacher to the student. Reinforcement and communication processes can do much to help the participant gain the necessary self-confidence.

6. There should be a constant *reevaluation* of the progress and achievement rate of the learner. Perhaps goals will have to be shifted upward or downard or programs modified, depending on situations. A continual evaluation of progress is a necessity.

These, then, are the principles of a sound achievement training program. They, and other principles and programs, have been described by McClelland (1972). If they are adhered to, the attitudes and performances of many students should improve dramatically. Achievement can be reflected primarily through an interactive process, and both the teacher and the learner need to be involved in such a way as to build a working relationship toward the establishment and realization of goals. The command, or dictatorial, process has inherent flaws in it. On the other hand, allowing the participant free rein in the decision-making process is also a frivolous activity. Yet, a fruitful relationship between the student and instructor can emerge with careful planning and thoughtfulness. These procedures, unfortunately, are not recognized, advocated, or utilized in a sufficient number of situations. It is to be hoped that the recognition of an achievement orientation will lead to specially designed programs to enhance motives and productivity.

Extrinsic and Intrinsic Motivation

Motivation stems from an internal or external source. When the origin of a drive is from within a person—that is to say, something is done for its own sake—it is *intrinsiically motivated*. Performance in a skill or participation in a sport is for personal reasons, namely joy, satisfaction, or skill development. Intrinsic motivation implies self-actualization and ego involvement. An *extrinsically motivated* person persists at an activity for the material gain received from it. Intensive study in a class is done, not so much to acquire knowledge, as to attain a high grade. Participation in a sport is oriented for the possible recognition and glory, instead of for comradeship, inner satisfaction, and achievement. Extrinsic motivation is sometimes interpreted as need-deficiency motivation.

From an educational and ideal point of view, intrinsic motivation is more desirable than extrinsic motivation. Unfortunately, because of cultural practices, we are frequently rewarded materially from childhood throughout life for demonstrating correct responses and acceptable behavior. We expect and become conditioned to rewards. Inner drive, though, is usually a more sustained and effective form of motivation. It should be acknowledged that, in many situations, both extrinsic and intrinsic factors operate, but with varying degrees of impact. Yet, if motivation from within is the primary source of a person's, say an athlete's, endeavors, participation will more than likely continue after the days of fanfare, hero worship and excitement are over.

A number of examples exists where nonexisting intrinsic motivation may be overcome by powerful extrinsic motivation. A person may not be intrinsically motivated to master a task but may overcome this indifference by becoming extrinsically motivated, such as in seeking a high grade in a class. Studies with industrial workers indicate that motivation to achieve is increased when there is a chance of attaining an extrinsic reward (money, approval of others, and so on) in the future.

Nevertheless, there is research and theoretical support for the contention that an individual who has a strong belief in control over personal destiny is likely to achieve better, placing greater value on skill and achievement. Intrinsic motivation, in this respect, is an extremely powerful influence on behavior. If an individual perceives personal control in a situation, and reinforcement depends on his or her own behavior, "internal control" is demonstrated, according to J. B. Rotter (1966). "External control" describes a situation in which it is thought that one's behavior is dependent on luck or chance. Expectations of reinforcement as a consequence of behavior and the locus-of-control construct of Rotter are necessary to consider in any attempts to explain behavior. Individuals differ in their attitude toward a situation, depending on its control by external or internal factors, and develop expectancies accordingly.

What of the concept of the presence of a generalized intrinsic motivation in certain individuals? Is it true that some people do try harder and use their potential more effectively in a variety of situations? Is there a general need to achieve and succeed or to avoid failure regardless of the task or the person's capabilities? Although such may be the case in some instances, research evidence by Bernard Fine (1972) does not bear these premises out. The relationship of predictor tests— including hand immersion in cold (5°C) water, the Cattell 120-A Test and 16 Personality Factor Test, the Maudsley Personality Inventory, and a biographical inventory—to criterion tests, anagrams, the digit symbol substitution test, screw sorting, and hand dynamometer performance was determined with various statistical analyses. Fine did not find any general motivational factor as an acceptable predictor of performance. A particular aspect of motivation may be related to any task and situation.

The relationship of task level of difficulty to intrinsic and extrinsic forms of motivation has been conceptualized by Margaret Clifford (1972). It can be observed in Figure 12-7 that, as task complexity increases, intrinsic motivation plays a more important role. She writes:

> The relationship between task complexity and the effectiveness of intrinsic and extrinsic motivation suggests that while only a limited amount of intrinsic motivation is

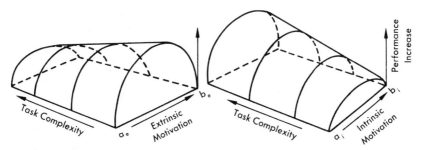

FIGURE 12-7. Relation of performance increase to task complexity and intrinsic and extrinsic motivation. (*From Clifford, M., Competition as a motivational technique in the classroom.* American Educational Research Journal, *Winter 1972, 9, 1, 123–137. Copyright 1972, American Educational Research Association, Washington, D.C.*)

associated with a simple task, a noticeable performance increase can be generated through extrinsic motivation. On the . . . [one] hand, a significant performance increase can be generated through extrinsic motivation. On the other hand, a significant performance increase on a highly complex task will be dependent upon intrinsic motivation.

In view of the typical problem-solving tasks students encounter, the model indicates that emphasis must be placed on intrinsic motivation. Educational researchers must attempt to systematically examine the effects of such intrinsic motives. This will involve the identification, measurement, and assessment of such factors as relevance of subject matter as perceived by the learner, need achievement of the student, tolerance for ambiguity, and optimum learning rates for individuals. The extent to which intrinsic motives can be developed, controlled, and manipulated is debatable. However, two points of concern appear evident: (1) learning of complex tasks is heavily dependent upon intrinsic motivation, and (2) too little applied educational research has been conducted to preclude the possibility of effectively manipulating factors related to intrinsic motives (p. 135).

Recent research points to another consideration. Extrinsic sources of motivation (e.g., rewards trophies, ribbons) that become associated with participation and performance and are expected in an activity may eventually undermine intrinsic motivation. These rewards are not contingent on personal performances related to personally established goals but are given for successful performance against an opponent or standard, or merely for participation, regardless of outcome. If the rewards are salient, the student becomes more concerned with rewards than the activity. Consequently, if the rewards are terminated, participation in an activity may also cease (Deci, 1975).

A point must be made here. If the goal of competition, in academics or athletics, is to aid the person in developing feelings of competence, and rewards are to be used effectively, they must be contingent on the personal achievement of the participant. Rewards allocated without regard to the quality of performance have little or no value because they do not arouse the intrinsic interest that becomes associated with effective control (Ross, 1976). A person who feels in control over performance will make internal attributions regarding that performance. Participation in that activity will continue because it is intrinisically interesting, it enhances self-concept, and it provides a means for self-testing in a task that will provide information about personal ability.

It seems plausible to conclude, then, that the development of intrinsic interest in an activity will cause an individual to continue participation in that activity. Extrinsic rewards given merely for participation may result in devalued behavior (Nisbett & Valins, 1972) and reduce future participation in that activity (Lepper & Greene, 1975). Subjective perception of competitive behavior in this case is that the behavior is less desirable and valuable in its own right (Nisbett & Valins, 1972). It has become a means to an end. If this is the case, intrinsic motivation decreases and interests wanes.

As Dorothy Harris (1977) has rightfully warned, we are still not clear about what the ideal ratio is for extrinsic and intrinsic sources of motivation in order to maximize a person's potential continuation in sport. Both types are important and have specific purposes. Ideally, all participants in sport will always be intrinsically motivated, but of course this is not the case. Perhaps, however, we can work more effectively in this direction.

It would be a mistake to suggest that all rewards have devastating effects on behavior and should be done away with. There are two major warnings here, as recognized by Daryl Siedentop and Gregory Ramey (1977). One concerns reinforcement programs and the other, what is conveyed to a performer when a reward is received.

Reinforcement or behavior modification programs are typically used to increase behaviors that have a low frequency or low probability of being emitted by a person. Reinforcers would be helpful in this regard. If administered properly, they would be withdrawn as behaviors are shaped in the desirable direction, perhaps leading to the development of intrinsic motivation for the particular activity.

If the nature of rewards controls people, the rewards should be questioned. But if they are informational and contingent on actual (quality) achievement, they could be effective. As Siedentop and Ramey write, ''The perception of attributing causality to oneself or to the controlling effects of external rewards may prove to be a very relevant issue,' (p. 60). Thus, how one perceives rewards, as controlling them or as supplementary reinforcement for what one knows already, must be considered.

Situational Techniques: Considerations for Training

As we ponder the many sources of motivation presented in this section of the chapter, and think of yet others to be discussed in the next chapters, it becomes obvious that a variety of techniques is available to the instructor to enhance the motivation of learners. The identification of various personal, societal, and activity considerations with regard to motivation is helpful in designing appropriate instructional and training strategies to increase the probabilities of optimizing each person's motivation and performance. The motivational properties of any activity and situation can be influenced through subtle or direct training techniques. The following list of considerations is by no means exhaustive; actually, it should be viewed as a summary of the key points made in this section of the chapter and to be discussed in Chapter 13.

1. *Rewards, praise, and reinforcers.* The use and effectiveness of these techniques have been addressed to some extent so far and will be treated in more detail in Chapter 13.

2. *Punishment and threat.* The use of these techniques can encourage motivation due to fear (not a very desirable educational approach).

3. The availability and provision of *knowledge of results,* with consideration for specifity, frequency, and type, with regard to performance will be addressed in Chapter 13.

4. *The establishment of personal goals and expectations.* Level of aspiration or performance expectancy is related to achievement. Many people can and do establish realistic and high performance goals; others do not. Because goal level will reflect past successes and failures in similar situations—and are, in turn, interpreted according to absolute or relative standards—it is quite necessary for individuals to view their performances within a realistic framework of personal development, potential, and the nature of each experience. By ensuring one's rational interpretation of each performance, there is less chance of poor performance in a future situation resulting from loss of motivation because of (a) overconfidence and an unrealistically positive interpretation of past performances; or (b) underconfidence and an unrealistically negative appraisal of past performances.

5. *The development and presentation of instructor objectives.* Students should be aware of the instructor's specific expectations.

6. *Competition against and cooperation with others* (to be discussed later).

7. *Instructor enthusiasm, leadership style, and the compatibility between teacher and student* as to communication style and belief in the teacher.

8. *Training programs and practice procedures.* Training programs and practice procedures should be *interesting and meaningful* to the students. "Enabling activities," those that will facilitate the progress of the person to realize goals oriented toward the future, constitute the contents or practice. If these activities are interpreted by the student as relevant to the achievement of his or her goals, motivation will be increased and practice sustained in an enthusiastic manner. Perhaps it might be a good idea for the teacher to explain to the learner the rationale behind certain training procedures, especially if it appears that some resistance might be exhibited. In an era where authority figures are being questioned more and more, and youth are encouraged to think, analyze, and question, a "do-as-I-say" attitude in learning situations does not work as universally as was the case years ago.

Enabling activities are only meaningful when perceived as such by those who must perform them. Intensity and duration of practice will be partially reflected by the favorable attitudes held by the learner toward the training procedures. An understanding of their importance encourages the student to practice conscientiously.

9. *Student participation.* The establishment of personal goals and training procedures can be effective.

10. *Intrinsic motivation.* It appears that the development of intrinsic motivation will lead to more satisfying, long-lasting results in motor performance. Feelings of fulfillment, expression, and involvement will probably inspire the typical learner to greater achievement over a longer period of time than participation for more materialistic gains. The preponderance of achievers most likely receive both internal and external benefits from their performances: one can achieve a sense of fulfillment as well as bask in the glories of fame and prestige. Nonetheless, favorable disposition toward the activity for personal, "idealistic" purposes would seem to be a strong and compelling force to continue conscientious training over a great span of time. In societies that seem to encourage the selection and demonstration of behaviors that depend on reward systems, it is difficult to sustain motivation and best performance. A heavy reliance on rewards to influence the nature and type of behaviors is not as desirable as the emittance of behavior that is self-generated for personally rewarding reasons. Figure 12-8 illustrates extrinsic and intrinsic sources of motivation.

Continual skilled performance may be defined in part as the ability to perform under self-regulation and direction rather than under the influence of external sources and environmental cues. It may also reflect a change from dependence on extrinsic sources of motivation to internally generated sources. Extrinsic incentives may operate effectively to affect the attitudes of someone toward an activity and to stimulate an interest in it. The motivation to train may also occur. But, ideally, the major source of action should change from extrinsic to intrinsic. Even

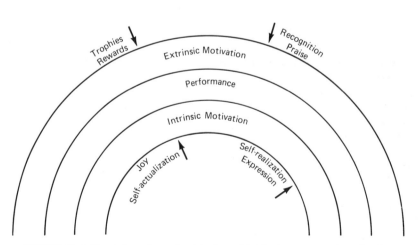

FIGURE 12-8. The interaction of extrinsic and intrinsic sources of motivation.

more ideally, the primary initial rationale for undertaking an activity would be because of its intrinsic value to the participant.

11. *Learner feelings of control over self and task outcomes.* A more ideal situation is when a learner's locus of control is internal rather than external. That is to say, he or she perceives to be in "command of the situation." Performances are viewed as being due to personal ability and effort, when appropriate, and are not due merely to luck or other factors that are not under the control of the learner.

12. Instructor development of *student confidence, security, self-worth, and self-concept.* The motivation for students to persevere and to achieve will depend on the kinds of reinforcement they have had and felt, relative to previous experiences. A positive and realistic image of oneself is related to motivation and performance potential. Teachers are often guilty of berating students, of being negative to them. Some students are emotionally tough and will respond sufficiently to the Darwinian approach, which imposes a survival-of-the-fittest model. Others are quite sensitive and can literally be destroyed by heartless teachers.

It is amazing to see so many potential achievers who do not perform according to capabilities because of a loss of motivation that was influenced by a loss of self-confidence. Positive reinforcement is a valuable tool for the dramatic improvement of one's self-image. Experiencing successes also helps immeasurably. Situations and learners should be compatible in that the possibility of achievement is present on various occasions. Achievement does not necessarily have to be evaluated in terms of accomplishments over others. Performance according to previous performances and potential can also indicate a form of personal achievement.

13. The provision of *knowledge of results* when appropriate. This information serves different purposes, one of them motivational.

14. *Student success.* Students should be provided with tasks they are capable of achieving, primarily against their own standards and capabilities, rather than against normative data. Students need nonthreatening experiences and failure-avoidance strategies.

15. *Student thinking, decision making, and responsibility for actions.* As M. V. Covington and R. G. Beery (1976) write: "In the long run, the success of student-centered instruction depends on strengthening the underlying skills of autonomy, originality, and independence of thought that sustain it, and, in turn, the exercise of these skills depends on the opportunity to use them" (p. 141).

16. *Individual student needs, feelings, and reactions.* No application of induced motivation can be made intelligently without regard for individual differences. There are general guidelines that can be most helpful in dealing with people collectively. But a sensitivity to dissimilarities among learners with respect to personalities, values, reactions to incentives and situations, and the like will enable the instructor to treat each individual as needed.

This list, although not conclusive, provides a sufficient basis for the consideration of alternative or supplementative approaches to motivation. The ultimate goal is for learners to possess the optimal motivation for each task (see Figure 12-9).

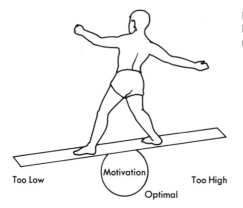

FIGURE 12-9. The delicate balance between motivation and performance.

Too Low   Motivation   Too High

Optimal

ATTENTION

The capacity of the learner to receive information or cues from the immediate learning situation and to encode, translate, store, interpret, and make appropriate decisions about motoric responses is influenced to a great extent by attentional processes, as described by Steven Keele (1973). Keele indicates that time is limited, with regard to the storage of information and its retrieval. Movements take time, also. Attention is associated with many aspects of information processing and performance, because attentional capabilities provide the framework for what we can do and how we do it.

The ability to attend selectively to cues and to maintain attention as necessary during an activity is a requirement of successful performance. The sequential and potential parallel active and ongoing processes, from input to output, were described in Chapter 6. However, the nature and importance of attention was alluded to but briefly then and deserves a much deeper analysis. Conceptual directions and research relevant to our understanding of attention and the processing of information will, therefore, be described in more detail here, as they influence the practicing of an act and contribute to the acquisition of skill in that act.

The Processing of Information

It is obvious that at anytime a few of the vast array of environmental and personal sources of information may be attended to by a learner/performer. These potential cues are not functional until they precipitate some behavior; or, in other words, they have been attended to. *Attentiveness refers to the readiness of a person to receive certain information and process it,* and this state may fluctuate at any time.

To some degree, a state of attention is associated with arousal states and degree of concentration, as pointed out by D. E. Berlyne (1970). However, he also distinguishes between those terms. For instance, at an extreme level of arousal, a person's attentiveness may be poor as a result of momentary changes in situational information. Concentration would refer to the extent of a person's attention, whether it be on a wide or narrow range of inputs.

The ability to exhibit prolonged concentration in activities of some duration often discriminates between successful and unsuccessful performers. Somehow, the learner must develop a state of ideal intermix between relaxation and intensity of effort. The balance is delicate. The highly skilled appear to reach this state without conscious effort. The beginner who tries to relax usually loses concentration and, paradoxically, becomes too tense when attempting to concentrate. Guidance and experiences lead to the preferred organismic state.

Although described for tennis in a popular publication (Gallwey, 1976), the state of relaxed concentration is a necessary condition for achievement in all tasks. Attention must be flexible and adaptable. At times it might be only on the ball, and at other times, a scanning ability may be desirable. The opponent's placement on the court, anticipation of his or her strategies, and a predetermined but adaptive personal response mode suggests the need for a wide band of focus. However, in its usual sense, attention is probably most associated with the term *selective attention*. The implication is that the human behaving system is maintaining a "weeding-out" process, or focusing on a restricted number of cues, or only on one, for that matter.

But it is important to remember that attentional processes operate sequentially in an activity, not only in preparation to a reaction to some stimulus event. Berlyne (1970) also suggests that there is attention in learning, attention in remembering, and attention in performance. More than likely, the beginner works hard at developing attentive processes; the advanced learner performs well as a result of having learned to use attentive processes without conscious direction.

Conceptual Orientations: Single and Multichannel Models

The area of attention was dormant for many years until rejuvenated in 1958 by the efforts of Donald Broadbent in his now classic book. He proposed a mechanical model of the single-channel concept, with human auditory attention perceived as a "Y." He suggested that although two pieces of information may enter the human system simultaneously, only one can funnel down the stem at any given time. W. B. Knowles (1963) supported Broadbent's views. In comparing a person to a multiplex communication system using a single channel to transmit messages from several sources to several destinations, Knowles (1963) suggests that:

So long as the channel is connected to a given source and a given destination, messages from other sources to the same or other destinations cannot be transmitted. The basic channel has a fixed capacity, but within this capacity overall rate of information flow can be maximized by proper coding and switching routines (p. 157).

Knowles' idea of switching is essentially the same concept referred to as gating in Broadbent's early works. In both instances, it is implied that attention may switch between input channels. A. B. Kristofferson (1967) has theorized that the switching is controlled by an internal "clock" that generates a succession of equally spaced points in time. Elaborating on the clock analogy, Kristofferson (1967) has postulated two major functions performed by the time points:

> They determine when attention can, but need not, switch from one input channel to another. And they also determine when messages which are in one stage of central processing can be transmitted to a subsequent stage (p. 93).

Within this conceptual framework, information is thought to be fed into the central processor via functionally independent channels whose boundaries are defined in terms of attention. Accordingly, the channel is thought of as "a set of all possible messages which can be admitted simultaneously into the central processor" (Kristofferson, 1967, p. 94). Whether a message may actually bypass the central processor seems to depend on the use that must be made of the information; this, in turn, depends on the nature of the task. A task that is highly automatic to the subject may not require attention, thus, in effect, circumventing the central processor. It is assumed that the organism processes information along independent channels that may be switched one at a time into a central processor. Second, on occasions when attention must switch channels, an increment of time is added to that necessary to process the message.

The limits of human information processing have most frequently been deliberated within the framework of the single-(limited) channel hypothesis. According to this premise, the execution of simultaneous tasks is maintained by time sharing the access to a central processing channel. Speculations vary as to the precise nature of the central limitation, but supporters of the single-channel hypothesis have generally indicated that there is a decrement in mutual task performance owing to the demands of the time-sharing situation (Brown, Tickner, & Simmonds, 1969; Colavita, 1974; Kristofferson, 1967; Lindsay, 1970; Noble, Trumbo, & Fowler, 1967).

On the other hand, certain investigators have conceptualized information processing within a different framework. Allport, Antonis, and Reynolds (1972) have forwarded evidence in support of a multichannel hypothesis that incorporates A. Triesman's (1969) notion of specific feature analyzers. The multichannel model, composed of a number of independent special-purpose processors operating *in parallel,* is said to accommodate simultaneous task performance to the extent that the requirements for the specialized processors do not overlap. Thus, the limits of information processing, according to this multichannel approach, are a function of the dissimilarity of the concomitant tasks involved.

Research Paradigms: Divided Attention

An analysis of primary task performance under varying levels of secondary task demands, or decisional stress, was the type of paradigm developed to resolve issues, in order to contribute to an understanding of information-processing capacities. A number of investigators have sought to assess the relative effects of a secondary loading task on primary task performance. Investigators have made use of an auditory shadowing task in analyzing the concomitant performance deterioration on a primary tracking task. Also, the performance of a tracking task has reduced the speed and accuracy with which subjects could read four visual displays. Pursuit rotor performance has declined proportionately to the intensity of secondary task (foot-pedal responses) demands. Specific perceptions related to car driving ability have been impaired in the presence of such secondary tasks as using a car phone.

Some investigators have attempted to interpret their findings within the single-channel framework. Noble et al. (1967) found that a secondary verbal task resulted in a marked interference with performance on an electronic tracking task, especially in relation to the timing involved. They contended that the interference rested not in the simultaneous processing of information but in the selection and implementation of the responses. This interpretation lent support to Adams' (1966) recasting of the one-channel mechanism as a decision mechanism that functions to resolve event uncertainty, but only to the extent that this resolution process involves the selection of a response.

Such concurrent response limitations have often been explained in terms of time switching. Reaction time to certain and uncertain auditory and visual stimuli led Kristofferson (1967) to suggest that decrements in performance were the result of the time required to switch between sense modalities. Reviews of intersensory processes have generally shown that subjects require time to learn how to process bimodal information, even when the secondary input operates in an accessory fashion. J. Halpern and A. E. Lantz (1974), studying auditory and visual information accessory input, reported that bisensory interference was particularly evident during the early stages of practice. These findings suggest that certain stages of performance may be particularly sensitive to the information-processing loading produced by the task, regardless of the nature of information, pointing to a limited human information-processing capacity.

Terminology in this area of research has been somewhat confusing. It is essential at this point to distinguish among task-demand situations and to clarify terms as they relate to our discussion. The task under investigation, and to which additional tasks are added, is usually referred to as a primary task. If the subject is instructed to avoid making errors on the primary task, the secondary task is called a subsidiary task. On the other hand, if the subject is instructed to aim for error-free performance on the secondary task at the expense of the primary one, the secondary task is called a loading task.

A loading task has been used as the distraction stressor for the primary task in a number of studies in order to analyze a fundamental dichotomy between the single-channel approach and the multichannel approach: the issue of whether the human system is a sequential or parallel processor of information when it must respond simultaneously to dissimilar tasks. In addition, the relative effects of high and low distraction stress on the learning of a primary task have been examined.

A simple summary of the single-channel model and the parallel processing

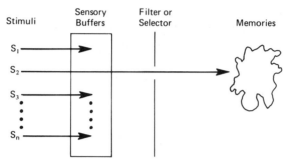

FIGURE 12-10. A schematic representation of single-channel or filter theory. Only one signal at a time gains access to the memory system. *(Keele, S. W., & Neill, W. T. Mechanisms of attention. In E. C. Carterette & P. Friedman (Eds.), Handbook of perception (Vol. 9). New York: Academic Press, 1978.)*

model has been illustrated by Keele and Neill (1978) and is reproduced in Figures 12-10 and 12-11. As we will see, research has been reported to support the existence of both models, depending on situations and task demands.

A. J. Marcel (1970) has analyzed the issue of whether the processes involved in memory search and recognition are carried out sequentially or in parallel. Most processing activities appear to involve sequential steps. However, Marcel (1970) states that "one may attend to events simultaneously if they are on two functionally separate channels, but not if they are on functionally the same channel" (p. 90). With practice or experience, possibilities improve for individuals to change from sequential to parallel processors. With recoding or thinking, two units of analysis may be treated as one unit.

Beth Kerr (1973) has summarized the dual task literature as well as the literature on conceptual orientations about capacity during different mental operations. Some operations apparently require processing capacity, others do not and can proceed in parallel form. Thus, depending on the operations required by subjects, support can be generated for a single-channel capacity model or a parallel processing model.

Human Processing Capabilities

As we have seen, processing capabilities depend on a number of factors, in spite of the limited capacity that individuals possess to function capably from moment to moment. For instance, when time sharing between tasks, performance worsens unless (1) one of the tasks is sufficiently automatized (it does not make any real attentional demands), or (2) one of the tasks does not contain arousal properties (it is not demanding).

There is an optimal level of arousal for perceptual selectivity, a sort of ideal band width for attention. In a sense, attention is controlled by arousal level. When cues are available and properly attended to, the human system is operating in an ideal manner. Although capacities are fixed, appropriate strategies for processing will overcome many limitations.

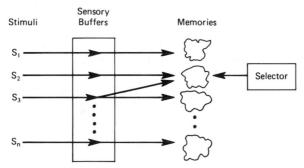

FIGURE 12-11. A schematic representation of parallel access of signals to memory followed by a mechanism that selects one activated memory or another. (*From Keele, S. W., & Neill, W. T. Mechanisms of attention. In E. C. Carterette & P. Friedman (Eds.), Handbook of perception (Vol. 9). New York: Academic Press, 1978.*)

The human system can be "loaded" with demands on the input side or on the output side, either or both of which will lead to longer reaction times due to greater processing demands. Consider, if you will, the number of stimulus alternatives or response alternatives that may be present in any task situation. The greater the number, the longer the reaction time. And if there is uncertainty as to the appropriate stimulus and appropriate response, times may be even longer. Figure 12-12 provides this relationship. A fast reaction time and quickness in movement are prerequisites for skilled performance in many instances. Figure 12-12 shows how the human system can become loaded and overloaded, with predictable response outcomes. E. Legge and P. J. Barber (1976) have indicated that response uncertainty (and selection) is twice as important as stimulus uncertainty (stimulus identification) in determining reaction time.

In a dual-task paradigm, Christopher Wickens (1976) concluded that limits of attention are more severe at the output than at the input stages of processing.

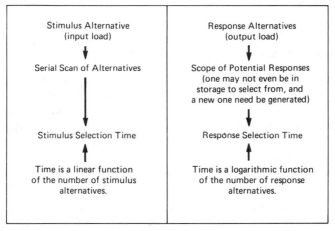

FIGURE 12-12. Time as a function of stimulus or response alternatives.

Thus, from another perspective, evidence is provided to emphasize that attention may influence perceptual and response processes differentially. As more is known about relevant factors, performance expectations will be predicted better and instructional procedures can be more sensitive to such human limitations.

Processing capabilities, as has been shown, depend on input, central monitoring or output demands, and the ability of the person to decrease attentional load through the use of appropriate strategies. Limits of attention will be reflected by the mental processes activated and needed for performance of one or more ongoing tasks.

INSTRUCTIONAL AND TRAINING TRADE-OFFS

Choices among procedural alternatives in instruction are often difficult to make. The instructor of skills has many potential decisions to make with regard to the conduct and organization of instructional procedures. In a number of cases, trade-off situations exist. In other words, something is gained and something is lost, depending on the alternative selected. An emphasis on speed versus accuracy in the practice of a skill is a good example of this. With increased speed, accuracy is usually diminished, and vice-versa.

In other situations, the trade-off may be time. Is it better to practice a skill continuously or with rests, or to have alternative skills interpolated throughout practice? Another type of trade-off has to do with the objectives of the training program and the learning strategy advocated. For instance, if the immediate speed of acquiring skill is important, a highly guided and directed type of instruction might be supported. If transfer and retention are of .consideration, perhaps a problem-evolving approach in the initial learning situation would be more desirable.

With these examples, we can see that the management of on-going practice is no easy matter. The topics to be addressed here have generally been investigated for many years and are no strangers to researcher and practitioner alike.

Management of Practice Sessions

Anyone interested in the most efficient means of skill learning must invariably consider the length of the practice sessions, their frequency in a given period of time, and the work-rest ratio within a practice period. The effective use of time, as defined by maximum productivity or skill development in minimum practice time, can be determined theoretically from the results of countless investigations found in the psychological literature.

Of course, many factors other than time allotment and distribution are involved in the eventual acquisition of a skill. Some factors are obvious and observable; e.g., the relative difficulty of the skill, the amount and quality of instruction offered, available facilities and equipment, and the capabilities and developmental status of the learner. Other factors are not so apparent and might include motivation and determination, emotional status, and mental readiness. All these factors operate in various combinations to affect the outcome of the administration of practice sessions.

Many of these variables are difficult to isolate and control. One aspect of the learning situation that can be directed by the instructor is the amount and distribution of time to be designated for the acquisition of a skill or a group of skills. Any teacher or coach is interested not only in providing a period of long enough duration for skill attainment, but also in apportioning the time so that it might bring the most desired immediate and future results. Attempts to improve learning efficiency in any field of activity must consider the problem of optimal spacing of training sessions and the spacing of skills or rest during a particular practice session.

Length and Spacing of Practice

What is the ideal length of practice periods and rest intervals? Although it would be satisfying to be able to propose a set answer, the problem is not so simple. Obviously, if the activity is a physically demanding one, attention to cues will diminish and learning in general will suffer as fatigue increases. In this case, the length of the session should be relatively short if maximum learning potential is to be realized.

The skill level of the performer is another consideration. Beginners normally have shorter spans of attention than advanced performers, and their motivation is very much more variable. Hence, as a general rule, practice periods may be increased in length (to a point) as skill is attained. Children usually sustain interest in a specific activity for briefer time periods than adults, and instructional periods should be weighed accordingly. These are but two of the commonsense approaches toward practice scheduling.

In one of the more novel experiments on practice schedules, C. G. Knapp and W. R. Dixon (1950) had two groups of college students learn how to juggle. One group juggled three balls for five minutes each day and the other group practiced fifteen minutes every second day until the criterion of successful juggling was met: one hundred consecutive catches. An analysis of the data indicated that the first group learned the task much faster, with one minute of practice in group I equal to one minute and eighty seconds of practice in group II. The investigators concluded from these results that learning a task such as juggling was enhanced by shorter practice and shorter rest periods. This and other studies support the belief in shorter practice and rest periods and, in general, practice extended over a longer duration of time.

From a practical standpoint, many educators wonder whether the semester or trimester college plan is best for the assimilation of knowledge. Similarly, physical educators are concerned with the relative effects of each plan on skill acquisition. I. F. Waglow (1966) observed the effects of a seventeen-week semester and a fourteen-week trimester on skill achievement in tennis, golf, and handball. Actually, 1,800 minutes of class time were devoted to each activity under the semester plan and 1,820 minutes were appropriated under the trimester plan. Even so, Waglow found a significant difference in favor of the semester plan for tennis and golf, but not for handball.

When examining the amount of learning of elementary school girls in a throwing-velocity task, over time (six weeks), Dean Austin (1975) noted that distributed practice resulted in a progressive learning curve and a significantly greater amount of learning than massed practice.

It would generally appear, then, that *gross motor skills can be learned more efficiently with shorter but more numerous sessions spaced over a longer time period.* Many studies can be found in which sports skills, prose, nonsense syllables, inverted alphabet writing, digits, mazes, concepts, symbols, aerial gunnery, typing, piano playing, and pursuit rotors have been used as learning tasks. Summarizing all this research, it is apparent that the optimal rest period necessary for the acquisition of verbal, written, or motor skills varies with the material used. Of twenty-four studies reviewed by this writer at one time under the topic of optimal rest intervals between practice periods, thirteen showed superior performance with a greater distribution of practice; eight studies indicated a preference for a rest interval somewhere in the middle of those used; and in three investigations no difference in performance was found with the various intervals employed.

However, these results are somewhat misleading, as what may have been a minimum rest between trials in one study may have been the maximum rest interval used in another. It is difficult to reach a conclusion, except perhaps that somewhere between too little rest and too much layoff is the desired condition for practice. Also, gross motor skills may be acquired better with more of a rest interval between practices than can other types of learning material, e.g., nonsense syllables and pursuit rotors.

In motor learning as in weight training, there seems to be a point of diminishing returns. Present evidence does not support the contention that five days a week of weight lifting is more effective in increasing strength than three days a week of lifting. Similarly, D. Massey (1959) found very little difference in the manner in which three groups performed on a stabilimeter (star-tracing) task as a result of their prescribed practices. One group practiced three days a week for five weeks, a second group practiced five days a week for five weeks, and a third group had only nine days of practice. On this particular task, nine days of practice were sufficient for skill acquisition, which means that actually sixteen of the twenty-five practice days that the second group had seemingly were wasted.

There are many ways in which practice and rest schedules can be altered. Yet, in most of the studies discussed here and even in research not mentioned in this section, interest has been directed primarily to immediate performance rather than to the ultimate retention of what has been learned. The next section, which deals with massed and distributed practice, also will include a number of investigations primarily concerned with the immediate effects of the varied practice schedules. Any conclusions on the relative effectiveness of various training procedures should be made after a review of the material on retention, to be presented later.

Massed Versus Distributed Practice

The distribution of time allotted for the learning of a specific skill has posed a serious problem to instructors, especially because there are usually many skills to be learned in a limited period of time. Ultimately, the instructor may utilize one of the following methods of practice. On the one hand, students could consistently and continuously practice the skill to be learned without any intermittent pauses. This method is termed massed practice. On the other hand, the students might learn the skill in shorter but more frequent practice sessions. These practice periods would be divided by rest intervals or intervals of alternate skill learning, a condition known as distributed practice. Is the continuous practice period more effective in skill acquisition and retention than one broken by spaced rest periods? Is it better to practice a task with very little interruption for rest or is rest beneficial to learning and performance? If pauses are desired, what are the optimal intervals between practice trials?

In attempts to improve learning efficiency in any field of activity, considerations must be given to the problem of optimal spacing of training sessions. Some instructors are in favor of teaching a skill in one session and having the students practice this skill repetitiously in the one period. Other instructors believe in requiring the students to practice different skills for a short duration at each meeting. The actual length of time devoted to the learning of a skill under massed and distributed conditions might be the same. However, under massed conditions the practice of the skill occurs continuously in one session, whereas the practice of this same skill under distributed conditions would be limited each session but practiced in a number of sessions.

The relative effectiveness of concentrating all practice or study into one session, as compared with dividing it into smaller units to occur at varying intervals of time, is not easily determined. Numerous studies have been completed in psychology on the distribution of practice effects on learning, the earliest in 1885 by Ebbinghaus. Unfortunately, very little work may be found in the experimental literature relating to the effects of distribution of practice on the learning and retaining of gross motor skills. Nevertheless, popular opinion is that short, frequent performances are more favorable and profitable to learning than long sessions crowded into a brief span of time. In a laboratory setting, R. B. Ammons (1951) had two groups of ten subjects perform thirty-six practice trials on the pursuit rotor. The massed practice group was not allowed any rest between trials, whereas the distributed practice group paused five minutes between trials. Distributed practice was favored under the various performance achievement criteria used by the experimenter.

In an athletic situation, Coleman Griffith (1932) noticed similar results. He had one group of basketball players continuously shoot a basketball for an hour, whereas another group shot three minutes and relaxed two minutes for an hour. The next day the procedures were reversed. Both groups shot about an equal amount of time; but when shooting with frequent rest periods, the men averaged 15 per cent more baskets than when shooting steadily.

These are but a sample of the investigations in this area of learning. Figure 12-13 typifies the relationship of massed and distributed practice effects.

In spite of the general findings indicating the preferability of some form of distributed practice over massed practice, leading theoreticians have had reservations in advocating this procedure. The reason for this is that in a number of recent studies in which measures of retention were employed, invariably no differences in performance were noted between massed and distributed practice groups. Yet, there is little reason to doubt the *superiority of distributed practice over massed practice for immediate performance* in a variety of tasks. It appears that performance is greater under distributed practice, for superior task scores to those found under massed practice are invariably reported in the research literature. Yet, this impression may be deceptive.

Skill retention is not favored so clearly under one practice condition. After a rest interval, tests of retention usually indicate a lessened dissimilarity in performance between groups trained under massed and spaced practice conditions. In other words, it appears that varied practice conditions, because of the temporary aspect of their influence, affect performance more than they do learning. Massed and distributed practice, when administered within reason, are probably approxi-

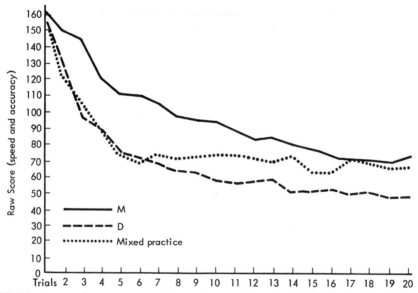

FIGURE 12-13. Performance comparisons of massed practice (M), distributed practice (D), and mixed practice on a stabilometer task. The massed-practice group had twenty consecutive trials, the distributed practice group was allowed a one-minute rest period between trials, and the mixed practice group had five trials of distributed practice and the remaining fifteen of massed practice. Notice how the mixed-practice learning curve assumes the characteristics of each practice method at the different points of the experiment. The distributed practice method is clearly more effective throughout the practice trials. (*From Lorge, I. Influence of regularly interpolated time intervals upon subsequent learning.* Teachers College Contributions to Education, *1930, 438.*)

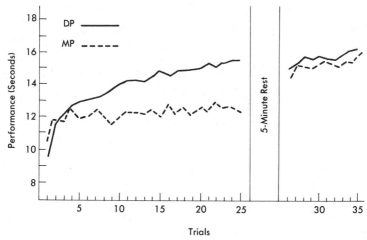

FIGURE 12-14. Performance curves for DP and MP groups. (*From Whitley, J. D. Effects of practice distribution on learning a fine motor task. Research Quarterly, 1970, 41, 576–583.*)

mately equally effective in promoting learning. If distributed practice primarily affected learning, the wide differences at the end of practice in favor of distributed practice would remain the same on later performance tests of retention.

Practice performance differences and retention comparisons can be seen in Figure 12-14, the data for which were collected by Jim Whitley (1970). A novel fine motor task involving foot tracking was administered to both groups of subjects. It is readily apparent that the differences and similarities between a massed practice (M) group and a distributed practice (D) group were in the expected direction.

Whole Versus Part Learning

Most skills can be taught in their entirety or broken down into parts. For example, the side stroke in swimming contains a coordinated leg pattern, a coordinated arm pattern, a breathing phase, and a relaxation stage. All these aspects of the stroke can be learned separately before the completed stroke is attempted, or the stroke can be practiced in its totality at the initial stages of learning.

The basketball lay-up is an example of another skill that can be learned by the whole method or in parts (the approach and dribble, the aim, the release, and the follow-through). Many times, it is not so easy to distinguish whole from part learning. *Whole* could refer to the sport itself, a skill in that sport, or even a part of that skill. In the latter case, when the arm stroke in the side stroke is taught so that each arm is practiced independently, that is an example of part learning. But if the arms are practiced as they coordinate with each other, it could be argued that whole learning is exemplified. It could also be argued that this is still part learning, because the complete side stroke is not being practiced. Therefore, it is possible to confuse the terms and what they label. One should view these terms as relative to each other and to the material learned. Broadly speaking, the problem concerns separate practice on each of several components, compared to practice on the whole task.

Some researchers have attempted to combine the features of both whole and part methods, creating whole-part and progressive-part methods. Whereas the part method implies equal practice or equal time devoted to the units, it is possible to practice the sequential parts with additional repetitions on weak units. The latter procedure allows the student to move from unit to unit only after each one has been mastered. The whole-part method, according to some researchers, may describe the situation wherein the learner views the desired end product and then practices each part until the skill is finalized. The progressive-part, repetitive-part, or continuous-part procedure requires the individual to practice already-learned units with each newly introduced unit. In other words, the subject practices one subtask, then the second subtask with the first, the third with the first two, until all subtasks are learned and performed together.

Psychologists generally agree that if a skill is relatively simple, the advisable procedure is to employ the whole method. More complex skills require some sort of breakdown. Although G. E. Briggs and W. J. Brogden (1954) found a superiority of whole over part practice on a complex coordination test, an analysis of their data suggests that the superiority of whole practice may disappear at high levels of task complexity. It is believed that if the learner is aware of the goal and how the final act should be executed, quicker insight will be gained into the problem. The parts will be more meaningful and will be more easily coordinated into the desired ultimate skill.

Researchers such as James Naylor and Briggs (1963) have distinguished two aspects of the task that might be considered before designating learning to proceed under part or whole conditions. *Task complexity* refers to the demands made on a person's memory and is a function of information processing. *Task organization* indicates the nature of the interrelationships of several task dimensions or components. A task has a low organization when there are only a few independent components comprising the task. The studies of these and other researchers suggest that part practice is more favorable for tasks of high complexity and low organization. When the organization is high, i.e., there is an increase of the component interaction, the whole method is preferable (see Figure 12-15).

Complexity in terms of task demands may be understood better by the following questions: How difficult does the learner perceive the task to be? How many things have to be thought about, to be remembered from previous related

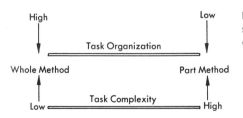

FIGURE 12-15. Part or whole practice as suggested against the criteria of task organization and task complexity.

experiences? To what extent is it possible to forget the task over time and, therefore, pose a challenge to the learner to remember it?

Because a highly organized task is one that contains a high degree of interrelationship among its components, it is necessary to be able to understand what interrelationship means. One criterion might be the sequence of movements involved. Another is the consideration for what the corresponding or opposing limbs (the entire body) are required to do at any one point in the execution of the task. Are many parts of the body involved or only a few? Are the arms working together or in different directions simultaneously? If the legs and arms are moving in similar patterns (e.g., the elementary backstroke), the task should be reasonably highly organized. With different patterns and other factors to consider (e.g., the crawl), the task becomes lowly organized. Thus, it can be seen that task organization, or interrelatedness of parts, is a function of (1) the sequence of movements involved and (2) the type, extent, and demands of the movements made at any one point in the task execution.

The use of the task organization–task complexity model for motor skills as shown in Figure 12-15 is highly speculative at the present time. There is difficulty with this paradigm when we start to think about sports skills (the tennis serve or golf swing) and realize that no skill will fit snuggly at one end of the continuum for either criteria.

Because it is sometimes difficult to establish where a skill would fall on the continuum, the same holds true for suggesting the application of whole or part instructional methods. At other times, there could be strong agreement on where a task can be placed in the paradigm. One of the cases where the most discrepancy lies is the golf swing. Where in the paradigm would you place it? The practical applications of the Naylor–Briggs model to physical education activities is described by Marion Johnson (1970). Furthermore, an attempt is made to define and discriminate among activity wholes and parts.

This problem of whole versus part learning is more complex for motor skills than for verbal materials. The fractionation of a task requires isolating components equal in difficulty and length, which is not easily done with typical motor skills. A survey of the research on physical activities indicates little preference for one method over the other. R. L. Wickstrom (1958) compared learning basic gymnastics and tumbling stunts by the whole method to the whole-direct repetitive method (similar to the progressive-part procedure, for the subjects practiced a part of a stunt and then moved on to the second part, combining both). He found little difference in the performances of the groups. In the teaching of sport skills, perhaps common sense might dictate which skills can be taught as wholes and which should be fractionated. Whole methods are to be advocated where possible, if for no other reason than efficiency, for as Wickstrom and other investigators have observed, whole-learning methods generally permit the student to reach a criterion in fewer trials than part methods.

It is difficult to generalize from task to task in favor of one particular method. Rather, it is more important to analyze what is to be learned. Perhaps the concepts of task complexity and task organization should be applied to the numerous motor activities for a more accurate indication of those skills that might be favored under whole- or part-learning conditions.

As a final thought, there is some opinion that more intelligent subjects are likelier to fare better under the whole method. F. J. McGuigan and E. F. Mac-Caslin (1955) collected data on rifle marksmanship for four days of firing at different yard markers. Groups were taught either under the whole method, which consisted of watching a demonstration and being instructed and practicing on all the subtasks together; or with the repetitive-part method, learning one subtask for firing, then the second at the same time with the first, and so on. Although the whole method yielded superior performance for all levels of intelligence in slow fire, a more challenging task, sustained fire, was learned more effectively under the whole method only by the subjects with above-average intelligence.

Sequential Order of Events: Serial Learning

In many real-life activities, a series of events must be completed in a predesignated order before an entire act is considered successful. If we once learned a list of words, we could be tested by the free recall method or tested for the recall of the exact sequence of the words in the original learning. For motor skill activities, invariably it is a specific serial order of events that must be executed. Psychologists have been able to control extraneous varibles to a great extent by studying the learning of lists of nonsense syllables, prose, and poetry. The learning of sequential materials, a particular order of parts comprising a whole, has been termed *serial learning*. When nonsense syllables are presented in random arrangement and subjects are allowed to recall them in any order they desire, studies have usually found the words at the end of the list to be most frequently recalled. However, when nonsense syllables are presented serially or organized material such as prose is learned, whatever was learned first is retained best, the last material is mastered second best, and the middle is last to be recalled.

Middle-learned material can be expected to be retained least well because of the negative influence of the preceding and succeeding learnings, among other factors. R. A. Magill (1976) attempted to determine whether similar findings would occur with a relatively simple motor task, a manual lever apparatus. The subjects had to learn three positions in serial order. Unexpectedly, the positions were learned best in the sequence presented to the subjects. If more positions had been required on each trial, we might speculate findings similar to the verbal literature.

Apparently, the level of recall of serial learning depends on a number of factors, notably the number of events or length of a word list, its structure and organization, and the organizational strategies used by the learner. A serial learning curve is most often a U-shaped curve that graphically depicts the existence of a primacy and recency effect. Proactive and retroactive inhibitory effects (negative transfer) seem to operate in traditional situations.

The bowing effect, or U-shaped curve, typically observed in verbal serial learning studies, is probably the result of the first and last learned items (primacy and recency) being somewhat isolated from interference effects. E. R. Harcum

(1975) and others have stated that the learner can take corrective measures to reduce interference, such as by constructing special memorial codes that reduce the number of possible alternatives. L. Postman (1963) has contended that recoding and rehearsal strategies can increase resistance to interference and maximize the effects of training.

In one of the few motor learning experiments, F. L. Hagenbeck (1978) used a curvilinear positioning apparatus in which subjects had to learn to move a lever to six serial positions. He was especially interested in the effects of particular learning strategies on the shape of the serial learning curve. Imagery, relevant labeling, and kinesthetic strategy groups showed the expected bowed serial acquisition curve during acquisition, indicating the primacy and recency effects. The irrelevant labeling and control groups exhibited a linear serial acquisition curve, indicating only a primacy effect. However, in tests of retention at five and sixty seconds later, the imagery group was most successful, followed by the relevant labeling group, in eliminating or controlling interference. In other words, Hagenbeck demonstrated support for the contention that a particular learning strategy can reduce interference. Apparently, organization is facilitated and an internal code is constructed. From a body-of-knowledge perspective, as well as for instructional and learning purposes, the effects of ordering materials and skills and improving the memory of the entire sequence need to be better understood.

Mental Versus Physical Practice

Active participation has traditional connotations, for we think of it as primarily emphasizing physical movement. Mental activity suggests inner conscious activation. Although no act is purely physical or solely cognitive, we will refer to such terms in their usual context for the sake of convenience in this section, in order to present research findings in which the relative effects of physical and mental practice on the learning of motor skills have been analyzed. Just how much activity is necessary, or to put it another way, to what extent can mental rehearsal be substituted for physical participation?

Time spent in overt (observable) physical activity may be replaced with verbal instructions and directions, films, viewing another's performance, reading material, and mental imagery or practice. The effectiveness of these techniques alone and in conjunction with actual physical involvement is of great interest to learners and instructors.

Numerous experiments support the contention that learning motor skills occurs with active overt practice and specific instruction. Evidence on ideal ratios of overt practice to other means of learning is conspicuous by its absence. There are many people who feel the only way to learn a motor skill is through active physical (overt) participation. The results of studies on covert (mental) practice serve to question this belief; and certainly the value of lecture, films, reading material, and the like cannot be denied. How much time should be devoted to any of these techniques as a replacement for activity?

Empirical evidence suggests that beginners profit more from overt involvement in the activity. One investigator who obtained contrary data, John Jones (1965), found that overt practice was not necessary for his subjects to learn a gymnastic skill, the hock-swing upstart. Covert practice was a sufficient condition for learning, and interestingly enough, undirected covert practice was found to be more effective than directed covert practice. Verbal and written instructions appear to be more beneficial and meaningful as an individual's skill level increases. This would be especially true with complex skills. Although there is no total substitution for participation, as the learner progresses, greater skill may be obtained when the activity is supplemented with various teaching aids, such as detailed verbal and written directions.

Mental practice is a form of passive learning in the sense that overt practice does not take place. In order not to offend those who would claim that the individual actively responds even during mental practice, it must be restated that this concept is indeed true. However, relatively speaking, the learner *appears* to be passive. *Mental* or *image practice* or *conceptualization* refers to task rehearsal in which there are no observable movements. Researchers have compared the effectiveness of learning tasks through actual physical practice with mental practice or a combination of physical–mental practice.

As far back as 1899, the question was raised as to whether gymnastic movements could be learned through covert practice even if they were not practiced overtly. The relationship of skill learning and muscle activity to conceptualization has been demonstrated in various ways in a number of experiments since that time. One of the earlier studies was completed by H. M. Perry (1939) in which he administered five tasks to his subjects, tasks that ranged from simple motor tasks to those demanding ideational and symbolic activities. The tasks were a three-hole tapping test, a peg-board test, a card-sorting test, a symbolic digit-substitution test, and a mirror-tracing test. Perry compared the effects of actual to mental practice on the performance of each task.

Mental rehearsal was found to yield significantly better performances on four of the five tasks than no practice at all. Physical practice was superior to conceptualization on three tasks; however, the mental practice group was favored on the peg-board task. Other researchers, in general, have obtained similar results. Typically, physical practice is better than mental practice, which, in turn, is better than no practice at all. L. V. Clark's (1960) subjects learned the Pacific Coast one-handed foul shot under conditions of physical and mental practice, and he found mental practice to be nearly as effective as physical practice.

In fact, E. Rawlings, I. L. Rawlings, S. S. Chem, & M. D. Yilk (1972) report the equally beneficial effects of mental and overt rehearsal on the learning of a pursuit rotor task. Three groups of female subjects participated in the study for ten days. The mentally rehearsed subjects pictured the apparatus (not in view) and imagined themselves performing the task without actually making the movements. In the first experiment, the overt and covert practice groups performed similarly after the ten days of practice and better than the no-practice group (see Figure 12-16). In the second phase of the study, with male subjects, the rest interval between trials was examined. As can be seen in Figure 12-17 the rate of learn-

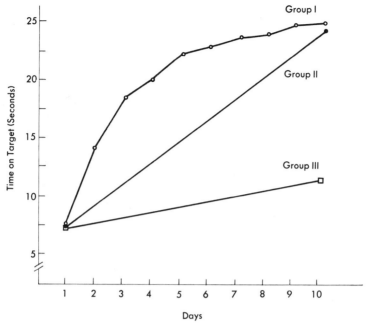

FIGURE 12-16. Mean total time on target for Days 1–10 for Group 1 (physical practice), Group 2 (mental rehearsal), and Group 3 (control). (*From Rawlings, E., Rawlings, I. L., Chem, S. S., & Yilk, M. D. The facilitating effects of mental rehearsal in the acquisition of rotary pursuit tracking.* Psychonomic Science, 1972, 26, 71–73.)

ing was fastest for group I. This group mentally rehearsed the task following each overt practice session, whereas the second group was engaged in a color-memory task following each overt practice session.

Other researchers, although noticing the significant beneficial effects of mental rehearsal, have not obtained such effective results from this form of practice. More in line with the general research findings in this area are the data obtained by W. E. Twining (1949), in which ring tossing was the skill to be learned. Three groups were involved, one that threw 210 rings on the first day and the twenty-second day; a second group that threw 210 rings on the first day and seventy rings each day from the second through the twenty-first day and 210 rings on the twenty-second day; and a third group that threw 210 rings on the first day, mentally rehearsed the skill for fifteen minutes daily from the second through the twenty-first day and threw 210 rings on the twenty-second day. The subjects, without practice, showed no significant learning. The subjects receiving physical practice improved 137 per cent. The subjects who had mental practice improved 36 per cent.

In investigations in which a third group is compared, one that is physically and mentally practiced, usual results indicate this method to be as effective as physical practice or slightly inferior to it. A combination of physical-mental practice is probably better than mental practice alone.

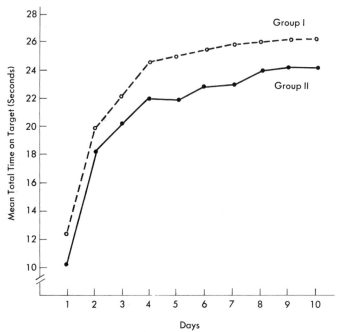

FIGURE 12-17. Mean total time on target for Days 1–10 for Group 1 (motor practice + mental rehearsal during rest period) and Group 2 (motor practice + color naming during rest period). *(From Rawlings, E., Rawlings, I. L., Chem, S. S., & Yilk, M. D. The facilitating effects of mental rehearsal in the acquisition of rotary pursuit tracking. Psychonomic Science, 1972, 26, 71–73.)*

Present-day investigators have attempted to come to grips with the many variables that might affect learning by mental practice. Some of these include the skill level of the learner on the skill to be learned, the novelty of the task, intelligence, kinesthetic sense, and ratios of physical to mental practice. Intelligence, for example, has a low correlation with various estimates of overt performance. Excellent summaries of the research on all topics related to mental rehearsal are presented by Alan Richardson (1967a,b).

Although it might be true that covert practice is only effective with tasks already overtly experienced by the learners, the question arises as to how it might formally be introduced effectively into a practice regimen that includes overt practice of a motor skill. In response, Singer and Witker (1970) designed an experiment to determine the point of introduction, in relation to overt practice, that covert practice might best facilitate learning (see Table 12-2) in a star tracing task. Four groups practiced mentally at various designated points during the overt practice context; the fifth group practiced without any mental rehearsal. The data were analyzed in various statistical ways, but no significant performance differences were found among the groups. As we can see in Figure 12-18, however, there appears to be a trend indicating some value of early introduction of mental rehearsal within the context of overt practice.

TABLE 12-2 Practice Schedules

Week	I		II		III		IV		V
Session	1	2	3	4	5	6	7	8	9
Group									
I	M	M	P	P	P	P	P	P	Posttest
II	P	P	M	M	P	P	P	P	Posttest
III	P	P	P	P	M	M	P	P	Posttest
IV	P	P	P	P	P	P	M	M	Posttest
V	P	P	P	P	P	P	P	P	Posttest

M = Mental Rehearsal
P = Physical Practice

(From Singer, R. N., & Witker, J. Mental rehearsal and point of introduction within the context of overt practice. *Perceptual and Motor Skills,* 1970, **31**, 169–170.)

Perhaps previous overt practice in more complex tasks facilitates the ease with which conceptualization takes place. It is quite difficult to envision the intricacies of an act unless one has had actual experience performing it, a hint that mental practice has more value with the highly skilled individual. A number of studies indicate that the novice gains faster with overt practice than with covert practice alone.

Another consideration is the ability level of the individual in a given task; that is, the person must have the necessary skill to perform the actions if instructions of any kind are to be valuable. Organized actions must correspond to verbal concepts. Words and concepts are only valuable in the motor learning situation to the extent that they can be translated into coordinated movements.

The learner must always have the correct task image in mind. For performance to improve, the individual probably has to have some match available—a match of the actual performance with an image of what the correct model is like. And there is a continual attempt to better performance until the image matches the model perfectly. The primary interest in the research reported here is how and to what extent deliberate mental rehearsal of a movement-oriented task affects the rate of learning and performance on it.

Aside from experimental data, empirical evidence indicates that almost all athletes subject themselves to some form of mental rehearsal before and even after competition. They constantly review, analyze, and conceptualize their performances, although usually in a less structured manner than has been employed in formalized experimentation. Nevertheless, at least one high school tennis coach has developed and implemented planned mental practice periods preceding and complementing the actual play of the athletes. Following one of these conceptualizing sessions, a player was overheard to comment, ''Hope I do in practice as well as I think!''

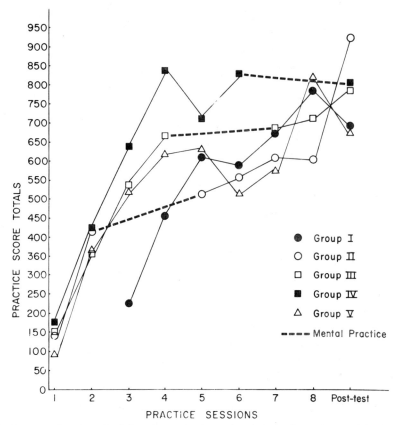

FIGURE 12-18. Practice schedules of mental rehearsal and physical practice combinations for different groups. (*From Singer, R. N., & Witker, J. Mental rehearsal and point of introduction within the context of overt practice.* Perceptual and Motor Skills, *1970, 31, 169–170.*)

An example of a structured program in sport has been developed by psychologist Richard Suinn (1976), who has worked with Olympic skiers. He calls his method visuomotor behavior rehearsal. This involves relaxation, the practice of imagery, and the use of imagery to help motor skill performance. Imagery is used to practice skills. Suinn reports great success with his technique. Exactly how mental rehearsal can be useful for all skill level performers in various activities has not been worked out yet, but the importance of cognitive processes in motor performance is becoming realized more and more.

Speed Versus Accuracy

When a motor skill is newly introduced to the learner, the instructor might have to decide whether it is best to practice this skill as fast as possible, as precisely as possible, or both. The right methodology can affect short-term as well as long-term success.

Many times the question is raised as to whether one should emphasize speed or accuracy in the early stages of learning. The tennis player might initially attempt to master accuracy in stroking by standing relatively still and concentrating on the stroke and the direction of the ball, or, practice could proceed under gamelike conditions, with the player striking the ball when constantly on the move, in and away from the net. The fencer might learn how to lunge by practicing slow, carefully calculated movements that emphasize form and accuracy; or, swift and agile movements associated with actual competition could be practiced.

When learning motor skills, accuracy has usually been emphasized first. However, there is evidence enough to justify that practice in sport should resemble game situations. Any skill should probably be rehearsed as it would be performed on the job or in the "real" situation. Many basketball players shoot well by themselves or even under lessened pressures of practice sessions. However, defensive hands in their faces, shooting on the move, game pressures, boisterous spectators, and other variables contribute to the downfall of these same players. Skill attainment implies the ability to adjust to changing conditions. Practice sessions that simulate contest situations will be more effective in preparing the performer for what to expect and for what is desired in these contests.

Two interesting experiments serve the purpose of emphasizing the need for practice to resemble ultimate desired performance. In one study, subjects had to lunge at a target (Solley, 1952). Solley found the group that emphasized speed in learning performed better when speed was the necessary factor for successful performance. Equal emphasis on speed and accuracy in practice yielded the most favorable results when both these factors were important to effective performance.

Ruth Fulton (1945) tested sixty college women on two tasks, tracing movements required on the Snoddy stabilimeter and a striking movement at a target. During training, one group of subjects was encouraged to speed, and other to attain accuracy. Early emphasis on speed for both tasks was more effective, as stronger transfer was noted of the speed set than the accuracy set. When an individual practices at a high speed and then attempts to attain accuracy along with the speed, the movement of the act does not have to be changed. However, low speed practice transformed to the greater speed demanded in competition requires a new movement, a change in body control. No negative transfer effects on accuracy resulted from early speed emphasis in Fulton's investigation. In interpreting her data for athletic skill learning, Fulton concluded that, where momentum is associated with effective performance, such as in tennis strokes, hammer throws, and golf strokes, an early practice emphasis on accuracy will be detrimental.

The dilemma of trade-offs in instruction occurs not only when considering emphasis on speed versus accuracy. In any trade-off situation where there are at least two alternative approaches, the instructor should weigh possible benefits against detriments. An extreme emphasis on speed negatively affects accuracy, and vice-versa. In some respects, if practice proceeds to reflect real condition performance expectations, no trade-offs have occurred. Learners should practice in conditions that are as realistic as possible. It is probably true that it is better in the long run for tennis beginners to practice the full stroke instead of a modified, slowed response. Situations should be created that will make adjustments easier from the learning conditions to the real performance conditions.

There are exceptions to this general proposal. First of all, certain students may demonstrate performance problems and hampered progress. It may be necessary to make a trade-off whereby the learner isolates particular task components and practices with slower movements. Learner difficulties may be remediated with an altered instructional approach. Second, it is not always practical or safe immediately to experience tasks under real conditions. Flying a plane, operating complex machinery, and other activities in which safety factors and costly equipment are involved suggest the initial use of simulated experiences.

We may also deduce from material presented in Chapter 7 on abilities that different abilities are related to stages of practice. In the Hinrichs study, accuracy was found to be more related to early achievement on the pursuit rotor task, whereas speed was more important at the latter stages. Thus, it would seem that the ability to perform accurate movements quickly will ultimately differentiate the highly from the lowly skilled. This notion is borne out in a practical sense from the data compiled by John Woods (1967) with beginning tennis players. Three different instructional programs led to the following conclusion:

> For a tennis skill which is deemed to require both ball velocity and ball placement accuracy simultaneously, the most desirable results were obtained by equal and simultaneous emphasis on both the velocity and accuracy variables. The second most desirable results were obtained by beginning with velocity and terminating with accuracy. The least desirable results were obtained by initial emphasis on accuracy followed by velocity (p. 141).

For practical research (using a ball throwing skill), the apparatus described by Robert Malina and G. Lawrence Rarick (1968) is recommended to assess speed and accuracy measurements.

Theoretical directions on the relationship between speed and accuracy of movement have primarily come from the efforts of Paul Fitts. The relationship of distance, speed, and accuracy is expressed in the following way:

$$T = a + b \, \log_2 \frac{2A}{W}$$

where:

T = duration of movement
A = amplitude of movement
W = width of the target
a and b = constants
$\log_2 \frac{2A}{W}$ = a measure of information required to select the tolerance range from the total range of movements

The duration of a movement is a function of the ratio of movement distance, or amplitude (A), to the specified target size, or width (W). As one varies the distance to be moved, for example, the duration of movement should not change if the target size has been altered by the same proportion. C. I. Howarth, W. D. A. Beggs, and J. M. Bowden (1971) have compared Fitts's formula with their own. Differences in equations are discussed, as is theory, to describe the decrease in accuracy at high speeds of performance, and vice-versa.

Drill Versus the Problem-Solving Approach

Different educational teaching philosophies have been emphasized at various periods in this century. The revolt against the traditional method of learning (concerned with course content) inspired learning not by mere repetition but through questioning and probing. Deweyism brought about consideration for individual differences in interests, rates of learning, and, in general, a problem-solving approach to learning. Lately, many experts on educational curricula have spoken out against so-called student-oriented courses in favor of teacher- or content-oriented course. The plea is for a return to traditional teaching methods. Whether material can be learned more effectively through drill and memorization or problem solving and probing is the current argument. Perhaps different material can be learned better under different conditions, and the goals of the instructor in the program and the favored learning strategies of the student should be considered in any situation. Drill and problem-solving differences in approaches may be noted in Figure 12-19.

What about a comparison of the application of these methodologies to motor skill learning? Drill has always been the basic means of teaching motor skills, primarily because it does provide results and possibly because it does not require much creativeness and ingenuity on the part of the instructor. Arranging a situation that encourages students to think, reason, and then act toward a goal is a method rarely practiced by instructors and coaches; hence, its merits are difficult to ascertain. However, it should be of interest to speculate on the effectiveness of drill versus problem-solving approaches with motor learners.

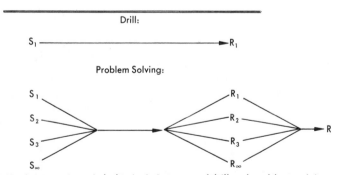

FIGURE 12-19. A comparison, in behavioristic terms, of drill and problem-solving methods. A specific response (R_1) is practiced to a particular stimulus (S_1) in the drill approach. In problem solving, a number of stimulus cues $(S_1 - S_x)$ are present in the learning situation and there may be a variety of acceptable responses $(R_1 - R_x)$, from which one (R) is selected by the learner.

The command technique is associated with a formal, structured environment in which learning is heavily guided toward specific outcomes. It is considered behavioristic (Singer & Dick, 1974) because strong control is exerted over the learner's method of progress. A common instructional approach to techniques of guided learning is the use of programmed learning. The program for this may assume the form of a machine or a book or may be an instructor who closely follows a predetermined instructional sequence. The programmed instruction approach encourages highly guided and reinforced responses. Skinner (1968), a pioneer in the development of programmed instruction, contends that it is easier to learn a skill correctly the first time than it is to undo past error-filled experiences. Programmed learning controls the learner through step-by-step progressions in order to obtain the desired behaviors.

In contrast, the discovery method approach to instruction allows the learner to experiment and to explore solutions to problems. The teacher presents the material to be learned in the form of a problem. The learner is encouraged to discover the way to accomplish the goal and solve the problem. He or she is not given the solution. The teacher may make suggestions in the form of questions, as well as make comparisons to past problem-solving experiences. Proponents believe that this method encourages reflective thinking, association, and self-direction.

There has been considerable attention given lately to exploration skills, especially by physical educators interested in educating elementary school-children. Instead of perpetuating traditional teaching methods, these teachers have attempted to guide youngsters to a greater awareness of factors associated with any activity: namely time, force, and space. The approach is such as to initiate individual creativity in mastering basic movement skills, those that underlie simple and complex sport activities in varying degrees. This rationale appears to be justifiable and the approach is refreshing. How effective the immediate and long-term results are in comparison with those of traditional teaching methods is a question unanswerable at the present time.

As to the athletic skills of older children, the drill method has the advantage of facilitating the execution of an act until it is habitlike. This method is fine for the high jumper, broad jumper, and diver, to name a few, who basically demonstrate a skill under the same static environmental conditions with each performance. Comparing this situation to the one faced by the tennis player, basketball player, and soccer player, we can observe that, in the former case, the environment is relatively stable; fixed responses not only are allowable, they are encouraged (see Chapter 1, again, for further discussion).

In the latter circumstance, environmental conditions are dynamic. Unpredictable stimuli require the performer to have a flexible repertoire of responses. If the player (say, the basketball player) becomes routinized in movements, an alert opponent will take advantage. The player who usually dribbles to the right side and invariably stops short to take a jump shot is easier to defend against than the player who is a threat to move in any direction and who varies shots. A team that is overcoached may reflect this practice in the following manner. The offensive pattern calls for the guard to dribble the ball toward the sideline and pass it to the forward and then move through the middle to the opposite side. From there, perhaps a few team patterns may be executed. A smart defensive team expects the guard's initial pass to the forward and intercepts one or two passes. The guard has been so trained to perform the same routine that proper adjustment is not made. Perhaps the player's as well as the team's play may disintegrate totally.

Players who have been exposed to diverse game circumstances, who are not overdrilled, will react more favorably to the unexpected. Drill has its function. It encourages a consistency in performance and a skillfully executed act. Obviously, certain skills must be developed before complex movement patterns can be elicited. But if coaches or physical educators merely *train* instead of *educate,* if they make robots of their pupils, they have done them a great disservice. Active youngsters must be able to reason quickly in challenging situations and have the abilities to express their thoughts. Involvement in an open skill environment (externally paced tasks) includes detection, discrimination, and recognition of the diverse conditions under which a person must perform. Inability to do this will affect the choice of plans to match the unique conditions and will lead to unsuccessful performance. Therefore, both drill and problem-solving approaches serve in meeting teaching and student goals.

Even in sports that demand a skill to be performed in a relatively predictable environment, the problem-solving method might promote the learning of more complex skills. When the student is introspective and does not only repeat an act continually without understanding what is happening, quicker insight may be gained into other relevant skills. Perhaps overall swimming objectives are taught more effectively when the beginner, with teacher guidance and supervision, is encouraged to think of means of propulsion through the water on the side, back, and front, and then to react in a supervised trial-and-error method. The drilled individual learns the skill but maybe nothing more; the individual who has to reason and learn in a loosely structured situation may learn the skill as well as water principles, confidence, safety, and ways of transferring elements to other strokes and water conditions. Figure 12-20 contains the schematic relationship of task classification and instructional approach.

There is no firm evidence to support a stand for the drill or the problem-solving approach to all types of motor skill learning situations and objectives. One

FIGURE 12-20. The relationship of instructional approaches to type of task. The scheme is not to suggest that only one approach can be used for the learning of a task. Many times both approaches contribute to skill mastery. However, drill is usually favored for tasks that are oriented toward self-pacing and problem solving for externally paced tasks.

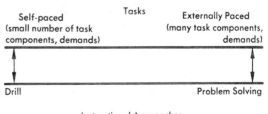

Tasks

Self-paced (small number of task components, demands)

Externally Paced (many task components, demands)

Drill

Problem Solving

Instructional Approaches

may assume the prerogative of conjecture, of course, to determine the values of each method. From an educational point of view, a problem-solving approach certainly is consistent with the philosophy of leading educators. From a skill learning point of view, arguments can be justified for either method. Perhaps, as was mentioned previously, to be considered at the onset is the nature of the skill, its relation to other material to be taught, and the objectives of the teacher.

In one of the few experiments on the topic, Carol Berendsen (1967) concluded in favor of the unstructured problem-solving method rather than a structured practice drill method for beginning female college tennis students. Although no differences in attitude scores or in performance were noted on final attained proficiency levels in basic tennis skills, the problem-solving students scored higher on the written test and on the combined written and skill tests.

Programmed Learning

Our society is so besieged with technological advancement and innovations, it is not surprising that some enterprising educators rebel against the traditional classroom learning situation. Because machines have substituted for human productivity and have been demonstrated to be more efficient in industry in certain cases, these educators suggest that machines can serve a similar purpose in education.

Actually, the concept of a teaching machine is by no means new. L. S. Pressey is credited for creation of a teaching machine in the 1920s and Skinner for streamlining it in later years. Skinner applied his laboratory research on reinforcement in learning to the device's design and is acknowledged as the leader in convincing the public of the machine's value, as well as influencing its widespread popularity. In its simplest form, the machine is constructed for individual usage, with the content of a course or course area presented to the learner in a simple-to-more- difficult sequence. The learner has to respond correctly to the questions and is informed by the machine as to the correctness of the answer. Proper responses permit the learner to advance through the material; complex and more difficult material is learned only after simpler material has been mastered.

Courses have to be programmed in a logical way. The material is presented in detail, step by step, ensuring progressive knowledge acquisition. The Skinner method encourages only correct responses, whereas the Crowder technique permits errors, operating under the philosophy that a learner may profit from his or her mistakes.

Wilbur Schramm (1964) has listed the essential characteristics of programmed learning:

1. An ordered sequence of stimulus items.
2. A response by the learner to each of the stimuli.
3. Reinforcement of the response by immediate knowledge of results.
4. Progression in small steps.

5. Practice consisting of mostly correct responses and few errors.
6. Learning proceeding in successively closer approximations to the desired objectives.

Presently, there are many types of teaching machines and programmed texts on the market. Some are relatively inexpensive but others, such as computer-assisted machines, can be quite costly. Basically, though, all these machines are geared to operate under certain accepted learning principles. One of these is the imparting of immediate knowledge of results, of reinforcing correct responses. Reinforcement, especially when directly following a response, is essential for learning. Obviously, a teacher faced with a number of pupils in a class cannot provide individual attention. Hence, another strong feature of the machine is that it permits students to work at their own pace and within their own abilities. Whereas the teacher must gear a lesson to the average learning speed of the class, programmed individualized units meet specific needs and abilities. There are other merits to teaching machines, but they need not be analyzed here. The use of computers and other media in education is increasing, and Figures 12-21, 12-22 and 12-23 illustrate some applicable situations.

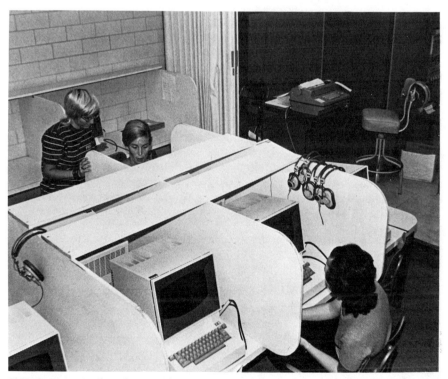

FIGURE 12-21. Students learning through a computer-managed course in which the material is programmed.

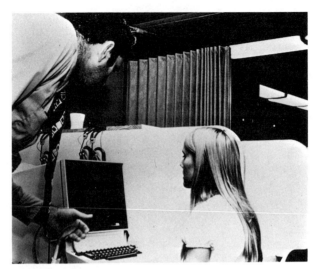

FIGURE 12-22. Instruction is being provided to a student in the use of a computer terminal for the learning of course material.

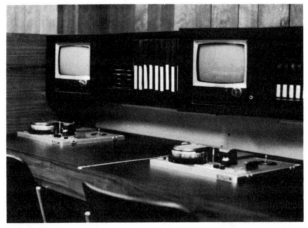

FIGURE 12-23. A resource center with appropriate media permits students to learn at their own preferred rates.

Of most concern with these machines, or programmed texts, is how well they educate students. Although research is not yet ample enough, nor experimental designs sufficiently sophisticated, to warrant any conclusive statements, results are most promising. A number of investigators, if not finding programmed material to be better learned than material taught by traditional teaching methods, have noted greater efficiency in the form of the time-saving benefits of the programmed method. As an example, J. R. Rawls, O. Perry, and F. O. Timmons (1966) found psychology course material to be learned at a substantial time saving

MOTOR LEARNING AND HUMAN PERFORMANCE

with a programmed group as compared to a lectured-to group. Although no significant difference was noted between the groups on a knowledge test administered at the end of the unit, a retention test given six weeks later favored the programmed group.

The advantages associated with these various devices have been derived when the material to be acquired was *not* in the motor skill area. This is understandable, for the content of most motor skills has yet to be programmed in a satisfactory manner. Programmed texts and teaching machines can be used, if desired, for the learning of information related to athletic skills. With regard to a particular sport, programs can be developed containing such matter as relevant physiological and mechanical principles, rules, strategies, and history. What about programming movement skills? Is it possible?

Neuman and Singer (1968) attempted to program beginning tennis skills in the form of booklet material. A programmed group of subjects was compared to a traditionally taught group at the end of the unit on various tennis measures. The data indicated the general skill level of the groups, as measured by the Hewitt Revised Dyer Backboard Tennis Test and a single elimination tournament, was similar. The traditionally taught group improved significantly in general skills, but the programmed group did not. The programmed group received better subjective scores on form than did the traditionally taught group. Because only fourteen periods of instruction elapsed, it is interesting to speculate on what the effects would have been of a longer duration of time. The early mastery of form, such as that produced by the programmed method, might facilitate the attainment of better skill and playing ability in the long run more than the traditional method.

In P. L. Leonard's (1970) study, with beginning synchronized swimming stunts, a self-instructional group was compared to a teacher-directed group in achievements at the end of eight lessons. Performances were similar between the groups. With golf, however, J. D. Adler (1967) found greater improvement for the group using programmed lessons than the group that received conventional lecture, demonstration, and practice instruction.

Possibly, the future will bring more sophisticated attempts at programmed instruction of motor patterns. These efforts would certainly coincide with those in industry and education. Although some people would replace teachers altogether with machines, most educators favoring programmed instruction view the teacher as playing an important role in individual guidance, along with the programmed material. The teacher is not to be replaced but is to be freed to devote more time to individual instruction and assistance.

Error-Free Versus Error-Full Learning

A logical next step in our discussion following "programmed learning" is to raise the question: Is it better to learn motor tasks with errors discouraged or encouraged? Can and should we learn from mistakes? Is it better to minimize the possibility of erroneous responses? A programmed learning approach encompasses the viewpoint that, indeed, errors (wrong responses) should not be experienced.

The learner is supposed to experience success continually. Errors merely lead to frustration, a lack of reinforcement, and a building up of undesirable responses. It is thought that when we learn errors, they will be repeated.

Yet, when we think of motor skills, common sense suggests that by experiencing alternate and nondesirable responses, the learner learns how to adjust accordingly in future related situations. Adaptive behavior is extremely important in the successful execution of many complex skills, especially those that involve a long sequence of movements to unpredictable stimuli. The major dilemma here is that, although the learner may benefit from mistakes in the future, practice must be guided effectively enough so that errors are not continually practiced and conditioned. It is much easier to learn new responses than to have to unlearn old ones before making the appropriate responses.

Interestingly enough, the value of permitting or even encouraging errors in the learning of motor skills is difficult to assess because of the paucity of research on the topic. Fortunately, a few recent studies provide some insights into the problem. Apparatuses have been designed in some cases to create error-free learning situations in perceptual and motor tasks by providing prompts, cues, guidance, and feedback. The programmed learning technique, especially used for verbal materials, is an excellent example of an approach to instruction and training geared to minimize errors. Dennis Holding (1970) attempted to determine whether subjects tend to reject the same errors in the course of learning and if the repetition of errors depends on a commitment to the learning of wrong responses in the early and formative stages.

A discrimination reaction timer with one of four pairings of red and green lights to be responded to by one of four keys was used with three groups of subjects. Some support for the idea that errors may be learned was reported. Furthermore, even errors that are not well learned may have long-term negative effects. The beneficial effort of errors on ultimate performance will probably occur in only one or two special cases, speculates Holding (1970), although his experiment was not designed, in terms of the task employed, to support the following statements.

> The idea of learning by one's errors may have some validity in the case where the structure of a task tends strongly to elicit specific erroneous responses; executing the incorrect responses will then offer an opportunity for extinction and amendment. Alternatively, learning by making errors may occur in circumstances where gaining extra information about the task depends upon executing a wide range of responses. In this case, making or being offered to make only the correct responses may deny the subject "knowledge of alternatives," with detrimental effects upon the acquisition of skill (p. 733).

Error-full learning is typical in most motor learning situations. That is to say, the trial-and-error learning method typically begins by allowing learners to make a variety of responses available in a given situation. The learner gradually acquires the appropriate responses to specified cues, if fortunate. As Dirk Prather (1971) indicates, a summary of the limited literature reveals that the errorless learning of simple tasks should be beneficial, especially if training is not restricted to a few trials. Consequently, he designed a study in which a complex task involved in flying was to be learned under error-free and error-filled methods. He did not find either method more superior in training on the task. The theoretical position that incorrect responses interfere with the learning of the correct response was not substantiated in his experiment. However, when teaching for transfer, error-full, or trial-and-error learning was superior to errorless training. Prather observed that the trial-and-error group seemed to be more actively involved in the learning situation and that the errorless group was more passive. Because most real-life situations require transfer abilities in complex tasks, it appears that the trial-and-error method should be advocated.

Investigations by Singer and Pease (1976, 1978) and Singer and Gaines (1975), in which a computer-managed novel serial manipulative task was used, revealed efficiency in time of learning in early learning trials under guided methods of instruction. The data in the Singer and Gaines study supported the trial-and-error (problem-solving) method for transfer effectiveness when the number of trials was determined by a criterion performance score, the first study in which it was employed as the dependent measure. Learning to criterion is more in line with competency-based approaches in the classroom. By providing criterion learning, an adequate similar amount of learning is achieved by groups trained with either technique. This provides an alternative approach to other research studies in which one looks at transfer as a function of initial learning task strategy.

Singer and Pease (1976) found significant differences favoring the discovery method for both retention and transfer. A third instructional condition that included a combination of the two contrasting strategies was demonstrated to be equal to the discovery learning condition in its effects on retention and transfer performance. The implications from these data indicate the importance of at least a partial discovery instructional methodology in a learning situation, should time factors not allow for the total use of discovery methods (trial and error).

The present state of the literature, although quite favorable in verbal learning situations to prompting and feedback devices (e.g., programmed instruction), indicates a tendency to support a learning-from-errors procedure with complex motor tasks, if positive transfer effects to other tasks are desirable. Where many alternative responses are possible, it is indeed possible, as Holding (1970) indicated, that the experiencing of errors may benefit the learning process in the long run, assuming that errors are not uniformly conditioned.

CHAPTER HIGHLIGHTS

1. Latest developments in the area of psychoinstructional design suggest the procedures and means of presenting content to learners—or, in other words, how to manage instruction more scientifically and systematically.

2. Practice should be of sufficient quality and duration to ensure the development of skill.

3. The goal of instruction and learning is to get learners to become self-sufficient and self-reliant.

4. Learners at different levels of skills demonstrate behavioral patterns unique to each level, and instructors need to orient their instructional procedures accordingly.

5. Students learn at different rates of speed, and it is extremely hazardous to predict final achievement levels on the basis of preliminary test scores.

6. Motivation influences selection of and preference for an activity, persistence at the activity, effort, and adequacy of performance relative to performance standards.

7. Level of performance, which is behavior in a particular situation, is the result of motivation (attitudes, feelings, expectancies) and capabilities (genetics, past experiences, and learning). It is important to note that motivation influences both present performance level and previous experiences and learning.

8. Four dimensions of motor activities may be considered in regard to motivation: complexity, physical demands, appeal, and meaningfulness. More complex activities require less arousal level than simpler ones for their execution, except when simple tasks are to be repeated over and over again. More arousal is needed for the execution of "physical tasks," those in which the mechanics of movement are relatively simple or else well learned, and power, speed, strength, or endurance are the primary bases for success. When activities are appealing, interesting, and meaningful to learners, motivation will be present to a more desirable degree.

9. Individuals vary in many dimensions, with implications for motivational considerations. Disscussed in this chapter was the relationship of motivation and performance, regarding such personal factors as (a) under- or overachievement; (b) level of aspiration or expectations in performance; (c) need to achieve; (d) need for social approval; (e) need to avoid failure or to avoid success; (f) level of anxiety; (g) future orientation, or personal goals; (h) internal or external locus of control; (i) extrinsic and intrinsic motivation; and (j) self-concept.

10. Various conceptual approaches to the study of motivation have resulted in different research paradigms, emphases, and conclusions. Behavioristic approaches tend to emphasize reinforcements and situational control over the learner. Humanistic approaches are oriented to more inner-directed and self-determined behavior: helping people to help themselves. Approaches in cognitive psychology emphasize personal expectations in performance and interpretations (attributions toward) of performance outcomes.

11. Achievement motivation programs are related to the cognitive psychology school of thought, as intrinsic motivation for an activity is encouraged. An attempt is made to reach the attitudes and thoughts of learners, to develop a sense of responsibility in learners.

12. Extrinsic versus intrinsic sources of motivation were identified, with the latter generally the more desirable of the two. Extrinsic (external) sources refer to material gains; intrinsic (internal) sources refer to material gains; intrinsic (internal) sources are associated with personal satisfaction.

13. In concluding the section on motivation, a number of situational considerations were mentioned, programs or activities an instructor could initiate to influence motivation. They included (a) the use of rewards and reinforcers; (b) punishment; (c) the use of knowledge of results of performance; (d) the establishment of learner goals and expectations; (e) the development and use of instructor objectives; (f) competition; (g) cooperation; (h) instructor enthusiasm; (i) effective leadership style and communication; (j) interesting and meaningful training procedures; (k) student involvement in goal setting, program development, and decision making; (1) the development of learners' intrinsic strategies; (m) learner feelings of control over self and over task outcomes; (n) learner's development of self-image, confidence, and self-worth; (o) the application of knowledge of results of performance outcomes; (p) successful learner experiences; and (q) increased student responsibilities in the learning program.

14. The capacity to process information at any stage depends, to a great extent, on attentional processes. Attention is related to such states as arousal and concentration, although distinctions can be made. The dominant concept of attention for many years was the single-channel model, although in more recent years, multichannel and other types of models have been proposed to describe human information-processing (attentional) capabilities. On the basis of studies dealing with divided attention (dual task or secondary task loading paradigms), it would appear that a number of human possibilities exist, depending on the attentional demands of simultaneously presented tasks.

15. Many instructional decisions, which have trade-off outcomes as to practice value, confront the instructor. Although there are many qualifiers, trade-offs and potential outcomes are as follows: (a) practice sessions should be briefer and distributed over a longer time rather than longer and concentrated over a shorter period of time; (b) massed practice and distributed practice often lead to similar retention performances, although distributed practice is superior to massed practice as to immediate effects; (c) whole practice is favored when tasks are relatively simple and well organized, whereas part practice should be used with tasks that are complex; (d) mental practice, without any overt practice, is more effective in learning a motor skill than no practice at all, although physical practice (with nondeliberate or deliberate mental intervention) provides best results; (e) emphasis on speed diminishes accuracy and emphasis on accuracy reduces speed in movement, and practice performance conditions should simulate testing situations as much as possible (e.g., if both speed and accuracy are equally important ultimately, both should be emphasized in practice; (f) when a sequence of events comprises the entire activity, the last and first learned usually are retained the best, although certain learning strategies may help to overcome the expected serial learning curve; (g) either instructional method, drill or problem solving can be effective, depending on training objectives; (h) programmed (self-) learning encourages independent and individual rates of work, although the learning of a motor skill may be equally effective under programmed as under traditional learning experiences; and (i) highly prompted learning is expedient when learning a task, but discovery learning may lead to better retention and transfer.

References

Adams, J. A. Some mechanisms of motor responding: An examination of attention. In E. A. Bilodeau (Ed.), *Acquisition of skill*. New York: Academic Press, 1966.

Adler, J. D. *The use of programmed lessons in teaching a complex perceptual-motor skill*. Unpublished doctoral dissertation, University of Oregon, 1967.

Allport, A. D., Antonis, B., & Reynolds, P. On the division of attention: A disproof of the single channel hypothesis. *Quarterly Journal of Experimental Psychology*, 1972, *24*, 225–235.

Ammons, R. B. Effect of distribution of practice on rotary pursuit "hits." *Journal of Experimental Psychology*, 1951, *41*, 17–22.

Austin, D. A. Effect of distributed and massed practice upon the learning of a velocity task. *Research Quarterly*, 1975, *46*, 23–30.

Berendsen, C. A. *The relative effectiveness of descriptive teaching and structured problem solving in learning basic tennis skills*. Unpublished master's thesis, University of Washington, 1967.

Berlyne, D. E. Attention as a problem in behavior theory. In D. I. Mostofsky (Ed.), *Attention: Contemporary theory and analysis*. New York: Appleton-Century-Crofts, 1970.

Birch, D., & Veroff, J. *Motivation: A study of action*. Belmont, Calif.: Brooks/Cole, 1966.

Briggs, G. E., & Brogden, W. J. The effect of component practice on performance of a lever-positioning skill. *Journal of Experimental Psychology*, 1954, *48*, 375–380.

Broadbent, D. E. *Perception and communication*. London: Pergamon Press, 1958.

Brown, I. D., Tickner, A. H., & Simmonds, D. C. V. Interference between concurrent tasks of driving and telephoning. *Journal of Applied Psychology*, 1969, *53*, 419–424.

Clark, L. V. Effect of mental practice on the development of a certain motor skill. *Research Quarterly*, 1960, *31*, 560–569.

Clifford, M. Competition as a motivational technique in the classroom. *American Educational Research Journal*, 1972, *9*, 123–137.

Colavita, F. Human sensory dominance. *Perception and Psychophysics*, 1974, *16*, 409–412.

Covington, M. V., & Beery, R. G. *Self-worth and school learning*. New York: Holt, Rinehart & Winston, 1976.

Davis, R. H., Alexander, L. T., & Yelon, S. L. *Learning system design: An approach to the improvement of instruction*. New York: McGraw-Hill, 1974.

Deci, E. L. *Intrinsic motivation*. New York: Plenum Press, 1975.

Fine, B. J. Intrinsic motivation, intelligence, and personality as related to cognitive and motor performance. *Perceptual and Motor Skills*, 1972, *34*, 319–329.

Fitts, P. M., & Posner, M. I. *Human performance*. Belmont, Calif.: Brooks/Cole, 1967.

Fleishman, E. A. A relationship between incentive motivation and ability level in psychomotor performance. *Journal of Experimental Psychology*, 1958, *56*, 78–81.

Fleishman, E. A., & Hempel, W. E. Changes in factor structure of a complex psychomotor test as a function of practice. *Psychometrika*, 1954, *19*, 239–254.

Fulton, R. E. Speed and accuracy in learning movements. *Archives of Psychology*, 1945, *300*.

Gagné, R. M. (Ed.). *Psychological principles in systems development*. New York: Holt, Rinehart & Winston, 1962.

Gagné, R. M., & Briggs, L. J. *Principles in instructional design*. New York: Holt, Rinehart & Winston, 1974.

Gallwey, W. T. *Inner tennis: Playing the game*. New York: Random House, 1976.

Griffith, C. R. *Psychology of coaching*. New York: Charles Scribner's Sons, 1932.

Hagenbeck, F. L. *Strategy utilization on the acquisition and retention of a serial motor task*. Unpublished master's thesis, Florida State University, 1978.

Halpern, J., & Lantz, A. E. Learning to utilize information presented over two sensory channels. *Perception and Psychophysics*, 1974, *16*, 321–328.

Harcum, E. R. *Serial learning and paralearning: Control processes in serial acquisition*. New York: John Wiley, 1975.

Harris, D. V. *Intrinsic motivation with implications for sport*. Paper presented at the NAPECW-NCPEAM Conference, Orlando, Florida, January 1977.

Heider, F. *The psychology of interpersonal relations*. New York: John Wiley, 1958.

Holding, D. H. Repeated errors in motor learning. *Ergonomics*, 1970, *13*, 727–734.

Howarth, C. I., Beggs, W. D. A., & Bowden, J. M. The relationship between speed and accuracy of movement aimed at a target. *Acta Psychologica*, 1971, *35*, 207–218.

Johnson, M. C. Gestalten practice pattern selection: Methodology and task structure. *Quest*, 1970, *14*, 56–64.

Jones, J. G. Motor learning without demonstration of physical practice under two conditions of mental practice. *Research Quarterly*, 1965, *36*, 270–276.

Keele, S. W. *Attention and human performance*. Pacific Palisades, Calif.: Goodyear Publishing Co., 1973.

Keele, S. W., & Neill, W. T. Mechanisms of attention. In E. C. Carterette & P. Friedman (Eds.), *Handbook of perception* (Vol. 9). New York: Academic Press, 1978.

Kerr, B. Processing demands during mental operations. *Memory and Cognition*, 1973, *1*, 401–412.

Knapp, C. G., & Dixon, W. R. Learning to juggle: I. A study to determine the effect of two different distributions of practice on learning efficiency. *Research Quarterly*, 1950, *21*, 331–336.

Knowles, W. B. Operation loading tasks. *Human Factors*, 1963, *5*, 151–161.

Kolb, D. A. Achievement motivation training program for underachieving high school boys. *Journal of Personality and Social Psychology*, 1965, *2*, 783–792.

Kolesnik, W. B. *Motivation: Understanding and influencing human behavior*. Boston: Allyn & Bacon, 1978.

Kristofferson, A. B. Attention and psychophysical time. *Acta Psychologica*, 1967, *27*, 93–100.

Legge, E., & Barber, P. J. *Information and skill*. London: Methuen, 1976.

Leonard, P. L. *A self-instructional unit for learning beginning synchronized swimming stunts*. Unpublished master's thesis, Southern Illinois University, 1970.

Lepper, M. R., & Greene, D. Turning play into work: Effects of adult surveillance and extrinsic rewards on children's intrinsic motivation. *Journal of Personality and Social Psychology*, 1975, *31*, 479–486.

Lindsay, P. H. Multichannel processing in perception. In D. I. Mostovsky (Ed.), *Attention: Contemporary theory and analysis*. New York: Appleton-Century-Crofts, 1970.

Maehr, M. Toward a framework for the cross-cultural study of achievement motivation: McClelland reconsidered and redirected. In M. G. Wade & R. Martens (Eds.), *Psychology of motor behavior and sport*, Proceedings of the North American Society for the Psychology of Sport and Physical Activity. Urbana, Ill.: Human Kinetics Publishers, 1974.

Magill, R. A. Order of acquisition of the parts of a serial-motor task. *Research Quarterly*, 1976, *47*, 134–139.

Malina, R. M., & Rarick, G. L. A device for assessing the role of information feedback in speed and accuracy of throwing performance. *Research Quarterly,* 1968, *39,* 120–123.

Marcel, A. J. Some constraints on sequential and parallel processing, and the limits of attention. *Acta Psychologica,* 1970, *33,* 77–92.

Massey, D. The significance of interpolated time intervals on motor learning. *Research Quarterly,* 1959, *30,* 189–201.

McClelland, D. C. What is the effect of achievement motivation training in the schools? *Teachers College Record,* 1972, *74,* 129–145.

McGuigan, F. J., & MacCaslin, E. F. Whole and part methods of learning a perceptual motor skill. *American Journal of Psychology,* 1955, *68,* 658–661.

Mosston, M. *Teaching physical education: From command to discovery.* Columbus, Ohio: Charles E. Merrill, 1966.

Naylor, J. C., & Briggs, G. E. *Long-term retention of learned skills: A review of the literature.* ASD Technical Report 61-390, U.S. Department of Commerce, 1963.

Neuman, M. C., & Singer, R. N. A comparison of traditional versus programmed methods of learning tennis. *Research Quarterly,* 1968, *39,* 1044–1048.

Newell, K. M. Knowledge of results and motor learning. *Journal of Motor Behavior,* 1974, *6,* 235–244.

Nisbett, R. E., & Valins, S. Perceiving the causes of one's own behavior. In E. E. Jones, D. E. Kanouse, H. H. Kelley, R. E. Nisbett, S. Valins, & B. Weiner (Eds.), *Attribution: Perceiving the causes of behavior.* Morristown, N.J.: General Learning Press, 1972.

Noble, M., Trumbo, D., & Fowler, F. Further evidence of secondary task interference in tracking. *Journal of Experimental Psychology,* 1967, *73,* 146–149.

Palermo, D. S., Castaneda, A., & McCandless, B. R. The relationship of anxiety in children to performance in a complex learning task. *Child Development,* 1956, *27,* 333–337.

Perry, H. M. The relative efficiency of actual and imaginary practice in five selected tasks. *Archives of Psychology,* 1939, *243,* 1–76.

Postman, L. Does interference theory predict too much forgetting? *Journal of Verbal Learning and Verbal Behavior,* 1963, *2,* 40–48.

Prather, D. C. Trial-and-error versus errorless learning: Training, transfer and stress. *American Journal of Psychology,* 1971, *84,* 377–385.

Rawlings, E. I., Rawlings, I. L., Chen, S. S., & Yilk, M. D. The facilitating effects of mental rehearsal in the acquisition of rotary pursuit tracking. *Psychonomic Science,* 1972, *26,* 71–73.

Rawls, J. R., Perry, O., & Timmons, E. O. A comparative study of conventional instruction and individual programmed instruction in the college classroom. *Journal of Applied Psychology,* 1966, *50,* 388–391.

Renshaw, S., & Postle, D. K. Pursuit learning under three types of instruction. *Journal of General Psychology,* 1928, *1,* 360–367.

Richardson, A. Mental practice: A review and discussion: Part I. *Research Quarterly,* 1967, *38,* 95–107. (a)

Richardson, A. Mental practice: A review and discussion: Part II. *Research Quarterly,* 1967, *38,* 263–273. (b)

Rogers, C. Feedback precision and post-feedback interval duration. *Journal of Experimental Psychology,* 1974, *102,* 604–608.

Ross, M. Self-perception of intrinsic motivation. In J. H. Harvey, W. J. Ickes, & R. F. Kidd (eds.), *New directions in attribution research: Vol. 1.* Hillsdale, N.J.: Erlbaum, 1976.

Rotter, J. G. Generalized expectancies for internal versus external control of reinforcement. *Psychological Monographs,* 1966, *80*(1).

Schramm, W. Programmed instruction today and tomorrow. In A. Foshay et al. (Eds.), *Programmed instruction.* Washington, D.C.: U.S. Dept. of Health, Education, and Welfare, 1964.

Siedentop, D., & Ramey, G. Extrinsic rewards and intrinsic motivation. *Motor Skills: Theory Into Practice,* 1977, *2,* 49–62.

Singer, R. N. Motivation in sport. *International Journal of Sport Psychology,* 1977, *8,* 1–22.

Singer, R. N., & Dick, W. *Teaching physical education: A systems approach.* Boston: Houghton Mifflin, 1974.

Singer, R. N., & Gaines, L. Effect of prompted and trial-and-error learning on transfer performance of a serial motor task. *American Educational Research Journal,* 1975, *12,* 395–403.

Singer, R. N., & Pease, D. The effect of different instructional strategies on learning, retention, and transfer of a serial motor task. *Research Quarterly,* 1976, *47,* 788–796.

Singer, R. N., & Pease, D. Effect of guided vs. discovery learning strategies on initial motor task learning, transfer, and retention. *Research Quarterly,* 1978, *49,* 206–217.

Singer, R. N., & Witker, J. Mental rehearsal and point of introduction within the context of overt practice. *Perceptual and Motor Skills,* 1970, *31,* 169–170.

Skinner, B. *The technology of teaching.* New York: Appleton-Century-Crofts, 1968.

Smyth, M. M. The effect of visual guidance on the acquisition of a simple motor task. *Journal of Motor Behavior,* 1977, *9,* 275–284.

Solley, W. H. The effects of verbal instruction of speed and accuracy upon the learning of a motor skill. *Research Quarterly,* 1952, *23,* 231–240.

Suinn, R. M. Body thinking: Psychology for Olympic champs. *Psychology Today,* 1976, *10,* 38–43.

Triesman, A. Strategies and models of selective attention. *Psychological Review,* 1969, *76,* 282–299.

Trussell, E. Prediction of success in a motor skill on the basis of early learning achievement. *Research Quarterly,* 1965, *39,* 342–347.

Twining, W. E. Mental practice and physical practice in learning a motor skill. *Research Quarterly,* 1949, *20,* 432–435.

Waglow, I. F. Effect of school term length on skill achievement in tennis, golf, and handball. *Research Quarterly,* 1966, *37,* 157–159.

Weiner, B. (Ed.). *Cognitive views of human motivation.* New York: Academic Press, 1974.

Weiner, B., & Walker, E. L. Motivational factors in short-term retention. *Journal of Experimental Psychology,* 1966, *71,* 190–193.

Welch, M. Prediction of motor skill attainment from early learning. *Perceptual and Motor Skills,* 1963, *17,* 263–266.

Welch, M., & Henry, F. Individual differences in various parameters. *Journal of Motor Behavior,* 1971, *3,* 78–96.

Whitley, J. D. Effects of practice distribution on learning a fine motor task. *Research Quarterly,* 1970, *48,* 576–583.

Wickens, C. D. The effects of divided attention on information processing in manual tracking. *Journal of Experimental Psychology,* 1976, *2,* 1–13.

Wickstrom, R. L. Comparative study of methodologies for teaching gymnastics and tumbling stunts. *Research Quarterly,* 1958, *29,* 109–115.

Woods, J. B. The effect of varied instructional emphasis upon the development of a motor skill. *Research Quarterly,* 1967, *38,* 132–142.

13 INSTRUCTIONAL AND TRAINING PROCEDURES: AFTER-PRACTICE CONSIDERATIONS

We now turn to factors that can occur following the execution of a specific act or a practice session that will have a bearing on strengthening that learning and subsequent learnings. As a reminder, many instructor-imposed or learner-generated events are difficult to isolate as only occurring prior to, during, or following a performance. For instance, motivational sources must be considered on all three occasions. However, discussions have been placed for convenience in these chapters dealing with practice, and overlap may be noted on occasion.

In this chapter, events that may be construed as reinforcers will be analyzed. Reinforcement theory has had a long history in behavioristic psychology, and the uses of rewards and punishments in the shaping of behavior have been studied extensively in many types of programs and even analyzed on moral grounds. Another major area of focus is augmented, or supplementary, feedback. This is the type of information that an instructor or some specially designed equipment can provide to the student about his or her performance in order to promote the acquisition of skill. Addressed will be questions surrounding when, how, and even if such information should be supplied to the learner.

Recent advances in cognitive and social psychology attest to the importance of understanding attributions to performance outcomes. Reasons that people give for their performances are linked with expectations and, in turn, can influence subsequent performance levels. We dealt with expectations and level of aspiration in Chapter 11, and expectations, attributions, and motivation in Chapter 12; the material in this chapter will be a continuation of that discussion, within the conceptual framework that attribution theory has provided.

Many skills and learning strategies are taught with the intention of transferability—that is, to promote the learning of future related activities. The transfer of training has been studied extensively, and the many considerations that need to be addressed will be, later in this chapter. One argument that has persisted for a century is the degree to which what we learn is specific to a particular act or experience and to what degree generalizability is a possibility.

Finally, the nature of retention and influences on it will be analyzed and described. Memory systems were first discussed in a conceptual framework in Chapter 6, and it would probably be wise for you to review that material before reading the section on retention in this chapter.

REINFORCEMENT

The term *reinforcement* refers to any event that increases the probability of the occurrence or maintains the strength of a particular act or behavior. For all intents and purposes, a reinforcer is a form of reward, and perhaps *reward* is a more general term than *reinforcement*. However, reinforcement has attained a specific meaning with regard to the classical and instrumental learning experiments designed by psychologists. In unique animal experiments, such scientists as Pavlov and Skinner have demonstrated the effect of a reinforcer on conditioning an act or directing behavior.

With reference to motor skill learning, any statement about reward also holds true for reinforcement. When learning a motor skill, the encouragement, praise, grade, or money awarded to a student after a correct performance serves as a reinforcer. These rewards reinforce the act; they tell the individual that what is being done is what is desired and that, possibly, further good performances will be rewarded in the same way. It has been found that immediate reinforcement is more effective than any delay in reinforcement. Association of a correct response with a given stimulus becomes strengthened with immediate reinforcement, for during any delay other activity occurs and the individual is apt to confuse which response is being rewarded.

Operant conditioning theory, as developed by Skinner and his followers and described briefly in Chapter 4, is based on the effect of reinforcement contingencies on the acquisition of desired behaviors. Programmed learning techniques, referred to in Chapter 12, also depend heavily on the use of immediate reinforcement.

Another aspect of reinforcement to consider is its ideal frequency. Although continual reinforcement may be preferable, it rarely occurs in real-life situations. A number of nonreinforced behaviors may occur before one finally is reinforced, and this number may vary from occasion to occasion. Because continuous reinforcement is relatively nonexistent in the learning of tasks, some form of intermittent reinforcement, either by design or naturally, may be available instead.

Experimentally, four types of schedules of reinforcement have been identified: ratio, interval, variable, and fixed. Because the type of reinforcement schedule may have a profound influence on behaviors, their formulation and potential effect are of great interest. Each schedule is briefly described in the following manner:

1. Ratio schedule: A set or fixed proportion of nonreinforced responses to reinforced responses; e.g., twenty to one.
2. Interval schedule: A predetermined amount of time before reinforcement occurs.
3. Variable schedule: Irregular reinforcements after a number of responses or an amount of time (applied to ratio or interval schedules).
4. Fixed schedule: Reinforcements regularly given after a constant period of time or number of responses (applied to ratio or interval schedules).

Actually, typical situations do contain a large amount of uncertainty in reward. The baseball batter does not get a hit every time at bat, but certainly one hit in three attempts (unpredictable in occurrence) is sufficient to act as a reinforcer. It is never known in advance when or what kind of hit will be made, but by achieving an adequate number of them, the athlete is continually motivated whenever it is time to go to bat. Variable-ratio reinforcement schedules occur in many other places, and are the rule, most notably the play in a slot machine, where one never knows when the payoff will be.

Variable-ratio reinforcements produce high and stable rates of responding, whereas variable interval schedules usually yield lesser values in lower forms of organisms. A variable reinforcement schedule, with its inherent uncertainty, is quite effective in shaping, maintaining, and elevating behaviors, as long as reinforcements come after a reasonable number of responses. This is not always the case, however, as evidenced by the unbelievable persistence a person may show with a slot machine without a payoff reinforcement.

Distinctions have been made between *positive* and *negative* reinforcers. Actually, positive reinforcement is usually defined in the same manner as the term *reinforcement* by itself, which was done in the first sentence in this section. A negative reinforcer is a stimulus that, when *removed*, results in an increased probability that the response will occur in the future. Negative, or *aversive*, stimuli, which reinforce when they disappear, can be a loud noise or any obnoxious event.

Some basic books on the topic of operant conditioning and reinforcement have been written by G. S. Reynolds (1968) and W. I. Smith and J. W. Moore (1966). Discussions center around concepts, terms, applications to the behavioral sciences, and uses in traditional learning programs as well as in therapy.

Success and Failure

In any given endeavor, the outcome will be viewed as relative success or failure, depending on the criteria for success. It may be recalled that personal success or failure depends on the level of aspiration, which in turn serves as a motivational force. The traditional concept of encouraging successes and avoiding failures in order to elevate motivation and at the same time improve performance is perhaps too simply stated. The relative effects of success and failure on motivation are much more complex than once believed.

John Atkinson (1957) has suggested the probability of motivation increasing or decreasing as a result of experienced success or failure. For example, the expectant probability of success with a task of intermediate difficulty is 0.5. For a difficult task, one of say a 0.2 probability of success, motivation steadily increases with repeated success until the probability of success is 0.5. Motivation after that point *decreases* as the probability increases to certainty (1.00). The probability of success is so high that there is no interest or incentive. Atkinson concludes that one should always look for new and more challenging tasks.

Atkinson considers another aspect of the problem when he writes on the results of repeated failure in an easy task (*p,* or expectant probability = 0.8). Motivation should *increase* with failure until the expectant probability has been lowered to 0.5; after that, the motivation should weaken. The motivation should lessen with the first failure on a difficult task. Success with simpler tasks increases motivation on subsequent, more difficult tasks; the level of aspiration rises with success.

The old assumption that success automatically increases motivation and that failure automatically decreases it is not always true, as has been shown by P. Brickman, J. A. W. Linsemneier, and A. G. McCareins (1976). On the other hand, not all research substantiates all of Atkinson's concepts about motivation. Nevertheless, there appears to be justification for a number of them. The difficulty of the task as it appears to the performer, as well as initial success with its undertaking, contributes to personal motivational level. Another consideration for probabilities and motivation is the anxiety level of the individual. An anxious individual confronts a new challenge with a probability of success different from a lesser anxious person. Fear of failure results in quickened loss of motivation.

Finally, the number of successful acts before failure occurs may affect performance in various ways. Bayton and Conley (1957) divided seventy-five college students into three groups and administered the Minnesota Rate of Manipulation Test to them. One group received five trials of success before experiencing failure; for the second group, failure came after the tenth trial; and the third group experienced failure after the fifteenth trial. Results indicate that early failure has an inhibitory effect on an experience. As success increases through time, subsequent failures increase motivation. After ten and fifteen successful trials, a shift to failure increased the level of performance, whereas this was not so after five trials.

An application of these results to the learning of motor skills would call for learners to experience as much success as possible in the early stages before failure.

Reward and Punishment, Praise and Criticism

Although there have been many methods developed to influence the motivational process, perhaps the most widely used in everyday situations fall into reward and punishment categories. Examples of rewarding good behavior and correct responses and punishing the undesired are so familiar to everyone that there is no need to list them here. However, the relative effectiveness of each, as demonstrated by practical experience and research evidence, deserves examination.

Thorndike influenced ideas on punishment through a good part of this century. At first, on the basis of experiments with animals, he concluded that reward and punishment had equal effects on behavior. He later modified this position, as evidence indicated reward to be a more stable and a stronger influence for desirable behavior than punishment. Skinner, working with rats, noted the more temporary and unpredictable effect of punishment. Punishment inhibits behavior, but wears off. Hence, it has a temporary effect unless it is administered continually. A punishment is supposed to decrease the probability of particular behavior occurring again in the future.

At the present time, psychologists and educators agree that of the two, it is better to take a positive approach to the learning situation. Praise, because it is specific to the act and informative, informs the person when the correct behavior is manifested. Punishment tells the person what not to do instead of what to do. After punishment, the desired response still has to be discovered. In our society, even the threat of the most dire consequences for antisocial behavior does not totally inhibit such acts. The implementation of threats, criticism, or pain, no matter how severe, does not always work. The effects of punishment are not consistent from individual to individual or situation to situation.

The ineffectiveness of punishment can be explained also by the usual delay between the time an act takes place and the administration of the punishment. Reward is almost always immediate; that is, the type obtained by the individual personally. The youngster may take a cookie from the jar without permission—and is rewarded. When mother discovers what has happened, perhaps hours later, the child is punished. The situation results in a conflict for the child.

Yelling and screaming at a child for performing a skill incorrectly may help in improving skill level, but it also may cause confusion, anguish, and resistant behavior. On the other hand, positive reinforcement for ideal or near ideal performances by praise and encouragement will probably be more effective in attaining hoped-for goals. The work of Skinner has demonstrated the heights one can reach in controlling and, hence, predicting behavior through constant reinforcements.

E. B. Hurlock (1925), although using addition problems as the task to be learned, demonstrated the relative effects of various incentives. Children in four groups were tested under four different conditions: praise, reproof, no comment, and ignored (but heard praise and reproof given to others). The praised group did best, the reproved group was second best, the ignored group third, and the no-comment group finished last.

Yet, it is possible that we truly do not know much about the properties of punishment and how it can be used effectively to shape behavior. James Johnston (1972) has surveyed the research literature dealing with punishment and has uncovered many myths and inaccuracies concerning its use. He has called for a better understanding of the relative merits of positive reinforcement and punishment and recommended that decisions be based on scientific evidence rather than on moral convictions. Recent evidence has shown punishment procedures to be quite effective in certain learning situations. For instance, K. L. Witte and E. E. Grossman (1971) administered a tactile form discrimination task to kindergarten children under three reinforcement conditions: reward only, punishment only, and reward and punishment. In terms of correct responses, the latter two conditions were equally effective, both being superior in results to the first condition. Apparently, punishment in this study resulted in a greater attentiveness on the part of the subjects. Orientation to the task was at a higher level. The motivational properties of punishment in this type of setting were ruled out in favor of an attentional hypothesis.

Extrinsic reinforcers have been demonstrated by Brent Rushall and John Pettinger (1969) to be highly effective in influencing the work output and training efficiency of members of an age-group swimming club, ages nine to fifteen. The subjects performed laps under different conditions: (1) no designated reinforcement, (2) coach's discouragement and comments, (3) candy reinforcement for each lap completed, and (4) money (one cent) reinforcement for each lap completed. The latter two conditions were equally effective and superior to the first two conditions in producing a greater distance of swimming attained by the subjects. Thus, the importance of reinforcement contingencies was established, at least for this age group and level of skill. Rushall and Pettinger (1969) have developed a model for the use of reinforcements to affect and direct behaviors. The stages suggested are

1. Define and list desirable and undesirable behaviors, noting their frequency of occurrence.
2. Structure the stimulus situation for teaching and controlling desirable behaviors.
3. Determine significant reinforcers and punishers.
4. Apply operant paradigms for behavior control.
5. Evaluate the effects of attempted control (p. 541).

Rushall and Daryl Siedentop (1972) have produced a book based on operant conditioning and reinforcement geared for physical educators and coaches. Theoretical discussion and practical implications are contained throughout the text. More recently, J. A. Dickinson (1977) developed a similar theme. In the format of Skinner, he has attempted to identify environmental contingencies of reinforcement and punishment that lead to participation in sports, as well as their effects on the acquisition of skills and other behaviors associated with sports.

A major issue in the use of rewards is their effect on controlling behavior versus providing directional information. Many proponents of the use of reward systems defend them on the basis of the second objective rather than the first one. If rewards are to be implemented in a training program, they should be gradually removed before long, or dependence on them may occur. In other words, the learner will participate for the receipt of rewards more than for the acquisition of skills and knowledge and personally meaningful and pleasurable experiences.

Societies differ in their value systems about the use of rewards. In the

United States, we are very reward conscious and directed. Sport is an excellent example of an extension of the overuse of reward systems for competition and winning. How can the situation be changed? Either a complete overhauling of the system is in order, or, at least, a more judicious deployment of rewards could be engineered.

AUGMENTED FEEDBACK (KNOWLEDGE OF RESULTS)

An early experiment contributing to the concept that practice alone does not always "make perfect" was one in which blindfolded subjects had to draw a line of so many inches. As they were never informed about how they were doing, the subjects did not improve in their performances. Many studies since then, in which a wide range of methods and materials have been analyzed, have tended to demonstrate the importance of knowledge of performance or the knowledge of the results of performance.

As we know, much information is usually available to the learner/performer of motor skills as a result of his or her efforts. This state of affairs has been termed response-produced feedback. We know it if the movement feels good and can see whether an object goes into a target. In such events as diving and gymnastics, more limited information is available. *Augmented,* or *supplementary, feedback* is necessary when an insufficient amount of information is available as a consequence of actions. The term *knowledge of results* (KR) appears in the literature quite frequently and has been used to describe feedback provided by an external source (the teacher) or through the learner's own efforts. For our purposes, we will refer to KR in the same way as augmented feedback.

Although feedback and KR have been used interchangeably in the research literature and in daily dialogue, they might be differentiated in the following way. Feedback is typically associated with self-regulated stimulation through movement and closed-loop control models. Sensory feedback control over behavior is, therefore, an internalized process. Knowledge of results is associated more with external sources of information that the learner can use in the next attempt at a task. Ina McD. Bilodeau (1969) has presented an excellent review of the research and acknowledges the confusion in the use of feedback and KR terminology. She favors the term *information feedback* to denote a stimulus presented by an external source during or after a learner's response. Such a term is analogous to the way KR is referred to. Perhaps, as Holding (1965) suggests, internal feedback and external feedback should be distinguished, with the latter applied to the term *knowledge of results*. We will use the terms as interpreted earlier in the paragraph.

We typically receive feedback when we perform most athletic skills. In performing a swimming stroke, if it does not feel right, we try to adapt and correct our movements. The quarterback who continually attempts to pass into a particular zone, only to find it well covered by defenders, adjusts the offense. The archer can see if the arrow is missing the target and can compensate accordingly in the next responses. From merely making a basket, serving in the proper court, or making a putt, we are informed if our response is correct.

There are other cases in which it is necessary for an outsider to provide relevant information. Sometimes we are not aware of what we do wrong to cause an inappropriate response. A violation of a mechanical principle, bad form resulting in inefficient performance, or other errors can be relayed to the performer by an instructor. Knowledge of results may or may not be useful, depending on the availability of sufficient feedback and the ability to evaluate and use it.

In practice for some sports or in actual competition, knowledge of results serves a definite purpose. If the fencer is not rewarded by a point when an opponent is legally touched, unnecessary adjustments may be made. Enjoyment and learning are hampered. The same holds true for fouls not called in a basketball game. The foul call informs the player that the referee knows that a rule has been violated, and no call permits the player greater freedom and perhaps more violations of other rules. Without knowledge of results, improvement cannot occur. Violations not called in practice severely limit the performance in a game, especially if the player is not aware when illegal acts are being committed.

Types of Knowledge of Results (KR)

The variety of forms that KR can assume is best expressed by Holding (1965). When KR (extrinsic, supplementary) is to be provided, considerations must be made for the type, as well as timing. Figure 13-1 illustrates these considerations. Certain tasks will dictate the limitations on the kinds of KR it is possible to provide to the learner. Other tasks provide more options. Channels and sources also should be considered. The best situation for the learner is to receive the optimal degree of information, so that he or she can profit from it in any situation. Too little will be of minor assistance and too much will flood the information channel capacity of the system. Redundancy in feedback can assist on some occasions as reinforcing cues for each other for the benefit of the learner. On other occasions, it is useless and a waste of energies. Thus, the whole question of augmenting feedback comes into question.

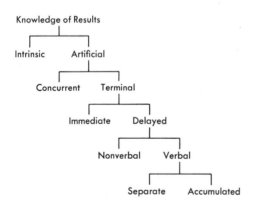

FIGURE 13-1. Different kinds of knowledge of results. (*From Holding, D. H.* Principles of training. *Oxford: Pergamon, 1965.*) Reprinted with permission of Pergamon Press, Ltd.

Considering the learner's abilities, skill level, and the task, when is there enough information present in the task and situation for the learner to use without any need for outside intervention and assistance? If additional information is to be supplied, what is the desired form, geared for which sensory channels, of what magnitude and duration, and in what temporal relation to the task?

Evidence conflicts with regard to the advisability of employing supplementary, or agumented, feedback, which in fact, is what KR usually represents. Equivocal findings indicate the nonutility of attempting to generalize too far, across all kinds of tasks, learners, and forms of augmented feedback. A more fruitful attempt would be to analyze situations more specifically, for obviously there are occasions when supplementary feedback is not only helpful, but a necessity for effective performance. The desirability of kinds of KR has been investigated under controlled conditions in which sources for KR are withheld from or added to learning situations.

The possible use of augmented feedback should be considered in relation to:

1. the substantiality and value of the feedback intrinsic to the task.
2. the skill level of the learner (need and ability to use kinds of feedback and KR).
3. the redundancy of cues and the kinds that are to be favored.

Theoretical interpretations of how feedback operates in motor behavior were alluded to in Chapter 5, especially in regard to the work of Adams and his proposed closed-loop theory. Does response-produced feedback merely affect momentary performance or a more permanent state of learning? In an attempt to answer this and related questions, Adams, Goetz, and Marshall (1972) had subjects practice under augmented or minimal feedback conditions with a self-paced positioning task. Visual, auditory, and proprioceptive feedback were examined in various contexts. The conclusions follow:

1. The acquisition of skill was directly related to the amount of feedback present.
2. Augmented feedback led to more effective performance than minimal feedback.
3. Response-produced feedback had a great impact on both learning and performance and should be central in theories of learning dealing with motor behaviors.

How precise should augmented information feedback be in order really to assist the learner? Obviously, the instructor has a variety of alternatives as to the degree to which specific feedback is provided to the learner. Frank Smoll (1972) attempted to resolve this issue. Using a duckpin bowling ball task, three different forms of feedback were provided to the subjects after each delivery: (1) quantitative feedback to 0.01 of a second, (2) quantitative feedback to 0.1 of a second, and (3) qualitative feedback (comments such as the delivery was too fast, too slow, or correct). Smoll concluded that the two quantitative feedback conditions led to superior performances, as compared to the qualitative method. The two quantitative methods did not differ in effect on performance. Sometimes, if KR information is too precise (Rogers, 1974) it can be detrimental to performance. Much depends on a person's ability to interpret and make effective use of the KR provided. The usefulness of precise KR is probably a function of a person's skill level; the more advanced the level, the more precise the KR can be. It does appear that there is an optimal precision level of feedback that yields the most favorable performances, and it should be in the direction of greater precision.

A distinction might be made between guidance cues and feedback, although they may, on occasion, refer to the same situation. Norman Gordon (1968) suggests that

> Guiding cues differ from feedback in that they are always present regardless of the subject's action, whereas feedback cues vary as a function of the subject's response, although they may be considered to constitute a form of intermittent guidance, as well. On the other hand, the provision of adding guiding cues designed to augment input cues can have the effect of altering feedback information if the nature of the guidance is such as to markedly affect responses (p. 24).

Gordon's data led him to conclude that augmented feedback benefited the learners. It increased motivation and enhanced attention to the appropriate cues. One of the dangers of supplementary information is too much reliance on it. In order to be of value later in task performance or in transfer tasks, such cues should be withdrawn at an appropriate stage of performance. It has also been demonstrated that motor performance levels (after reasonable skill has been achieved) can be maintained when KR is withdrawn (Newell, 1976). In other words, it is important in the earlier stages of learning.

Research and Theoretical Considerations

Research on the topic of knowledge of results is too vast to be presented here; the reviews by Adams (1978) and Newell (1976) should be of value to the interested reader. Among the issues raised are two questions: (1) Is the intertrial interval more important than the knowledge of results delay? (2) Will a delay of KR have the same effect on all types of tasks? The postknowledge of results interval during the acquisition of skill is of theoretical as well as practical import with regard to time delay and intervening activities. Three important factors should be considered with regard to KR:

1. The effects of varying time durations before KR is given.
2. The effects of various interpolated activities in the KR delay interval.
3. The relation of length of time as well as activity with motor tasks of varying complexity.

It makes sense that there should be an optimal period following the execution of an act that KR will be of value. However, much evidence indicates that the delay alone of KR does not affect the acqusition of motor skills. Further research has been initiated to determine the effects of interpolated activity during the KR-delay interval. Although it seems reasonable to hypothesize that interference would occur during this period with the administration of activities, such has not usually been proved to be the case. The learner appears to learn a simple motor task adequately, whether or not a simple interpolated activity is administered. This is true when it is either similar or dissimilar to the one being learned, between each response and the time KR is provided.

With regard to the post-KR interval, or the legth of time that expires from the provision of KR to the next response, some researchers have investigated delay periods of from one, two, five, ten, twenty, or thirty seconds. In general, it appears that one second is not sufficient time for KR to be processed effectively. However, several researchers have indicated different periods of time as being ideal or else of no effect on performance. Experimentally, the paradigm illustrating the relationships of responses, KR, and delay periods would be as drawn in Figure 13-2.

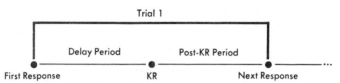

FIGURE 13-2. Relationship of a response, delay period for the provision of knowledge of results, and the delay period from KR to the second response.

Interpolated activities have assumed a variety of forms and their effects on learning and performance do not lend themselves easily to any generalizations. The post-KR interval has been filled with verbal tasks or unique motor tasks. Because most of the research evidence is based on rather simple motor tasks, the value of KR at a particular interval of time or the effects of interpolated activities are difficult to assess for complex tasks. Nevertheless, the post-KR interval is of importance to consider because of the fact that the learner processes the information or results received concerning the previous response and then makes a decision about how to respond in the next response. Yet, little is known about the relation of this interval to the processes involved in acquiring a motor skill. One of the more recent attempts at examining interpolated activity and time-delay factors in a KR experiment has been reported by Magill (1973). Tracking, positioning, reaction time, and complex tasks and the role of feedback have been discussed by John Annett (1969) in one of the chapters of his book.

Robert Ammons (1956) summarized the earlier research on knowledge of results and states eleven empirical generalizations:

1. The performer usually has hypotheses about what is to be done and how to do it, and these interact with knowledge of performance.
2. For all practical purposes, there is always some knowledge of performance available to the human performer.

3. Knowledge of performance affects rate of learning and level reached by learning.
4. Knowledge of performance affects motivation.
5. The more specific the knowledge of performance, the more rapid the improvement and the higher the level of performance.
6. The longer the delay in giving knowledge of performance, the less effect the given information has.
7. In the case of discontinuous tasks where knowledge of performance is given, small intervals between trials are generally better for learning that are longer ones.
8. When knowledge of performance is decreased, performance drops.
9. When knowledge of performance is decreased, performance drops more rapidly if trials are relatively massed.
10. When subjects are not being given supplementary knowledge of performance by the experimenter any longer, the ones who maintain their performance level probably have developed some substitute knowledge of performance.
11. When direct (supplementary) knowledge of performance is removed, systematic "undershooting" or "overshooting" may appear in performance (pp. 281–293).

Reinforcement, Motivation, and Augmented Feedback

Augmented feedback can serve to motivate, regulate, direct, and/or reinforce behaviors. The informational properties of knowledge of results will, depending on the task and the learner's capabilities, guide or cue ongoing movements in the continuous task or influence the next repeated response in discrete tasks. As far as motivation is concerned, augumented feedback may encourage or discourage performance efforts. Learned responses may be activated and sustained, alternative responses may be developed, and, in general, a more favorable performing and learning climate will exist. Perhaps it can be suggested that feedback be classified in three categories, depending on the main intent:

1. Information feedback: used for comparison purposes to correct errors.
2. Rewarding (reinforcing) feedback: little information present, helps shape behavior in certain directions
3. Motivating feedback: influences attitude to continue practicing the task.

Feedback, or KR, if theoretically pure, would be necessary either to improve or to maintain performance levels on occasions. Yet, the primary value of KR is in the earlier learning trials, as research indicates that performances in a number of tasks can be sustained following the withdrawal of KR. Many times supplementary feedback, although not really necessary for regulation in task performance, will possess reinforcing and/or motivating virtues, shaping and motivating behaviors. Activity is thereby attended to more seriously, conscientiously, and in a persevering manner. Merely saying to the learner that the performance was good or bad, although not very helpful for detailed analysis of behavior, can be an encouraging or discouraging form of feedback information.

A most unusual approach to the topic of reinforcement is provided by Joseph Nuttin (1968). He analyzed the relative effects of rewards and punishments from a series of personally directed studies to challenge Thorndike's law of effect. Of importance here is that Nuttin emphasized that rewards and punishment provide error information in many motor tasks. Thus, the informational value serves to cue the learner for specific stimuli and particular responses.

In a series of studies in which Roger Black was involved (e.g., Slayton & Black, 1971), similar effects of knowledge of results and reinforcement have been noted in resistance to extinction. That is, subjects provided with such information tended to persist longer at their tasks than those subjects who were controlled. Rewards or KR tend to strengthen an instrumental response; withdrawal leads to extinction of that response. The apparatus used was the pursuit rotor. The data were interpreted as suggesting that "the role of schedule of KR in determining resistance to extinction on a pursuit-rotor task is completely analogous to the role of schedule of reinforcement in instrumental conditioning" (Slayton & Black, 1971, p. 112).

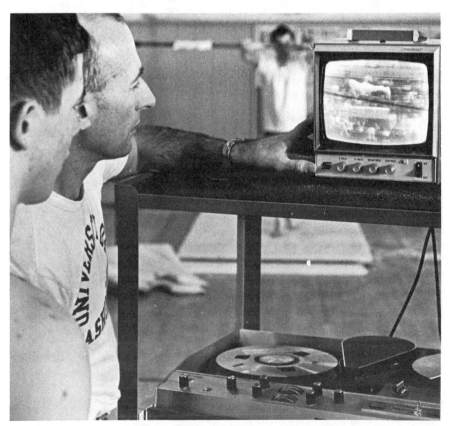

FIGURE 13-3. Coach and performer review the athlete's routine seconds after its completion. (*From Ampex Corporation; 401 Broadway; Redwood City, California.*)

In all the discussion on KR, however, it can readily be deduced that cues can possess a variety of psychological properties. The serious scholar can easily be exasperated in any attempt to isolate functions. The use of videotape in an instructional setting is a good practical example in which a particular medium may possess reinforcement, motivational, and feedback properties (see Figures 13-3 through 13-6 for examples in physical education and sport).

ATTRIBUTIONS

Following performance in an activity, it is fairly typical not only to appraise its quality and effectiveness, but also to make personal evaluations as to the caus-

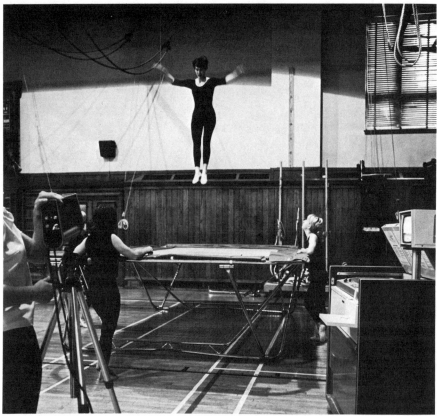

FIGURE 13-4. A young woman is being recorded on videotape as part of a gymnastics class. After going through her performance, she is immediately able to see herself on the television receiver, which is part of the portable Videotrainer at left. With videotape recording, students are given a chance to analyze their performance and correct their errors. (*From Ampex Corporation; 401 Broadway; Redwood City, California.*)

MOTOR LEARNING AND HUMAN PERFORMANCE

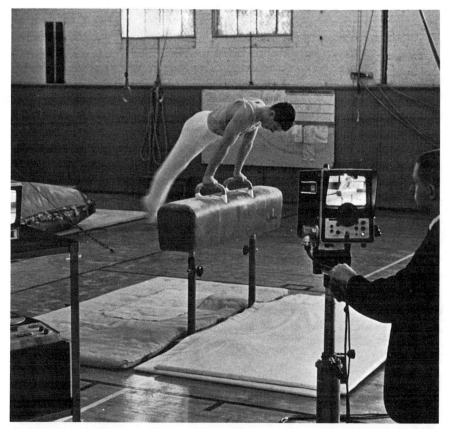

FIGURE 13-5. A member of a gymnastics team performs a routine on a sidehorse. His routine is picked up by a television camera and recorded on a videotape recorder as part of a meet with the University of Illinois. Each team competed on its own campus, with an impartial panel of judges viewing the video tapes of both teams to render its decision. It was the first such meet ever held. Illinois was the winner, 180.65 to 173.10. (*From Ampex Corporation; 401 Broadway; Redwood City, California.*)

ative factors. The evaluations, or reasons, are termed attributions. Often, sports figures are asked by sports reporters, "To what do you attribute your magnificent performance?" A typical answer might be, "Lucky, I guess." Or, "To hard work." Other responses may be offered, as well.

It was demonstrated briefly in Chapter 11 how attributions are related to future performance expectancy levels; in Chapter 12 it was demonstrated how cognitive psychology has offered attribution theory, a motivational theory, to explain the behaviors of individuals. In this section of the book, we will go into much greater detail about attributions, what causes them, who causes them, under what conditions they are created, and their potential influence on motor performance.

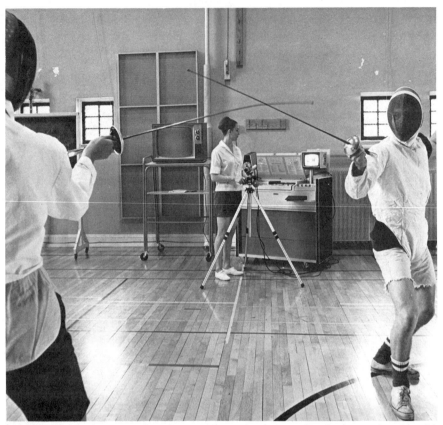

FIGURE 13-6. Students view their fencing form and style immediately after performing with an assist from a Videotrainer system. (*From Ampex Corporation; 401 Broadway; Redwood City, California.*)

Theory

The basic assumption of attribution theory is that behavior is determined to some degree by personal perceptions and an understanding of current events. Importance is placed on the personal beliefs regarding the causes and subsequent expectation of performance outcomes. Causes for perceived success or failure in an act have been described by Bernard Weiner (1974) in a two-dimensional classification scheme. Ability and effort, two possible attributions, are considered to be internal. Task difficulty and luck, two other possible attributions, are external factors. These are the four major attributes that have been identified and examined in the research, although additional ones also have been conceived recently. The notion of internal and external factors, or locus of control, relates to the earlier work of Rotter (described in Chapter 12).

Furthermore, ability and task difficulty are viewed as relatively stable factors, whereas effort and luck are relatively unstable factors. Table 13-1 provides this matrix. Different attributions, with regard to locus of control, result in differential affective responses. Stability perceptions produce differential expectancy shifts.

TABLE 13-1 Classification Scheme for the Perceived Determinants of Achievement Behavior

	Locus of Control	
Stability	Internal	External
Stable	Ability	Task difficulty
Unstable	Effort	Luck

From Weiner, B. (ed.). *Achievement motivation and attribution theory.* Morristown, N.J.: General Learning Press, 1974.

This matrix has been expanded by Weiner and others to explain more behavioral tendencies, but it will suffice for our purposes as the heart of attribution theory. Performance in any situation may be as much influenced by such activated processes as by external stimuli in the environment.

Relationship to Expectations and Performance

Cognitive motivational theory may offer a theoretical base for the partial explanation and prediction of performance in motor skills. Given certain information, such as success or failure, persons probably make attributions to causal elements that may influence later achievements. If success feedback is experienced, individuals will probably make attributions to internal factors of ability and effort; under failing conditions, attributions are probably directed toward task difficulty.

In the learning of motor tasks, as contrasted with cognitive learning (unless computer-managed instruction is utilized), feedback for performance evaluation purposes is invariably available in some form. Therefore, the effect of performance feedback on attributions, expectations, and subsequent performance can be monitored continually in a learning situation.

Furthermore, high and low achievers presumably have different perceptions of responsibility for task outcome. The high-need achiever believes success is due to both ability and effort and that failure is the result of lack of effort. The person low in achievement need ascribes no particular attributional preference for success but believes that failure is due to lack of ability.

These disparate perceptions of responsibility in persons classified as high and low in need achievement under conditions where success or failure are experienced may have important implications for understanding motor performance and learning and the application of effective instructional techniques. For example, high-need achievers are reported to be more persistent after failure (Weiner, 1965), and this has been interpreted as due to the application of increased effort expenditure (Kukla, 1972).

The relationship between attributions and expectancies may also provide explanations for motor performance, especially if attributions are to stable factors. Researchers using cognitive tasks have revealed that attributions to the factors of ability and task difficulty have a greater effect on expectancy shifts than attributions to the unstable factors of luck and effort. Expectancies of future performance have also been shown to influence performance in certain cognitive tasks. It is possible that attributions, expectancies, and performance may be related in some definite manner (see Figure 13-7). For example, a successful performance may be attributed to stable, internal factors, which in turn influences expectancies for future performance by raising the level of aspiration, which in turn produces a greater degree of persistence and effort resulting in a change in performance. Feedback concerning performance failure may encourage or discourage subsequent performance, depending on whether failure is viewed as an indication that more effort is required to master a task of greater than expected difficulty or if failure is viewed as the result of personal limitations (Brickman & Hendricks, 1975; Brickman et al., 1976; Roth & Kubal, 1975).

Cognitive interpretations of motor behavior may provide an insight into performance, where task outcomes influence both attributions and consequent striving for the goal. Attribution theory and the attributional theory of performance appear to have linked other cognitive theories into a scheme whereby the outcome of performance can be more readily interpreted.

However, in the majority of studies, a post hoc analysis of performance data has been provided. On-going analyses of attributions and expectancies during the learning of task, where subjects are given repeated success and failure experiences, have not been made. However, there have been recent attempts to examine the effects of bogus feedback on performance, considering such variables as self-acceptance, in the context of cognitive dissonance theory (Bartz, 1975); ego-involvement also, within the framework of cognitive dissonance theory (Iso-Ahola, 1976); and trait anxiety and sex, in the context of drive theory (Martens, Gill, & Scanlan, 1976). Repeated analyses may offer a more reliable index of these cogni-

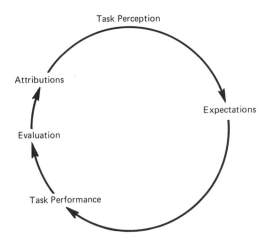

Task Perception

Attributions

Evaluation

Task Performance

Expectations

FIGURE 13-7. The conceptual relationship of attributions, expectations, and performance. (*From Singer, R. N., & McCaughan, L. Motivation effects of attributions, expectancy, and achievement motivation during the learning of a novel motor task.* Journal of Motor Behavior, *1978, 10, 245–254.*)

tive operations and can be done easily in motor learning situations. An attributional analysis during skill acquisition may assist in understanding the persistence and intensity of persons with differential achievement dispositions and aid in the prediction of performance in competitive situations.

In one of the few recent motor behavior studies on the topic (Singer & McCaughan, 1978), several cognitive motivational theories including achievement motivation, attribution theory, and an attributional theory of performance, were linked to explain and predict psychomotor performance. Sixty high- and sixty low-need achieving male high school students were randomly placed into success and failure feedback conditions, and performance scores on a lever-positioning apparatus were assessed. Following each block of performance trials, fictitious feedback in the form of success and failure information was given, and then each subject completed attribution and expectancy questionnaires. Neither high- or low-need achievers made disparate attributional ratings, but the situational effects of success and failure supported attribution theory. Success feedback elicited internal attributions among the subjects, whereas subjects receiving failure experiences externalized attributions. Expectancies for future performance improved more following success than after failure and were generally predicted by attributions to stable elements. Although trends were present, performance scores were unaffected by these cognitive beliefs. However, a significant prediction of performance was obtained when stepwise multiple regression procedures were used with constant error as the criterion variable. The factors of expectancy and luck significantly predicted performance. However, no firm basis for prediction should be assumed because only a minor proportion of true variance was accounted for by these variables.

This study is reported as a step in the direction to untangle the many situational and personal variables that can conceivably operate and interact in any learning/performance situation. Perhaps different procedures and a different task would have led to some alternative conclusions. However, at the present time, some advisable manipulations in performance situations might be as follows: (1) successes should be maximized, related to individual ability levels. This will lead to the development of an internal locus of control. Furthermore, attributions for performance will be made to the internal factors of ability and effort. (2) An emphasis on effort evaluations should be made rather than win-lose, success-failure, evaluations. This might encourage continuance at an activity. With this in mind, Weiner (1975) has made a plea for rewarding the effort put forth in competitive athletics. An effort evaluation of the athlete's performance in relation to personal ability should lead to enhanced self-concept through participation in competitive athletics.

TRANSFER OF TRAINING

That there have been many references so far to the transference of instructional and training methods and materials to skilled performance. This particular section contains direct reference to the concept of transfer, in theory and practice.

Almost all of learning is based on the concept of transfer. *Transfer* implies the influence of a learned task on one to be learned or the utilization of strategies in a new situation related to the one in which they were learned. School curricula and educational theory reflect the realization of and need for formal education that will carry over into life's experiences and chosen occupations. Is it not true that the purpose of education is to prepare an individual to live more effectively within oneself and within society? If we believe in this meaning of education, then we must accept the fact that behaviors may be transferable from one situation to another, depending on similarities and other variables.

Transfer training implies practice not only for present use, but also for future application. It is to be hoped that what is learned in one context can be carried over to another context. In a sense, then, transfer training is learning for later situations. Exactly how transfer takes place and what is transferred has been the subject of many investigations and the inspiration for theoretical speculation. Also, it is important to remember that transfer can be thought of in two ways: between activities and within an activity. *Lateral transfer* (task to task) is usually investigated by researchers to determine the influence of learning capabilities from one task or area to another task or area. *Vertical transfer* (within task) is the concern of psychoinstructional designers; where subordinate tasks are designated as prerequisites for higher-order learning in the same activity.

Measurement

Typically, experimental procedures employed in studies of transfer assume two forms. In the first case, an experimental group learns task A, the control group rests, and both groups are tested on task B. The difference in performance between the groups on task B, if any, would be due to the effect of learning task A.

	Task A	Task B
Experimental group	Learns	Learns
Control group	Rests	Learns

One of the weaknesses in the design in this table is the possibility that the groups were not equated at the start of the experiment. This problem may be overcome by pretesting the groups on the eventual task to be learned. If too much testing practice is given at this time, there is the danger that the potential influence of one task on a second task will be concealed.

	Task B	Task A	Task B
Experimental group	Tested	Learns	Learns
Control group	Tested	Rests	Learns

Transfer from one task to another task or from one situation to another situation will depend on the relationship between their stimuli and the responses demanded of the individuals. Such psychological terms as stimulus generalization and response generalization are appropriate to this discussion. Stimulus generalization explains the condition such that when a particular response is learned to a stimulus, similar stimuli will evoke the same response. In response generalization once a response has been learned to a given stimulus, the stimulus will cause similar responses to be elicited. It stands to reason that we can learn to associate the same response to a given range of stimuli (stimulus generalization) as well as a range of responses to a particular stimulus (response generalization). These terms will be discussed intermittently within the context of the material in this section.

C. E. Osgood (1949) has attempted to show S–R relationships and to predict task-to-task transfer effects. Figure 13-8 depicts the Osgood Transfer Surface, a theoretical transfer model. It illustrates that, after a specific response is learned to a given stimulus, S_1–R_1, maximum interference—hence, negative transfer—occurs when a completely new response has to be learned to that stimulus, S_1–R_2. As the stimulus gradually changes, until it is completely different from the first one, and the response also, S_2–R_2, there is zero transfer. A new stimulus that requires an already learned response, S_2–R_1, results in zero transfer, although any relationship at all between these stimuli will result in positive transfer in behavior.

Although the Transfer Surface does a good job explaining and predicting transfer relationships, it does not take into account some potential influencing variables. One of these is the amount of training on the first task, S_1–R_1. More practice yields better transfer effects, for it is observed that little training results in broad generalization transfer and more training in sharper generalization transfer.

The Surface recognizes the possibility of transfer of training effects as being zero, negative, or positive. *Positive transfer* ocurs when prior learning promotes present learning, and *negative transfer* infers an inhibitory effect of prior learning on immediate learning. *Zero or no transfer* takes place when former learning has no effect on the learning of an immediate task. It would not be difficult for any of us to remember instances in which all three conditions have occurred. There is an interesting relationship between amount of transfer, type of transfer, and amount of pretraining. It has already been stated that specific transfer is enhanced by more prior-task training; but, in addition, it is probable that negative transfer will occur with little practice, whereas extensive practice will encourage more positive transfer.

Learning to hit a fast-pitched baseball might be considered as $S_1 - R_1$. Assume that the ballplayer then will try to learn how to pull the ball (swing earlier), which is a variation of R_1. The stimulus remains the same, but the response is slightly altered. We will probably expect some degree of positive transfer, perhaps some negative influence, with the ultimate transfer effect being either sightly positive or zero. Now suppose that the response to be mastered is a bunt. This response is quite different from the original one. If the batter has been conditioned to swing away at a pitched ball and now has to learn to bunt, interference between responses will probably occur (as predicted by the Osgood Surface).

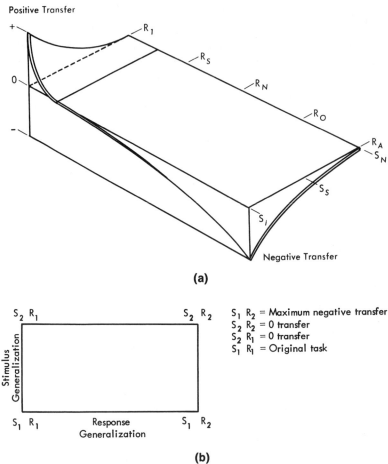

FIGURE 13-8. (a) The Osgood Transfer Surface. The medial planes represent effects of zero magnitude, response generalization is represented along the length, and stimulus generalization along its width. R_1 original or extremely similar response, S_1 original or extremely similar stimulus, R_S to R_A increasingly different responses, S_S to S_N increasingly different stimuli. The Surface may be used to find another task in relation to the original one to predict the extent of transfer as well as the presence of negative or positive transfer. (*From Osgood, C. E. The similarity paradox in human learning: A resolution.* Psychological Review, *1949, 56, 132–143.*)

(b) Osgood Surface modified. As the second response R_2 to the same stimulus S_1 becomes more unrelated to R_1, maximum interference occurs. As the stimulus is gradually changed at the same time the response is until the condition S_2–R_2 occurs, less interference is present. When the response remains the same but the stimulus gradually changes until S_2–R_1 is reached, positive transfer effects decrease until no transfer is present.

Returning to the baseball scene, and S_1–R_1 as the original task, let us modify the stimulus. If a curve ball instead of a fast ball is thrown, and the same response as before is desired, positive transfer should occur. However, the more the stimulus is changed, the less positive the transfer. If an underhanded softball throw is

MOTOR LEARNING AND HUMAN PERFORMANCE

the new stimulus, the batting behavior of the individual may little resemble that which was demonstrated with the pitched baseball, thereby revealing little, if any, in the way of positive transfer effects.

Whenever one performs in and reacts to a new situation, to a certain extent, respnses will reflect previous experiences. Sometimes it is desirable to perform similarly as before, sometimes not. In experimental situations, the investigator can determine, through statistical analysis, any significant positive or negative transfer effects.

Conditions Affecting Transfer

There are numerous conditions associated with, and which may potentially affect, the transfer effects of one task to another. Probably the most important of these is the *similarity* between the tasks. A greater resemblance between task elements, between their respective stimuli and responses, will result in the greatest amount of transfer. For instance, Ammons, Ammons, and Morgan (1958) trained their subjects on varying speeds of the pursuit rotor. Transfer effects were found to be proportional to the similarity between the speed rates of any two tasks. As in our discussion on this matter, especially the reference to the Osgood Transfer Surface, the probable negative and positive transfer effects are indicated when certain variables are present.

The *amount of practice* on the prior task has already been shown to be related to the amount and nature of transfer expected. More practice on a task that might positively influence performance on a second task will result in performance in the expected direction. Even experience with elements or components of a task can facilitate the learning of it (Vincent, 1968). Subjects practicing on specific perceptual components of motor skills showed the advantage of this experience when compared to control subjects. *Motivation* to transfer skill or knowledge from one situation to another situation is yet another consideration.

It is also possible that the *method of training* may have some bearing on the transfer effectiveness. In recent years, a few investigators have looked into the matter of whole-versus-part learning methods and their relative efficiency in facilitating transfer. In one experiment, Briggs and Waters (1958), using simulated aircraft control dynamics, found that it was important to practice the whole task if the highest transfer potential is to be realized. Part practice does not integrate component skills. For transfer purposes, the authors recommend that the whole task be simplified rather than fractionalized. Briggs and Naylor (1962) tested their subjects for transfer on a three-dimensional tracking task learned under different practice methods. The whole and progressive part methods were equal and significantly better than the pure part and simplified whole methods for transfer effectiveness.

Intent of transfer is yet another factor of influence. If the instructor indicates the elements common to two tasks and provides the basis for insight and understanding, the learner will probably make greater use of what has been learned on the prior task when it comes time to perform a related second task. In other words, greater assistance is provided when skills are taught with the intention of transferring over to other skills.

Referring back to skills with a certain degree of relationship, it is of interest to speculate whether positive or negative effects will occur between such activities as tennis and badminton, baseball and golf, and basketball and volleyball. Let us use tennis and badminton as an example. They are both racket sports involving the striking of a projectile. Eye–hand coordination is extremely important in both sports, as is agility and quickness of movement. It might be hypothesized that outstanding ability in one of these sports should render the individual highly successful in the other sport. However, there are other considerations. Badminton strokes are made with a highly flexible wrist, whereas a tennis ball is usually stroked with a firm wrist. A tennis ball has altogether different characteristics than does the badminton shuttlecock. It might, therefore, be argued that high skill in one activity would hinder the learning of the other activity.

Although task similarities encourage related movement patterns, this response generalization is not always desirable. Response generalization promotes initial skill acquisition, but it is response distinction that is important at the highly skilled levels of performance. The precision and accuracy of a given task distinguish it from that which is required in other tasks. So, in a sense, response generalization is the opposite of skill. Response generalization infers generalized movements common between two tasks, whereas skill requires precision movements.

The attempted development of theoretical relationships between sports leaves much to be desired because of the complexity of these activities. When dealing with simple tasks, elements may be identified with much greater ease. Exactly how much transfer occurs from athletic skill to athletic skill is, thus, difficult to ascertain, especially if the entire context of their usage is considered.

Often, *general principles learned in problem solving* will transfer favorably from situation to situation (Ausubel, Novak, & Hanesian, 1978). Judd's experiment in 1908 on learning the principle of shooting at targets submerged underwater, as well as other studies, demonstrated the carry-over effect of learning strategies, problem-solving capabilities, adaptive abilities, and the like.

Learning to Learn

Another aspect of the learning function, often neglected, is the transfer that occurs from merely learning materials similar in nature. When materials or tasks undertaken are alike, improvement results just from learning how to learn them. One has to learn how to take multiple-choice written tests, how to lift weights, or how to solve psychomotor tasks.

Learning how to learn involves learning the technique of attacking a problem of a particular kind. The individual acquires the appropriate *set,* and reduces general stimuli to specific cues. After repeated experience with the same type of tasks, after attentive adjustment is established, greater learning always occurs.

The psychologist most associated with calling this phenomenon to the attention of all those concerned with learning is Harry Harlow. Harlow (1949), working with monkeys, gave them different discrimination problems to solve. At first, the monkeys took a long time to learn the problems, but as they tackled more problems, there was a decrease in solution time. Therefore, learning how to learn something is necessarily a partial explanation of how one task transfers over to another similar task.

Bilateral Transfer

There is considerable evidence to indicate the transference of electrical activity and skilled movements from one part of the body to another. Physiologically, it has been demonstrated that mental activity causes electrical stimulation of the areas of the body being thought about.

The contributions of Cook (1933a, 1933b) to that area of study he called cross-education provided early evidence about the transfer of a skill learned in one part of the body to another. Transfer was found to be greatest to the muscle group opposite and symmetrical; it was least to the muscle group opposite and unsymmetrical to the practiced limb. Even strength can be transferred from a trained to an untrained limb. G. A. Logan and A. Lockhart (1962) report contralateral transfer of strength from the knee extensors of the trained leg to the knee extensors of the untrained limb.

Thus, in any act, there is a tendency for response generalization. Activity that is overt and apparently body specific has an overall effect on the individual. Internal activity is constantly going on during our periods of wakefulness, and it appears as if the interwoven complexity of the nervous sytem permits motor patterns to be learned from practiced to unpracticed limbs.

Task Difficulty

If the ultimate objective is skill in a particular activity, the instructor may proceed in one of three ways: (1) students can be guided from easy to more complex steps, thus providing the learners with initial success and satisfaction in the activity; (2) skill(s) can be taught directly; or, learners may have to overcome the extreme difficulties of the task(s) before undertaking the precise task(s), thus operating under a complex-to-easy task procedure.

Theoretically, it makes good sense to build up to a particular objective, to master simple skills before learning more difficult ones and to gain the satisfaction that is supplied with successful attempts. Obviously, a person should be able to show the greatest achievement when attempting simple tasks. Contrarily, theoretical support could be mustered for the teaching of skills from the complex to the simple. When one confronts the more difficult task first, if it is not unreasonably complex, a progression to the easier tasks should bother the learner very little because the harder task contained all the elements of the simple ones. It appears that there may be a conflict over the desirability of introducng simple skills as opposed to complex ones when teaching for transfer. There is yet another alternative to the problem. If achievement on a particular skill is wanted, and perhaps it is of mediocre difficulty, should it be taught directly? Because of the specificity nature of skill learning, transfer from skill to skill, no matter how related they are, may not occur in the most efficient manner.

Skinner, as we have noted is one of the leading promoters of the teaching machine, and he has introduced the theory of shaping behavior. It is actually based on the concept of transfer of training from the simple to the more difficult. A sequence of events leads to the desired outcome, with the progressive transfer system increasing the probability of a correct response.

D. A. Lordahl and E. J. Archer (1958), in two pursuit rotor experiments, varied task difficulty by manipulating target rotation speed or the radius of the target orbit. Direct practice was better than transfer practice. There was slightly more positive transfer when training from the simple to the complex than vice-versa in one of the experiments, whereas there were no differential transfer effects from an easy or more complex task in the other experiment.

Baker, Wylie, and Gagné (1950) had subjects follow a signal on a target by turning a crank handle. Response rates were changed for each of four tasks. Training on a faster rate of speed produced more transfer to perform at the slower rate than vice-versa. The investigators concluded, therefore, that a greater amount of transfer occurs when task I is relatively difficult and task II relatively easy. C. G. Gibbs (1951), utilizing a handle-winding task and a steering task, declared that the greatest transfer from a difficult to an easy task occurred when the same kind of ability was required in both tasks. However, he warns that an increase in task difficulty will not necessarily cause the most rapid rate of learning, as there is an optimum range of task difficulty.

In most cases, direct practice on the task of concern leads to the most favorable results. However, changes in task practice, whether from easy to hard or vice-versa, may produce beneficial effects on performance. Richard May and Pam Duncan's (1973) data indicate that there may be an optimal amount of change in difficulty for best total performance. An intermediate degree of change led to most favorable results in a puzzle-block skills task. Changes in task difficulty may promote attention to relevant aspects of the task, especially where identifying and isolating important stimuli is important. Those authors wrote that, "It might be useful to consider a task continuum along which amount of cognitive versus motor involvement is scaled. The greater the cognitive component, the more changes in difficulty may facilitate performance. With maximal motor involvement, changes in the problem might disrupt or inhibit performance" (p. 128).

That extreme transfer practice subjects generally do poorer than central transfer practice subjects is a notion upheld by the data collected by S. D. Leonard, E. W. Karnes, J. Oxendine, and J. Hesson (1970) using a pursuit rotor. With the criterion task set at 45 revolutions per minute, those subjects who practiced at 40, 45, and 50 revolutions per minute performed better than those at 30 and 60 revolutions per minute.

As R. H. Day (1956) points out in summarizing the studies concerned with the effect of the difficulty of initial and final tasks on transfer training, there are inconsistencies from study to study in defining difficulty and discrepancies among experimental results. Difficulty of a task can be affected by manipulating stimulus or response variables. With regard to the response situation, Day concludes that there is a greater degree of transfer from a difficult to an easy condition than the reverse.

Singer (1966) designed an investigation to study this problem using archery skill with physical education activities. Three classes of students practiced under different conditions: class A learned and practiced archery at the 10-yard line; class C began at the 40-yard line; and class B started at the 25-yard line. The three groups were then tested on the 25-yard line. When testing for transfer, no significant difference was observed in the transfer effects from practice on an easier task (class A), as compared to the transfer effects of a more difficult task (class C), in comparison to precise distance practice (class B). Ultimate success, as measured by the Columbia Junior Round, indicated no significant difference between the groups—task proficiency was not affected by the initial learning technique.

The matter of which level of skill to begin with is hard to resolve. Immediate reward and satisfaction are certainly important, but so is the time element. It appears as if many present-day writers are in favor of learning a more difficult skill directly, rather than through lead-up activities. Many also favor progression from the more difficult to the simple rather than the opposite way. Perhaps the teaching method should reflect the instructor-student objectives. If what is desired is the development of a perfected act (in a stable stimulus environment), then possibly, complex skills should be practiced first. If the technique is not as important as being aware of relevant cues and understanding the situation (in a changing environment), possibly, as Barbara Knapp (1964) suggests, the learning should progress from the simpler situation.

Adaptive Training

Support for the belief that practice should proceed from easier to more difficult task demands is found in the newly popularized concept of *adaptive training*. Thus far, the interest has lodged in mastering equipment requiring the involvement of perceptual and motor behaviors. Equipment has been developed as training devices that provide automatic adjustments according to problem difficulty and the person's level of performance. With improvement, the difficulty of the task is varied and increased. In the adaptive approach, the learner's errors are maintained at a constant level as task difficulty varies.

The contrasting approach is to set the task at a specified operational level so that the performer's errors are free to vary. The roots of adaptive training rest in an individualized approach to skill mastery, with concepts apparently somewhat allied to programmed learning techniques. In the most informative article on the topic prepared so far, Charles R. Kelly (1971) indicates the limitations of traditional training programs:

1. Group instruction makes it extremely hard to be sensitive and to vary tasks according to each student's level of performance.

2. Automatic training devices contain preprogrammed tasks and do not consider the person's level of performance and rate of progression.

Figure 13-9 demonstrates the distinction between fixed and adaptive training. The feedback loop in the adaptive model serves to change the task demands as a consequence of the learner's level of performance. Fixed training is not as sensitive as adaptive training. It is a closed-loop approach. Machine-controlled adaptive training contains three unique elements:

1. A means for measuring performance.
2. An adjustable feature of the task or problem which changes in difficulty (the adaptive variable).
3. Adaptive logic, which automatically changes the adaptive variable as a function of performance measurement.

Training automatically becomes harder as skill progresses. Three training systems are illustrated in Figure 13-10. Graph A illustrates a fixed difficulty system that is not sensitive to learners' progress. In graph B, one example of an adaptive model, the task becomes more complex with skill acquisition. The change is not as dramatic as in graph C. In this case, the performance measurement remains constant throughout training. One variable would ideally change systematically with adaptation and, therefore, is the recommended procedure. System error is stated at the beginning of training, which the learner must meet. The system adapts to the difficulty level of the task and the ability level of the person.

Training devices and systems can be effective when carefully devised, when the difficulty level of the task is geared for the individual and not fixed. The magnitude of errors made is indicative of task load. The efficiency of the adaptive approach has been shown when compared to the success demonstrated in training on the criterion, or final, task itself, or when arbitrary levels of increasing fixed difficulty are used. Of course, in a group setting where individualized approaches

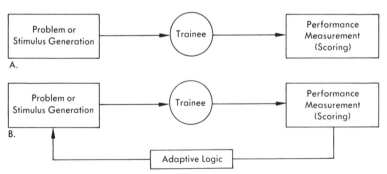

FIGURE 13-9. Fixed versus adaptive training. (A) Fixed (preprogrammed) training. (B) Adaptive training. (*From Kelley, C. R. Fundamental problems. In J. J. McGrath & D. H. Harris (Eds.), Adaptive training.* Aviation Research Monographs, *1971, 1, 1–35.*)

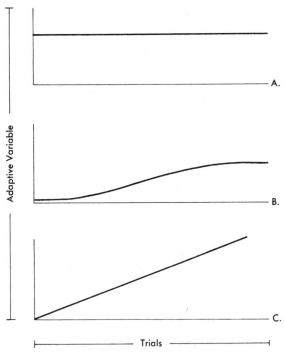

FIGURE 13-10. System change with learning. (A) Fixed difficulty system. (B) Adaptive system 1. (C) Adaptive system 2. (*From Kelley, C. R. Fundamental problems. In J. J. McGrath & D. H. Harris (Eds.), Adaptive training.* Aviation Research Monographs, *1971, 1, 1–35.*)

to training are impossible, the mean level or constant level for a number of individuals during practice provides the best compromise training technique. But the adaptive approach provides the best indicant in the form of reliable measurements of learner progress.

The adaptive variables that might be manipulated include modifications in the simulated environment, stress presence, augmented information, display changes, or task demands. The adaptive variable should systematically affect the difficulty of the task. A logical progression indicates which variable should be manipulated to move the task from simple to difficult. The logic employed in the system is of paramount importance. This may depend on precise mathematical equations or commonsense adjustment rules. The concepts show much promise for the intelligent planning of individualized training programs.

Theories of Transfer

The transfer effect of learning certain skills or matter precludes the learning of anything new. Actually, nothing a person learns is truly completely new. Everything undertaken has been seen and done before, only in different forms and shapes. What we learn and the speed of acquisition depend on positive and negative transfer situations and their interaction effects.

Examine, for instance, the situation in which a person learns the sport of tennis for the first time. One does not really start at a zero level of skill. Past experiences, such as in batting, catching, or throwing a ball, will transfer over to this activity. Previous experiences in racket games, examples of which are ping-pong, squash, and badminton, will influence tennis skill acquisition. Experiences in games that require quick and sudden movements, depth perception, alert reactions, strategy, and the like, will also have an effect.

How can we explain and predict the nature of transfer through theory? How is the concept of transfer, as well as the abundant research evidence to date (only partially reviewed in this chapter), to be incorporated into a theory?

Perhaps the first theory of transfer, which was in existence for many years prior to the twentieth century, is the *formal-discipline theory*. It no longer has any support from educators who have even casually reviewed the research evidence. At one time, the transferability of mental functions was considered to be wide in scope. The faculties of the mind were supposedly developed through specific courses, and these courses were not taught for their content but for their general mind-strengthening ability. It was felt that such mental functions as logic, concentration, reason, and memory could be developed in this manner.

Through the efforts of the great pioneer psychologist Thorndike in the earlier part of this century, the formal-discipline theory was discredited. One cannot train the mind in a general sense from particular courses or training. Course work abilities do not necessarily transfer over to practical situations. Instead, Thorndike proposed the *identical-elements theory,* based on his belief in learning by association (S–R theory). To Thorndike, transfer between two tasks or situations was only as effective as the number of elements common to them. The definition of an element is a question continually raised. When the term *element* is narrowly interpreted, it leads to more rejection of the theory; and alternatively, more generalized interpretation results in greater acceptance.

Compare the theory to one termed *generalization theory*. In contrast to consideration for specific stimuli or specific information, generalization theory encompasses the transferability of principles and problem-solving situations. As we now know, evidence conflicts as to the validation of this theory. However, classroom teachings are often based on the premise that an individual can transfer matter learned in these ways to other situations. This theory is probably most consistent with educational philosophy. It, like the identical-elements theory, has its proponents and doubters.

Among the other theories proposed is the *transposition theory* by the Gestaltists, but this and others need not be presented here. Suffice to say that the numerous theories in existence to describe learning phenomena indicate at least some experimental support. Research findings may often be interpreted in various ways, thus resulting in the possible formulation of a number of theories from the same data.

RETENTION: FACTORS AND PROCESSES

Motor skills are often learned with the intention of successfully performing them at a later date. Although immediate performance is also a consideration, written or skill tests and athletic contests are examples of occasions when later recall or recognition of what has been learned is demanded. Retention, or long-term memory, may depend on a number of factors, namely the nature of the task, its meaningfulness to the learner, the time lapse between the original learning and recall, interpolated activities, and the conditions under which the task was learned. Let us examine such factors, as well as prominent theories describing this aspect of the learning process.

Retention and forgetting are terms used to describe the same process. Whereas *retention* refers to what is remembered and can be determined by measuring the difference between the amount originally learned and the amount forgotten, the amount *forgotten* is equal to the amount learned minus the amount retained.

In the preceding section we discussed the nature of transfer of learning. Adams (1969) has suggested a distinction between learning and retention. Presumably, of interest in transfer studies is the influence of prior learning on a new task, whereas retention studies are concerned with variables that govern the persistence of learned behaviors. This may not be a totally true picture. One of the factors that influences the retention of a particular once-learned task is the positive or negative transfer effects of the intervening experiences. Learning and retention will be the net result of a number of negative and positive effects of previous experiences. Transfer effects can indeed be prominent in the observation of retention, at least in the real world. Obviously, laboratory conditions can be developed to control for each factor. In any event, retention is inferred from behavior after a certain period of time has elapsed from previous practice, as depicted in Figure 13-11.

Normally, we might expect to find a decrease in retention with the passage of time in which there is no practice, but research results indicate that this is not always the case. A number of studies have demonstrated that the retention curve does not always drop rapidly following the postrest learning period but instead continues to rise. This improvement instead of a decrement in the recall of a task after a period of rest has been termed *reminiscence*. It appears that certain practice conditions may be more advantageous for reminiscence than others.

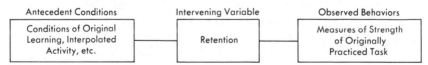

FIGURE 13-11. The conceptual status of retention treated as an intervening variable. (*From Adams, J. Retention: Nature, measurement, and fundamental processes. In M. H. Marx (Ed.), Learning: Processes. New York: Macmillan, 1969. Reprinted with permission of Macmillan Publishing Co., Inc.*)

Methodology of Retention Experiments

Three measures generally have been used in investigations concerned with retention. These include recognition, relearning, and recall. *Recognition* is the method so often used in written testing, an example of which is the multiple-choice test. A *recall* score is informative in that it indicates how much or how well something is remembered.

A *relearning* score is determined in the following way. The number of trials the subject needs to relearn a task—for example, 12 is subtracted from the number of trials it originally took to learn it to a particular criterion—say, 15. The figure obtained, 3, is placed over the original learning trials, 15, and this results in a *savings score*. In this case, the savings score, otherwise known as the *retention score,* is 20 per cent. Conversely, the forgotten score would be 80 per cent. In terms of their retention effectiveness, recognition is best, whereas recall results in the poorest performances.

When testing for retention two methods have been employed. In older studies, repeated tests were used on the same subjects, in order to measure retention at various intervals after the completion of practice. This procedure has been rightfully attacked, for each test influences the next test and becomes but another form of practice. This flaw in experimentation undermines the effectiveness or desirability of such a method. A designation of the subjects into subgroups, after the practice periods are over, to be tested at different times for retention, adds precision to the experiment. This desired method requires the investigator to have an ample number of subjects at the beginning of his study.

The purest measure of the retention of a once-learned skill is a one-trial test at a later date. With more than one trial, relearning occurs quickly. Unfortunately, a one-trial test of retention may not be very reliable, for performance measures are prone to fluctuate from trial to trial and occasion to occasion. In addition, because retention scores usually represent the differences between scores at the termination of practice and at a later date, an accurate assessment of initial learning is necessary. The criterion of initial learning is about as difficult to agree on as an appropriate test of retention. Some aspects of this problem are addressed by Richard Rivenes and Martha Mawhinney (1968).

Short-Term and Long-Term Memory

To retrieve information accurately and repeat performances during some time period following an initial experience indicates the quality of the retention, or long-term memory ability of the individual, with regard to particular tasks. If behavior is considered to be reflected by an information-processing system, then the way we receive, discriminate to select, rehearse, and in general, hold on to material in storage for later usage is worthy of our understanding. In Chapter 6, distinctions and relationships between two memory systems were described in which the human system was analyzed according to the subsystems that contributed motor performance and skill acquisition. Some of the major points will be amplified here.

Information, if it is to be long lasting, must pass through the short-term memory system (STM) into the long-term memory system (LTM). And if it is not appropriately rehearsed and registered, this information will "float out" of the STM system.

Information-processing theorists inform us that we have a limited channel capacity. Whether it has to do with distinguishing among various sensory inputs or deciding among choices of cues, there is just so much information that can be handled at one time. Overloading the channel capacity by attempting to rehearse too much material can result in information that will not be used and, therefore, will be wasted. Or, too much noise in the channel can distort and confuse the processing functions. The capacity of the STM system, or memory span, is probably larger than once was thought, as capacity usage can be improved on with the activation of the appropriate strategies.

There is disagreement with regard to the capacity of LTM storage. It apparently cannot store every isolated experience, piece of information, or representation of isolated skill. There must be some organized storage system that reduces this need and yet allows us to emit appropriate behaviors on many occasions.

Besides the *appropriate amount* of input at any one time, *exposure time* will also affect STM and LTM processes. In order for information to proceed from STM to LTM, a reasonable exposure time for rehearsal, coding, and imagery is necessary. A number of verbal learning experiments point to twenty or thirty seconds as optimal, but there is little agreement for motor tasks. Adequate rehearsal time permits the organization of materials and effective registration.

Also, *interpolated* activity has been thought to affect the STM process. Interfering or rehearsal-preventing activities present immediately after exposure to some learning situation impede STM. An excellent overview with a model of STM and LTM is described by Richard Atkinson and Richard Schiffrin (1971). The processes involved in STM are given prime importance because of their consequences. Control processes must be optimized for effective STM. These include overt or covert repetition or rehearsal of material, coding, imaging (verbal input transcribed to visual images), decision rule formulation, and organizational schemes, retrieval strategies, and problem-solving techniques. They vary from person to person and task to task. But the subject has control over the processes selected in STM, as contrasted to the permanent structural components of LTM.

STM is the transient process; LTM constitutes the permanent storage. Of course, what is meant by permanency is debatable. There are arguments favoring the concept that permanent memories exist, but that failure to reproduce behaviors lies in a poor retrieval system or inadequate set. On the other hand, there are those who believe that memory traces gradually fade out of storage. Data obtained by Schiffrin (1970) suggest that memory failure is the result of an inadequate memory search during retrieval, rather than a fading out of the memory trace.

There is also issue over what is actually stored, or remembered. More than likely, an internalized model of rules or patterns of actions is available upon the appropriate signal. The right selection will depend on previous experiences, the current situation, and retrieval capabilities.

The terms *primary memory* (PM) and *secondary memory* (SM) *stores* have been used interchangeably with the terms *short-term* and *long-term memory storage systems*. As Norman (1976) indicates, information is rehearsed in the PM store and may or may not be advanced to the SM store. Rehearsal is extremely important in increasing the likelihood of this passage. Figure 13-12 shows the interaction of three key systems: acquisition, memory, and decision. Once information goes into PM, it is either forgotten after immediate usage or else enters SM. Actions (decisions) will reflect biases, situational impedence (noise, error), strategies, and the strength of the memory and ability to retrieve relevant items. Theory suggests that much attention should be paid to ways of transferring important information from the primary to the secondary store. As Steven Keele puts it (1973): "Memory does not simply reflect whatever impinges on the senses. Stored material undergoes a series of transformations and abstractions. Storage [for STM] is quite brief, ranging approximately one second for visual and tactual inputs to perhaps twenty or so seconds for the kinesthetic system" (p. 29).

LTM is relatively immune to forgetting. To improve the functions of LTM, Keele suggests rehearsal, organization, and imagery. So far we have discussed a two-stage approach to memory: STM and LTM. From a biochemical framework,

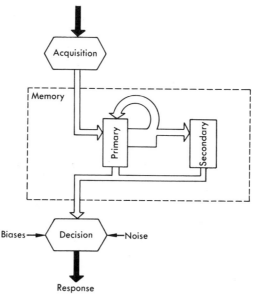

FIGURE 13-12. Interactions among the three different processes affecting the subject's actions in a memory experiment. In the acquisition process, the sensory input is encoded for the memory process. Items in primary memory are rapidly forgotten, whereas items in secondary memory can be retained for long periods of time. In the decision process, the output of the memory is combined with the subject's biases to determine a response. Noise can be considered to enter the process at this point. (*From Norman, D. A. Memory and Attention. New York: John Wiley, 1969.*)

Ward Halstead and William Rucker (1968) feel that a two-stage model is too simple. They propose another phase of memory, an intermediate phase, which "holds information during the period while the dynamic trace is dissipating and the permanent or consolidated trace is still being constructed" (pp. 39–40). Furthermore, they suggest that neurons produce special proteins that help to record a memory trace. RNA (ribonucleic acid) is proposed as responsible for LTM, although evidence is unclear about the specific role of RNA in memory consolidation. Writing from a neurological perspective, J. Anthony Deutsch (1968) suggests that certain memory disorders can be attributed to a lowered efficiency of impulse transmission across synapses. Special drugs may help to remediate this circumstance.

Karl Pribram (1969) believes that neurophysiologically that there is substantial evidence to believe that memory occurs according to the principle of the *hologram.*

> In a hologram the information in a scene is recorded on a photographic plate in the form of a complex interference, or diffraction, pattern that appears meaningless. When the pattern is illuminated by coherent light, however, the original image is reconstructed. What makes the hologram unique as a storage device is that every element in the original image is distributed over the entire photographic plate. The hypothesis is attractive because remembering or recollecting literally implies a reconstructive process—the assembly of dismembered mnemonic events (p. 73).

Pribram believes that the organizer for complex events involves the association areas of the cerebral cortex. These areas exert control on inputs by way of other structures in the brain. However, they are responsible for providing a major part of the organizing process involved in memory. Perspectives from psychology, physiology, neurology, and biochemistry provide a more complete picture of the operation of memory as it affects behavior.

Practice Methods

Most investigators concerned with varying the practice-rest ratios have been interested primarily in the immediate acquisition of the tasks, whereas few have extended their investigations to observe retention effects of the practice conditions. This point was emphasized earlier in the chapter.

In line with the research evidence are the findings from an experiment that are depicted in Figure 13-13. Although initial differences are small, there evidently is a critical point at which massed practice inhibits and worsens performance, whereas distributed practice appears to be continually beneficial. A test one week after the termination of practice indicated little difference between the groups. A survey of research investigating retention effects after a period of at least twenty-four hours from the final moment of practice indicates little difference between groups as a result of whole or part practice methods.

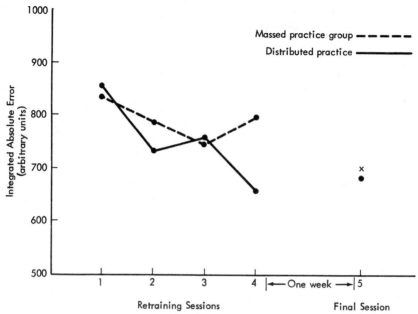

FIGURE 13-13. Effect of different retraining programs during retraining and after a further one-week rest. The subjects were tested on a tracking task. (*From Fleishman, E. A., & Parker, J. F., Jr. Factors in the retention and relearning of perceptual-motor skill.* Journal of Experimental Psychology, *1962, 64, 215–226.*) Copyright 1962 by the American Psychological Association. Reprinted by permission.

Reminiscence

Reminiscence is the opposite of forgetting, for it is the phenomenon in which performance increases after a rest interval and is, therefore, attributable to rest. Reminiscence also is believed to occur only when the task has been partially learned. Reminiscence was not isolated as separate from the distribution effects of practice until the work of P. B. Ballard (1913). He read passages from "The Ancient Mariner" for fifteen minutes to elementary school children and then required them to write all that could be remembered. The students were then divided into smaller groups and were tested from one to seven days later. The reminiscence peak was found to be greatest after a two-day delay, as the students remembered more at that point than immediately after the reading.

Since the publication of Ballard's study, researchers have manipulated numerous variables in order to determine the effects on reminiscence. Reminiscence may depend on a number of factors, such as the type of learning technique employed, type of subject matter, degree of mastery before rest, type of practice (degree of distribution), and length of the rest interval. Reminiscence in motor learning studies has not received a great deal of attention, but it is interesting to speculate about its existence and the processes that contribute to it.

Gross motor skills have been of concern in some studies, but the nature of the designs and the tasks employed make it difficult to state definitely how reminiscence works. M. C. Fox and V. P. Young (1962) instructed two groups of students for periods of six weeks and nine weeks in badminton skills. The students were tested after six weeks and twelve weeks of no practice on a wall volley test and short serve test. No reminiscence was noticed on the short service test. The group instructed for nine weeks did significantly better after six weeks than the group given six weeks of instruction, but there was no difference between the groups after twelve weeks. The former group regressed, while the latter group improved and displayed the effects of reminiscence. Evidently, the additional three weeks of instruction did not contribute to long-term retention.

B. J. Purdy and A. Lockhart (1962) tested subjects one year after they had learned five novel skills, e.g., ball toss and foot volley. These investigators discovered that 89 per cent of the subjects displayed reminiscence in one or more of the skills, an incidence of reminiscence much higher than found in other studies. It is difficult to generalize how long after the termination of practice performance increases—and if, indeed, it will increase. The method used most in measuring reminiscence is a comparison of skill demonstrated after a specified interval of time with the amount displayed at the end of formal practice. Thus far, it appears that studies yield inconsistent results as to the optimal rest period following practice for reminiscence.

Research also indicates that the method of distributing practice might reflect greater or lesser degrees of reminiscence. It seems that the relative massing of practice trials will afford the greatest amount of reminiscence, which, in turn, will result in a similar performance or in a performance slightly below that of a distributed practice group. A possible explanation is that, at the immediate conclusion of practice, the distributed practice usually yields a superior performance; however, after a rest period, the distributed group performs less effectively, the massed group better, and, therefore, ultimately both are approximately equal.

The traditional explanation of reminiscence is associated with inhibition theory, where rest presumably allows the dissipation of reactive inhibition, a transient inhibitory potential that builds up within a person as a result of continuously responding in a task with little or no rest. Such suggestions were made by Clark Hull in the 1940s and still have appeal, especially to classical behaviorists.

Another point of view has been expressed in recent years that has great appeal but insufficient research support at the present time. It is associated with activiation theory. Possibly, reduced performance following massed practice is due to a diminished activation level and subsequent rest, and the administration of additional task trials or a test resulting in reminiscence, or improved performance, is a consequence of the return to a more optimal arousal level. Some studies have shown the beneficial effects on reminiscence from interpolated activity situations geared to increase a subject's activation level. For instance, the data from David Hammond's (1972) two experiments were in accordance with the arousal theory explanation of reminiscence. A visual stimulus (a 1,000-watt light flash) or a cold temperature stimulus (hand immersion in water at 10°C) provided during rest after massed practice on a pursuit rotor led to a significant reminiscence effect. Reminiscence is also a function of ability level (Eysenck & Gray, 1971), as high-ability individuals demonstrate greater reminiscence effects.

Learning Tasks

As a general rule, it can be stated that gross motor skills are retained for many years at a higher skill level than any other learning materials, such as fine motor skills and prose. We may have last performed on a bicycle when twelve years of age, but even after an eight-year layoff, cycling ability would be extremely high. Compare this situation with a passage memorized from a poem or from history, learned years ago and not practiced for a long period of time. Would you expect to recall the passage with the same degree of accuracy that you demonstrated on the bicycle? Of course not.

The long-term retention permanence of motor skills was demonstrated in a series of experiments undertaken by Edgar Swift at the beginning of the twentieth century. Swift (1906), using himself as the subject, learned to type over a fifty-day period. Two years elapsed before he touched a typewriter again, and it took him only eleven days to reach the same proficiency he had attained after fifty days. Swift (1905) had two subjects practice keeping two balls going with one hand, one ball being caught and thrown while the other was in the air. After rest periods of more than six hundred days, retention tests indicated that the subjects in all but two instances performed better than they had at the close of regular practice. Employing the same skill (ball juggling), Swift (1910) practiced for forty-two days and then waited six years before attempting the skill again. It took him only eleven days to relearn the act and demonstrate a performance equivalent to that at the end of the original practice.

More specifically, within the motor skill domain, continuous tasks are retained better than discrete tasks, even after long periods of no practice. Riding a bicycle and swimming are examples of continuous tasks; a test of reaction time constitutes a discrete task. Apparently, least interference from the experiencing of other activities occurs with continuous tasks. They are usually overlearned (overpracticed), they contain kinesthetic cue characteristics that aid in immediately arousing memory traces, and errors can be corrected quickly. Discrete motor learning tasks and verbal tasks may be less well remembered than continuous motor tasks because the factors primarily mentioned do not operate as favorably in this category of behavior.

An important consideration as to what is retained is the meaningfulness to the learner of what is learned. Nonsense syllables are forgotten very quickly (compare the learning cuves in Figure 13-14). Some prose is retained longer than other prose, depending on its meaningfulness, not only logically, but also in importance to the person. Motor skills, especially to children, are held high in personal worth, and efforts to achieve are intensive and extensive. There is a relative permanence to the meaningful material that we learn.

Although motor skills are generally retained better than other types of learned material, the more abstract they are, the more the retention curve resem-

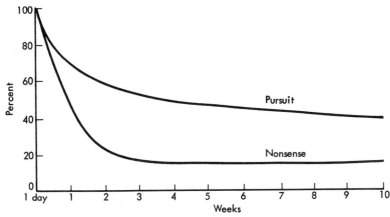

FIGURE 13-14. Retention comparison of verbal material (nonsense syllables) and a motor skill (pursuit rotor). (*From Leavitt, H. J., & Schlosberg, H. The retention of verbal and of motor skills.* Journal of Experimental Psychology, *1944, 34, 404–417.*) Copyright 1944 by the American Psychological Association. Reprinted by permission.

bles that of verbal or written matter. For instance, Adams and Dijkstra (1966) had their subjects learn a motor task that required mastering the positioning of sliding elements on a bar. Retention was tested in intervals ranging from 5 to 120 seconds. The results fundamentally agreed with the findings of verbal research on STM: that rapid forgetting occurs with the passage of time, but the performance becomes more stable with reinforcement.

There is a danger in comparing the retention of verbal and motor tasks. Methods and measures differ in each situation. There is really no pure way of establishing and comparing the capacities of people to retain verbal and motor tasks. For instance, in many verbal tasks a person is asked to recall, without any prompts or cues. When asked to ride a bicycle or swim, the person can recognize old cues once surrounded by a familiar situation. In other words, retention testing seems to be generally biased in favor of motor skills over verbal tasks.

Dean Ryan (1962) tested eighty men after three, five, seven, and twenty-one days had lapsed from practice on stabilometer and pursuit rotor skills. Little or no loss in performance was found on the retention days tested, and the pursuit rotor skill was retained better than that of the stabilometer. Ryan was interested in extending the retention periods to determine the lasting effects of a once-learned motor skill. In a second study, Ryan (1965) gave eleven initial learning trials on the stabilometer to his subjects, who were divided later into three groups to be tested three months, six months, and one year after the termination of practice. There was no significant difference on the first retention trial for all three groups; all showed a loss in proficiency. A longer nonpractice period resulted in more trials being needed to regain the earlier proficiency.

Once again, unusual motor tasks will not be retained as well as the familiar ones, for example, in sports skills. Everyday experience and empirical evidence support the notion of the long-lasting effects of once-learned athletic skills. Explanations for this phenomenon may lie in one or all of the following suggestions. It may be due to the relative importance motor skill achievement has to the individual. Perhaps it occurs because of the total body effort intellectually and physically needed to perform an athletic skill successfully. Athletic skill retention can also be explained by simply examining the number of hours devoted to its learning, as compared to the time spent in learning a literary passage. Whereas a child may allocate a few hours for memorizing a poem, he or she plays softball incessantly. Is it any wonder, then, that the greater number of S–R occurrences in the athletic situation result in superior retention?

Overlearning

How much should a task be practiced for it to be learned sufficiently? The rub in this question is the word *sufficiently*. Perhaps the question should be restated to read: How much practice is necessary for the greatest amount of retention (assuming this is what is desired)?

All things being equal, the amount of initial practice is directly related to the amount retained, as retention has been demonstrated to be higher when the task is learned well. Partially learned material is forgotten faster than mastered material. Of course, it would be extremely difficult to know when the skill is learned well enough and the individual has had enough practice. But, as Fleishman and Parker (1962) have demonstrated, the most important factor in retention is the initial level of proficiency. These investigators practiced their subjects on a highly complex tracking task over a six-week period. Other interesting results of the study were that (1) the amount of verbal guidance during practice had no effect on retention; (2) massed and distributed practice effects did not differ on a retention test given one week after practice; and (3) retention on this motor task was quite high, even after a rest period of twenty-four months.

Retention will be enhanced even more if the skill is overlearned. *Overlearning* refers to practice provided on a task after it has been learned according to some criterion. The criterion in many psychological studies dealing with the learning of written material is one perfect recitation. If precise experimental control is wanted, the number of trials it takes the subject to achieve the criterion measure is recorded. The researcher can then arbitrarily provide the subject with more practice trials on the task; by dividing this figure by the original number of practices, the percentage of overlearning is derived. Invariably, studies concerned with overlearning find that greater practice beyond the learning criterion results in better retention performances.

Merrill Melnick (1971) conducted one of the few investigations in the overlearning area with a motor learning task, balancing on a stabilometer. Subjects received 0, 50, 100, or 200 per cent overlearning. Retention tests were given one week or one month later. Absolute retention (immediate recall) was measured on the basis of the subjects' score on the first retention trial, whereas relative retention was arrived at with a per cent of saving score based on the ratio of trials taken for initial mastery and trials taken on the retention test to reach a criterion. The absolute retention measure showed retention intervals to be favored by overlearning, with the different overlearning percentages approximately equally as effective. Relative retention scores led to one major difference: 200 per cent overlearning was significantly better than 0 per cent in the one-month retention test.

There is some practical concern as to who are the best retainers, fast or slow learners. If a person acquires skill quickly, will it also be retained at a high level of proficiency? Early studies showed that fast learners were better retainers than slow learners. However, a weakness in testing procedure was that both types of learners had the same number of learning trials. The fast learners retained more because they learned more initially. Later studies have usually demonstrated that, if all the subjects have to reach an initial learning criterion regardless of the number of practice trials, the slow learner will score higher on retention tests. This could be explained by the overlearning effect.

An exception to the notion that fast learners are at a disadvantage when compared to slow learners in retaining learned tasks is reported by Melnick, Lersten, and Lockhart (1972). Three groups of subjects were formed on the basis of the speed (number of trials) with which they achieved a criterion score on a balance task. Retention scores were similar among the groups. The fast learners, those who took a relatively small number of trials to reach criterion, were not apparently handicapped in the retention test one week later. However, it should be pointed out that, between the initial learning trials and the retention test, all subjects were provided with 100 per cent overlearning practice. Coupled with a task ceiling effect—thirty seconds on any trial is maximum performance—it is possible that the additional practice allowed the "fast" learning group to have enough practice on this particular task to confound the retention test scores. Nevertheless, the problem is worthy of further study, for the implications are great for understanding retention theory and for practical implications in practice arrangements for learners who initially acquire skills at different rates of speed.

Proactive and Retroactive Inhibition

The things we typically learn are not isolated, but rather fall into sequential patterns of various learning materials. Because of this, the learning and retention of a particular response might very well be affected by what is learned, especially of a related nature, before and after training on the response. Going a step further and translating this to psychological terms, if a specific response is desired for a given stimulus (S_1–R_1) and a second response is learned for this same stimulus (S_1–R_2) either before or after S_1–R_1 occurs, interference in retention of S_1–R_1 will be observable.

Proactive inhibition refers to the negative effect one learned task has on the retention of a newer task. *Retroactive inhibition* describes the condition when a recently learned task impairs the retention performance of an older learned task. Generally, experimental designs to measure proaction or retroaction are as follows:

PROACTION

Groups	Prior Learning	Desired Learning	Recall
Experimental	Task B	Task A	Task A*
Control	None	Task A	Task A

RETROACTION

Groups	Original Learning	Interpolated Learning	Recall
Experimental	Task A	Task B	Task A*
Control	Task A	Rest	Task A

*Although task A recall is desired, task A and task B responses will conflict.

Proactive inhibition has been investigated considerably less than retroactive inhibition and, at one time, was thought to be less of an influence on retention than retroactive inhibition. However, what is true of one condition is usually true of the other. It does not matter whether related tasks are learned before or after the desired learning task; inhibition of varying degrees will occur on retention tests. With retroaction, the desired response has been weakened by the second learned response; but in proaction, it is the first competing response that has been weakened by the learning of the desired response, the second one.

Forgetting is thought to occur because of a competition of responses, and certainly this is the case in proaction and retroaction. We live in a verbal world and learn many, many words in a lifetime. Retroaction and proaction are constantly building up, causing, relatively, much and rapid forgetting. Motor skills are not forgotten quickly, mainly because there are not that many to learn, many are unique, and they are practiced at great length. In learning to ride a bicycle, one has to adjust to such factors as balance and gravity. Bicycle riding will not be unlearned, for there are no competing responses to this situation. It should be remembered, though, that negative transfer can occur in motor skill learning, and anytime S_1 is presented after R_1 and R_2 have become associated with it, there is the danger of conflict.

Theories of Retention and Forgetting

It is usually felt that forgetting is a decline in performance caused by the passage of time. However, experimental evidence points to the fact that ultimate retention will be more dependent on the intervening events than on time, per se. Greater activity brings about the development of competing response tendencies, thus resulting in a higher degree of forgetting.

Experimentally, this idea is verified by holding the time period constant between the last original learning trial and the recall test but varying the amount of intervening activity. If time alone is responsible for forgetting, the recall scores should be the same, regardless of time spent in activity. But this is not the case. If four groups had learned certain material and were tested after twenty-four hours on a retention test, with group A allowed only two hours of activity during this rest period, group B four hours of activity, group C twelve hours, and group D actively responding for the entire twenty-four-hour period, performance on the recall test could be predicted. The least active group during the retention period would do best on the recall test, and the most active group would perform worst of all.

One can gather from this discussion that we should be able to retain more after sleep than following waking activities. Whether something, once learned, is ever truly forgotten is open to question. Freud's work, as well as that of others interested in psychoanalysis, indicates not only that early life experience and behavior are important in determining later life behavior, but also that many childhood experiences can be recalled under emotional recall situations. Things learned can be retained better under more favorable learning situations and more efficient learning techniques. Currently, major advances are being made in the memorization of written and verbal material through coding techniques. However, the process of forgetting is still not well understood, from either psychological or physiological viewpoints.

How can we explain what is retained and the strength of this later performance? Theorists representing different schools of thought approach the matter in various ways. E. L. Walker (1958) believes that high arousal during the associative process (practice) results in greater permanent memory. Koffka (1935), a leader in Gestalt psychology, states that a greater organization of the stimulus trace results in less probability of its weakening over time. Broadbent (1958) writes that perceptual filters operate during attempted retention, and recall will occur if the correct channel is monitored and monitored at the right time. These concepts are still being explored.

Interesting theories have been advanced to explain performance during and after massed and distributed practice. McGeoch (1961) has reviewed numerous theories and categorizes them as follows: work theories, perseveration theories, and differential forgetting theories.

Differential forgetting theories, according to McGeoch, generally handle massed and distributed practice effects by stating that during practice a subject learns incorrect and conflicting responses as well as correct ones. Because the conflicting associations are probably less well learned than the appropriate responses, the conflicting ones will dissipate with rest at a faster rate than during practice. Therefore, according to the theory, learning will take place faster during distributed practice because the incorrect responses will have had an opportunity to drop out more quickly than under massed practice conditions. However, there are theoretical limitations on the desirable length of the rest interval.

Reminiscence can be explained in a similar manner: rest intervals provide an opportunity for dropping out or forgetting wrong associations that are less strongly favored than the right ones and, hence, are forgotten more rapidly. Under this theory, massed practice would probably be expected to yield a greater reminiscence effect than distributed practice.

Perseveration theories tend to hold that some activity persists in the individual after the termination of practice, therefore resulting in the learned response becoming more strongly fixated than it was previously. Neural processes presumably perseverate for a considerable time following learning. Distributed practice permits the setting-in process to proceed with minimal interference, whereas massed practice would not allow enough time to permit this activity to occur.

Work theories generally state that the act of repeating a response tends to build up either a loss of interest, boredom, physical fatigue, or mental fatigue. The interfering processes presumably disappear with rest, and the more permanent learned responses supposedly remain.

Hull's (1943) theory, based on a theoretical construct called *reactive inhibition,* is most representative of the work theories and probably has encouraged more investigations in the area of massed versus distributed practice than any other theory. Hull postulates that two inhibitory processes occur when responses are made, reactive inhibition (I_R) and conditioned inhibition (S^IR). I_R is temporary by nature and dissipates with time, whereas S^IR is relatively permanent. With increased practice, the temporary work decrement increases and explains the poorer performance of subjects learning under massed practice conditions. By the same token, distributed practice permits I_R effects to disappear more easily; hence, the superior performance of distributed practice subjects. Also, reminiscence is described as occurring when the I_R effects have been rendered ineffective as a result of rest from repeating the desired responses.

However, Hull's work theory holds that, over a long time interval, reactive potential diminishes. Supposedly, reactive inhibition disappears after ten to twenty minutes of rest, resulting in increased performance at that time. Some writers are of the opinion that perhaps I_R lasts for a day or even a week. Even if it lasted for a month, there is no logical explanation of why the disappearance of I_R should result in an eventual superior performance for massed practice subjects than for distributed practice subjects. Considering that all subjects had experienced the same number of practice trials, the associated strength for the habit should at best be equal under massed and distributed conditions.

Some investigators have applied Hull's basic concepts to motor skill learning, more specifically, rotary pursuit learning. G. A. Kimble (1949) calls his theory a "two-factor theory of inhibition." Proponents of this theory state that, in many studies, especially those employing motor tasks, rest periods are too short to allow for the dissipation of the majority of the reactive inhibition. Figure 13-15 illustrates how pursuit rotor performance would fit into this theory.

When a subject learns under relatively massed practice, an inhibition develops that hinders performance rather than learning. Therefore, performance would be weaker under massed conditions than under distributed practice because the inhibition dissipates rapidly with rest. Precisely what the optimal rest period is for superior performance has been disputed, as a result of the findings of various

MOTOR LEARNING AND HUMAN PERFORMANCE

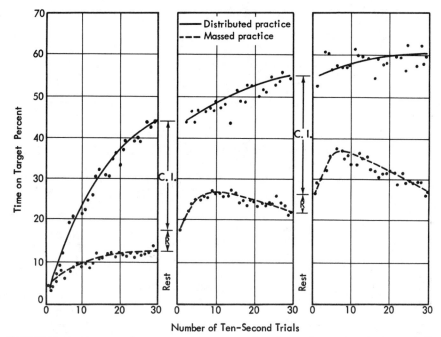

FIGURE 13-15. Motor performance as it represents learning and retention during and after massed and distributed practice conditions and according to Hullian theory. Pursuit-rotor performance varies markedly with the spacing of the trial, or practice, periods. Each dot represents the average time-on-target during a 10-second period. The upper curve shows the performance of subjects who were allowed a 30-second rest pause between each 10-second trial. The lower curve shows the performance of subjects denied such a rest. Both groups were given two 10-minute rest periods. The improvement in performance shown by the massed-practice group immediately following the 10-minute break is called reminiscence (R), which is believed to be a measure of reactive inhibition accumulated during massed practice. The major depressant on scores of the massed-practice group, however, is conditioned inhibition (CI). (*From Eysenck, H. J. The measurement of motivation.* Scientific American, *1963, 208, 130–140.*) Copyright © 1963 by Scientific American, Inc. All rights reserved.

studies. Most likely, inhibition affects performance rather than what is learned.

Perhaps the amount of effort exerted by the subject in learning will have its effects on performance (Ellis, 1953). More effortful behavior might result in a greater amount of I_R present and, therefore a greater need to cease activity. Effortfulness would depend on the physical energy required for the learning of the task and the length of time without rest while practicing.

The fact that greater overall bodily effort is required for the mastery of athletic skills, in contrast to learning nonsense syllables or rotary-pursuit tasks, may be one of the reasons why reminiscence has been demonstrated after twelve or more weeks of no practice of athletic skills. Massed practice would theoretically be less effective with the learning of gross motor skills than other learning materials because of the effort involved. On the same explanatory grounds, reminiscence should then be greater after practicing these gross motor skills.

Factors Contributing to Retention

At this point, from the material presented on retention, we can generalize about those techniques or procedures that favor increasing probabilities of high retention. Some scholars (e.g., Stelmach, 1974) have developed some of the following ideas to a much greater extent than is presented here.

1. Material should be well organized for the benefit of the learner, so there will be ease in internally organizing it for storage and retrieval purposes.
2. Material should be perceived by the learner as meaningful.
3. Material should be learned well (overpracticed).
4. Competing activities should be minimized, from time of practice to test of retention.
5. Time lag from practice to retention should not be too long, or else some related task experiences should occur in the interval.
6. Material should be presented in such a way as to be compatible with the information-processing abilities of the learner, considering transition from STM to LTM.
7. Retention tests should encourage the opportunity for the person to reorient.
8. The use of covert rehearsal or observation of others performing the task in the rest interval can be beneficial.

CHAPTER HIGHLIGHTS

1. The use of reinforcers as a powerful means of shaping behavior has been recognized for many years, with consideration for type, schedule, and frequency of reinforcers. Their use is especially favored with those learners who do not seem to have much of an interest in learning a motor activity. Rewards are favored over punishments.

2. Augmented, or supplementary, feedback (knowledge about performance or the results of performance) should be considered when there is insufficient information available to the learner in the situation. Supplementary feedback may be provided during or immediately after performance, after performance at some designated time period, and in various forms. It may serve not only as information to guide the learner, but as a source of motivation or reinforcement, as well.

3. People make attributions (perceived causes) of their performance outcomes; these, in turn, can influence their expectations for achievement when confronted with the same situation in the future. Internal causations are generally more desirable than external ones, as stable (task difficulty and ability level) attributes are preferable to unstable (energy expended and luck) attributes. Experiences should be established that lead to more successes, more objective attributes, and, in turn, better performances.

4. Learning is built upon previous learnings; hence, transfer potential exists from them for most of the things we attempt to learn. Previous learning may positively or negatively influence present learning, and much depends on situational similarities, response similarities, and personal understandings, perceptions, and motivation. Specific topics of interest covered in this chapter included: (a) the learning to learn phenomena, whereby learners improve in situations by learning how to take a test; (b) bilateral transfer, where students are shown to improve in the use of a nontrained limb as a result of learning a task with the use of a corresponding limb; (c) task difficulty, where it is usually demonstrated that it is better to progress from simple to more complex tasks in most activities but sometimes is more effective to proceed from more to less difficult tasks; (d) adaptive training, where the nature of a task is continuously modified as skill is acquired in it, thereby maintaining task difficulty as a constant; and (e) theories of transfer, which usually range from the notion of task specificity to generality possibilities.

5. Retention of once-learned material was discussed in relation to many factors. Short-term and long-term memory relationships were examined (see also Chapter 6 for further information) as to how information can be stored and retrieved more effectively at a later date. An interesting phenomenon termed reminiscence, which denotes improvement in later performance due to rest or nonpractice, has been observed on occasion. It probably is primarily a function of the conditions surrounding the initial practice and resultant depressed performance.

Meaningful practice on meaningful tasks increases retention probability. Overlearning a task—i.e., beyond a criterion—will lead to better retention. Continuous tasks have been found to be retained more effectively than discrete tasks. That which has been learned prior to (proactive) or after (retroactive) the learning of a task can have an inhibitory effect on its retention. Theories and research indicate that the passage of time without practice and competing response tendencies will lower retention potential.

References

Adams, J. A. Retention: Nature, measurement, and fundamental processes. In M. H. Marx (Ed.), *Learning: Processes*. New York: Macmillan, 1969.

Adams, J. A. Theoretical issues for knowledge of results. In G. E. Stelmach (Ed.), *Information processing in motor control and learning*. New York: Academic Press, 1978.

Adams, J. A., & Dijkstra, S. Short-term memory for motor responses. *Journal of Experimental Psychology*, 1966, *71*, 314–318.

Adams, J. A., Goetz, E. T., & Marshall, P. H. Response feedback and motor learning. *Journal of Experimental Psychology*, 1972, *92*, 391–397.

Ammons, R. B. Effects of knowledge of performance: A survey and tentative theoretical formulation. *Journal of General Psychology*, 1956, *54*, 279–299.

Ammons, R. B., Ammons, C. H., & Morgan, R. L. Transfer of skill and decremented factors along the speed dimension in rotary pursuit. *Perceptual and Motor Skills*, 1958, *11*, 43.

Annett, J. *Feedback and human behavior*. Baltimore: Penguin Books, 1969.

Atkinson, J. W. Motivational determinants of risk-taking behavior. *Psychology Review*, 1957, *64*, 359–372.

Atkinson, R. C., & Shiffrin, R. M. The control of short-term memory. *Scientific American,* 1971, *216,* 2–10.

Ausubel, D. P., Novak, J. D., & Hanesian, H. *Educational psychology: A cognitive view.* New York: Holt, Rinehart & Winston, 1978.

Baker, K. E., Wylie, R. C., & Gagné, R. M. Transfer of training to a motor skill as a function of variation in rate of response. *Journal of Experimental Psychology,* 1950, *40,* 721–732.

Ballard, P. B. Obliviscence and reminiscence. *British Journal of Psychology Monographs Supplements,* 1913, *2.*

Bartz, D. W. Self-acceptance and disconfirming feedback as influences upon performance of a gross motor skill. *Journal of Motor Behavior,* 1975, *7,* 251–257.

Bayton, J. A., & Conley, H. W. Duration of success background and the effect of failure upon performance. *Journal of General Psychology,* 1957, *56,* 179–185.

Bilodeau, I. M. Information feedback. In I. M. Bilodeau (Ed.), *Principles of skill acquisition.* New York: Academic Press, 1969.

Brickman, P., & Hendricks, M. Expectancy for gradual improvement and reaction to success and failure. *Journal of Personality and Social Psychology,* 1975, *32,* 893–900.

Brickman, P., Linsenmeier, J. A. W., & McCareins, A. G. Performance enhancement by relevant success and irrelevant failure. *Journal of Personality and Social Psychology,* 1976, *33,* 149–160.

Briggs, G. E., & Naylor, J. C. The relative efficiency of several training methods as a function of transfer of task complexity. *Journal of Experimental Psychology,* 1962, *64,* 505–512.

Briggs, G. E., & Waters, L. K. Training and transfer as a function of component interaction. *Journal of Experimental Psychology,* 1958, *56,* 492–500.

Broadbent, D. E. *Perception and communication.* London: Pergamon Press, 1958.

Cook, T. W. Studies in cross-education: Mirror tracing the star-shaped maze. *Journal of Experimental Psychology,* 1933, *16,* 144–160. (a)

Cook, T. W. Studies in cross-education: Further experiments in mirror tracing the star-shaped maze. *Journal of Experimental Psychology,* 1933, *16,* 769–700. (b)

Day, R. H. Relative task difficulty and transfer of training in skilled performance. *Psychological Bulletin,* 1956, *53,* 160–168.

Deutsch, J. A. Neural basis of memory. *Psychology Today,* 1968, *2,* 56–60.

Dickinson, J. A. *A behavioral analysis of sport.* Princeton, N.J.: Princeton Book Co., 1977.

Ellis, D. S. Inhibition theory and the effort variables. *Psychology Review,* 1953, *60,* 383–392.

Eysenck, H. J. The measurement of motivation. *Scientific American,* 1963, *208,* 130–140.

Eysenck, H. J., & Gray, J. E. Reminiscence and the shape of the learning curve as a function of subjects' ability level on the pursuit rotor. *British Journal of Psychology,* 1971, *62,* 199–215.

Fleishman, E. A., & Parker, J. F. Factors in the retention and relearning of perceptual-motor skill. *Journal of Experimental Psychology,* 1962, *64,* 215–226.

Fox, M. C., & Young, V. P. Effect of reminiscence on learning selected badminton skills. *Research Quarterly,* 1962, *73,* 386–394.

Gibbs, C. B. Transfer of training and skill assumptions in tracking tasks. *Quarterly Journal of Experimental Psychology,* 1951, *3,* 99–110.

Gordon, N. B. Guidance versus augmented feedback and motor skill. *Journal of Experimental Psychology,* 1968, *77,* 24–30.

Halstead, W. C., & Rucker, W. B. Memory: A molecular maze. *Psychology Today*, 1968, *2*, 38–41.

Hammond, D. Effects of visual and thermal stimulation upon reminiscence in rotary pursuit tracking. *The Irish Journal of Psychology*, 1972, *3*, 177–84.

Harlow, H. F. The formation of learning sets. *Psychological Review*, 1949, *56*, 51–65.

Holding, D. H. *Principles of training*. Oxford, England: Pergamon Press, Ltd., 1965.

Hull, C. L. *Principles of behavior*. New York: Appleton-Century-Crofts, 1943.

Hurlock, E. B. An evaluation of certain incentives on school work. *Journal of Educational Psychology*, 1925, *16*, 145–159.

Iso-Ahola, S. Motivational effects of outcome feedback on motor performance. *Journal of Motor Behavior*, 1976, *8*, 267–276.

Johnston, J. M. Punishment of human behavior. *American Psychologist*, 1972, *27*, 1033–1054.

Keele, S. W. *Attention and human performance*. Pacific Palisades, Calif.: Goodyear Publishing Co., 1973.

Kelley, C. R. Fundamental problems. In J. J. McGrath & D. H. Harris (Eds.), Adaptive training. *Aviation Research Monographs*, 1971, *1*, 1–35.

Kimble, G. A. An experimental test of a two-factor theory of inhibition. *Journal of Experimental Psychology*, 1949, *39*, 15–23.

Knapp, B. *Skill in sports: The attainment of proficiency*. London: Routledge & Kegan Paul, 1964.

Koffka, K. *Principles of Gestalt psychology*. New York: Harcourt Brace Jovanovich, 1935.

Kukla, A. Foundations of an attributional theory of performance. *Psychological Review*, 1972, *79*, 454–470.

Leavitt, H. J., & Schlosberg, H. The retention of verbal and motor skills. *Journal of Experimental Psychology*, 1944, *34*, 404–417.

Leonard, S. D., Karnes, E. W., Oxendine, J., & Hesson, J. Effects of task difficulty on transfer performance on rotary pursuit. *Perceptual and Motor Skills*, 1970, *30*, 731–736.

Logan, G. A., & Lockhart, A. Contralateral transfer of specificity of strength training. *Journal of American Physical Therapy Association*, 1962, *42*, 658–660.

Lordahl, D. A., & Archer, E. J. Transfer effects on a rotary pursuit task as a function of first-task difficulty. *Journal of Experimental Psychology*, 1958, *56*, 421–426.

Magill, R. The post-KR interval: Time and activity effects and the relationship of motor short-term memory. *Journal of Motor-Behavior*, 1973, *5*, 49–56.

Martens, R., Gill, D. L., & Scanlan, T. K. Competitive trait anxiety, success-failure and sex determinants of motor performance. *Perceptual and Motor Skills*, 1976, *43*, 1199–1208.

May, R. B., & Duncan, P. Facilitation on a response-loaded task by changes in task difficulty. *Perceptual and Motor Skills*, 1973, *36*, 123–129.

McGeoch, J. A. *The psychology of human learning*. New York: David McKay, 1961.

Melnick, M. J. Effects of overlearning on the retention of a gross motor skill. *Research Quarterly*, 1971, *42*, 60–69.

Melnick, M. J., Lernsten, K. C., & Lockhart, A. S. Retention of fast and slow learners following overlearning of a gross motor skill. *Journal of Motor Behavior*, 1972, *4*, 187–193.

Newell, K. M. Knowledge of results and motor learning. In J. Keogh & R. S. Hutton (Eds.), *Exercise and sport sciences reviews* (Vol. 4). Santa Barbara, Calif.: Journal Publishing Affiliates, 1976.

Norman, D. A. *Memory and attention.* (2nd ed.). New York: John Wiley, 1976.

Nuttin, J. *Reward and punishment in human learning.* New York: Academic Press, 1968.

Osgood, C. E. The similarity paradox in human learning: A resolution. *Psychological Review,* 1949, *56,* 132–143.

Pribram, K. H. The neurophysiology of remembering. *Scientific American,* 1969, *220,* 73–86.

Purdy, B. J., & Lockhart, A. Retention and relearning of gross motor skills after long periods of no practice. *Research Quarterly,* 1962, *33,* 265–272.

Reynolds, G. S. *A primer of operant conditioning.* Glenview, Ill.: Scott, Foresman, 1968.

Rivenes, R. S., & Mawhinney, M. M. Retention of perceptual motor skill: An analysis of new methods. *Research Quarterly,* 1968, *39,* 684–689.

Rogers, C. Feedback precision and post-feedback interval duration. *Journal of Experimental Psychology,* 1974, *102,* 604–608.

Roth, S., & Kubal, L. The effects of noncontingent reinforcement on tasks of differing importance: Facilitation and learned helplessness. *Journal of Personality and Social Psychology,* 1975, *32,* 680–691.

Rushall, B. S., & Pettinger, J. An evaluation of the effects of various reinforcers used as motivation in swimming. *The Research Quarterly,* 1969, *40,* 540–545.

Rushall, B. S., & Siedentop, D. *The development and control of behavior in sport and physical education.* Philadelphia: Lea & Febiger, 1972.

Ryan, E. D. Retention of stabilometer and pursuit rotor skills. *Research Quarterly,* 1962, *33,* 593–598.

Ryan, E. D. Retention of stabilometer performance over extended periods of time. *Research Quarterly,* 1965, *36,* 46–51.

Shiffrin, R. M. Forgetting: Trace erosion or retrieval failure? *Science,* 1970, *168,* 1601–1603.

Singer, R. N. Transfer effects and ultimate success in archery due to degree of difficulty of the initial learning. *Research Quarterly,* 1966, *37,* 532–539.

Singer, R. N., & McCaughan, L. R. Motivational effects of attributions, expectancy, and achievement motivation during the learning of a novel motor task. *Journal of Motor Behavior,* 1978, *10,* 245–254.

Slayton, A. J., & Black, R. W. Effects of knowledge of results and amount of stimulus change on "resistance to extinction" on a perceptual motor task. *Psychonomic Science,* 1971, *22,* 111–112.

Smith, W. I., & Moore, J. W. *Conditioning and instrumental learning.* New York: McGraw-Hill, 1966.

Smoll, F. L. Effects of precision of information feedback upon acquisition of a motor skill. *Research Quarterly,* 1972, *43,* 489–493.

Stelmach, G. E. Retention of motor skills. In J. Wilmore (Ed.), *Review in exercise and sports sciences, Vol. 11.* New York: Academic Press, 1974.

Swift, E. J. Memory of a complex skillful act. *American Journal of Psychology,* 1905, *16,* 131–133.

Swift, E. J. Memory of skillful movements. *Psychology Bulletin,* 1906, *3,* 185–187.

Swift, E. J. Relearning a skilful act: An experimental study in neuromuscular memory. *Psychology Bulletin,* 1910, *7,* 17–19.

Vincent, W. J. Transfer effects between motor skills judged similar in perceptual components. *Research Quarterly,* 1968, *39,* 380–388.

Walker, E. L. Action decrement and its relation to learning. *Psychological Review,* 1958, *65,* 129–142.

Weiner, B. The effects of unsatisfied achievement motivation on persistence and subsequent performance. *Journal of Personality,* 1965, *33,* 428–442.

Weiner, B. (Ed.). *Achievement motivation and attribution theory.* Morristown, N.J.: General Learning Press, 1974.

Weiner, B., & Sierad, J. Misattribution for failure and enhancement of achievement strivings. *Journal of Personality and Social Psychology,* 1975, *31,* 415–421.

Witte, K. L., & Grossman, E. E. The effects of reward and punishment upon children's attention, motivation, and discrimination learning. *Child Development,* 1971, *42,* 534–542.

14 SOCIAL AND PERFORMANCE FACTORS

In this last chapter, we turn our attention to the learner when learning/performing is influenced by considerations of group dynamics and social interaction. People often train and ultimately perform tasks under social rather than isolated conditions. To learn or perform against, with, or in front of other people is obviously not the same as when no one else is present. There are some predictable behavioral outcomes under these differential conditions, and we will see what they are.

Similarly, individuals may find themselves in environments more or less conducive to practice and learning. Temperature, altitude, lighting, noise, and many other factors impinge on one's potential to learn and perform. In addition, fatigue or pain may arise as a result of learning-working-performing conditions. Perseverance at and improvement in motor activity are partially associated with the ability to withstand either state. Prior to performance, prolonged sensory restriction or sleep deprivation may take its toll on motor performances, too. Any of the four conditions—sensory restriction, sleep deprivation, fatigue, or pain—can lead to temporary performance decrements. In order to impact negatively on learning, too, these conditions must be fairly severe and persistent.

Finally, attitudes toward activity selection and continuance often reflect cultural values. A society, "the big environment," shapes the interests and behaviors of its members. Unique achievements in various types of motor skills may be associated with particular countries or regions in countries. Although not discussed in this chapter, it is also recognized that family, friends, and influential others impact on a person's interest and potential success in particular activities.

SOCIAL FACTORS

Others are often involved in some way in the learning of skills. A learner is guided by an instructor, learns with other students, may be in competitive and/or collaborative-cooperative circumstances, and may even have to perform in the presence of observers. Is learning or performance worsened, improved, or maintained when it occurs in a social context, in contrast to when one is alone? To answer this simple question, complex analyses must be made. Consideration must be given to the nature of the learner and reactivity tendencies, the activity, the skill level of the learner, and how the social conditions are arranged.

From another perspective, training conditions must be designed to promote performance in the actual testing condition. Interestingly enough, although many performance tests require collaborative activities, training programs are geared to individual experiences. The limited research available for perusal is suggestive of the more desirable training conditions to fit the testing conditions. We will address this issue first, to be followed by the ones mentioned earlier.

Team and Individual Training

In typical learning situations, learners are trained to acquire personal skills as they relate to a task. Learners are not often given experiences in interaction skills, although those skills may be required in the future in order to share responsibilities and work in complementary roles on the same task. In other words, the learners eventually may have to function as part of a team.

Teams and small groups, as distinguished by R. Glaser, O. J. Klaus, and K. Egerman (1962), possess unique characteristics. *Teams* have the following characteristics: (1) they are relatively rigid in structure, organization, and communication pattern ; (2) the task of each team member is well defined; and (3) the functioning of the team depends on the coordinated participation of all or several individuals.

In contrast, *small groups* differ in that they generally: (1) have an indefinite or loose structure, organization, and communication pattern; (2) have assignments that are assumed in the course of group interaction rather than designated beforehand; and (3) yield a product that can be a function of one or more of the group members involved, depending on the quality and quantity of the members' participation.

The military and the sports world are both concerned with team operations and personnel who have to perform cohesively toward common goals. However, whatever limited research there is available on the topic of team training and evaluation has primarily evolved from the military sector. For example, the subjects in William Johnston's (1966) experiment had to execute coordination skills demanded in a simulated radar-controlled aerial intercept task. No difference was found if the skills were individual or team taught, but the investigator suggests that the tasks in his study required much more teamwork than those used in other studies. In apparent agreement with the sentiments expressed throughout this book on the importance of practice conditions closely resembling testing conditions is the conclusion to Johnston's report: when the transfer task is characterized by team activity, it appears desirable to train potential team members in a team context rather than individually so that the necessary team skills can be developed. Of course, many times, basic skills have to be taught first to people individually.

The lack of transfer and predictability from skills performed alone to those performed in a group is further demonstrated in a series of studies published by Andrew Comrey (1953, 1954). Subjects were tested individually and in pairs on hand-manipulation taks associated with the Purdue Pegboard Assembly Task. Less than half of the group performance variance could be predicted from individual performance on a similar kind of task. Evidently, individual skill alone is not enough to predict success in a group task, for there are other variables to be considered. A warning from the results of these studies is that people should not always be paired on the basis of individual abilities because group performance does not depend on individual scores.

Training procedures will vary, depending on objectives—if the task is to be performed in established and simplified situations or in nonpredictable and more complex situations—and on a number of other factors. In a recent extensive study of the literature, directed for military usage, but of general interest as well, H. Wagner, N. Hibbits, R. D. Rosenblatt, and R. Schulz (1977) summarized their findings as follows: "(1) Team training is a necessary addition to individual training for tasks which require interaction and other 'team skills.' (2) Effective team training can occur only if the team members enter the training situation with the individual skill competencies that are needed. (3) The team context is not the appropriate location for initial acquisition of skills by individuals. (4) Performance feedback is critical to team as well as individual acquisition of skills'' (p. 17).

Competition

Competition is a strong motivating device. Two common forms are competing against one's own standards and against the performance of others. There is a strong feeling that learning does not occur without the presence of some type of competition. Competition can be associated with the following activities:

1. Performance against established group norm standards.
2. Performance against personal standards.
3. Performance alone against another person.
4. Performance within a group but against other members of the group.
5. Performance within a group againt other groups.

Numerous investigations and empirical observations lend support for the contribution competition makes to personal motivation and, subsequently, to performance. Typically, performance levels improve when the situation is a competitive one, especially if the task is not so complex as to cause the individual to falter under the stress. Well-learned skills should be performed with usual or higher-than-usual proficiency.

However, there is some concern about the overall beneficial effects of subjecting children and young men and women to constant competitive situations (e.g., Roberts & Russell, 1977). Although many circumstances in life foster competitiveness, many others require cooperation. When working with or against people, performances are obviously subject to change. Many educators favor the practice of teaching motor skills primarily in a cooperative situation rather than in a situation that fosters extreme competitiveness. It appears that the real issue surrounding competition is the extent to which it should be emphasized or deemphasized.

Competition elevates the arousal level within the organism, and to the extent that it causes it to be optimal for the task at hand and the skill level of the person, it possesses merit. We might expect that competition differentially affects higher and lower anxiety learners, to the advantage of those having lower anxiety. Logic and theory would support this notion. But Rainer Martens and Dan Landers (1969) did not find this to be true. A coincident timing task was administered to extreme scoring subjects on the Taylor Manifest Anxiety Scale. Competition did not interact with anxiety to affect performance differentially.

Although it is true that competition enhances arousal (e.g., physiological parameters such as heart rate; see Evans, 1972), a corresponding improvement in motor performance may not be observed. Evans, as well as some other investigators, has not demonstrated expected relationships between physiological parameters of performance scores. The inverted U-shaped hypothesis was not supported, in that the predicted relationship between arousal (obtained in heart rate) and incremental or decremental performance in a competitive situation was not found. Such evidence may imply weaknesses in the theory or in experimental methodology.

Contradictory results with different motor tasks within the same study have been reported by Clyde Noble, J. E. Fuchs, D. P. Robel, and R. W. Chambers (1958). Two motor tasks were learned under isolated and social conditions. Pursuit rotor performance was not affected by the number of subjects in a group. However, the social competitive situation stimulated greater increments in performance than did isolated practice in a discrimination reaction-time task. Figure 14-1 contains the learning curves derived from the data acquired in the discrimination reaction-time task. Perhaps unique task demands interact with various learning environments (e.g., social versus isolated) to produce task-specific results.

Cooperation

Invariably, data from relevant experiments have indicated the superiority of competitive and cooperative ventures over a no-incentive situation. Because so many conditions contain both competitive and cooperative elements, it is not easy to decide which one is more effective in facilitating learning. In team sports and partner games, the performer has to learn how to play cooperatively as well as to express a desire for defeating the opponents. It would appear that pure competitive measures are more effective than cooperative ventures in motivating performance. This is especially true with young children. Competition is more easily learned than cooperation. Cooperation involves greater degrees of maturation and intellectual involvement. Joint ventures presuppose a sublimation of some personal drives and desires and require that certain understandings be transmitted to children. When comparing group versus individual performance, there is evidence that co-

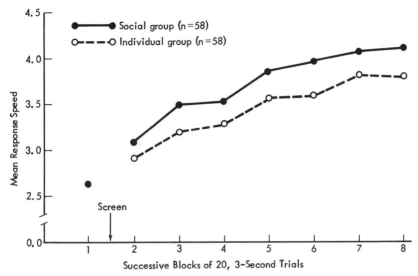

FIGURE 14-1. Acquisition curves of speed in discrimination reaction under individual (partitioned) versus social (nonpartitioned) conditions of practice. (*From Noble, C. E., Fuchs, J. E., Robel, D. P., & Chambers, R. W. Individual versus social performance on two perceptual-motor tasks.* Perceptual and Motor Skills, *1958, 8, 131–134.*)

operative efforts may be more efficient. N. Weyner and D. Zeaman (1956) analyzed data obtained from groups of two and four subjects run as teams and individual efforts on pursuit rotor performance. It was found that by numerically increasing the team members, better performances were attained

Group interaction can be a more powerful positive influence on performance than an individual effort. An implication is that working in small groups provides a pooling of learning that benefits performance. Also, merely performing tasks in the presence of others serves as a social motivator. An example of the small-group approach lies in the teaching of swimming skills by pairing off students to assist each other.

Disregarding task peculiarities and learner characteristics, it does appear that social group settings can be quite favorable to learners. This is especially true when (1) their knowledge and abilities are positively related to the topic; (2) they are a cohesive unit that can work and communicate together; (3) they are not passive but actively offer assistance, reinforcement, and feedback; (4) they compete against each other within the group; and (5) the size of the group is reasonable (Singer, 1972).

Social Facilitation Theory

The effects of others on the behavior of one was formulated into a testable hypothesis by Robert Zajonc (1965). His article, "Social Facilitation," is widely referred to in present-day literature dealing with social situations and behavioral effects. Actually, either facilitating or impeding effects on learning and performance can be noted when the subject is in the presence of another. And Zajonc's model predicts performance accordingly.

Remaining in the drive theory (Hull-Spence) tradition, Zajonc speculates that social presence increases the level of arousal (motivation) within a performer. In turn, response preferences are emitted. When the dominant responses in the repertoire of responses are correct ones, as is the case with the skilled performer, social presence should be of benefit to the individual. Conversely, if the dominant responses are incorrect ones (exemplified early in learning), the social presence effect should be detrimental. In other words, dominant responses tend to be activated under the stress of the social presence, thereby influencing the quality of the response. The learning process of difficult activities should be negatively affected under social presence conditions. Once high levels of proficiency are reached, performance should be facilitated. These thoughts are summarized in Table 14-1.

TABLE 14-1 Social Facilitation Theory*

Stage I Early Learning	Stage II High Skill Level
Response possibilities: Wrong is dominant	Response possibilities: Right is dominant
Social Presence Effect: Detrimental	Beneficial

*There is a greater probability of making a wrong response early in learning a complex skill with social presence than making a right one at high skill levels.

The typical test of the Zajonc hypothesis is through two types of social presence mediums: (1) coaction and (2) spectators. In the first situation, people are actively engaged in similar activities (cooperating, competing, observing each other, and so on). In the second situation, an audience views the behaviors of one or more performers. Presumably, both forms of social interaction should result in the same effects on an individual performing (although, as we shall see shortly, Bird's (1973) data do not support this contention).

Although data taking exception to aspects of Zajonc's theory have been published, by and large a good deal of support exists. A practical interpretation of the theory follows. Learn a complex motor task under solitary conditions, and when a reasonable level of achievement is obtained and the individual is prepared for the stress of social presence, he or she should not only bear it, but perform better as a result of it. A good overview of the social facilitation literature, with implications for motor behavior, has been developed by Dan Landers and Penny McCullagh (1976).

Coaction

Any discussion of the way individual behaviors are shaped by competition and cooperative training programs, or by being involved in an activity simultaneously with other individuals, refers to the effects of coaction. The presence of coactors implies that an individual is working in a social context. As we have seen, individual performance may very well be influenced by such a situation.

In a typical coaction experiment, subjects working in the same type of activity independently, but next to each other, are compared in their individual performances with those who work in isolated environments. Data generated with lower forms of organisms support the hypothesis that coaction situations generally stimulate greater activity than solitary conditions. Productivity with already learned behaviors is increased. The social facilitating effects of coaction environments are predictably more likely with familiar tasks than with less familiar and difficult ones. The negative effects of coaction, in the form of nondesirable stress, may operate to depress individual performance in the initial learning stages of complex tasks.

Coaction settings often arouse individuals to greater performance levels. This may be due to the motivational aspects of the situation. The benefits of coaction, in this case individuals actively, independently, and simultaneously engaged in the same task, have been reported by Anne Bird (1973). The subjects in this investigation performed either a manual dexterity task or a hand-steadiness task. Of the three groups of subjects that were formed, one performed alone, a second performed in a coaction situation, and the third performed in the presence of a passive audience. Essentially, Bird's results were as follows: (1) in hand steadiness, the solitary group did not differ significantly in performance from the other two groups, although coaction produced better scores than did the audience situation; and (2) in manual dexterity, the solitary and audience groups performed similarly and the coaction group achieved significantly higher scores than the other two groups.

The data are illustrated in Figures 14-2 and 14-3. Social situations evidently affect individual performances differentially, according to (1) type of task and (2) type of social situation. Coaction effects and audience presence effects were not similar in both tasks. But, generally speaking, coacting subjects performed well in both activities.

The simpler the task, the more likely dominant responses will be correct. P. J. Hunt and J. M. Hillery (1973) observed that coacting subjects made fewer mistakes than isolates as they performed on a simple maze task. The opposite was true with the complex maze task, as can be seen in Figure 14-4. The data support the social facilitation hypothesis.

However, merely attempting to assure the dominance of a correct response in a task does not necessarily result in expected beneficial coaction effects. A. V. Carron and B. Bennett (1976), using four-choice reaction-time tasks, found no differences in performance level or performance consistency of groups trained under coaction or isolated conditions, regardless of habit strength (dominant cor-

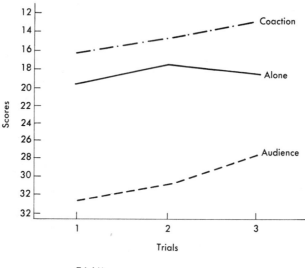

Trial Means:

Alone: 19.73, 17.63, 18.67

Audience: 32.47, 30.93, 27.63

Coaction: 16.27, 14.97, 13.00

FIGURE 14-2. Trial performance on the hand-steadiness task. (*From Bird, A. M. Effects of social facilitation upon female's performance of two psychomotor tasks. Research Quarterly, 1973, 44, 322–330.*)

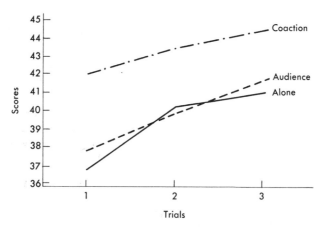

Trial Means:

Alone: 36.70, 40.10, 40.90

Audience: 37.74, 39.77, 41.60

Coaction: 41.97, 43.33, 44.37

FIGURE 14-3. Trial performance on the manual dexterity task. (*From Bird, A. M. Effects of social facilitation upon female's performance of two psychomotor tasks. Research Quarterly, 1973, 44, 322–330.*)

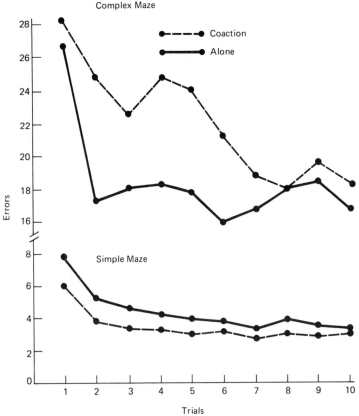

FIGURE 14-4. The effects of coaction and task difficulty on performance at a maze. (*From Hunt, P. J., & Hillery, J. M. Social facilitation in a coaching setting: An examination of the effects of learning over trials.* Journal of Experimental Social Psychology, *1973, 9, 563–571.*) Copyright 1973 by Academic Press, Inc. Reprinted by permission.

rect response or incorrect response). Experimental artifacts, explained by the investigators, may have contributed to these surprising findings. These explanations, and many more, help to show the obstacles that need to be overcome in order to "purify" the research dealing with social factors.

Audience Effect

It has been nearly everyone's experience to know individuals who can demonstrate a high degree of skill proficiency when performing alone or in the comfortable confines of a practice situation but who disintegrate during actual competition and in front of an audience. There also are people whose performance improves under this circumstance. Because of the complexity of the human organism and the degree to which a skill may have been learned, the presence or absence of spectators may seem to have unpredictable effects on different people.

Returning to social facilitation theory, there are indications that the presence of others might prove to be detrimental if the skill, especially a more complex one, is in the early stages of being learned. A skill well learned and demonstrated for viewers should be executed in a consistent and stable manner. Highly developed skills are less affected by distractions.

So far we have discussed social facilitation theory in a general way, excluding such factors as task complexity, individual anxiety and motivational levels, and the composition of the audience. There are many examples in the real world where people practice their art by themselves, to be performed later in front of others. Athletes, actors and actresses, dancers, musicians, educators, politicians, and others are required on occasion to perform in front of others. For experimental purposes, the situation must be much more controlled and, therefore, contrived in order to examine spectator effects. Having a small group of passive (neutral) spectators in close proximity to a subject watch that subject learning and performing a task is a typical study in the skills area.

In one such investigation, Martens's (1969) data upheld social facilitation theory. When subjects were initially learning the task in front of an audience, they performed more poorly than subjects learning alone. Once the task had been learned fairly well, subjects in front of spectators performed better than those performing in isolation. Furthermore, subjects performing in spectator presence were more consistent in their responses. Differences between the groups in performance can be observed in Figure 14-5.

A paradigm for subjecting social facilitation theory to scientific investigation can be arranged in the following way. Singer (1970) formed four groups of subjects, with each tested on two occasions under one of the following conditions:

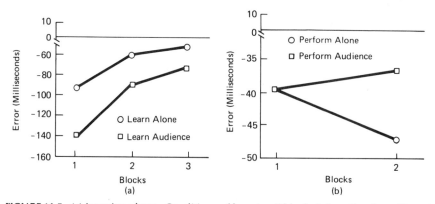

FIGURE 14-5. (a) Learning phase: Conditions of learning X blocks interaction for arithmetic error. (b) Performance phase: Conditions of performance X blocks interaction for arithmetic error intravariance. (*From Martens, R. Effect of an audience on learning and performance of a complex motor skill. Journal of Personality and Social Psychology, 1969, 12, 252–260.*) Copyright 1969 by the American Psychological Association. Reprinted by permission.

spectators–no spectators, spectators–spectators, no spectators–no spectators, no spectators–spectators:

Learning Trials	Performance Trials
Spectators	Spectators
	No Spectators
No Spectators	Spectators
	No Spectators

Block I trials are considered learning trials. Block II trials are considered performance trials; that is, the skill level of the subjects is considered to be reasonably high at this point.

The performer's anxiety level may interact with audience presence or absence, producing a number of possible outcomes. Evidence is reported in an investigation by Cox (1966). The effect of only the experimenter, mothers, teachers, peers, and strangers on primary-grade children with varying anxiety levels performing a marble-dropping task was studied. Low-anxious boys showed better performances in general and high-anxious boys showed poorer performances in the presence of people. Interestingly enough, when only the experimenter was present, low anxious boys showed response decrements, while the high-anxious group improved.

Because the presence of others provides some stress to the learner, the situation may be more disruptive to anxious persons. There are some contradictory data on this position, but there are other data and logic to support it. Consideration for kinds of tasks (e.g., motor or verbal, simple or difficult), age level, sex, techniques for the measurement of anxiety, and other variables may help to explain discrepancies. Meanwhile, it appears that more anxious individuals will probably respond more sensitively and fully to stressful conditions, and that social facilitation theory can explain these behaviors.

Level of motivation affects the social facilitation of behaviors that have been well learned. A lever-pulling task was administered by James Sorce and Gregory Fouts (1973) to subjects alone or with an audience present (the experimenter). Three motivational groups were formed according to changes in skin conductance between baseline and the first experimental condition. It was found that the high motivation group performed more slowly than the low or medium motivated groups in the presence of a spectator. No differences in performance among the motivational groups occurred without an audience. Perhaps if someone is operating at a high motivational level, audience presence increases motivational level past the optimal point.

One of the outstanding attributes of the superior athlete is the ability to perform specialty skills in a consistent, highly skilled manner, apparently disregarding the tension-filled atmosphere of stadiums or gymnasiums full of spectators. Is this performance trait transferable to other situations? Are these individuals, after learning entirely new skills in private, able to perform in the same efficient manner, with the same success, before an audience?

In order to provide some insight into the problem, Singer (1965) attempted to determine the effect of spectator presence on athletes and nonathletes performing a novel motor task. A stabilometer, requiring balance ability, was the task practiced by the subjects alone on one day and in front of a group of spectators the next day. The athletes represented various sports at Ohio State University and were acknowledged as being among the better athletes at that university.

In front of the audience, the nonathletes were observed to perform significantly better than the athletes. Apparently, there was no positive transfer effect for the athletes, who were used to displaying their motor abilities before spectators. Possibly, athletes are more sensitive to having people watch them perform and feel uncomfortable before a group demonstrating a skill at which they are not extremely competent. Even when practicing alone, the athletes did not show superior balancing ability. In fact, although not significant, the nonathletes generally displayed superior performance to the athletes throughout the practice trials. The specificity with which we learn appears to be verified by the inability of those athletes to transfer the balance needed and developed for their particular sports to the task used in this study. Figure 14-6 contains the performance curves of the two groups, alone and before spectators. Thirty-second time trials were administered to the subjects; a decline in the curves indicates better performance.

The social influence on motor performance is certainly an area in need of extensive research. Because of the many confounding variables acting on any situation involving the learning and performing of skills in a social context, many researchers have avoided attacking the various aspects of the problem. Because we usually do not learn or perform our skills in an isolated situation, any learning

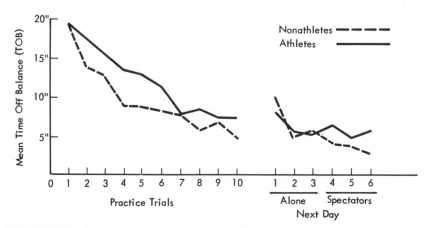

FIGURE 14-6. Performance comparison between athletes and nonathletes before and during presence of spectators. (*From Singer, R. N. Effect of spectators on athletes and nonathletes performing a gross motor task.* Research Quarterly, *1965, 36, 473–482.*)

MOTOR LEARNING AND HUMAN PERFORMANCE

principles must be modified to consider each individual, with his or her unique emotional qualities and dominant personality features, as well as the environment surrounding the activity.

Social presence, considering a number of variables, probably works in the following way. Simple tasks demanding physical energy, repetition, power, strength, or endurance are probably benefited by social presence. Social presence conditions stimulate behavior. For many of these events, the person has to be extremely motivated to mobilize the body's resources. However, until they are well learned, motor skills requiring complex coordination, finely executed movements, and intense concentration can be impaired easily by the presence of an audience. The demonstration of any skill, once developed to a high degree of proficiency, should be favorably affected by an audience. Certainly, skilled behavior is not expected to be disrupted by the presence of others. Excellence in skilled movement implies control and self-directed use of emotions.

The more reactive audience adds to the possible effect on an individual's performance. Assuming its reinforcing and motivating properties, the audience should raise the drive level of the person. Dominant responses, right or wrong, probably tend to be emitted even more when an active audience, rather than a passive audience, is on the scene. Contrary to expectation, the best skilled athletes in various sports are infrequently affected by crowd behavior. Their performances are relatively stable, consistent, and predictable. They have learned how to perform effectively under all kinds of conditions. That is why they are labeled skilled.

For the average person, working in a motivated state is necessary for a reasonable performance yield. Every task requires that an ideal level of motivation be expressed by the learner. When the highest level of motivation is operating, audience presence can overstimulate and impair muscular coordination. The highly skilled athlete is able to control emotions to work in a favorable way in his or her behavior in front of spectators. What of the athlete who does well in practice but cannot match personal performance during the contest? If skill is defined as the ability to execute proper spatially and temporally timed responses to appropriate cues under varying environmental conditions, the "practice athlete" is obviously not highly skilled. One must learn to perform in front of spectators. Experience and emotional adjustments are the necessary remediation.

Social presence may be distracting, as well as motivating, but it inevitably produces some effect on behavior. We must not forget that the performer is in a position of evaluation and appraisal when demonstrating in front of spectators (Jones & Gerard, 1967). The attitudes and anxieties of the performer to being critically observed indicate sensitivity to the situation. Familiar and friendly audiences tend to make the average individual more comfortable, whereas unknown and even unseen audiences can have a deleterious effect on performance.

If subjects are self-conscious, they are more likely to suffer under social presence conditions. Gymnasts who are concerned about how they appear to the spectators viewing the contest are likely to score more poorly than gymnasts who concentrate on execution and form.

PERFORMANCE FACTORS

Besides social factors, other conditions in the learning environment can affect performance conditions. In this section, we will primarily analyze *performance* variables, those that may temporarily diminish performance results but, in fact, may not be of major consequence in learning. Then again, any factor that is severe enough or perseveres for a while could conceivably lead to poor practice conditions and, ultimately, little, if any, learning.

A variety of situational occurrences could influence the learner/performer in a number of ways. The "normal" functioning human system can be *temporarily* impaired, resulting in subpar performance. Some of the variables of possible negative influence on performance are examined here, notably, sense restriction, sleep deprivation, fatigue, and pain. Other variables are discussed elsewhere in this book. Also, such variables as injury to a body part or feelings of ill health can temporarily slow down the system. They are not treated any further here, however, because their effects on performance are too obvious. First of all, alternative working circumstances need to be recognized in terms of variations and potential impact.

Working Conditions

Work output is related to the environment: temperature, noise, lighting, and the like. Many studies have been undertaken in industrial psychology to determine optimal working conditions. It would stand to reason that there is an optimal environment for learning and performing motor tasks. The literature is too extensive to report here, so one investigation is presented as an example.

Various heat-stress environments were created and subjects' performance recorded on a tracking task and a reaction-time task, with a peripheral stimulus presented simultaneously. The temperatures under each condition were 84.9°, 88.4°, and 89.8°F. The subjects performed in one of these environments as well as in a comfortable environment. N. Z. Azer, P. E. McNall, and H. C. Leung (1972) found that the 89.8°F. environment created a significant deterioration in tracking and an increase in reaction time. Performances worsened with prolonged exposure to heat stress, as might be expected.

Although motor learning researchers have generally not addressed such variables and their influence on learning and performance, these variables are of major concern in real-world learning environments. Hence, they have attracted the attention of applied psychologists. Environmental factors, peripheral yet relevant to the performance activity, cannot be discounted in their potential influence on task learning, task persistence, and level of performance. The scientific study of work leads to a more effective design of appropriate environmental conditions.

Ergonomics is the name given to the science of work. Attempts are made to reduce the burden on the person as he or she attempts to perform. Time and motion studies are geared toward this objective. Fatigue and impairment are net results of unsuitable working conditions, and factors that contribute to these constraints need to be identified and reorganized. O. G. Edholm's book (1967) provides a good overview of this area and of work output as related to various regulated and nonregulated environmental conditions.

Effects of Fatigue

Fatigue can be caused by excessive and strenuous work. The ability to resist fatigue, partly because of the physiological and fitness state, as well as the psychological framework, of the person, enables one to perform motor tasks continuously and effectively. Recall the human behaving system proposed in Chapter 6. It appears that fatigue can influence mechanisms as they operate from the input of information to the output of some behavior.

A variety of interpretations, explanations, and definitions of the term *fatigue* have been offered by laymen and scholars. Physiologists usually offer one perspective, psychologists another. It is not unusual to associate the fatigue effects of muscular work with physiological processes. This is an oversimplistic interpretation, however. Writing for many years on the topic of fatigue, S. Howard Bartley (1968) prefers an extremely broad interpretation of the term: "Fatigue is an experienced state of discomfort, aversion, and inability to perform, otherwise known as tiredness or weariness. The term applies to the total individual (the organism-as-a-person) and not properly to an organ or tissue" (p. 345).

When fatigue states are reached in the performance of most motor tasks, muscle discomfort is usually apparent. Extreme exertion or prolonged activity result in disrupted behavior. Performance becomes erratic and impaired. There is an interruption of control and a loss of efficiency. Irregularity in timing is observed. The person realizes that to proceed further with the task is impossible; the task demands are too great. In fact, we can view fatigue as the result of an *overload* on the system and *boredom* as the result of an *underload* on the system.

The solutions for overcoming fatigue depend on the task and the person. Rest may be the answer for many activities. Drugs such as amphetamines (pep pills) may work on occasion. Increased effort, motivation, and stimuli can help to overcome fatigue. Changing tasks (completely different), attitudes, or attention may assist in combating fatigue. Practice in fatiguing situations will aid the person in becoming adjusted to performing under such conditions; a state of performance resistance to fatigue will develop.

The human system behaves—that is, movements are enacted—after information is received, those signals are perceived, and decisions about them are made. Apparently, fatigue primarily affects the central processes involved between information receipt and the initiation of movement. In tasks heavily laden with a perceptual component, less attention is paid to task-relevant signals. Externally paced tasks require immediate recognition of cues that might occur in an unpredictable fashion. Impaired attention and perception will negatively influence behavior. An inability to perform coordinated and well-timed movements will disrupt both self-paced and externally paced tasks.

One area of concern for skill instructors is the degree to which fatigue can be expected to inhibit learning and make performance erratic. Although there is an assumption on the part of many that fatigue disrupts learning and performance, this may not always be the case. The body may be stressed through continuous local activity (an arm, for example) or through general activity involving many muscles in different sites. Tasks may primarily involve strength, endurance, speed, or accuracy. It may be expected, according to directions indicated in the research, that

1. General body activity and moderately high fatigue will impair performances requiring strength, endurance, and, on occasion, rapid movements; accuracy or balance performance may not be affected (see Figure 14-7 for an illustration of the latter case).
2. Fatigue caused by one task does not necessarily influence the learning and performance of a subsequent task (e.g., Welch, 1969, showed that heavy fatigue caused by a step-up test did not impair performance on three coordination tests; Brzezinska, 1970, reports that there is no generalization of fatigue between unrelated tasks; fatigue caused by one task does not spread to other tasks, except in cases where there are common factors).
3. General, light, fatiguing exercise may on occasion aid the learning of a motor task, perhaps serving as warm-up or causing an increased concentration on the learning task (e.g., Benson, 1968, noted that learning to juggle was enhanced when subjects practiced in a fatigued state).
4. For many tasks, moderately high fatiguing activities will impede performance rather than learning; that is, learning is occurring all the time, but fatigue temporarily depresses performance, thereby producing lower levels of achievement

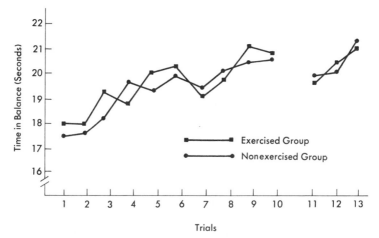

FIGURE 14-7. Performance on a stabilometer for groups exercised on a treadmill or nonexercised. No differences in performance were noted between the groups. Reprinted with permission of author and publisher from: Bartz, D. W., and Smith, L. E. Effect of moderate exercise on the performance and learning of a gross motor skill. *Perceptual and Motor Skills*, 1970, *31*, 187–190.

(e.g., Schmidt, 1969, observed that balance performance worsened under fatigue but improved considerably without fatigue).

5. Severe exercise will be detrimental to both learning and performance (e.g., Carron, 1972), demonstrated the long-lasting effect of extremely fatiguing bicycle ergometer work in impairing balance on the ladder-climb task).

The influence of exhaustive exercise on learning can be proposed through consolidation theory, suggest Robert Hutton, James Stevens, and Faith Stevens (1972). It is thought that continued neural activity associated with an event goes on until a memory trace is established (consolidation). If the trace is vulnerable during the consolidation period, as thought, any sudden and strong stimuli can conceivably disrupt the trace. Vigorous exercise introduced immediately after a learning event may be one of many examples of stimuli providing an impedance to memory consolidation. Although Hutton et al. embrace the theory, their data are quite preliminary, and the theory itself represents primarily an extrapolation from research with variables other than fatigue.

Instructors must determine the optimal period of time students should spend learning skills before fatigue effects would make that time wasteful. Common sense is perhaps one of the best indicators of when a person is too tired mentally or physically to receive any value from continued practice. Although there are times when performance may suffer slightly under minor conditions of fatigue, ultimate learning does not. Under excessive fatigue, it is quite difficult for the learner to be attentive to new cues and new material. The returns of the practice of pushing the learner when he or she is too tired are slight and, consequently, this practice is regarded as undesirable. Furthermore, the learner may practice erroneous responses that will have to be unlearned at a later date. Consideration must also be given to safety factors and the danger involved in the execution of a particular task, especially if the performer is extremely weary.

Pain

Pain, or at least an individual's perception of it, will usually have some bearing on the performance of skills. Physiologically, pain mechanisms are quite similar for all people. The ability to detect painful stimuli may operate in the same way we gain information related to vision, taste, and movement: specialized sense receptors have specific functions, and pain receptors are activated when painful experiences are present. Another point of view is that pain encompasses so many stimuli that it cannot be related to a single sense modality. Advocates of this concept suggest that intense stimulation activates nonspecific receptors and that pain patterns emerge instead.

Beyond the activation of pain receptors is the person's psychological attitude to the pain situation. Previous experiences influence the ability to cope with pain. Furthermore, pain thresholds also may be related to genetic factors. Experimental research and empirical observations suggest that some persons are able to withstand pain more than others. This situation may be related to an individual's pain threshold, conditioning factors related to previous experiences, and motivation to overcome the pain. Pain tolerance is related to a host of variables.

The ability to withstand pain is beneficial in demonstrating high levels of task proficiency under adverse conditions. Although physiological mechanisms and chemical substances can contribute to the curtailment of activity, conscious mental behavior operates to influence behavior as well.

For certain endeavors, namely verbal tasks or tasks involving exceptional amounts of attention, vigilance, and appropriate perceptions for accurate, fast responses, an ideal state of arousal seems to be desirable. However, when pain, fatigue, and physical endurance are occurring during practice and must be tolerated for achievement, it is possible that a mentally alert, sensitive state would be a disadvantage for the organism. The direction of thoughts, the conscious state, during such activity might enable an individual to be more or less tolerant of circumstances.

It is generally accepted that cerebral involvement and arousal level can affect autonomic functions. Adrenalin secretion and skin conductance, as well as subjectively estimated arousal level, can diminish with repeated trials on a perceptual conflict test. This habituation response is commonly seen in cardiorespiratory responses to repeated administration of treadmill or ergometer work bouts. It has been suggested that, in some cases, control of arousal level can be accomplished by assigning subjects objective, cognitive tasks to be carried out during test administration (Brown, 1966; W. E. Collins, G. H. Crampton, & J. B. Posner, 1961). Similar procedures have been said to exert a regulatory influence on the reduction of blood oxygenation of well-trained athletes during breath holding (Yegerow, 1965). Whether this, in fact, occurs or whether the differences in breath-holding time were a result of the subjects being predictably variable in their ability to withstand the discomfort of breath holding is a moot point; however, it is important that different conscious states may bring about different responses as a result of cerebral-autonomic interactions.

The ability to endure appears to reside in the willingness to withstand the pain experienced, a result of the accumulation of noxious metabolites in the working muscles (Dorpat & Holmes, 1955). Athletes often report that feelings of pain can be suppressed during endurance work by diverting their attention away from the exercise bout. However, this has not been supported by experimental evidence. Paradoxically, it has been shown that, generally, as pain appears, more effort is exerted (Evans & McGlashan, 1967). This increased effort would then bring about a greater production and accumulation of metabolites and, concomitantly, more pain, a cycle that would continue until the quit point was reached. It seems that it must be very difficult to maintain diversionary cognition during these latter stages of performance, but that may be a key to enhanced task execution, insofar as endurance is concerned.

With the current popularity of long distance running, penetrating analyses are being made of reasons why people run, and in fact, what they think about their attempt to endure the event. W. P. Morgan (1978) has described runners as associators or dissociators. In other words, the sensory input from the working joints, muscles, lungs, and heart can be paid attention to or ignored during running. Each strategy can be effective for certain purposes. Morgan recommends that the average jogger should use dissociation at first, but later, should imitate the elite runners, who seem to be able to use an associative strategy effectively.

The ability to endure pain and fatigue may not be related only to the person's training state and the nature of the task, but to personality variables, as well. For instance, the relationship of extraversion and the ability to withstand pain have been the topic of a few studies (Levine, Tusky, & Nichols, 1966; Lynn & Eysenck, 1961). It has been hypothesized that individuals who score high on an extraversion personality trait should have greater levels of pain tolerance than individuals who score low on extraversion.

Some researchers have examined the relationship of pain tolerance and participation in athletic activities. In one such study (Ryan & Kovacic, 1966), contact sport athletes, noncontact sport athletes, and nonathletes were compared and observed in their ability to tolerate induced pain. A definite relationship was found, with contact sport athletes demonstrating a better ability to withstand pain. Perhaps they learn to tolerate pain as a result of their previous experiences. Willingness and ability to tolerate pain are associated with type and extent of athletic participation.

Perhaps there are persons who are pain reducers or pain augmenters (Petrie, 1967). Individual perception in a situation would be related to these characteristics. The augmenter is one who amplifies the intensity of perception of pain; the reducer is one who does the opposite. Internally based motivation and previous experiences are thought to be related to pain tolerance. Conjecturing, a contact sport athlete might accept more pain, because of being used to it, and knowing the consequences will be of no great significance. Noncontact athletes, and especially nonathletes, might not be familiar with absorbing extreme pain in an activity and therefore be apprehensive of the potentially damaging effects.

Although athletes often perform better than nonathletes in contrived pain situations, pain threshold has by no means been determined as a general phenomenon to the variety of pain sources or parts of the body involved. Pain can evidently limit behavior in some human systems and not in others. Training to become used to pain and to perform in spite of it is useful in elevating performance, providing damage to body tissues is not an issue.

Sense Restriction

In order to maintain a state of alertness (in a particular activity), an individual must not restrict the senses and perceptual activity preceding the time of performance. Sense restriction or deprivation data lead to the conviction that one needs varying sensory stimulation to function adaptively (Neff, 1965). Research is still not sufficient in this area, at least in practical situations, but there is evidence to indicate the negative results of a nonvariable sensory environment. Although researchers talk about sensory deprivation, in fact, the perceptual processes are considerably less active than under normal conditions, as we will see by the design of the experiments in this area.

W. H. Bexton, W. Heron, and T. H. Scott (1956) studied twenty-two male subjects during a three-day isolation period. The subjects were confined to cubicles where they were restricted in their daily activities and therefore experienced decreased variations in their sensory environments. They were subjected at different periods to cognitive tests (e.g., multiplying, completing series of numbers, and making words from jumbled letters). The subjects were found to suffer from increasingly impaired intellectual ability and even suffered from visual hallucinations the longer they were under the experimental conditions.

The findings of this study emphasize the need for varying stimuli to keep us aroused and mentally active. Although cognitive tasks were employed in the study described above, we might very well expect similar findings in motor tasks. When one is restricted to a bed for several days because of illness or injury, acuity impairment in attempting skills performed prior to the situation is commonly discovered. This may be due to a non-stimulating sensory environment. The bedridden state might influence actual structural changes, such as in muscle tissue (atrophy), which might also slightly impair motor performance, depending on the length of confinement and the complexity of the skill to be performed.

One of the few sense restriction studies dealing with perceptual and motor skills was undertaken by Jack Vernon, T. E. McGill, W. L. Gulick, and D. K. Candland (1959). Subjects in this study were isolated and deprived of sensory stimulation for twenty-four, forty-eight, or seventy-two hours. The five tests administered were color perception, depth perception, pursuit rotor, mirror drawing, and rail walking. The subjects were tested prior to isolation, upon release, and twenty-four hours afterward. Among the interesting findings, indicating the different but somewhat consistent effects of sense deprivation on the different tasks, were that

1. color perception was especially impaired when confinement was forty-eight and seventy-two hours.
2. depth perception was not affected under the imposed conditions.
3. pursuit rotor performance was only negatively affected when confinement lasted forty-eight hours.
4. mirror tracing performance, when speed to traverse was the dependent variable, was similar to pursuit rotor performance.
5. rail walking was especially negatively effected after seventy-two hours isolation.

In this study, as has been found in others, the detrimental influence of sense deprivation was rather short-lived. Recovery in performance was reasonably good twenty-four hours after confinement was over.

The role of activity and exercise in counteracting perceptual loss has been studied by Zubek (1963). In comparing groups of subjects confined to a chamber for a period of one week, he determined that even a few exercise periods a day seemed to eliminate many of the impairments produced by perceptual deprivation. Other research findings on the effects of sense restriction on perceptual and motor activities have been conflicting because of varying methods of experimentation. As a point of interest, in other studies since the pioneering one of Bexton, et al., reported earlier, such pronounced detrimental effects of sense restriction have not been found. Some results even indicate an improvement in certain functions as a result of sensory deprivation. However, it appears that a variety of perceptual and motor functions may be susceptible to impairment as a function of sensory restriction, but the range of effects does not seem to be as great as was believed.

A good summary of the literature is offered by John Corso (1967). He states that the effects of

> sensory deprivation on perceptual motor performance will depend upon both the duration of the confinement and the nature of the specific task imposed. For most subjects, the maximal change in performance occurs at the end of a forty-eight-hour confinement period. . . . The results indicate that difficulty is experienced in performing new perceptual motor tasks in a sensory-deprived environment, but the question of disruption of old motor responses (excluding handwriting) has not been posed and should be investigated. The evidence also indicates that the disruptive effects of sensory deprivation on perceptual motor behavior are of relatively short duration; additional studies are needed to determine the specific forms of the recovery functions (p. 574).

The study of attention and alertness, called vigilance, has indicated that as a subject views the same stimuli, attentiveness decreases. Vigilance studies have been performed under a wide range of experimental conditions, mainly in order to determine pilot and military effectiveness during those times when concentration is important for long periods in which a specific, unsuspecting stimulus may suddenly appear. The person must monitor and detect infrequent, random, and low intensity events. Under such conditions, it is desirable to provide an environment that will maintain the human behaving system at a reasonable level of functioning. Even a novel stimulus will improve the subject's alertness. The baseball outfielder who rarely has a ball hit in that direction may be less alert than the third baseman who has been bombarded frequently with shots.

Situations similar to that for the baseball outfielder are piloting a plane under conditions of extended confinement, driving a car on a superhighway, or reading, studying, or listening to lectures for prolonged periods of time. Performance seems to decline with time as a person is subjected to too much monotony and repetition. Boredom and inattentiveness result. An important function of the instructor is to provide conditions that improve stimulation and motivation.

Sleep Deprivation

An individual needs to be properly energized and rested for productive outcomes. Personal physiological and psychological factors interplay with task characteristics and suggest the ideal amount of rest needed for each person to perform and endure, according to task demands. We can easily think of military, industrial, agricultural, athletic, and other motor activities in which rest and sleep are sharply constrained because of situational factors. The obvious practical questions are the following: To what extent does sleep deprivation impair motor performance? How much sleep loss can the individual overcome? With which tasks?

A review of the literature has been published by P. Naitoh and R. E. Townsend (1970). As might be expected, performance becomes more variable and ultimately worsens if sleep deprivation continues long enough. Performance will be a function of such variables as

1. task characteristics and demands (e.g., difficulty, duration, and the refined movements associated with a complex cue display).
2. the state of the organism (e.g., motivation, personality, and adjustment to the imposed sleep deprivation condition).
3. the duration of the sleep deprivation period.
4. the testing conditions.

Most of the research seems to cover the circumstance where subjects are deprived of sleep for a set period of time and then are tested in various performance measures. In this design, the effects will probably run similar to those found in sense deprivation studies. George Holland (1968) used a similar design, except that he trained his subjects on the tasks of interest for four weeks. He examined the consequences of one night's sleep derivation on the performance of a jump test (quickness and accuracy in moving through a pattern with a series of hops and steps), a manipulation test (a pattern similar to the jump test, scaled down, requiring the hand movement of a stylus), and a bicycle work performance test. The loss of sleep did not affect scores on the jump test or the manipulation test. Work output on the bicycle showed a significant decrement. Holland conjectures that these tasks may have been too short term and brief to tax the attention span of sleep-deprived subjects.

Another approach is to reexamine performance work and rest ratios without sleep or to work continuously without sleep. Earl Alluisi (1969) recommends the synthetic-work technique to assess output during extended periods of work. A job or work situation is created in which a number of tasks are administered to subjects for continuous practice over days and weeks. Various work–rest schedules over time with different tasks reveal one's ability to sustain performance. Alluisi and his colleagues have attempted to answer questions related to a person's capability to sustain activity without sleep over extended time durations. One such approach is described by Ben Morgan, Bill Brown, and Alluisi (1970). They report that "in evaluating men's endurance within the continuous-work situation, one is forced also to consider man's typical circadian rhythms [diurnal rhythms— physiological data such as pulse rates, axillary temperatures, etc., as related to time of day], his activities during the rest portions of the schedule, and the effects of his sleep-wakefulness cycles and habits on performance," (p. 22). The researchers conclude that

> Performance during the forty-eight hours of continuous work was greatly influenced by the circadian rhythm. The first performance decrements occurred after approximately eighteen hours of work; during the early morning hours of the first night, average performance decreased to approximately 82 per cent of baseline performance. During the first half of the second day of work, performance improved to about 90 per cent of baseline, but decreased again during the night to approximately 67 per cent of baseline. All measures of performance indicated that the recovery of performance was complete (to baseline levels) following the twenty-four-hour period of rest and recovery (p. iii).

Continuous work is more demanding than distributed work schedules and, consequently, will show more obvious impairments. Performance decrements are more pronounced with more complex or strenuous activities. Recovery of performance is usually found to be fairly complete following one night's sleep, thus suggesting the transient nature of the effects of sleep deprivation conditions. It might be speculated that people can be trained to perform without as much sleep as they think they need to be in a state of readiness. As Alluisi (1969) points out, people can follow a work–rest schedule of four hours of work and four hours off work for very long periods of time without noticeable deleterious effects on performance.

CULTURAL INFLUENCE

Preferences for and successes in various endeavors are strongly influenced by the family, peer groups, the community, and society. The types of activities participated in by parents influence a child's selection. So does the reinforcement given by parents to a child's behaviors. Among other findings, Eldon Snyder and Elmer Spreitzer (1973) state that their data indicate the role family influence plays in sports socialization. Family influence variables were predictive of sports involvement for both sexes.

The size of the family and even birth order are related to different family member characteristics and activity pursuits. The family exerts a powerful influence in shaping activity interests and individual drive for accomplishment. Social and economic class barriers are difficult to break down when individuals tend to enter occupational levels similar to those of their fathers. There are identifiable characteristic attitudes and values associated with certain social classes. Thus, the social system tends to place constraints on the human system, and these are manifested in a variety of behaviors.

Similarly, as part of the immediate system, one's friends will direct tendencies to like certain activities and dislike others. Need to achieve in them will be associated, in part, with perceived peer expectations or pressures. Mechanical skills, performing artistry, or athletic skills may be developed to some extent through family, peer, social class, and environmental influences.

Countries and their respective cultures may differ in representative values and supported activities. This point is quite apparent in sport and physical training. Popular sports vary from one country to another, and even from one community to another. Respect for physical fitness and discipline can also be shown to vary according to cultural influence. Members of a particular society tend to instill in other members an attitude to behave in a common, accepted way. We are "shaped" by our culture in every way by the recognition of status symbols, reward systems, authority structure, child-rearing practices, and the like. The society and its structure encourage certain behaviors and discourage others. Although many of us like to think in terms of freedom of choice and independence, it is difficult to conceive of any individual whose behaviors have not been molded by social pressures, obvious or subtle.

CHAPTER HIGHLIGHTS

1. Social interactive forces can influence learning and performance differently than when a person undertakes a task under isolated conditions. Competition, cooperation, coaction, and the presence of others (audience effect) constitute social factors of major interest. They have arousal properties that can lead to increased performance under many conditions. But if the task is complex and not well learned, such social factors can elicit worsened behaviors on the part of the individuals. Social facilitation theory describes this chain of events.

2. Environmental factors, such as noise, temperature, lighting, and altitude, can influence performance one way or another, depending on their deviation from the optimal and an individual's experiences under such conditions.

3. Fatigue and pain, if in excess, can produce performance and learning deficits. If in moderation, they may temporarily inhibit performance but not learning. Learner capability of dealing with these conditions will obviously influence reactions to them.

4. Sleep deprivation and sensory restriction will temporarily impair performance if of long enough duration. Behaviors should be more appropriate when conditions are returned to normal.

References

Alluisi, E. A. Sustained performance. In E. A. Bilodeau (Ed.), *Principles of skill acquisiton.* New York: Academic Press, 1969.

Azer, N. Z., McNall, P. E., & Leung, H. C. Effects of heat stress on performance. *Ergonomics,* 1972, *15,* 681–691.

Bartley, S. H. Fatigue. In *International encyclopedia of the social sciences.* New York: Macmillan, 1968.

Bartz, D. W., & Smith, L. E. Effect of moderate exercise on the performance and learning of a gross motor skill. *Perceptual and Motor Skills,* 1970, *31,* 187–190.

Benson, D. W. Influence of imposed fatigue on learning a jumping task and a juggling task. *Research Quarterly,* 1968, *39,* 251–257.

Bexton, W. H., Heron, W., & Scott, T. H. Effects of decreased variation in the sensory environment. *Canadian Journal of Psychology*, 1956, *8*, 70–76.

Bird, A. M. Effects of social facilitation upon females' performance of two psychomotor tasks. *Research Quarterly*, 1973, *44*, 322–330.

Brown, J. H. Modification of vestibular nystagmus by change of task during stimulation. *Perceptual and Motor Skills*, 1966, *22*, 603–611.

Brzezinska, Z. Generalization of fatigue in activity and vigilance. *Polish Psychological Bulletin*, 1970, *1*, 32–38.

Carron, A. V. Motor performance and learning under physical fatigue. *Medicine and Science in Sports*, 1972, *4*, 101–106.

Carron, A. V., & Bennett, B. The effects of initial habit strength differences upon performance in a coaction situation. *Journal of Motor Behavior*, 1976, *8*, 297–304.

Collins, W. E., Crampton, G. H., & Posner, J. B. Effects of mental activity on vestibular nystagmus and the electroencephalogram. *Nature*, 1961, *190*, 1964–1965.

Comrey, A. L. Group performance in a manual dexterity task. *Journal of Applied Psychology*, 1953, *37*, 207–210.

Comrey, A. L., & Deskin, G. Group manual dexterity in women. *Journal of Applied Psychology*, 1954, *38*, 178–180.

Corso, J. F. *The experimental psychology of sensory behavior*. New York: Holt, Rinehart & Winston, 1967.

Cox, F. N. Some effects of test anxiety and presence or absence of other persons on boys' performance on a repetitive motor task. *Journal of Experimental Child Psychology*, 1966, *3*, 100–112.

Dorpat, T. L., & Holmes, T. H. Mechanisms of skeletal muscle pain and fatigue. *A. M. A. Archives of Neurology and Psychiatry*, 1955, *74*, 628–640.

Edholm, O. G. *The biology of work*. New York: McGraw-Hill, 1967.

Evans, F. J., & McGlashan, T. H. Work and effort during pain. *Perceptual and Motor Skills*, 1967, *25*, 794.

Evans, J. F. Resting heart rate and the effects of an incentive. *Psychonomic Science*, 1972, *26*, 99–100.

Glaser, R., Klaus, D. J., & Egerman, K. *Increasing team proficiency through training: The acquisition and extinction of a team response*. Technical Report AIR B64-5/62, American Institutes for Research, May 1962.

Holland, G. Effects of limited sleep deprivation on performance of selected motor tasks. *Research Quarterly*, 1968, *39*, 285–294.

Hunt, P. J., & Hillery, J. M. Social facilitation in a coacting setting: An examination of the effects of learning over trials. *Journal of Experimental Social Psychology*, 1973, *9*, 563–571.

Hutton, R. S., Stevens, J. L., & Stevens, F. The effects of strenuous and exhaustive exercise on learning: A theoretical note and preliminary findings. *Journal of Motor Behavior*, 1972, *4*, 207–216.

Johnston, W. A. Transfer of team skills as a function of type of training. *Journal of Applied Psychology*, 1966, *50*, 102–108.

Jones, E. E., & Gerard, H. B. *Social psychology*. New York: John Wiley, 1967.

Landers, D. M., & McCullagh, P. D. Social facilitation of motor performance. In J. H. Wilmore (Ed.), *Exercise and sport science reviews* (Vol. 4). Santa Barbara, Calif.: Journal Publishing Affiliates, 1976.

Levine, R. M., Tusky, B., & Nichols, D. C. Tolerance for pain, extraversion, and neuroticism: Failure to replicate results. *Perceptual and Motor Skills*, 1966, *23*, 847–850.

Lynn, R., & Eysenck, H. F. Tolerance for pain, extraversion and neuroticism. *Perceptual and Motor Skills*, 1961, *12*, 161–162.

Martens, R. Effect of an audience on learning and performance of a complex motor skill. *Journal of Personality and Social Psychology*, 1969, *12*, 252–259.

Martens, R., & Landers, D. M. Effect of anxiety, competition, and failure on performance of a complex motor task. *Journal of Motor Behavior*, 1969, *1*, 1–10.

Morgan, B. B., Brown, B. R., & Alluisi, E. A. *Effects of 48 hours of continuous work and sleep loss on sustained performance.* Army THEMIS contract, Interim Technical Report No. ITR-70-16, 1970.

Morgan, W. P. The mind of the marathoner. *Psychology Today*, 1978, *11*, 38–49.

Naitoh, P., & Townsend, R. E. The role of sleep deprivation research in human factors. *Human Factors*, 1970, *12*, 575–585.

Neff, W. D. *Contributions to sensory psychology.* New York: Academic Press, 1965.

Noble, C., Fuchs, J. E., Robel, D. P., & Chambers, R. W. Individual vs. social performance on two perceptual-motor tasks. *Perceptual and Motor Skills*, 1958, *8*, 131–134.

Petrie, A. *Individuality in pain and suffering.* Chicago: University of Chicago Press, 1967.

Roberts, G. C., & Russell, D. G. The forgotten factor: Psychological processes of competition. *Australian Journal of Sports Medicine*, 1977, *9*, 38–43.

Ryan, E. D., & Kovacic, C. Pain tolerance and athletic participation. *Perceptual and Motor Skills*, 1966, *22*, 383–390.

Schmidt, R. A. Performance and learning a gross motor skill under conditions of artificially induced fatigue. *Research Quarterly*, 1969, *40*, 185–190.

Singer, R. N. Effect of spectators on athletes and nonathletes performing a gross motor task. *Research Quarterly*, 1965, *36*, 473–482.

Singer, R. N. Effect of an audience on performance of a motor task. *Jounal of Motor Behavior*, 1970, *11*, 88–95.

Singer, R. N. Social facilitation. In W. P. Morgan (Ed.), *Ergogenic aids and muscular performance.* New York: Academic Press, 1972.

Snyder, E. E., & Spreitzer, E. A. Family infuence and involvement in sports. *Resarch Quarterly*, 1973, *44*, 249–255.

Sorce, J., & Fouts, G. Level of motivation in social facilitation of a simple task. *Perceptual and Motor Skills*, 1973, *36*, 572–576.

Vernon, J. A., McGill, T. E., Gulick, W. L., & Candland, D. K. Effect of sensory deprivation on some perceptual and motor skills. *Perceptual and Motor Skills*, 1959, *9*, 91–97.

Wagner, H., Hibbits, N., Rosenblatt, R. D., Schulz, R. *Team training and evaluation strategies: state-of-the-art.* Technical Report 77-1, Human Resources Research Office, February 1977.

Welch, M. Specificity of heavy work fatigue: Absence of transfer from heavy leg work to coordination tasks using the arms. *Research Quarterly*, 1969, *40*, 402–406.

Weyner, N., & Zeaman, D. Team and individual performance on a motor learning task. *Journal of General Psychology*, 1956, *55*, 127–142.

Yegerow, A. S., cited by Puni, A. T. Problem of voluntary regulation of motor activity in sports. In F. Antonelli (Ed.), *Proceedings of the first international congress of sports psychology.* Rome, Italy, 1965.

Zubek, J. P. Counteracting effects of physical exercises performed during prolonged perceptual deprivation. *Science*, 1963, *142*, 504–506.

Zajonc, R. B. Social facilitation. *Science*, 1965, *149*, 269–274.

15 EPILOGUE

The study of motor learning, as we have seen, can take many directions, cover a variety of topics, and range from the theoretical to the applied. The primary intention behind the writing of this book was to reveal the contemporary status of the field of motor learning from research and practical perspectives. The approach was all-encompassing. The size of the book and the number of issues and topics attest to this observation.

People have different reasons for reading a book like this: it may be mandated reading for a course or courses in motor learning, or it may be selected by option. Certain topics probably have been of more interest than others, depending on one's concerns and the manner in which the material was presented. Whether scanned quickly or labored over studiously, it is hoped that the book has fulfilled a need to increase the information base about motor learning in one source while it generated interest in and enthusiasm for selected topics.

Writing this book has become more difficult with each edition, much to my surprise. After completing this third edition, and reflecting on the ten-year interim between it and the first, I am amazed about and overwhelmed with the many learning factors that must be considered, the ever-expanding body of knowledge, and the difficulty in presenting the information accurately, adequately, and appropriately. On top of this, you, the reader, and I, the writer, have had to come to grips with theoretical, methodological, and practical perspectives.

We have traversed the field, beginning with an introduction to terminology and a general orientation. Research methodology and laboratory equipment unique to the study of motor learning have been discussed. This material, along with chapters dealing with theoretical orientations to the way learners learn and perform, has served as a foundation for understanding the research and practical considerations in the area: (1) the nature of the learning process (similarities among people), (2) factors that contribute to learner differences in acquiring and maintaining skill, and (3) instructional approaches that reveal a sensitivity to the many variables that may influence learning.

Consequently, we have had to become familiar with information derived from a variety of sources. Psychological and other literature have been presented in which experimental, differential, and theoretical approaches were used to analyze personal characteristics, developmental factors, social and environmental variables, and instructional techniques that might contribute to a positive change in behavior.

Thus, no simple deductions could be made about the learning of motor skills. Rather, when people interact with situations to acquire and perform complex skills, we are more aware of the many factors that might be considered for the improvement of instruction and learning conditions for learners in general and for those who should receive special attention.

If we examine the immediate past and the present to project into the future, what can be speculated about developments in motor learning? First of all, there is every indication that scholarly activity will continue to increase, in a range on the continuum from highly conceptual and "pure" research to the derivation of practical guidelines for learners and instructors. That range also will include topics of interest, for they have continued to expand and become more diverse as more scholars and teachers have become concerned with motor learning.

Motor behaviors are fascinating to study, as they may also provide information about the way cognitive processes work. Movement skill can be assessed with great precision. It can be measured repeatedly. Classical and contemporary reaction-time paradigms, for instance, have been ingeniously designed by investigators to make inferences about mental operations that might occur in sequence or overlap during performance. Consequently, movements are studied not only by motor learning specialists for their own particular reasons, but by cognitive psychologists as well, in order to learn more about cognitive processes. This trend will probably be sustained.

Researchers will continue to ask more penetrating questions, work in more solid conceptual directions, improve experimental designs and methodology, and develop a more substantiative body of knowledge about motor behaviors. Those concerned with instruction and training will find more useful information in the literature and implement their own practical research programs in an attempt to upgrade the quality of instruction and instructional settings.

Conceptually speaking, we need more answers about what occurs within the learner/performer. What directs what, and how? As issues sharpen between centralists (motor program control) and peripheralists (feedback control), neurophysiological and psychological evidence will be integrated more fully, unique research paradigms developed, and new tasks used. We should become more aware of the role of cognitive processes in the acquisition and retention of motor behaviors. And, associated with this topic, is the need to understand how and which strategies will assist learners in maximizing their potential to use their limited attentional and working capacities.

Methodologically, there are questions that need to be raised about the assessment of learning. What should represent a learning score? Which of the many potential available dependent measures should be selected, under what conditions, and why? Furthermore, by simulating real-world activities, can computers and other equipment be made more useful to those who study motor behaviors? Can and should experiments be standardized more in order to attempt to obtain consistent results for deriving "laws" of behavior? Or is a variety of procedures and tasks within investigations on the same topic the healthy way to go to obtain useful inferences about behavior?

The issues to be resolved and the topics to be studied appear to be endless. Although the trend has been toward better-defined topics and refined methodology, there is always the necessity to integrate material, to understand phenomena, from a global perspective. Such responsibility need not always rest on the shoulders of instructors, or "practical" researchers. Researchers who consider themselves "purists" might also take note. The ability to make intelligent interpretations of and broaden applications from data often depends on the knowledge base of the investigator, his or her depth and breadth.

We now end our journey, at least temporarily. Although this book is now concluded, we must all realize that the text is not a terminal point but a beginning point. It is for me. I hope it is for you.

Selected Annotated Student References

Adams, J. A. *Learning and memory: An introduction.* Homewood, Ill.: Dorsey Press, 1976. A general overview of the field of learning; standard contemporary topics are presented, with scientific evidence and practical applications.

Annett, J. *Feedback and human behavior.* Baltimore: Penguin Books, 1969. A convenient source that covers the parameters of feedback (knowledge of results).

Bell, V. L. *Sensorimotor learning.* Pacific Palisades, Calif.: Goodyear Publishing Co., 1970. A simplified, general introduction and overview of research findings related to motor learning and applied to physical education.

Berlin, P. (Ed.). A symposium on motor learning. *Quest,* 1966, 6. This edition is dedicated to attacking aspects of motor learning with contributions from leading physical educators.

Bernstein, N. *The coordination and regulation of movements.* Oxford, England: Pergamon Press, 1967. Contains a collection of papers, translated from Russian to English, that demonstrate Bernstein's perceptivity in formulating concepts about human movement from a cybernetic point of view.

Bilodeau, E. A. (Ed.). *Acquisition of skill.* New York: Academic Press, 1966. A highly sophisticated attempt by psychologists to interpret extensive research related to aspects of motor skill acquisition.

Carron, A. V. *Laboratory experiments in motor learning.* Englewood Cliffs, N.J.: Prentice-Hall, 1971. Twenty-three experiments, along with techniques in experimentation, are presented.

Connally, K. J. (Ed.). *Mechanisms of motor skill development.* New York: Academic Press, 1970. This is a scholarly multidisciplinary approach—probably the best source for materials on developmental factors and motor skills.

Covington, M. V., & Beery, R. G. *Self-worth and school learning.* New York: Holt, Rinehart & Winston, 1976 (paperback). With an emphasis on cognitive motivational theory, theory and practice are interwoven, and very meaningful suggestions are made about how to improve students' confidence and motivation in the classroom.

Cratty, B. *Movement behavior and motor learning.* Philadelphia: Lea & Febiger, 1973. This book provides excellent resource material related to human movement and learning.

Cratty, B. *Teaching motor skills*. Englewood Cliffs, N. J.: Prentice-Hall, 1973. This is a practical approach toward teaching motor skills, based on research and theory.

Cratty, B. J., & Hutton, R. S. *Experiments in movement behavior and motor learning*. Philadelphia: Lea & Febiger, 1969. Twenty-five experiments are presented, with an attempt to communicate simple experimental designs, statistics, and information on motor learning.

DeCecco, John P. *The psychology of learning and instruction*. Englewood Cliffs, N.J.: Prentice-Hall, 1968. (See particularly Chapter 8, "The Teaching and Learning of Skills.") This is a practical approach to effective teaching, including models, a body of information, and guidelines.

Deci, E. L. *Intrinsic motivation*. New York: Plenum Press, 1975. Research and theory are delved into, as the nature of intrinsic motivation is explored, developed, and influenced by various factors.

Dickinson, J. *Proprioceptive control of human movement*. London: Lepus Books, 1974. This is a comprehensive multidisciplinary approach to the study of proprioception.

Drowatzky, J. N. *Motor learning: Principles and practices*. Minneapolis: Burgess, 1975. This is an introductory book dealing with the learning process, the learner, and types of tasks.

Ellis, H. C. *Fundamentals of human learning, memory, and cognition* (2nd ed.). Dubuque, Iowa: William C. Brown, 1978. This vast introductory overview is of the entire field of learning from every point of view.

Estes, W. K. (Ed.). *Handbook of learning and cognitive processes* (4 vols.). Hillsdale, N.J.: Erlbaum, 1975–76. Excellent theoretical and technical material concerning contemporary issues and areas in cognitive psychology are presented, although much of it has special implications for serious scholars of motor learning.

Fitts, P. M., & Posner, M. I. *Human performance*. Belmont, Calif.: Brooks/Cole, 1967. One's ability to perform tasks is treated in information-processing form.

Gagné, R. M. *The conditions of learning* (3rd ed.). New York: Holt, Rinehart & Winston, 1977. A classic in the field, this book shows the relationship of the process of learning to the design of better education.

Gagné, R. M. (Ed.). Learning and individual differences. Columbus, Ohio: Charles E. Merrill, 1967. Topics related to individual differences are discussed, many of them of particular interest to the physical educator.

Gurowitz, E. M. *The molecular basis of memory*. Englewood Cliffs, N.J.: Prentice-Hall, 1969. The nature of memory is handled from such areas as neurology, biochemistry, and psychology.

Hilgard, E. R., & Bower, G. H. *Theories of learning*. Englewood Cliffs, N.J.: Prentice-Hall, 1975. This is a well-written, interesting presentation of the works of the leading learning theorists of the twentieth century.

Holding, D. H. *Principles of training*. Oxford, England: Pergamon Press, 1965. Although primarily written for industrial psychologists and workers, there is much material of relevance here to anyone concerned with motor skills.

Hyden, H., Lorenz, K., Magoun, H. W., Penfield, W., & Pribram, C. H. *On the biology of learning*. New York: Harcourt Brace Jovanovich, 1969. This is book is a collection of essays by acknowledged scholars on the neurophysiology and biochemistry of learning.

Jones, J. C. *Learning*. New York: Harcourt Brace Jovanovich, 1967. This paperback is written for teachers; it deals with the practical application of learning research.

Keele, Steven W. *Attention and human performance*. Pacific Palisades, Calif.: Goodyear

Publishing Co., 1973. Although the author claims it is introductory, dealing with information processes associated with attention and memory, the book is fairly advanced.

Kintsch, W. *Memory and cognition* (2nd ed.). New York: John Wiley, 1977. Many current topics in cognitive psychology (e.g., memory, thinking, concept formation) are described, and implications can be drawn for understanding the cognitive aspects of motor learning.

Klahr, D. (Ed.). *Cognition and instruction.* Hillsdale, N.J.: Erlbaum, 1976. Although this covers cognitive psychology research related to problems in instructional design for the learning of cognitive material, implications can easily be made for the learning of motor skills.

Knapp, B. *Skill in sport: The attainment of proficiency.* London: Routledge & Kegan Paul, 1964. This book on motor learning is written expressly for physical educators.

Kolesnik, W. B. *Motivation: Understanding and influencing human behavior.* Boston: Allyn & Bacon, 1978 (paperback). This is a practical approach to motivation, with all points of view given fair representation, so the reader comes away with a comprehensive overview of the different interpretations of motivations and techniques to implement programs to enhance motivation, performance, and achievement.

Krawiec, T. S., & Chaplin, J. P. *Systems and theories of psychology* (3rd ed.). New York: Holt, Rinehart and Winston, 1974. This is a comprehensive treatment of the evolution of systems and theories of psychology.

Lawther, J. D. *The learning and performance of physical skills* (2nd ed.). Englewood Cliffs, N.J.: Prentice-Hall, 1977. Written by a physical educator, this paperback offers general material regarding learning and physical education.

Legge, D. (Ed.). *Skills.* Baltimore: Penguin Books, 1970. This includes many classic papers, primarily from the English approach, with the emphasis on industrial problems, information processing, experimental psychology and the like.

Legge, D., & Barber, P. J. *Information and skill.* London: Methuen, 1976 (paperback). Higher-order topics related to the processes underlying skill are presented in an interesting and scholarly manner.

Lockhart, A. S., & Johnson, J. M. *Laboratory experiments in motor learning.* Dubuque, Iowa: William C. Brown, 1970. Twenty experiments are suggested in simple experimental form.

Logan, F. A. *Learning and motivation.* Dubuque, Iowa: William C. Brown, 1970. For the beginning student of learning, classical and standard areas of study and research are presented.

Maggio, E. *Psychophysiology of learning and memory.* Springfield, Ill.: Charles C Thomas, 1971. The author offers interesting perspectives in the area of psychophysiology.

Massaro, D. W. *Experimental psychology and information processing.* Chicago: Rand McNally, 1975. Within an information-processing framework, standard and contemporary topics are treated in an interesting and comprehensive manner.

Marteniuk, R. G. *Information processing in motor skills.* New York: Holt, Rinehart & Winston, 1976. This is an overall basic view of the processes involved in the learning and performance of skills.

Marx, M. H. *Learning: Interactions.* New York: Macmillan, 1970. The author shows the interrelationships between behavior changes (learning) and certain variables (motivation, perception, concept formation, and personality).

Marx, M. H. *Learning: Processes.* New York: Macmillan, 1969. A number of sections on aspects of learning by different authors, culminating in one on motor behavior, are offered.

McGeoch, J. A., & Irion, A. L. *The psychology of human learning.* New York: David McKay, 1952. Although an early publication, this is a classic in the field.

Norman, D. A. *Memory and attention.* New York: John Wiley, 1976. An introductory information-processing approach, this book is written in an interesting and informative manner.

Norman, D. A., & Lindsay, P. H. *Human information processing: An introduction to psychology.* New York: Academic Press, 1977. This is a comprehensive introductory book on many topics associated with cognitive psychology and information processing.

O'Connor, K. *Learning: An introduction.* Glenview, Ill.: Scott, Foresman, 1971. Elementary coverage of the standard topics in the psychology of learning is made.

O'Neil, H. F. (Ed.). *Learning strategies.* New York: Academic Press, 1978. Learning strategies are discussed from such perspectives as cognitive psychology, artificial intelligence, behavior modification, and motor learning.

Oxendine, J. B. *Psychology of motor learning.* New York: Appleton-Century-Crofts, 1968. Written by a physical educator, this is a text for a couurse in motor learning.

Rarick, G. L. (Ed.). *Physical activity: Human growth and development.* New York: Academic Press, 1973. This multidisciplinary scholarly approach is devoted to the study of physical activity and children.

Robb, M. D. *The dynamics of motor skill acquisition.* Englewood Cliffs, N.J.: Prentice-Hall, 1972. A cybernetic approach to motor learning, this book easy to follow, with many practical examples.

Rushall, B. S., & Siedentop, D. *The development of behavior in sport and physical education.* Philadelphia: Lea & Febiger, 1972. This book is a mix of theoretical bases of operant conditioning, reinforcement principles, and teaching and coaching situations in which behaviors can be effectively modified.

Sage, G. H. *Introduction to motor behavior: A neuropsychological approach* (2nd ed.). Reading, Mass.: Addison-Wesley, Inc., 1977. Authored by a physical educator, one of the leading features of this book is the emphasis on the neuropsychology underlying motor behavior, although it encompasses many areas.

Sahakian, W. S. (Ed.). *Psychology of learning: Systems, models, and theories.* Chicago: Markham Publishing Co., 1970. This is a compilation of papers of those who contributed greatly and distinguished themselves in the development of learning theory.

Schmidt, R. A. *Motor skills.* New York: Harper & Row, 1975. This is an advanced introductory book to the study of human behavior, stressing underlying processes.

Sidowski, J. B. (Ed.). *Experimental methods and instrumentation in psychology.* New York: McGraw-Hill, 1966. Designed for the advanced student of learning, this comprehnsive book describes experimental methods and instrumentation used in the major areas of psychology.

Singer, R. N. (Ed.). *Readings in motor learning.* Philadelphia: Lea & Febiger, 1972. Major topical areas containing interesting and outstanding efforts by leading scholars are discussed.

Singer, R. N. *The psychomotor domain: Movement behavior.* Philadelphia: Lea & Febiger, 1972. Major disciplines and specialty areas are covered in the psychomotor domain, with each scholar demonstrating the kind of work currently going on and unique to each area.

Singer, R. N., Milne, C., Magill, R., Vachon, L., & Powell, F. M. *Laboratory and field experiments in motor learning.* Springfield, Ill.: Charles C Thomas, 1975. Comprehensive coverage of contemporary topics, with a description of how to build or where to buy apparatus, many references, and explanations of learning curves, measurement, and statistics.

Skill learning and performance. *Research Quarterly,* 1972, *43.* This issue contains a number of interesting scholarly articles on the topic of skill learning.

Smith, W. I., & Rohrman, N. L. *Human learning.* New York: McGraw-Hill, 1970. A simple book, largely self-instructional and semiprogrammed.

Snelbecker, G. E. *Learning theory, instructional theory, and psychoeducational design.* New York: McGraw-Hill, 1974. Describes contemporary and historically important learning theories within the framework of scientific research and practical educational situations.

Stallings, L. M. *Motor skills: Development and learning.* Dubuque, Iowa: William C. Brown, 1973. Emphasis on current models and concepts in skill acquisition, with many implications for improving the teaching/learning situation.

Stelmach, G. E. (Ed.) *Information processing in motor control and learning.* New York: Academic Press, 1978. This book presents coverage of contemporary topics, such as new motor control models and theoretical issues related to conscious mechanisms in movement control, motor programming, and knowledge of results.

Stelmach, G. E. (Ed.). *Motor control: Issues and trends.* New York: Academic Press, 1976. Nine topics are addressed with special concern for closed-loop theory, schema theory, and the concept of motor programs.

Tarpy, R. M., & Mayer, R. E. *Foundations of learning and memory.* Glenview, Ill.: Scott, Foresman, 1978. Introductory coverage to standard topics in the psychology of learning.

Thatcher, R. W., & John, E. R. *Functional neuroscience, vol. 1: Foundations of cognitive processes.* Hillsdale, N.J.: Erlbaum, 1977. Such topics as arousal and attention, emotion, information representation, and memory are analyzed with regard to neuroatomical, biochemical, and neurological systems information, with special concerns for information-processing and higher cognitive functionings.

Travers, R. M. *Essentials of learning* (4th ed.). New York: Macmillan, 1977. This book contains an analysis of the results of research on learning, with special implications for students in education.

Welford, A. T. *Fundamentals of skill.* London: Methuen, 1968. This is a sophisticated reference, emphasizing psychophysics, information processing, and experimental psychology.

Welford, A. T. *Skilled performance: Perceptual and motor skills.* Glenview, Ill.: Scott, Foresman, 1976. This book contains principles related to skills; it is heavily oriented toward research findings and an information-processing theoretical approach.

Whiting, H. T. A. *Acquiring ball skill: A psychological interpretation.* London: G. Bell, 1969. This is an excellent source for semisophisticated treatment of psychological research applied to the learning of athletic skills.

Woodworth, R. S., & Scholsberg, H. *Experimental psychology.* New York: Holt, Rinehart & Winston, 1954. This book, truly a classic, presents fundamental materials on a wide range of topics.

Woolridge, D. E. *The machinery of the brain.* New York: McGraw-Hill, 1963. This book offers a beautiful analogy of brain and computer, with material interestingly presented for the beginner.

AUTHOR INDEX

A

Adams, J. A., 24–25, 26, 113–114, 121, 124, 128, 352–353, 373, 413, 444, 457, 458, 479, 487, 495
Adler, J., 439, 444
Albert, I., 370, 373
Alexander, L., 380, 444
Allport, A., 412, 444
Alluisi, E., 522, 523, 524, 526
Alvares, K. M., 214–215, 220
Ammons, C., 471, 495
Ammons, R., 419, 444, 459–460, 471, 495
Annett, J., 459, 495
Anshel, M., 359, 373
Anthony, W., 341, 373
Antonis, B., 412, 444
Archer, E., 474, 497
Arnold, J., 370, 373
Asmussen, E., 239, 262
Atkinson, J., 244, 262, 331, 373, 452, 495
Atkinson, R., 139, 177, 481, 496
Attneave, F., 105, 128
Austin, D., 418, 444
Ausubel, D., 327, 373, 472, 495
Azer, N., 514, 524

B

Bachman, J. C., 204
Bahrick, H., 37, 49, 60, 79
Bairstow, P. J., 207, 220
Baker, B., 315–316, 324
Baker, K., 338, 373, 474, 496
Ballard, P., 484, 496

Bandura, A., 278, 291, 344, 373
Barbe, W., 259, 262
Barber, P., 415, 445
Barrett, M., 342, 376
Barsch, R., 309–310, 323
Bartlett, F. C., 152, 177
Bartley, S., 515, 524
Bartz, D., 466, 496, 516, 524
Battig, W., 337, 362–363, 373
Bayton, J., 452, 496
Beach, F., 298–299, 323
Beals, R., 228, 262
Bechtoldt, H., 195, 219
Beecher, H., 368, 373
Beery, R., 409, 444
Beggs, W., 433, 445
Belbin, E., 45, 49
Belbin, R., 45, 49
Belmont, J., 280, 291
Bender, P., 284, 291, 293
Bennett, B., 507, 525
Benson, D., 516, 524
Berelson, B., 24, 26
Berendsen, C., 436, 444
Berger, R., 187, 220
Berlyne, D., 276, 291, 410–411, 444
Bermudez, J., 246, 263
Bernstein, N., 112–113, 128, 280, 291
Berry, G., 246, 263
Beutler, L., 257–258, 262
Bexton, W., 520, 521, 525
Biederman, I., 361, 373
Bilodeau, E. A., 27
Bilodeau, I., 27, 455, 496
Birch, D., 390, 444

535

Inhelder, B., 278, 293
Isaac, P., 93, 95
Isaacson, R. L., 160, 178
Ismail, A., 237, 238, 263
Iso-Ahola, S., 466, 497

J

Jacobs, P., 253, 263
Jaeger, M., 170, 179
Jagacinski, R., 93, 95
Jaynes, J., 298–299, 323
Jensen, A., 268–269, 292
John, E. R., 147, 178, 180
Johnson, G., 342, 375
Johnson, H. W., 30–31, 49
Johnson, M., 423, 445
Johnson, W., 300, 323, 502, 525
Johnston, J., 453, 497
Johnston, W. A., 502, 525
Johnston, W. L., 228, 262
Jokl, E., 287, 292, 319, 323
Jones, B., 170, 178
Jones, E., 513, 525
Jones, H., 316, 318, 323
Jones, J., 426, 445
Jones, M. B., 213–214, 220
Jones, T., 315–316, 324
Jordan, T., 362, 375
Judd, C., 342, 375

K

Kagan, J., 300, 324
Kahneman, D., 142, 178
Karlin, L., 362, 375
Karnes, E., 474, 497
Karvonen, M., 323
Kaspar, J., 312–313, 324
Kay, H., 104, 106, 128
Kaye, R., 365, 375
Keele, S., 118–119, 121, 122, 128, 151, 153, 165, 166, 170, 178, 410, 414, 415, 445, 482, 497
Keller, F. S., 39, 49
Kelley, C., 475–476, 477, 497

Kelso, J., 154, 166, 170, 178, 180, 348, 362, 375, 377
Kephart, N., 31, 49, 237, 263, 307–308, 311–312, 323, 324
Kerlinger, F., 82, 95
Kerr, B., 414, 445
Kershner, K., 312, 323
Kihlberg, J., 323
Kimber, D. C., 145
Kimble, G., 492, 497
Klaiber, E., 314–315, 323
Klapp, S., 121, 129, 151, 152, 153, 166, 178
Klatzky, T., 348, 375
Klaus, D., 502, 525
Klein, R., 362, 376
Knapp, B., 18, 27, 475
Knapp, C., 417, 445, 497
Knowles, W., 411, 445
Kobayashi, Y., 314–315, 323
Koekela, A., 323
Koffka, K., 90, 95, 491, 497
Kolb, D., 401, 445
Kolesnik, W., 389–390, 445
Koppenaal, L., 151, 178
Kovacic, C., 519, 526
Krahenbuhl, G., 250, 251, 262
Krasner, L., 368, 376
Krathwohl, D. R., 6, 26, 27
Kreit, L., 359, 375
Kristofferson, A., 412, 413, 445
Kroll, W., 63, 80
Kubal, L., 466, 498
Kukla, A., 465, 497

L

Laabs, G. E., 170, 178
LaBerge, D., 140, 142, 179
Landers, D., 344–345, 375
Landers, D. M., 506, 525
Lane, J., 246, 263
Langley, L. L., 203
Lantz, A., 413, 445
Laszlo, J., 207, 220
Leavell, L., 145
Leavitt, H., 487, 497
Legge, E., 415, 445

Murphy, M., 273, 291
Mussen, H., 300, 324

N

Nacson, J., 170, 178, 179
Naitoh, P., 522, 526
Nanda, H., 65, 80
Naylor, J., 422, 423, 446, 471, 496
Neff, W., 519, 526
Neill, W., 121, 122, 129, 414, 415, 445
Neisser, U., 137, 138, 179
Nelson, G., 289, 292
Nelson, R., 233–234, 263
Neuman, M., 89, 95, 439, 446
Newell, K., 276, 282, 293, 458, 497
Newman, R., 359, 376
Nichols, D., 519, 525
Nideffer, R., 371, 376
Nierenberg, R., 166, 180
Nisbett, R., 406, 446
Nissen, M., 362, 376
Noble, C., 315–316, 324, 504, 505, 526
Noble, M., 361, 377, 412, 413, 446
Nofsinger, M., 234, 263
Norman, D., 139, 140, 141, 179, 482, 498
Noro, L., 323
Novak, J., 472, 495
Nuttin, J., 461, 498

O

Oliver, J., 238, 263
Olson, E. A., 210, 221
Olson, M., 362, 375
Osborne, T., 269, 293
Osgood, C., 469, 470, 498
Oxendine, J., 474, 498

P

Paillard, J., 116, 129, 160, 179
Paivio, A., 278, 293
Palermo, D., 396
Parker, J., 339, 340, 376, 484, 488, 496
Parsons, O., 246, 263

Pascual-Leone, J., 283, 293
Payne, L., 321, 323
Pease, D., 441, 447
Penfield, W., 146, 179
Penman, K., 346–347, 376
Perry, H., 426, 446
Perry, O., 438–439, 446
Petrie, A., 519, 526
Pettinger, J., 454, 498
Pfeiffer, E., 79
Phillips, L., 246, 263
Piaget, J., 278, 293, 298, 324
Pick, A., 277, 293
Pick, H., 361, 376
Pomeranz, D., 368, 376
Posner, J., 518, 525
Posner, M., 98, 102–103, 104, 128, 129, 362, 376, 384, 444
Postle, D., 385–386, 446
Postman, L., 425, 446
Poulton, E. C., 16–17, 20, 27
Powell, F., 70, 73, 74, 80, 117–118, 129
Prather, D., 246, 263, 440, 446
Pribram, K., 117–118, 129, 483, 498
Pronko, N., 286, 291
Purdy, B., 485, 498

R

Radler, D., 307, 324
Rajaratnam, N., 65, 80
Ramey, G., 406, 447
Rarick, G. L., 432, 446
Ravizza, R., 299, 324
Rawlings, E., 426–427, 428, 446
Rawlings, I., 426–427, 428, 446
Rawls, J., 438–439, 446
Renshaw, S., 385–386, 446
Reynolds, G., 451, 498
Reynolds, P., 412, 444
Rhodes, F., 359, 376
Rich, S., 351–352, 374
Richardson, A., 428, 446
Rivenes, R., 480, 498
Roach, E., 311–312, 324
Robbins, M., 309, 323, 324
Robel, D., 504, 505, 526

Stephenson, J., 356, 377
Stephenson, R., 195, 198, 220
Sternberg, S., 209, 221
Stevens, F., 517, 525
Stevens, J., 517, 525
Stevens, S. S., 223, 263
Suinn, R., 429, 447
Summers, J. J., 153, 166, 178
Swets, J., 92, 96
Swift, E., 486, 498

T

Talland, G., 286–287, 293
Tanner, J. M., 224, 264
Taub, E., 166, 180
Taylor, J., 251, 252, 264
Temple, I., 138–139, 180
Templeton, A., 228, 264
Thatcher, R. W., 147, 180
Thomas, J., 62, 80, 283, 284, 292, 293
Thompson, C. W., 209, 219
Thorndike, E., 85–86, 96
Thornton, J., 253, 263
Thurston, L. L., 33, 49
Thurstone, T., 238, 264
Tickner, A., 412, 444
Timmons, E., 438–439, 446
Tolman, E. C., 9
Townsend, R., 522, 526
Travers, R., 20, 27
Travis, R. C., 203, 221
Treisman, A., 142, 180, 412, 447
Trumbo, D., 361, 377, 412, 446
Trussell, E., 352, 377, 388, 447
Tucker, L., 66, 80
Tucker, W., 223, 263
Tudor, J., 284, 293
Tulving, E., 150–151, 177
Tusky, B., 519, 525
Twining, W., 427, 447

U

Ulrich, L., 361, 377
Usselman, L., 79

V

Vachon, L., 70, 80
Valins, S., 406, 446
Vernon, J., 520, 526
Veroff, J., 390, 444
Vincent, W., 471, 498
Vogel, W., 314–315, 323

W

Wade, M., 275, 293
Waglow, I., 417–418, 447
Wagner, H., 503, 526
Walker, E., 399, 448, 491, 498
Wallace, S., 170, 180, 377
Wallis, E., 360, 374
Warren, D., 361, 376
Waters, L., 471, 496
Weaver, W., 104, 129
Weibell, F., 79
Weiner, B., 166, 180, 399, 401, 448, 464, 465, 499
Welch, M., 215, 221, 352, 377, 387, 388, 447, 516, 526
Welford, A., 107–108, 129
Weyner, N., 505, 526
Whiting, J. A., 108–110, 129, 313, 320–321, 324, 356, 377
Whiting, J., 332–333, 373
Whitley, J., 421, 447
Wickens, C., 275, 282, 293, 415–416, 448
Wickens, D. D., 393
Wickens, T., 139, 177
Wickstrom, R., 423, 448
Wiebe, Vernon, 206, 221
Wiener, N., 110, 129
Wilberg, R. B., 227, 264
Williams, H., 138–139, 180, 227, 264, 321, 324
Williams, M., 370, 373
Witker, J., 428, 429, 430, 447
Witte, K., 454, 499
Wood, C., 249, 250, 264
Woods, J., 432, 448
Wooldridge, D. E., 158, 180
Worthen, B., 341, 377

Wozniak, R., 281, 294
Wright, E., 360, 377
Wylie, R., 338, 373, 474, 496

Y

Yegerow, A., 518, 526
Yelon, S., 381, 444
Yilk, M., 426–427, 428, 446

Young, V. P., 485, 496
Youngen, L., 211

Z

Zajonc, R., 505–506, 526
Zeaman, D., 505, 526
Zimmerman, B., 278–279, 294
Zubek, J., 520–521, 526

SUBJECT INDEX

M

Massed vs. distributed practice, 419–421
Measurement of learning considerations
  accuracy (error), 60–63
  dependent measure(s), 59–63
  duration of study, 58–59
  learning score, 63–69
  response magnitude, 60
  speed of response, 60
  task selection, 52–53
  types of tasks, 54–56
Memory
  depth of processing vs. multi-store approach, 150–151
  short-term and long-term 146–151
  see also Retention
Mental vs. physical practice, 425–430
Mentally retarded, 237–239
Model of motor behavior, Chapter 6
  arousal, 144–146
  effectors, 161–163
  feedback, 164–167
  long-term memory store, 138–141, 146–151
  mechanisms, processes, and strategies, 169–172
  motor program selection, 151–153
  movement generator, 153–154
  movements, complex, 158–161
  movements, simple, 154–158
  perceptual mechanism, 141–143
  sensory store, 137–138
  short-term memory store, 146–151
Modeling, *see* Demonstrations
Models, *see* Theories and Models
Motivation, 388–410
  achievement motivation, 401–403
  behavioristic approaches (reinforcements, rewards), 398–400
  cognitive psychology approaches (attributions and expectations), 400–401
  effects on learning and performance, 391–392
  extrinsic and intrinsic, 403–406
  interpretations and explanations, 389–391
  humanistic approaches (self-fulfillment), 400

  optimal level, 393–394
  personal variables, 394–398
  situational techniques: considerations for training, 406–410
  task considerations, 393–394
  task selection, 329
Motor ability, 184–186
Motor capacity, 184–186
Motor development tests, 311–314
Motor educability, 184–186
Motor fitness, 184–186
Motor task classifications
  continuous, serial, and discrete, 19
  gross and fine, 13–21
  habitual and perceptual, 18–19
  object and person motion, 13–16
  open and closed, 16–17
  self-paced and externally-paced, 16–19
Movement speed, 208–212
  movement time, 208–212
  reaction time, 208–212
  reflex time, 208
  response time, 208

N

Need to achieve, *see* Personality
Neo-Piagetian theory, 283–285
Neurological problems and performance, 175–176

O

Overlearning (overpractice), *see* Retention

P

Pain, 517–519
Perception, 229–234
  description and definitions, 229–230
  figural aftereffects, 233–234
  personal factors, 230–232
  psychophysics, 232–233
Perceptual handicaps, *see* Handicaps
Perceptual-motor training programs, 304–311

general descriptive models, 99–104
   Cratty's three-level theory, 101–102
   the Fitts-Posner model, 102–103
   Gentile's model, 103–104
   Henry's memory drum theory,
     100–101
information processing models, 98–99,
   104–110
   Welford's model, 107–108
   Whiting's model, 108–110
mathematical and statistical models,
   90–91
performance models, 91–94
   signal detection, 92–94
   vigilance, 92
peripheral vs. central control issues,
   119–123
values and criticisms, 82–83
Touch, 228

Transfer of training, 467
   bilateral transfer, 473
   conditions, 471–472
   measurement, 468–471
   task difficulty, 473–475
   theories, 477–478

V

Values and attitudes, *see* Personality
Vision, 226–228

W

Warm-up, 335–336
Whole vs. part learning, 421–424
Working conditions, 514–515